CHILD PSYCHIATRY

CHILD PSYCHIATRY

Fifth Printing—1947

By

LEO KANNER, M. D.

Associate Professor of Psychiatry
The Johns Hopkins University
Baltimore, Maryland

With PREFACES *by*

ADOLF MEYER, M. D., LL. D.

Henry Phipps Professor Emeritus of Psychiatry
The Johns Hopkins University
Baltimore, Maryland

and

EDWARDS A. PARK, M. D.

Professor Emeritus of Pediatrics
The Johns Hopkins University
Baltimore, Maryland

Springfield · Illinois · U. S. A.

CHARLES C THOMAS · PUBLISHER

CHARLES C THOMAS • PUBLISHER
BANNERSTONE HOUSE
301-327 EAST LAWRENCE AVENUE, SPRINGFIELD, ILLINOIS

Published simultaneously in Canada by
THE RYERSON PRESS, TORONTO

First Printing, June, 1935
Second Printing, February, 1937
Third Printing, May, 1942
Fourth Printing, January, 1946
Fifth Printing, April, 1947

Printed in the United States of America

PREFACE TO THE FIFTH PRINTING

The fate of textbooks can rarely be predicted with any degree of certainty. It was especially difficult to foresee the fate of a text dealing with a subject which is taught officially in but few colleges and universities.

The more gratifying was, therefore, the reception given to *Child Psychiatry* from the time of its first publication to the present day, when a fifth printing is made imperative by continued demand.

Even more heartening is the observation that the book has come to serve not only as the accepted standard text for graduate instruction, but is also used widely as a guide and reference by all those who are actively interested in shaping the character of children. It has been recommended by reviewers in journals for teachers, social workers, psychologists, physicians, and directors of recreational centers.

At this particular period of our country's history, education for stability and sturdiness is recognized more than ever as an essential requirement. It is my sincere hope that this volume may continue to do its part in spreading the knowledge of children's behavior difficulties and the means of correcting them.

L. K.

Baltimore, Maryland

PREFACE

BY

ADOLF MEYER, M.D.

Henry Phipps Professor of Psychiatry
The Johns Hopkins University
Baltimore, Maryland

In the sixteenth, seventeenth and eighteenth centuries the occidental world had become man-conscious and in an unprecedented way aware of man's particular place in nature. It was natural that with Rousseau and Pestalozzi the child attained a status of new importance, not only in education but in the whole conception of the development and health of the human being. The nineteenth century laid the foundations for pediatrics and also for the naturalization of psychology, and the twentieth century is making the health and growth of the child one of the most active and fruitful fields of progress. Child study established new standards and conceptions and made important contributions toward a new conception of both objective and subjective psychology. One of the developments of this child psychology is child psychiatry, which gives the personality of the child a vital status and calls for valuable reorientations in education and social and medical thought and practice. Much of it proves to be organization of common-sense in dealing with the rank and file of childhood disorders; but on this is built a great deal of conscientious work on the general health and technical problems, which has too readily been looked upon as either "merely physical" or "merely educational." Child psychiatry is finding itself more and more on a safe and broad middle-of-the-road course between the extremes of reluctance and of excess of zeal. Like any strongly human field to-day, it has the fate of overpopularization and exploitation for literary and other purposes, while physicians are apt to be either too conservative or too eager and as impatient as the public.

The close neighborly relations of pediatrics and psychiatry at the Johns Hopkins Hospital gave an opportunity for coöperation, that, with the help of the Josiah Macy, Jr. Foundation, allowed Dr. Leo Kanner to organize the work of which the present volume is the natural product. A respect for the objective facts open to study and to practical work and a determination to maintain a balanced perspective and a mind open to the growing accumulation of experience and methods are the leading principles of the collaboration undertaken.

It was clearly realized that there were two real difficulties to be overcome: In the first place, the scientifically trained person's fear that the common-sense of everyday life has to be replaced, if one is to be on safe ground, by totally new methods, which then too often want to limit themselves to physics and chemistry and physiology and rigid statistics; and, on the other hand, there threaten oversystematizations in new endeavors in psychopathology, feeding on a similar disparagement of common sense with its propaganda of exclusive salvation by startling novelty of concepts and topics. It was deemed wisest to give child psychiatry all the rights and obligations of trained common-sense intent on using also the rapidly accumulating experience, but in constant contact with pediatric workers, and determined to maintain balanced conceptions.

The principles are those of a psychobiologically oriented psychiatry. The aim is to give equal consideration to the normal assets and to the special problems arising among the facts and factors of the child's life, to grant proportionate attention to the situation and to the special organs and functions in the total picture, and to give to what appears to be susceptible of adjustment a prominent position in the perspective. It is not necessary and not desirable as a general policy or in such a presentation as follows to put the emphasis on what is not likely to be sound practice and material of concern except in the hands of a few specially trained and privileged workers. Without oversystematization, the outstanding chapters give both setting and perspective and a total conception, which we hope will ring true to the experience of the workers in the field and be a helpful part of the ground for natural development in pediatrics.

I trust that this volume, one of the results of the enterprise, will be helpful in the creation of a wholesome working together of pediatrician and psychiatrist and the nurses and the parents. It is a practical outcome of the whole-hearted working together of the contributing agencies, Dr. Edwards A. Park and his staff, the Josiah Macy, Jr. Foundation, the Rockefeller Foundation, Dr. Stewart Paton, and the psychiatric group under Dr. Kanner's leadership. It will, we trust, prove a dependable orientation and a safe foundation and setting for all that active and creative investigative spirit which will gradually sift the more venturesome but not always well digested appeals to public and specialistic imagination. The book will serve as a safe starting point and an incentive to proceed from what is well tried to the ever new ground to be conquered.

PREFACE

BY

EDWARDS A. PARK, M.D.

Professor of Pediatrics
The Johns Hopkins University
Baltimore, Maryland

IN THE FAST changing medicine of today the pediatrician remains the grand example of the general practitioner. Though primarily an internist, he finds himself in turn dermatologist, otologist and neurologist. Moreover, of all classes of physicians the pediatrician is perhaps most nearly the ideal, since of necessity his work is so preëminently concerned with preventive medicine. He enters the home to advise in regard to the preservation of health as often as to meet the problems of disease. He discusses school work, clothing, companions, habits of exercise and sleep as well as diet and protection against the contagious diseases.

Because the pediatrician has this intimate family relationship and these special responsibilities, it is to him that the problems of abnormal behavior first come. In the struggle which the child wages continually for his place under the sun, the pediatrician holds the strategic position, for he is the only trained observer on the field. He alone has the chance to encounter personality difficulties in their incipiency. In the past we pediatricians have not been accustomed to regard the healthy development of the child's personality as our responsibility. With the continued growth of knowledge concerning the child the pediatrician can no longer escape this obligation; no one else is in the position to assume it. *Mens sana in corpore sano* is for him in particular both precept and goal.

If, then, the pediatrician is to fulfill his function completely, he must understand the child through and through as a living, acting, feeling, choosing being. He must be able to pick out reactions which are unhealthy and to know that they are fraught with ultimate danger, while scarcely more than tendencies or trends. He must be able to gauge the intelligence of the child and to estimate the emotional make-up, in order to be able to judge the capacity for healthy development. Since the fault lies as often in the environment as in the child, the pediatrician must understand also parents, teachers, and all those surrounding the child. Finally, like all general practitioners he must know himself well enough to be able to judge when to attack the problem in person and when to seek for aid.

This book of Dr. Kanner's points out to the pediatrician the personality difficulties of children. It gives him the knowledge of their structure and intrinsic and extrinsic relationships and shows him how to investigate and analyze them. It supplies a point of view, a method, a way of thinking. It also furnishes the principles of treatment and, therefore, a way of acting.

The book leads the pediatrician through a terrain which was not well mapped and clearly defined in his mind. In this terra incognita he was apt to wander and become lost or, perhaps, he refused to enter it at all.

The problems presented by the child may be complex enough! As compared to those of the adult, however, they generally are simple. The brevity of experience, the ignorance of life, the simplicity of thought tend to make the personality difficulties of children, particularly of young children, readily ascertainable and explicable. Dr. Kanner's book is written on the assumption that the common behavior disturbances of children are within the grasp of the pediatrically trained mind and with the belief that the pediatrician is the one to recognize them at the very beginning and to prevent their development. Dr. Kanner's book is not based on imaginary children; it is the outcome of the study of large numbers of actual children as they happened to come before him in the outpatient department and wards of the Harriet Lane.

The book is full of wisdom and common sense. No other book is quite like it. It brings to the pediatrician much needed aid.

TABLE OF CONTENTS

PART ONE

FIRST SECTION: THE BASIC PRINCIPLES

SECOND SECTION: EXAMINATION AND DIAGNOSIS

THIRD SECTION: THE PRINCIPLES AND AIMS OF PSYCHIATRIC TREATMENT

Part Two

FIRST SECTION: PERSONALITY DIFFICULTIES FORMING
ESSENTIAL FEATURES OR SEQUELS OF PHYSICAL
ILLNESS

SECOND SECTION: PERSONALITY DIFFICULTIES EXPRESSING THEMSELVES IN THE FORM OF INVOLUNTARY PART-DYSFUNCTIONS

THIRD SECTION: PERSONALITY DIFFICULTIES EXPRESSING
THEMSELVES CLEARLY AS WHOLE-DYSFUNCTIONS
OF THE INDIVIDUAL

INTRODUCTION

In November, 1930, under a special grant of the Josiah Macy, Jr. Foundation, psychiatric consultation service on a full time basis was established at the Harriet Lane Home for Invalid Children, the Pediatric Department of the Johns Hopkins Hospital and University in Baltimore. The main object of the experiment, as outlined by Dr. Adolf Meyer in collaboration with Dr. Edwards A. Park, Dr. Stewart Paton, and Dr. Ludwig Kast, was an "investigation of the rank and file of patients in the pediatric clinics for the formulation of psychiatric problems, the mastery of which should be made accessible to the pediatrician to serve him as the psychopathological principles in dealing with children."

It is obvious that the first task encountered by the psychiatrist privileged to undertake this highly important work was one of orientation, finding and elaborating a suitable avenue of practical activity, and sounding himself as well as the pediatric staff for a minimum of mutual understanding as a firm basis for further coöperation. It was especially desirable to have, and to be capable of conveying, a clear grasp of the current views and controversies with regard to the personality problems arising during the period of the early development of the growing individual. So many schools of thought in the realms of medicine, psychology, education, and criminology have in the recent past heaped their attention upon the child, that the resulting doctrines and claims had to be sifted carefully as to t'.eir objectiveness, validity, and actual usefulness. An active service field had to be created for first hand contact with patients in need of psychiatric study and handling, for the purpose of teaching, for the working out of a worthwhile research program, and with the aim of giving concrete demonstrations rather than general theoretical discussions.

The White House Conference on Child Health and Protection in 1930 has brought out considerable evidence of a great deal of bewilderment and uncertainty on the part of many participants, due mainly to the too largely theoretical and propagandist type of attack, the overspecialized tendencies of many psychiatrists, and the lack of perspective of some of the younger and older practitioners in matters going beyond ordinary medical methods. A somewhat unhealthy and often belligerent attitude has been assumed by raising the question of competency, which gave rise to assurances made by some psychiatrists, pediatricians, neurologists, psychologists, educators, and social workers, that the members of the respective profession or specialty alone—and no one else—has a right to deal with the behavior difficulties of children. Out of this theoretical rather than factual rivalry grew a desire for a narrow delimitation of the functions of each group, with the result that questionnaires sent out to selected representatives brought forth a confused and confusing medley of opinions, assertions, claims, and denunciations.

It is evident that an emphasis on contrasts rather than common interests has not contributed to a clarification of the problem. Fortunately for the creation of a sense of understanding and coöperation, the history of pediatrics offers a striking resemblance to certain aspects in the evolution of modern psychiatry. Pediatrics developed in the midst of medical specialization according to specific organs or organ systems (ophthalmology, rhinology, otology, cardiology, urology, gastro-enterology, neurology, etc.), or according to certain diseases (syphilology), or according to certain technical modes of examination and treatment (roentgenology, surgery, orthopedics, etc.). The pediatrician had a hard struggle attempting to establish himself and gain recognition among the members of all those specialities because he had the courage to introduce something that was not the consideration of just an organ or a group of symptoms or a technique. The age factor of growth and development became the paramount issue in the formation of his particular branch. The discovery was made that the child is, after all, not just a mere miniature adult but that he presents features altogether his own, owing to his being a child.

Pediatrics is a comparatively recent branch of medicine. For the past half century, the science of medical care and prophylaxis of childhood has made admirable progress in many directions. A comparison between the modest, rudimentary attempts of Thomas Phaer's *Boke of Children* (1544) and the modern pediatric textbooks gives one an overwhelming impression not unlike the amazement derived from a consideration of the breathtaking changes made during the same period in the technical sciences. Assisted by the advances in the other medical branches, pediatrics has perceptibly reduced the rate of infant and child mortality and has made this world a much safer place for the child.

It is perhaps not a mere coincidence that at the same time when pediatrics has reached its maturity and general recognition, interest in the young individual has gained a tremendous momentum in other quarters. Psychiatrists, psychologists, and sociologists alike have become aware of the fact that the child offered a new and exceedingly fertile field for research. A wealth of observations, theories, speculations, and practical measures has created a vast literature and given rise to an almost worldwide movement which may still be said to be in its beginning. The child has become a center of psychologic and sociologic interest with such an increasing rapidity that the pediatrician, proceeding with equal speed in the building up and broadening of his specialty, has hardly had the time and opportunity to orient himself in the bewildering mass of new material, offered mostly in a vocabulary for which he was not adequately prepared. In recent years, however, there has been more and more of a mutual approach. With increasing frequency voices have been raised in the discussion of the question as to whether and how the new insight gained of children's behavior could be incorporated in pediatric practice.

Child psychiatry had previously been looked upon as belonging entirely to the realm of psychiatry, just as child psychology and sociology were held to be the concerns of no other discipline than these two sciences. There was, on the other hand, not the slightest hesitancy in making preventive inoculation a common pediatric practice, even though it was primarily not evolved by the child specialist. The ophthalmologist finds it natural that the pediatrician has the right and duty to treat the usual uncomplicated conjunctivitis or blepharitis, and fundus examination has justly become a routine pediatric procedure, without creating any sense of rivalry or raising any question of competency. In a similar sense, the pediatrician feels in a growing degree the need of acquiring sufficient psychiatric understanding to treat the rank and file of personality problems of his little patients. Child psychiatry, thus, would cease to be the object of the psychiatrist alone. Its methods of examination and treatment and prophylaxis would, as pediatric psychiatry, also become one of a number of branches of the science of pediatrics.

The setting up of the age factor as the basis of the pediatric specialty begins to be broadened to include mental growth with at least the same justification as the development of bones and other tissues. It is felt more and more clearly that even the most careful investigation of the corporal structures and their normal and pathological functions must be supplemented by the realization of their integration in the form of a living and behaving personality. It is hardly surprising that this recognition is gradually leading progressive physicians to turn for assistance to the psychiatrists, who for a little more than a generation have made it their conscious and persistent task to emphasize the need of studying the individual as a whole and in his relations to his environment.

But the effort to obtain helpful psychiatric orientation threatened to be blocked by several obstacles, some of which were pointed out clearly and fairly by the eminent pediatrician, Joseph Brennemann, in a paper which bore the seemingly ominous title, *The Menace of Psychiatry* (*American Journal of the Diseases of Children. 1931, 42, 376–402*). The author justly took issue with the present unfortunate and often enough unskilful over-popularization of certain brands of "psychiatry," with the exclusive use and improper evaluation of certain tests, and with the claims of certain speculative psychiatric schools giving to the outsider the impression of "a confusion of theory and authority." He looked forward optimistically to the advent of "the pediatric psychiatrist or the psychiatric pediatrician" as the "obvious solution," and felt that "there is much evidence that he is in the making."

One difficulty confronting physicians who look for information about the psychopathology of childhood is the absence of a text which could serve them as a guide and reference book and make them acquainted with the principles of unbiased and practical common-sense work with the personality problems of their little patients. There exist, to be sure, a number of treatises and monographs and even a few textbooks which deal with "mental diseases" of children or with "the nervous child." But some of them have become antiquated in the light of the recent advances made in psychiatry. Others are concerned only with definite disease entities (real or artificially construed) and neglect completely the rank and file of behavior disorders not directly referable to nosographic units. Still others attack the whole subject with the prejudices and rituals dictated by certain psychiatric "schools." Another group is interested in the "functional" disorders only.

It seems fair to give a list of pioneer works devoted to child psychiatry.

Books written by psychiatrists and neurologists:

Emminghaus, Hermann. Die psychischen Störungen des Kindesalters. Tübingen. 1887.

Moreau de Tours, Paul. La folie chez les enfants. Paris. 1888.

Ireland, W. W. The Mental Affections of Children. Idiocy, Imbecility, and Insanity. Edinburgh. 1898.

Manheimer, M. Les troubles mentaux de l'enfance. Précis de psychiatrie infantile. Paris. 1899.

Strohmayer, W. Vorlesungen über die Psychopathologie des Kindesalters für Mediziner und Pädagogen. Tübingen. 1910.

Scholz, L. Anomale Kinder. Berlin. 1912.

De Sanctis, Sante. Neuropsichiatria infantile, patologica e diagnostica. Roma. 1925.

Homburger, A. Vorlesungen über Psychopathologie des Kindesalters. Berlin. 1926.

Sachs, B., and L. Hausman. Nervous and Mental Disorders from Birth Through Adolescence. New York. 1926.

Ziehen, Th. Die Geisteskrankheiten im Kindesalter, einschliesslich Schwachsinn und psychopathische Konstitutionen. Zweite Auflage. Berlin. 1926.

Cimbal, W. Die Neurosen des Kindesalters mit besonderer Berücksichtigung von Lernschwäche und Schwererziehbarkeit. Berlin und Wien. 1927.

Books written by pediatricians:

Rachford, B. K. Neurotic Disorders of Childhood. New York. 1905.

Guthrie, L. G. Functional Nervous Disorders in Childhood. 1907.

Cameron, H. C. The Nervous Child. Fourth Edition. London. 1929.

Benjamin, E. Grundlagen und Entwicklungsgeschichte der kindlichen Neurose. Leipzig. 1930.

The present volume, which is the first textbook of child psychiatry in the English language, is offered as an attempt to cover the entire field of children's personality disorders on a broad, objective, unbiased, and practical basis. It has grown out of everyday contacts with pediatricians, consultation work in a large pediatric clinic and dispensary, collaboration with private practitioners and the various child-caring agencies of the community (schools, orphanages, hospitals, welfare groups, courts, custodial and correctional institutions), and teaching activities at the Johns Hopkins University School of Medicine. It is intended primarily for physicians and medical students but is also meant to be of help to all those interested in children's behavior problems: social workers, psychologists, sociologists, educators, juvenile court workers, etc.

I am deeply moved to express my gratitude to the Josiah Macy, Jr. Foundation for the financial aid which has made the beginning of this work possible, the Rockefeller Foundation for taking over the full support of the enterprise and Drs. Adolf Meyer, Edwards A. Park, Stewart Paton, and Esther L. Richards for their continued inspiration, encouragement, and advice.

PART ONE
FIRST SECTION
THE BASIC PRINCIPLES

CHAPTER I

THE PREVAILING METHODS OF STUDYING AND HANDLING CHILDREN'S PSYCHIATRIC PROBLEMS

THEORIES, hypotheses and speculations have always existed in medicine and both furthered and hindered its development. Psychiatry has always had its share of theories, from the time of belief in demoniac possession up to the present date. In our own time, we are confronted with an unprecedented *embarras de richesses*. What usually happens is that a few valuable and concrete new facts are uncovered, which may well be added to the treasury of substantial knowledge of the functions of man. But on the basis of a small number of concrete observations gigantic systems have been erected, with formulae undertaking to explain immediately everything that ever happens or may happen to, or within, or between human beings. For the representatives and followers of the various schools it is an easy task to apply their specifically gaged rods to whatever problems they are called upon to tackle, even if there is frequently enough a need of employing Procrustean methods. To the disinterested outsider the spectacle of several groups each claiming to hold the sole key to the understanding of human nature and to the treatment of its ills may seem highly entertaining. But the psychiatrically untrained physician with a keen desire to help his patients intelligently is easily in danger of giving up his search for information and turning his back to the "menace of psychiatry," if he is surrounded by so many contradictory claims with strange vocabularies and often ceremonious techniques.

What are the outstanding current theories?

The physically-minded practitioner will perhaps be partial to the idea of *focal infection* which a few years ago captivated the medical world. The teaching that abscessed teeth, infected tonsils, inflamed appendices and gall bladders constitute a potential and sometimes actual danger to their possessors and therefore should be adequately treated, is undoubtedly a decided contribution to good hygiene and prophylaxis. But it was made the starting point of a system according to which all mental difficulties were said to be rooted always in some focal physical disturbance.[1] Such an attitude would, if generally accepted, tend to do away with the desire to study the personalities of abnormally reacting individuals, make psychiatry superfluous, and leave behavior disorders entirely to the surgeon's knife and the dentist's forceps. The laudable call for prompt recognition and treatment of locally circumscribed areas of infection with their possible effects on the total organism should not, however, make one develop an amnesia for a large variety of other, equally and often much more potent, factors.

[1] Cotton, H. A. The Defective Delinquent and Insane. Princeton and London. 1921.

The slogan of "focal infection" has recently been losing a great deal of its original appeal. But the physician who feels under obligation to explain all human activity, however complex it be, in terms of diseased organs only, is given another choice. In myxedema and cretinism with striking defect in the development of the mental faculties, the *glands of internal secretion* were found to be of considerable etiologic significance. The psychic accompaniments of exophthalmic goiter are well known to every physician. The study of endocrinology has furnished us with data, the theoretical as well as practical importance of which is truly inestimable. But here again the undoubted need of including these facts in one's occupation with the human being has led certain enthusiasts to proclaim the ductless glands and their products as the one and only unrivaled source of all functions of man. They have been presented to the public as the "glands regulating personality" and the "glands of destiny." Most of this, says Lurie,[1] "is fiction, or at best a gross exaggeration of facts. But from the few kernels of wheat that can be separated from the chaff, we find that disturbances in the function of the ductless glands may produce changes in the personality make-up of the individual of such a nature as to prevent him from making normal reactions and hence from making normal adjustment to his environment." Even to this cautious formulation one may add the remark that there is often, particularly in the child, a physiological fluctuation of endocrine functions, that there are wide individual variations within the limits of the normal, and that slight deviations from the average may at times indeed be causative or contributing factors in the etiology of faulty adjustment, but in other cases incidental or one of a group of several expressions of a difficulty anchored in the total personality. At any rate, the assignment of a monarchic rôle to the endocrinopathies in dealing with complex human performances must appear to the objective investigator as one-sided as the idea of an all-momentousness of an infected tooth or a supposedly guilty sigmoid.

Much more than the sites of focal infection and the internal secretions, *the central nervous system* has lent itself to attempts at a hypothetical hitching up of all modes of human behavior with more or less clearly outlined areas. It would lead too far to discuss here the localizing or otherwise neurologizing schemes of Bechterev's reflexology or the Pavlovian excitation, irradiation, and inhibition concepts or the numerous other tendencies along similar lines. They signify earnest endeavor combined with admirable cleverness, with imaginative and inventive genius, with industrious experimental work in well-equipped laboratories. They have resulted in substantial additions to the storehouse of our knowledge of the reactions of animals and man.

Even the most naïve localization hypotheses have gotten away from the idea that every "element" of feeling or thought is represented by a special cell or group of cells in the brain. But there still exists a strong tendency to speak in terms of a sex center, an anxiety center, or other similar centers, which have never been objectively demonstrated. Man is, con-

---

[1] Lurie, Louis A. The Relation of Endocrinopathic States to Conduct Disorders of Children. American Journal of Psychiatry. 1929, 9, 285–305.

sequently, reduced to a "thinking machine" in which these mythological brain centers have the leading rôle. It is not so much the human being in his entirety, according to these views, but a certain localized area in the central nervous system that is influenced by outside stimuli and by the working of the other areas in the direction of the production of, let us say, an anxiety attack. It is, of course, unquestionable that the central nervous system plays a very important part in any form of performance. If I raise my arm, a number of things happen, to be sure, in the precentral gyrus, in the pyramidal tract, in several muscle groups, in the circulatory system, in the respiratory organs because of a change of the intrathoracic volume, etc. But we must not forget that the raising of my arm may have been caused by a large variety of facts and deliberations. I may have raised it to make a donation to a beggar or to pay the storekeeper for something that I have purchased. I may have raised it unintentionally as accompaniment, which may be more or less habitual with me, of an emphatic statement. Or I may have, in this manner, greeted an acquaintance in the street. Even so much as a sneeze, and more so the successful suppression of a sneeze, will involve much more than just a center or any number of centers and organs; the entire body posture may be affected; even consciousness may be suspended for a brief moment. The presence or absence of witnesses may have a great deal to do with the mode of reacting. The sneeze may be anticipated with pleasure or a feeling of irritation. Any number of complications may occur, which can never be expressed in terms of centers alone. In hysteria, as a matter of fact, the usual stimuli may fail to evoke a sneezing response and yet result in the accompanying hyperemia of the conjunctivae.

Of particular importance in dealing with children is the theory developed in recent years by *the Orton[1] school.* Orton and his pupils deserve high credit for recognizing the significance of obvious or suppressed lefthandedness as possible contributing factors in certain cases of reading difficulty and stuttering. Subtle tests have been worked out by them for the detection of dextral, sinistral, and ambidextrous tendencies. No one can afford to disregard the insight gained through these studies. But few can afford to subordinate their desire for objective concreteness to the wholehearted acceptance of a fascinating yet unproven hypothesis, based on the idea of an existing *conflict between the two brain hemispheres:* "The principle of cerebral dominance, the clinical application of which has been so efficacious, posits a physiological substratum in the determination of right laterality of motor leads. It conceives as existing a center of chief dominance in the left cerebrum which exerts a dynastic influence over the right cerebrum to insure concerted but unequivocal action. When there is no sufficiently dominant gradient of activity present in either hemisphere, or when such is resident but not heeded in the right hemisphere, what I conceive to be the pathophysiological subsoil of the essential speech dysfunctions obtains." (Travis.)

[1] Orton, S. T. Word-Blindness in School Children. Archives of Neurology and Psychiatry. 1925, 14, 581–615.
Travis, Lee Edward. Speech Pathology. A Dynamic Neurological Treatment of Normal Speech and Speech Deviations. New York and London. 1931.

A new impetus, a new set of facts, a comparatively new mode of approach, and a new school arose from Watson's experiments with infants, carried out largely at the Psychology Laboratory of the Henry Phipps Psychiatric Clinic and based to a considerable extent on Pavlov's work with the conditioned reflex. A justified feeling of astonishment has ushered the investigator into his field of activity: "Will you believe the almost astounding truth that no well trained man or woman has ever watched the complete and daily development of a single child from its birth to its third year? Plants and animals we know about because we have studied them, but the human child until very recently has been a mystery. Radium has had more scientific study put upon it in the last fifteen years than has been given to the first three years of infancy since the beginning of time." Watson made careful observations of infants leading to a better knowledge of the very first manifestations of emotional reactions and the educational possibilities of their control in relatively uncomplicated laboratory settings. One has a right to appropriate the results of Watson's objective experiments in one's armamentarium of child study. They represent tests and findings which may be duplicated by any observer anywhere. But Watson drew theoretical conclusions and built up a system of psychology which he called *Behaviorism;* his psychology is, in a sense, not really a psychology. For, in reducing every human performance to a purely and exclusively neurophysiological relation of stimulus and response, in flatly refusing to work with the concept of consciousness, in proceeding on the assumption that all men are born alike and, if properly conditioned, could be reared to become Shakespeares or Beethovens or criminals, in reversing the medieval and pre-medieval animistic awe of the "soul" into complete apsychism or even psychophobia, in disregarding any data of introspection, he deprives his "biological rebirth" of any semblance of a psychological approach. It is characteristic and significant for those who deal with children's personality difficulties that in his programmatic books[1] the intelligence factor is not even alluded to by implication.

Chronologically, Watson's behaviorism and the focal infection and endocrine theories were preceded by the foundation of a psychological system which has greatly influenced the general psychological trends of our generation. At a time when psychiatry was in danger of stagnation in a rigid static-descriptive nosography, at a period when cellular pathology was the last word and ultimate refuge in accounting for any mode of human ailments, Freud's recognition of dynamic principles in the development of hysteria marked a brave and fruitful departure from all and every previous tradition. Moreover, his frank approach to the problems of sex, shunned until then with unreasonable prudishness, opened new avenues to the understanding of human nature and its evolution. These two accomplishments by the founder of *the psychoanalytic school* are sufficient to secure for him a place of lasting appreciation among the students of man's relations to man. This historically significant and psychologically inestimable departure from the then ordinary classificatory preoccupations carried Freud

[1] Watson, John B. Psychology from the Standpoint of a Behaviorist. Philadelphia and London. 1919.
Watson, John B. Psychological Care of Infant and Child. New York. 1928.

and his disciples gradually into transcendental realms so removed from the concrete and objective substrata, that on the soil of the psychological gains inaugurated with so much ingenuity grew a not less ingenious, but highly speculative, if not poetical, metapsychological structure. In it, man is endowed with that which is commonly spoken of as consciousness, with an unconscious in which are lodged the repressed sexual desires sacrificed in infancy and childhood to the needs of acculturation, and with a fore-conscious acting as a sort of "censor" and mediator between the conscious and unconscious. Every human activity is promptly referred to a supposed dominance of open or repressed sexual drives, setting up a constant inter-action and often a conflict between the ego, the superego, and the libido. In all this everchanging flow, the libido remains a constant factor among variables, since to each individual is attributed a "fixed amount" of it, which may be used up, sublimated, or converted into psychotic symp-toms, as the case may be. Every dream or symptom becomes a wish-fulfilment of a sexual nature which, if not apparent in the manifest content, may be unmasked through analytic interpretation of its inherent sym-bolism.

Occupation with adult patients with reconstruction of memories through the methods of "catharsis" and "free associations" has led the psycho-analysts to build up retrospectively a system of infantile sex evolution be-ginning with intrauterine or at least natal narcissism, or self-love, indulging in satisfaction of the different "erogenous zones," over the much discussed "family drama" in the form of the Oedipus complex, over bisexuality and homosexuality, to end with the final heterosexual adjustment as the normal adult pattern. It is most important to know that this whole scheme had been fully established before any child was ever approached by the psycho-analyst. When it was done, the ready-made measuring rod was simply applied to the child "as if" the theories obtained from the adult with a good deal of analogy and speculation had been proved beyond doubt to be ob-jective, substantial facts. Thus, the teachings of infantile sexuality and the Oedipus complex were not derived from the study of children but wilfully bestowed upon them *a priori*.[1]

[1] The following is a list of some of the more important psychoanalytic publica-tions dealing with children:

Bernfeld, Siegfried. Die Psychoanalyse in der Jugendbewegung. Imago. 1919, 5, 283–289.

Freud, Anna. Einführung in die Technik der Kinderanalyse. Leipzig-Wien-Zürich. 1927.

Freud, Anna. Psychoanalysis of the Child. In Handbook of Child Psychology, edited by Carl Murchison. Worcester. 1931, pp. 555–567.

Friedjung, Josef K. Was hat Freud der Kinderheilkunde gebracht? Kinder-ärztliche Praxis. 1931, 2, 289–292.

Hug-Hellmuth, H. von. Aus dem Seelenleben des Kindes. Eine psychoanaly-tische Studie. Zweite Auflage. Leipzig und Wien. 1921. (Schriften zur angewandten Seelenkunde, No. 15.)

Jung, C. G. Über Konflikte der kindlichen Seele. Jahrbuch für psychoanalytische und psychopathologische Forschung. 1910, 2, 33–58.

Klein, Melanie. Die Rolle der Schule in der libidinösen Entwicklung des Kindes. Internationale Zeitschrift für Psychoanalyse. 1923, 9, 323–344.

Alfred Adler seceded from the psychoanalytic school at a comparatively early period of its development. His *Individualpsychologie*,[1] emerging from Freudian principles, has developed into an independent doctrine which has had a tremendous influence particularly in the field of education. It rejects the idea of an absolutistic tyranny of sex over man, refuses to juggle with one-sidedly interpreted symbols, and endeavors to approach individual problems from the safer port of the underlying objective data with careful elaboration of the actual complaint. A study of *organ inferiority* led Adler to the observation that there seems to exist a tendency to compensation or over-compensation on the part of an inferior organ or organ system. This observation was broadened into the teaching that personality difficulties have their roots in a *feeling of inferiority and insecurity* derived from physical handicaps and from clashes with the environment which interferes with the person's need of self-assertion and exaggerated will to power. Adler comes to view behavior disorders of children as attempts at over-compensation for deficiencies, supplying the child with tools which are intended to make him the center of attention and to govern the family. No observer of growing or adult individuals can get away from the fact that these statements are based on the solid ground of factual material and have to be taken seriously into account in the evaluation and constructive treatment of disturbances in which they are found to be at work. But here again one is confronted with the desire, so characteristic of all the psychological systems discussed so far, to make this undeniable and valid contribution the starting point of a "nothing but"-attitude, subordinating all other factors encountered in the picture to an assumed all-momentousness of the "inferiority complex."

During the last decade, the study of personality functions has been enriched by the discovery of the so-called *eidetic phenomena*. They are most clearly summarized by Klüver: "E. R. Jaensch in Marburg must be credited with having been the first one systematically to attack the problem of eidetic imagery in children. EI (eidetic images) or, to use the German equivalent, *Anschauungsbilder*, are subjective visual, auditory, etc., phenomena which assume a perceptual character. An eidetic individual, after having been asked to look attentively at an object, is able, with eyes open or closed, to 'see' this object again. This is possible either immediately or after a certain lapse of time, even after the passage of several years. These eidetic phenomena, as 'images of hallucinatory clearness', are seen *'im buchstäblichen Sinne'* (in a literal sense); they are seen in the sense that after-images are seen. Although the stimulus object may be reproduced with almost photographic fidelity, EI as a rule differ from the original stimulus object with respect to color, form, and the number of details. They differ from hallucinations in that the eidetic individual does not believe in

Klein, Melanie. The Psychoanalysis of Children. London. 1923.

Morgenstern, Sophie. La psychanalyse infantile. L'Hygiène Mentale. 1928, 23, 158–169.

[1] Adler, Alfred. The Practice and Theory of Individual Psychology. Translated by P. Radin. New York. 1924.

Wexberg, Erwin. Individualpsychologie. Leipzig. 1928.

Wexberg, Erwin. Handbuch der Individualpsychologie. München. 1926.

the objective reality of the phenomena but recognizes their subjective character; they differ from memory-images in that the phenomena are really seen. These EI, it is pointed out, are not of pathological nature but must be considered as phenomena in 'normal and healthy' persons."[1]

Eidetic imagery is very frequent in children and young people and usually disappears in puberty. From this it was concluded that the eidetic type of vision represents the ontogenetic source ("unitary type") of perception, that there exists a "latent" or "overt" eidetic period as a "normal" phase of childhood.

The investigators soon felt that they could separate two more or less distinct features. Persons of the B or Basedowoid type are capable of vivid visualization of objects they are thinking about, of producing and banishing the images at will, of changing their colors and their position in space. People of the T or Tetanoid type cannot voluntarily evoke or suppress the images and it is only with considerable effort and after a long time that they may succeed in obtaining any alterations; they are said to be the kind of individuals who tend to "neuropathy," whereas individuals of the B type are disposed to "psychopathy." Since the people in general did not please the examiners with the presentation of clear cut types, BT and TB combinations were added to suit all subjects. The founders of the "school" have, true to form, not failed to make intellectual and emotional reactivity, achievements or failure in certain school subjects, ethical attitudes and the formation of certain ideals dependent on eidetic imagery. The cult of trying to influence the EI with specific drugs (Anhalonium Lewinii, calcium in the T type) has led to disappointment even of the most ardent adherents of the Marburg school. It must, however, be conceded that a few original factual observations may indeed lend themselves for practical utilization in the education of a properly selected number of children.

We have, thus far, tried to give a brief review of the outstanding current "schools," each of which holds out the assertion, unencumbered by the claims of its neighbors, that it alone preaches the true and infallible gospel of understanding and treating the child. They all have in common the urge to create a sort of universal language which should eliminate the use of all other tongues, but if viewed together, they offer a dissonance differing in nothing from that of the Tower of Babel. The choice of any of them, if one really wishes to choose, becomes a matter of faith rather than critical scientific balancing of demonstrable facts. We must, after all, meet individuals and situations as they are, in their manifoldness and relativity and plasticity, not as a rigid dictatorial system postulates them to be. At least in this connection, it may be well to draw a line between science and creed.

A survey of the prevailing methods of the study, treatment, and prevention of children's behavior disorders would be very incomplete, indeed, if it failed to include a movement, now international in scope, which since its inauguration in 1908 has grown into a conspicuous feature of our public life. Its inception was marked by the activities of Clifford W. Beers,

[1] Klüver, Heinrich. The Eidetic Child. In Handbook of Child Psychology, edited by Carl Murchison. Worcester. 1931, pp. 643–668.

an energetic and enthusiastic graduate of Yale University, who had recently
recovered from a major psychotic condition and decided to devote his life
and organizing talent to the amelioration and prevention of mental illness.
Adolf Meyer, then in New York, suggested upon his request for a suitable
name to be employed in connection with such efforts a term which in the
course of time has become a household word of the English and, through
literal translation, of all civilized languages, the term *mental hygiene.* The
movement was ushered in by Beers' book, *A Mind That Found Itself,*
the foundation of the Connecticut Society for Mental Hygiene (1908), and
the formation of the National Committee for Mental Hygiene (1909).
It culminated in 1930 in the famous first International Congress of Mental
Hygiene in Washington, D. C., to which the governments of more than
fifty countries sent their delegates. The Committee established an increasing number of Child Guidance Clinics in the various communities which
were expected to assume the financial responsibilities as soon as their
practical usefulness seemed to be sufficiently demonstrated.

Collaboration with practicing physicians has always been one of the leading items in the program; but, due to a number of understandable factors,
the approach has unfortunately not been a mutual one. The medical profession has viewed with unconcealed suspicion the fact that, in the enthusiastic and worthwhile efforts to interest the general public, the helpful
concept of mental hygiene was suffered to be abused for unscientific propaganda by medically untrained people who had little more to offer than just
their enthusiasm devoid of substantial contents. Sentimentalization, over-
popularization, feeding of an undigested terminology to naïve laymen, and
leaning towards one or the other "school," all these factors acted as de-
terrents keeping the physician away from the movement. They should not,
however, make one unmindful of the general interest that has been created
and of the actual contributions that have been made by the mental hygiene
movement which is with us to stay and from the coöperation with which
both the practicing physician and the members of the group could derive
a great deal of benefit.

CHAPTER II

THE PRINCIPLES OF AN OBJECTIVE PSYCHOBIOLOGY
AND PSYCHOPATHOLOGY OF CHILDHOOD

"FROM time immemorial the physician has been urged to treat not only the diseased organ or the condition, but also the patient. And of late years we have learned to realize that indeed some disorders can be explained, and treated, as abnormal and unhealthy ways of the person rather than as disorders of any one special organ. . . . Every medical teacher gives some advice on this topic of doing justice to the personality; oftenest, and probably too often, he feels that the talent for dealing with personality must be inborn and cannot be hammered in by any training.

"Of late years the difficulties in the total unified adjustment and behavior of our patients have been more and more reduced to intelligible processes: defects of development, intellectual, affective, or conative, improper use of the assets, etc. Instead of mere vague ideas, of something requiring special handling, we have today a growing body of facts in the way of habit disorders, harmful substitution and the like, which must be heeded in helping the patient to reach his best ground. How can the student be helped to command these facts most quickly? We teach him physics and chemistry and biology and physiology. Who teaches him the elements of those reactions which we call behavior and mentation? He enters this field with confused and confusing notions; how is he to straighten them out?"

These questions were asked by Adolf Meyer[1] and answered by him in many years of patient and persistent effort. If, in this chapter, we base our presentation on his teachings, it is not because we want our readers to become acquainted with, and adopt, just another of the existing "schools" of psychological thought or psychiatric technique. It is rather for this reason that we find in objective psychobiology the following features, for which one looks in vain in the fashionable doctrines:

Freedom from any mystical concepts.
Unwillingness to consider any selected group of facts as all-important or solely valid in the study of personality.
Readiness to accept from any worker or any "school" that which has been satisfactorily proved to be a factual contribution.
Working with concrete, objectively demonstrable facts obtained in an unprejudiced, critical, and self-critical manner.
Dealing with the individual as a psychobiological unit within a changeable- and changing-environment.

[1] Meyer, Adolf: Objective Psychology or Psychobiology with Subordination of the Medically Useless Contrast of Mental and Physical. The Journal of the American Medical Association 1915, 65, 860–863.
Kanner, Leo: The Significance of a Pluralistic Attitude in the Study of Human Behavior. Introduction to Some of the Leading Principles of Dr. Adolf Meyer's Objective Psychobiology. Journal of Abnormal and Social Psychology. 1933, 28, 30–41.

Recognition of the multiplicity of factors potentially and actually at play in interpersonal relations.

Melioristic utilization of the assets found in maladjusted individuals, for the betterment of the condition.

Using a terminology which can be made accessible to, and understood by, everyone whose capacity for clear, logical thinking and common sense has not been blunted by one-sided preoccupations.

Simplicity without an attempt at simplification.

Practical applicability in the sense of sober scientific work, which can be taught and learned, rather than an "art" or a "gift from Heaven" mysteriously bestowed upon a chosen few.

In recent years, due largely to the influence of Meyerian thought, one has become accustomed to speak of the individual (or child) "as a whole." Everyone, including philosophers, physicians, and psychologists, has in everyday life hardly ever failed to deal with people as units, as "individuals" in the etymological sense of this word. Nevertheless, attempts at theoretical formulation have had a conspicuous inclination either to "divide" the "individual" or else to eliminate with a rather drastic eraser undeniably present features with which the very same people did not hesitate to deal in their practical contact with human beings. To be more specific, we refer as examples of the first category to the animistic and vitalistic schools.

Animism is the oldest, most primitive, and still most widely spread form of accounting for the fact that man not only moves, eats, drinks, eliminates, sees, hears, smells, etc., but also thinks, feels, loves, hates, and is capable of giving verbal expression to his reasoning and emotions. Animism postulates a bipartition of man into body and soul or even a tripartition into body, soul, and mind. The soul enters its host at birth and stays there until death and, according to the more naïve conceptions, it may, even in the course of this union, detach itself from its container and go out on adventures during sleep or in an epileptic grand mal attack. The soul is looked upon as a separate, independent entity which may have existed long before the formation of its corporal frame, or is created at the moment of the union; after the final separation, it may lead a continued existence in Heaven or Hell, or Hades, or Walhalla, or reach the eternal bliss of Nirvana, or migrate about from body to body in a state of metempsychotic nomadism. The physician can do little, if anything, to the activities, "good" or "bad," of such a soul, which has been "treated" by the priest or the exorcist or the entranced medicine man or, post mortem, by the spiritualist in accordance with the established beliefs.

Vitalism differs from animism in that it does not insist on the workings of a substantial "soul." It holds that the living organism is activated by a "vital force," an "élan vital," or an "entelechy." The division of the individual into a somatic constituent and something different, more or less alien and imponderable, which nevertheless acts and drives and motivates, is strictly maintained. Thus we again have a dualism, in which the one component may be studied objectively with regard to its morphology, physiology, and structural pathology, and the other can be reached through speculation and dialectics only.

The last two or three centuries have witnessed an increasing tendency towards unification of man, who was until then assumed to be made up of two (or three) distinctive compartments. The resulting *monistic doctrines*, however, have mostly fallen into the other extreme of annihilating either "matter" or "mind," because they did not know how to combine them satisfactorily. This gave rise to a wide span of theories, ranging from pure idealistic panpsychism to coarse materialistic apsychism. Matter, on the one hand, was reduced dictatorially to particles of "mind-stuff," or to an "incidental aspect, an inadequate presentation of reality in our sensation." On the other hand, consciousness was either declared to be non-existent, or, at least very prematurely, tied up with the brain in the same sense as the whistling sound issuing forth from the steam engine or the shadow thrown by the moving parts of a machine or the squeaking noise made by the axle of an insufficiently greased cartwheel.

Of late years, a compromise has been attempted between the dualistic principle of interaction between body and soul and the monistic tenets of a dominance or sole existence of either "mind" alone or "matter" alone. We refer to the school of *psychophysical parallelism*, which assumes a coincident but otherwise not interdependent, "parallel" running together of a mental and physical aspect. Thus, a sort of pseudo-monism was created, which is not at all concerned about the "How" of the coincidence.

This very condensed review may at first glance impress the reader as an unnecessary and cumbersome digression in a discussion of children's psychiatric problems. It is nevertheless essential for an understanding of what we really mean when we speak of the *child as a whole*. It is evident that, when confronted with the complaint of temper tantrums or hypochondriasis, we can expect very little practical benefit from trying to attack a detachable soul, a vital spark, the brain cells from which thoughts are supposed to emanate, or a physical or mental "aspect." We have, furthermore, not been told by the founders and expounders of the various theories what sort of evolution, if any, the soul or entelechy or vital spark undergo before the individual in whom they roam has reached maturity. It is an interesting historical curiosity that none of these philosophical systems seems to have been bothered by the problems of mental development in the early years of life. The soul being something ready-made and capable of expressing itself as soon as the child has acquired completely the capacity of speech, it is not surprising to find that both in medical and educational thinking any behavior disorder was believed to be either merely physical—in that case drugs, electric current, hydrotherapy, etc., were administered—or merely the manifestation of a moral short-coming of the soul, of "badness," which called for "punishment." For the neurologizing schools it was somewhat easier to account for the developmental psychic differences between children and adults; immature brain centers must result in immature behavior. Yet how are we to influence a postulated center, the location and even existence of which is most uncertain?

We can, however, and do in everyday life, satisfactorily work with human beings as they appear before us, as acting, behaving, talking individuals of flesh and blood. We know that, independent of the person's volition and state of awareness, various organs and groups of organs continually perform their physiological, closely interrelated functions. We also know that the same person, whose heart muscle contracts and expands rhythmically, whose liver secretes bile, whose hair and nails grow when shortened, in his entirety acts and plans and calculates, is awake or asleep, recalls things of the past and looks forward to the future. It is this totality of the behaving organism that we refer to when we mention a name or use a personal pronoun. The "behavior" itself consists of meaningful muscular activities, which may be supplemented by vasomotor, pilomotor, and secretory manifestations, in the form of gestures, emotional expressions, and verbal (spoken or written) utterances; these overt performances are accompanied, preceded, and followed, by a more implicit, not so directly accessible, mode of behavior (thinking, feeling, remembering, being unable to recall, silent reading, etc.).

The normal structures of the organs and tissues which make up the individual's body and are similar or practically identical in the average persons of the same sex and age, are studied by the anatomist. The normal part-functions of these organs, which are more complicated and subject to greater variations and fluctuations, are the subject of the physiologist, who makes full use of the insight gained through anatomical knowledge. The abnormal structures and part-functions are the domain of the pathologist, who, in turn, avails himself advantageously of what anatomy and physiology have taught him. In each instance, it has become necessary to evolve different methods of investigation. The whole-functions, that is, the overt and implicit behavior of the individual, which are of still greater complexity and variability, are reached by the psychobiologist, who must be prepared to use the data furnished by the other investigators, developing at the same time his own methods of research. Psychobiology is, therefore, together with morphology, physiology, and pathology, a fundamental basis and branch of the science of medicine.

When we speak of dealing with the child as a whole, we have in mind a psychobiological approach to the whole-functions, or "behavior," of the growing individual. We become aware of the fact that the very moment that we recognize behavior, both overt and implicit, as a function of the total organism, the confusing contrast between body and mind, between physical and mental, no longer exists or need disturb anyone. "Mind" is not viewed as a mystical entity nor as something radiating from any number of cerebral cells, but as that with which we are actually confronted when listening to a violinist, quizzing a student, or witnessing an outburst of anger: the integrated whole-functions of a total personality.

Child psychology thus becomes an objective and concrete study of the mentally integrated individual during the natural progress of maturation. Instead of speculating about how the soul or the élan vital or the mental aspect might possibly behave itself in the years between birth and adolescence, it is more scientific to observe carefully the performances of the developing child during the successive stages or periods of mental integration or personality formation. These stages, which form a gradual continuity, are marked by the time factor (age) and the correlated evolution of accessory species-determined integrating factors, such as locomotion, speech, socialization, and pubescence. Viewing the growing individual as an integrated unit is the first step in the direction of a practical and objective psychobiology of childhood.

If, with this attitude as a background, we are confronted with a temper tantrum, a hypochondriacal complaint, enuresis, or stuttering, we are no longer driven to grope for a purely "organic" interpretation in the sense of wanting to influence the difficulty by the administration of drugs alone or by blaming the wetting always on a "weak bladder" or the like; nor do we have to forget for a minute that urination is a function of the kidneys and bladder or that the larynx and certain groups of muscles are involved in stuttering. Every behavior disorder, just as every normal behavior of any kind, is surely "physical" in the sense that it originates in, and is carried out by, an organism of flesh and blood. But the distinction between part-functions and whole-functions of the individual brings home an appreciation of the psychobiological nature and features of behavior, which must be studied and treated with psychobiological insight and methods.

What are these psychobiological methods?

A child is brought to the physician's attention with a complaint. This may consist of a lesion of the skin, an exanthematous condition, otitis media, whooping cough, or constant blinking. It will, in every case, become necessary to obtain a careful history of the onset of the difficulty, the mode and circumstances of its first appearance, its development up to the time of the consultation, and the therapeutic attempts already undertaken. This will be followed by a thorough examination of the child, resulting in the physician's reformulation of the complaint offered by the parent in a manner which would enable him to recognize clearly the problem and to make plans for the treatment. This reformulation we speak of as "diagnosis."

The complaint may be of such a nature that it does not involve the child's personality in the least, beyond the desire on the part of the patient, the family, or both, to have it corrected: a furuncle, a sprained ankle, uncomplicated varicella, the transient results of casual overeating. In these cases, prompt attention to the local or, in the instance of chicken-pox, the general condition will do full justice to the entire situation, though even here the need of staying away from school for a few days or weeks, over-solicitude on the part of the parents, or the desire to soothe the child's discomfort by taking him into the mother's bed may, or may not, more or less perceptibly enter into the situation.

There is a vast range between these disorders and such complaints in which the patient's personality is very obviously and conspicuously in the foreground, as in temper tantrums, hypochondriasis, obsessive thinking, persistent daydreaming, masturbation, excessive restlessness, truancy, or stealing. In order to do equal justice to these and similar, sometimes not so strikingly personality-determined difficulties, one would have to study carefully the child's personality.

In doing so, one would, to be objective, not wish to approach the patient with the ready-made formula of "badness," "just imagination," "Oedipus complex," or "feeling of inferiority." One would not immediately want to satisfy himself with "diagnostic" reformulations, which, without a sufficient acquaintance with the facts, may mean nothing or anything, such as "neuropathic constitution," "psychopathic inferiority," or "neurotic child." One would much rather wish to gain a concrete knowledge of all the possible facts and factors which may be at play, in order to be capable of actually remedying the condition for which help is being solicited.

After a satisfactory answer to the question: "What is the complaint?," the next logical step will be to ask: "Who is the child that presents this complaint?"

A brief biography (personal history) will be the best and most solid preparation for an analytic study of the patient's personality functions.

It will be followed by a thorough physical examination, the main purpose of which will be not a fishing for the site of "focal infection" nor for the one organ which could be made fully responsible, but a careful registration of the findings.

Knowledge of the patient's intellectual endowment will enable us to learn of the relation that exists between that which he is actually capable of grasping and doing and that which his environment (the family, the teacher, the playmates) expects him to comprehend and to achieve. It will help to tell us what use the child really makes, and has been taught to make of his intellectual assets. It will furthermore give us a valuable clue to the therapeutic possibilities, particularly to the problem as to what mode of approach one should most advantageously choose in the direct work with the child.

The child's emotional life and habits are of equal importance for the sizing up of the difficulty. On the basis of concrete examples, one will have to determine how, in the course of the patient's existence, love, hate, fear, anger, disappointment, etc., have found expression and become potent in the formation of his character and especially in the evolution of the specific complaint or complaints under consideration.

The child's principal aversions and predilections, urges and drives will be an object of our interest and inquiry.

In addition, we shall have to make ourselves thoroughly familiar with the features of the patient's environment and its possible, direct or indirect, connections with the difficulty to be treated.

Psychobiology and psychiatry deal to a very large extent with interpersonal relations between men. Ideal mental health may be described as consisting of a maximal ability of, plus best opportunity for, getting along with people, without the interference of inner conflicts or external frictions, in a manner that would make for full mutual satisfaction on a constant give-and-take basis. *Man is not only a biological, but also a highly differentiated sociobiological unit.*

Study of the environment does not presuppose any unusual theoretical preparations which might well deter the physician from psychiatric work with the individual child. It simply calls for an elaboration of the complaint in the light of the actual manner in which the patient gets along, and is taught to get along, at home, at school, with the playmates, and with the community at large. One soon learns to appreciate the difficulties with which the neglected, pampered, or too rigidly disciplined child may be confronted. One soon becomes aware of the rôle which a neighborhood bully, "sissified" clothes as object of ridicule among the schoolmates, or an unsympathetic teacher may play in determining the trend of a child's behavior.

A great deal has been made in recent years of an artificially construed controversy between those who hold that "environment" is the sole determinator of human behavior and others who maintain that everything can be satisfactorily explained by "heredity." Remaining, as we have decided to do, on the firm soil of objective observation, we do not have the urge to make dogmatic statements in the abstract, but are rather inclined to study in each case the facts for what they are worth, obtaining information about the reactions and personality trends of the antecedents with their possible bearing upon the complaint, making allowance for constitutionally determined characteristics wherever we find them to be at work, and making ourselves acquainted with that which the "milieu" has contributed.

Psychobiology is a *pluralistic* science. It is anchored in the multiplicity and variety and changeability of facts and occurrences found in real life and makes use of them in the practical work with patients, unencumbered by hypotheses or dogmatic postulates. It includes the physical, intellectual, conative, affective, and situational features and any really existing combinations in the scope of its unbiased work with any personality difficulty of adults or children.

Psychobiology is a *genetic-dynamic* science. Starting with the "Here" and "Now" of the complaint, it goes back to its origin and evolution and possible projections into the future, working with factual material with its concrete geographic and chronological implications, and studying the personality development of the child in the light of its environmental setting.

The psychobiologist and psychopathologist advocates a *melioristic* attitude. He is, to be true, far from holding out Pollyannish promises of doing away with mental illness in the course of a generation or two, nor does he deceive himself into believing, or making others believe, that perfection of the one or other method will, at our present state of knowledge, accomplish the miraculous feat of transforming personalities or healing all individual or social woes. But he does insist on making constructive use of the assets found in any child or any environment, without having to discount the existing limitations. No condition is so "hopeless" but that a worthwhile attempt could be made for its amelioration.

The objective psychobiologist and psychopathologist, finally, has a dread of terminological strait-jackets. He therefore prefers a reformulation of the complaint (diagnosis) in terms of what the examination has actually shown to be the outstanding problem, to the need of subscribing to certain rigid psychiatric "disease-entities." This would be particularly difficult in dealing with the rank and file of children's behavior disorders. We recognize, however, in the vast variety of personality problems certain similarities which may, for the purpose of better orientation and mutual understanding, be grouped together as related reaction-tendencies or reaction-patterns.

With these principles for a general background, the physician needs no longer be bewildered by a "confusion of theory and authority," by the idea that psychiatry is an art which must be "had" and cannot be acquired, and by developing an "inferiority complex" in the face of something which he has thought to be beyond his reach.[1]

[1] Kanner, Leo. Supplying the Psychiatric Needs of a Pediatric Clinic. American Journal of Orthopsychiatry. 1932, 2, 400–406.—Psychobiological Work with Children's Personality Difficulties. Ibid. 1934, 4, 402–412.

EXAMINATION AND DIAGNOSIS

CHAPTER III

GENERAL CONSIDERATIONS WITH REGARD TO PSYCHIATRIC EXAMINATION OF CHILDREN

IT IS ADVISABLE to have a separate, well ventilated room, in which a selected group of unbreakable and easily cleaned toys, suitable for both sexes and different ages, is available and kept with necessary sanitary precautions. While the children are awaiting their turns, one may unobtrusively observe their mode of getting acquainted, their reaction to the separation from the parent (usually the mother), and their choice and handling of playthings.

If the child is more than two years of age, the parents and the patient should be interviewed *separately*. This is desirable for various reasons. The main purpose is to avoid any discussion of the child's difficulties in his presence. The mother is often apt to quote diagnostic terms obtained through reading or from previous medical, osteopathic, or chiropractic consultations or from some supposedly enlightened relative or neighbor. How much harm may be done in this manner, was perhaps best demonstrated by a thirteen-year-old, slightly retarded girl who was wheeled into the office in an attitude of extreme weakness and helplessness and with the most pitiful facial expression that can be imagined. When questioned as to her complaint, she stated whiningly: "I have an auriculo-valvular disease." She did have a functional systolic murmur (in addition to other findings). The family physician had, years before, in her presence spoken of the possibility of her having an "auriculo-valvular disease," a "diagnosis" which, in conjunction with the attending parental apprehensions, had made a chronic invalid of the child. Many such instances could be prevented if the rule of separate interviews could be generally adopted in pediatric practice.

Just as the child's presence is undesirable when the complaint, the personal history, and the social background are obtained, so the parent's witnessing of the direct, physical or psychiatric, examination may seriously limit its usefulness. There is the mother who, in the course of the intelligence rating, will try to "help" her offspring by supplying the answer before one is sure whether or not, or in what form, the patient would react to the task, by giving signs, by nodding or shaking her head behind the physician's back, or by offering prolific excuses and "explanations" whenever she notices or expects a failure. There is the mother who goes away with the feeling, which she will not fail to broadcast, that the doctor was too rough with the child or too unskilful while struggling to get a good look at the pharynx or at the eyegrounds or while taking blood for the Wassermann test. There is the mother who will keep asking for reasons why this or that test is given and wish to be supplied with a vocabulary which she could parade at the next meeting of her bridge club. There is the child who will be handicapped in his responsiveness by the fear of instantaneous or later parental censorship of his performance.

The very act of separation may be of great importance for the evaluation of the entire situation. There may be reluctance and even resistance on the part of the mother, the child, or both. Many are the parents who declare outright that it would be utterly impossible to do anything with the patients in their absence; and then one finds the child very coöperative and well behaved. Many are the children who hold on to the mother's skirt and react to persuasion with crying or even with typical temper tantrums. Others enter the office, hands in their pockets, whistling, trying to appear indifferent, or looking about in the room with an attitude of genuine or assumed nonchalance. Others again are so timid that a great deal of encouragement is needed to make them feel comfortable.

The interview with the parent will best begin with a question for the complaint or the complaints and for a report of the onset and development of the present illness. The child's environment will then be inquired into, with due consideration of the family history, changes of residence, economic conditions and social status, illnesses and reaction tendencies of the individual members of the household. It is advisable to record concrete names and dates and places. The remark, found in so many histories, "F.L.&W." for "Father living and well," contains much less information than the entry: "Father, John Smith, age 45 years, carpenter, out of work for the past two months, has saved up enough to live on his own resources for about four more months, but worried considerably about the future; healthy, except for occasional colds which he takes very seriously, always fearing pneumonia; completed sixth grade at 14 years; had enuresis until six years of age; very conscientious, fond of his children, leaving their training largely to the mother, but getting upset over their slightest misbehavior."

The personal history will supply all the essential facts from the child's birth until the date of the consultation. Particular caution is indicated with regard to the evaluation of the early developmental data, the onset of dentition, walking and talking; we had, in our case material, an opportunity to compare the parents' statements concerning these items with the information given out previously by the same people to the referring pediatrician, and in many instances, in children who had been followed regularly in the dispensary since the first months of life, the actual data were also available to serve as reliable checks. It was found that in at least one-sixth of the cases there were considerable discrepancies sufficient to discourage reliance on the latest information. This is especially true in the case of unintelligent parents or those blessed with large families. But one is occasionally surprised to find the same uncertainty in otherwise well-informed mothers of only two or three children. From time to time, one hears the remark: "I am sorry that I cannot remember these things. I had it all written in a book, but it was lost."

It cannot be emphasized enough how important it is to enter specific chronological dates as well as significant accompanying factors. One often finds in the case record the entry: "He (or she) has had measles, chicken-pox, pertussis, mumps." It is much more helpful to know the exact ages at which these illnesses occurred, their duration, any serious complications of a physical or psychological nature, the resulting loss of school attendance with possible repetition of a grade, etc. Changes of residence, conspicuous fluctuations in the family's economic situation, the child's reactions to sickness, to travel, to success and failure, to praise and reprimand, to visits away from home, should have their place in the record.

Even after the most painstaking history, it is advisable to ask the informant if she (or he) feels that anything has been omitted. Sometimes additional facts are obtained, which may prove of value in the final reformulation of the complaint and in the therapeutic plan. Thus, in one case of a restless boy with mild tics, who was handicapped by the worries of an over-solicitous mother and by considerable interference on the part of neighbors and friends (who felt that he had tuberculosis, that there must be something wrong with his mind, that his "sallow complexion" reminded them of that of his father who died of carcinoma), it was learned that an uncle had offered to pay his tuition at an excellent boarding school; the treatment could instantly be planned along these lines, much to the patient's advantage.

After all this information has been obtained, the mother may be temporarily dismissed, and the child interviewed. In our cases, where the physical examination had been performed previously by the referring pediatrician, we could immediately proceed with the psychiatric investigation. It was found best to begin with the intelligence rating. The child who, in expectance of a discussion of his behavior difficulties, may have been tense or reluctant or even hostile, relaxes soon and becomes more comfortable if confronted with questions which to him seem irrelevant and more in the nature of an interesting game. The patient is, as it were, taken off his guard. One has, without making him aware of the fact, an opportunity to observe his appearance, his quality of responsiveness, his alertness or dullness, his composure or lack of composure, his attention or lack of attention, the nature of his twitchings or stuttering, his vocabulary, his degree of preoccupation, his display of effort, and many other features.

For the rest of the mental status, the complaint and the information received from the parent will serve as a valuable guide. One will want to know whether the child is aware of his difficulties and what is his attitude towards them, what are his ideas of parental, school, and church authority, his relation to siblings and playmates, his fears, worries, and wishes. One will inquire, very tactfully and discreetly, into the form and sources of his sex information. One will ask for his interests and hobbies, his aversions and hatreds. All this must be done in a vocabulary fully adapted to the patient's grasp.

The following outline is intended to serve as a guide for a comprehensive psychiatric case history. We have found it convenient to drop the usual separation of "Complaint" and "Present Illness"; we list in the complaint section all those data which are offered as having any bearing on the difficulty or difficulties for which examination is requested, with a chronological record of the onset, first manifestations and circumstances under which they appeared, development, and present status of each problem.

Outline of a Psychiatric Case Record History taking

History number:
Name:
Age:
Address:
Referred by whom?

Complaint:

As formulated by the referring physician, the parents, the school teacher, etc. Onset and evolution of the difficulties.

Family and social history:

Father: name, age, occupation, health, education, personality traits, habits, economic status, disciplinary methods.

Mother: name, maiden name, age, health, education, personality traits, habits, disciplinary methods, number of pregnancies. Do the parents live together or are they separated?

Siblings, in order of birth (recording also miscarriages, stillbirths, and dead children): name, age, health, grade and progress in school, personality traits, behavior difficulties, habits of each.

Other members of the household (relatives, boarders, domestic help).

Interpersonal relations in the home. History and content of parental dissensions. Has either of the parents been previously married? If so, what was the cause of the separation? Were there any children; what are their names, ages, personalities?

Family history of serious illness, especially tuberculosis (contact with the patient?), malignancies, chronic heart and kidney diseases, metabolic and endocrine disorders, nervous and mental difficulties, alcoholism and use of drugs; peculiar individuals; suicides; conflicts with the law; unusually successful persons, etc.

Home conditions: House or apartment? If house. is it owned or rented? How many rooms? Sleeping arrangements. Type of neighborhood and relation to neighbors. How long has the family lived in the present residence? Previous locations.

The family's income: History of unusual financial success or reverses changing the social situation and outlook. Effects of unemployment.

Family contact with social agencies.

Family recreations: Entertainments at home. Movies. Athletics and sports. Intellectual, religious, civic interests and activities.

Personality features of foster-parents, step parent, as the case may be. Attention to illegitimacy and guardianship.

Personal history:

Date, place, and mode of birth. Full term or premature? History of early feeding.

Developmental data: Holding up the head. Sitting. Standing. Walking. First words. First sentences. Control of bowels. Control of urination. Acquisition of independence with regard to dressing, crossing the street, avoidance of danger.

History of illness (at what age? any complications? mild or severe? duration? sequelae?), convulsions, operations, and injuries, always with exact dates and essential features. One should always ask for reasons for tonsillectomy and circumcision.

History of habit formation and home management: Eating, sleeping, studying, playing, sex habits, nailbiting, thumbsucking, and parental attitudes towards them.

Personality traits (always illustrated by concrete examples) of aggressiveness, shyness, unusual attachments (one-sided or mutual?), irritability, restlessness, sensitiveness, whining, tendency to withdrawal, day-dreaming, jealousy, generosity, cruelty; selection of playmates.

Distribution of work, recreation (what sort?), rest, and sleep over the twenty-four hour period.

School record: Kindergarten data. Name of school, and grade now attended. How many years in each grade? Subjects offering especial interests or difficulties to the child. Changes of schools and their effects. Distance of the school from the home. Behavior in the classroom and on the playground. Sunday school report.

Physical status:

General make-up. Height, weight, temperature. Results of systematic examination. Hearing and vision. Dental condition. Laboratory findings (blood count, tuberculin, Wassermann tests). Other tests as indicated in the individual case. Complete neurological status. Scars from operations. Menstrual history.

Mental status:

Behavior upon entrance and during interview.
Intelligence test and reaction thereto.
Complaint as formulated by the child.
Attitudes towards parents, siblings, playmates, school, church, authority in general.
Special wishes, fears, frustrations, obsessions, etc.

Diagnostic reformulation:

With avoidance of doubtful terminology. Summary of assets and liabilities.

Treatment:

Work with the child, the family, and the community.

Follow-up notes.

At the completion of the examination, the child is sent back to his toys and the mother again interviewed. In this second conference, the nature of the difficulty is discussed with her. It is very essential that the disclosure of the factors at work should be made with the greatest possible tact, in a form understandable and acceptable to the parent and inviting full coöperation. It is hardly necessary nor is it desirable, and in many instances it is outright harmful to speak to the family in terms of the I.Q. Latin or Greek diagnostic terms will either mean nothing to the mother or frighten her unnecessarily. It is important to bear in mind that, with the rare exception of parents hostile to their children, the average father and mother always try to give their offspring the best care in the best manner known to them. If, in the course of the investigation, their management of the patient has been found faulty, their criticism on the part of the physician should never be arrogant or offensive. Constructive, detailed, and comprehensive advice as to what should be done after the consultation is more to the point and gives better results than the practice, unfortunately not so uncommon as it should be, of berating the parents, even if they seem to deserve it, for mistakes made previously due to lack of knowledge, or for the sake of convenience, or in order to keep peace with a dictatorial mother-in-law. Generalities should be avoided; they confuse the mother and may give rise to misunderstandings and unpleasant misquotations.

CHAPTER IV

THE COMPLAINT FACTOR

THERE exists, as we have pointed out, a considerable number of methods of dealing with the psychopathology of childhood. The one will attack the behavior problems of children with a battery of concepts elaborated by the psychoanalytic school and attempt to interpret and treat them on the basis of infantile sexuality. Another group is bound primarily to view every type of maladjustment from the pedestal of the inferiority complex. Again to others, the theory of focal infection, the endocrinopathies, or eidetic imagery seem to serve as an ever-valid open sesame. Some people take up mental hygiene with the express purpose of preventing delinquency and full-fledged psychotic reactions in later life; though this is doubtless a laudable goal, worthy of every means of encouragement and support, the insistence on envisioning the worst makes one think of the pediatrician or internist who would view every occurrence of "tummy-ache" or vomiting in a child from the angle of precluding the later development of gastric carcinoma.

Independent of any such attitudes, with which the child is received at the very moment when he enters the office, an increasing number of workers has felt the need of gathering the facts and data involved in the individual case, before reaching any conclusions with regard to mechanisms and prognostic predictions and therapeutic programs. These workers feel that you must primarily know exactly what you want to measure, before you can proceed to apply any sort of meter or gage. They somehow cannot, when confronted with a sleepwalking child, restrict their curiosity to the universal fact that the patient has a male and a female parent and that there may exist some form or other of sexual cravings, in the broadest meaning of this word. They shudder, when dealing with a temper tantrum, at the debatable postulate that what you really want to do is to reduce the future population of psychopathic wards and penitentiaries. They prefer to start with the actual problem with all its essential implications and complications, as it presents itself at the time of the first interview, with proper consideration of the genetic-dynamic aspects as well as of the projections into the future.

In doing so, one immediately becomes aware of the important rôle which the complaint assumes as the starting point and central focus in the work with any psychiatric difficulty of a child. The realization of its significance has forced itself upon one's mind especially in a setting where there was an opportunity to gather the complaints as expressed not only by the parents and the patients themselves, and occasionally by school teachers, social workers, and members of the Juvenile Court, but also in every instance by the physician who has referred the child.

Any attempt at a formulation of the rank and file of psychiatric problems has to revert inevitably to the nature, sources, content, wording, and spirit of the complaint, the great diagnostic classificatory, therapeutic, and educational values of which are based on the following considerations:

It was found that any translation of the complaint into the examiner's abbreviated terminology was apt to result in a net loss of highly important leads and insights. The finest and most detailed description of a feeding problem will be incomplete if it does not include the over-solicitous mother's repeated interpolations, "Doctor, for God's sake, do tell me if I am going to lose my boy!", or another parent's untiring assertions, "There is nothing good in the child. . . She is the slowest child in the whole world . . . She is twice as slow as the slowest child in the world. . . I couldn't even think of trying to train her. . . She has made a nervous wreck of me. . . A person has got to have cast iron nerves to be around the child." The best account of the type, onset, frequency, and handling of enuresis is wanting if it does not contain the introductory remarks made by an indifferent gum-chewing type of woman, "Oh, I don't know. Kidney trouble, I guess. I don't know why the doctor wanted you to see him. It ain't so bad. You see, his little sister does the same thing, so I let them sleep together. They'll get over it all right. Oh, what time is it, doctor? I ain't got much time. I promised a friend of mine to meet her at the movies."

In every instance, the first question addressed to the informant should be, *"What is the complaint?"* Later, it is best supplemented by the query, *"Are there any other complaints?"* After this, the examiner takes over the lead in order to obtain in a more organized and systematic form the facts and details not given spontaneously by the complainant. The answers should be recorded verbatim. It may be argued that, under these circumstances, one is often apt to get a somewhat scrambled account of the difficulty, with numerous insertions and casual side-remarks, but it was found that just those insertions proved to be not less helpful and at times even more valuable than the plain statement that the child blinks his eyes or bites his fingernails or would not eat his breakfast. It is these side-remarks that often reflect quite eloquently the parental attitudes and expectations; they may throw a light on prevailing superstitions and popular lore. A colored child was referred for psychiatric consultation because of supposed somatic hallucinations, when in reality she had adopted a neighbor's suggestions that her classroom headaches might be caused by worms inside the body. The mother of a white girl asked for treatment of her child's night terrors because she had lost a powerful amulet given her by a witch doctor. It is these side-remarks which occasionally direct one's attention to iatrogenic, or physician-determined, conditions. This happened in the case of a boy whose mother was told, while pregnant with him, that it was going to be "either you or the baby," and when the child was born asphyctic, that he would not live long. It further occurred in the case of a ten-year-old boy with attacks of shortness of breath, whose doctor told the parents that his asthma, diagnosed by him at the age of one year, was bound to recur later in life.

An example, selected at random, may serve to illustrate the value of the routine practice of recording the complaint literally. In answer to the question, "What is the complaint?", the mother of a seven-year-old girl stated:

She don't sleep good. She kicks in her sleep. Her teeth is so bad. I had one of them pulled. She don't want nothin' to eat. All she wants is somethin' sweet. She's awfully nervous. She bites her finger-nails. When she gets excited, she just gnaws and gnaws. She's on the go all the time. She won't sit down two minutes. She don't mind very good. I don't like to holler at her but scold her because she bites her finger-nails and gets so nervous. She wants to go to school all the time but I wouldn't let her go until I find out what's the matter with her. My little brother lives with me. He is four years old. The two kids fight a great deal over toys and candy. Her eyes is bad, too. I took her to the movies one day and she said her eyes was bad. Everything went dark. She kept rubbin' them. That's the only time she complained. She's always eatin' between meals. She loves cake and candy. I'd rather give it to her than hear her bawl. She loves all kinds of stuff. She likes greens and cabbage and everything. She won't go to bed unless I go with her. She's scared to go in a dark room by herself. She's been that way ever since she has had scarlet fever. She's afraid of doctors. She's afraid they are going to stick needles in her. She kicks her legs up and screams. She would tear up the house if she don't get what she wants. I give her anything she wants. If I haven't got it I borrow it. She's always whining or cryin' about something. When she meets strangers she bites her finger-nails and gets so nervous. She fights and hits animals. She killed a little tame rabbit she had. My sister is going to have a baby. She asked about it. We told her that a stork is going to bring it. Now she wants to see the stork when it comes.

This report needs, of course, further elucidation. But the wealth of information which it affords within the span of a few minutes, the vivid picture it gives of what goes on at home, the impression it conveys of the mother's own personality, furnishes significant leads and places us right in the midst of the total situation.

Whenever possible, both the father and mother should be interviewed. This may throw additional light on the factors involved in the complaint. It is not insignificant to observe how two temperamental parents, disagreeing about the father's exact age, work up a spirited battle in front of the interviewer, in which mutual accusations bring out features that had previously been shrewdly concealed by the couple. A great deal was learned from the man who, much to his wife's displeasure, described her methods of spoiling the child, whereupon she retaliated by interrupting his denial of alcoholic habits with the remark, "You better go ahead and tell the doctor how drunk you were last Sunday and what you did to me and the children!" We are led into the midst of the home atmosphere by the father who would snatch from his wife the answer to any question put to her with the somewhat impatient introduction, "Now, doctor, if I may speak for my wife. . . ." We cannot afford to omit in the record a father's plea to have the child psychoanalyzed and the mother's correction that what is really needed is a determination of her offspring's inferiority complex.

The child's own contribution to the complaint is, of course, also solicited, always in the absence of the parents, Again, a wealth of telling material is thus added to the entire picture. There is the boy who, after his confidence has been gained, explains his initial lack of coöperation by telling how indignant he was when he found that he was taken to the hospital instead of to his aunt's, as the mother had told him; the very fact that the mother had thought it necessary to deceive him made him fear an operation or at least admission to the wards. There is the stable, intelligent boy who good-naturedly excused his mother's alarm over his being a "feeding problem" when all he did was to leave the carrots in his soup; the parents, devouring the terrorism of some of the popular literature, had rushed for psychiatric help. There is the lad whose vivid account of a scene at home speaks for itself: "My father don't hit me hard because I run away. Then we run around the dining room table. He says, 'Wait till you come here to eat,' but when I come in, my mother won't let him hit me. Next day he forgets about it." A mother comes with all signs of consternation because the child's many complaints make her think of them as symptoms of some very severe malady; she mistrusts the family physician who does not take them seriously. This is what the child has to say about himself:

Sometimes I have a pain in my right knee, and today, in the street car, I was putting my hand on the bench and it shakes all over. And then I have got a pain in my feet, right in the arch. And then I have pains in my head (points first to the left, then to the right temple). In school, this morning, it looked like the examples on the board came right in front of my eyes. Sometimes in my stomach I have pain right around here. When I walk about three or four blocks, I have the pain, and I have to stop. Then I have pains in my elbow right here when I shoot marbles. My eyes, right under here, hurts, only when I go to bed and lie down. When I lie down, it will be there for an hour. Then I have pains under here (axilla) when I write in school. I get a pain where this bone is behind my ear. I get it sometimes when I bend over my head. Pains in my wrist right there; as soon as I fix something it will hurt. Right under my knee in my left leg— pain like needles, go through here and come up here—that's the way it feels like. That's about all. Sometimes after I have eaten I am so hungry as if I hadn't eaten anything for a week." And then comes a very remarkable spontaneous addition: "My father has all the pains that I have. It is God's will. God wants us to suffer in this life so we'll be happy in the next."

Such examples could be quoted *ad libitum*. In fact, every case examined furnishes an adequate illustration of the orienting value of the complaint and its formulation by the family, the child, and any other sources of information.

In our particular setting of close contact with the staff of a large pediatric clinic, the complaint has proved to be of considerable educational and self-educational significance. Every patient is first seen in the ward or dispensary and, if any psychiatric problem arises, sent to us for consultation. In each instance, a clear statement of why the child is referred is expected of the pediatrician. At the beginning of our collaboration, most of these statements were vague and hasty and often a mere play with terms, such as neuropathic, neurotic, constitutionally inferior, or mentally retarded child, with the underlying idea that such a "diagnosis" more or less cleared the referring physician of any further interest in the issue. As a result of continued working together and on the basis of growing experience, the assistants, internes, and students have learned to concern themselves with the actual concrete facts of the difficulty in question and to in-corporate them in their requests for consultation. Thus, the so-called refer slips came to serve as a helpful and telling measure of the result of our teaching endeavors as well as of the pediatricians' degree of insight into psychiatric problems. At present, practically all of these notes contain a clear account of the difficulty, with a serious and often successful effort to size up the situation, without hiding behind a doubtful and ill-understood terminology.

One of the principal advantages of the complaint is that it lends itself for a systematic grouping of the many items and difficulties dealt with in child psychiatry. On perusing so excellent a presentation as Homburger's *Psychopathologie des Kindesalters*, one is struck by the lack of any organ-ization of the material; chapters on night terrors, enuresis, suicide, and the status of the neglected child succeed each other in a rather disconnected fashion. Ziehen's division into psychoses with and without intellectual de-fect does not take the rank and file of behavior problems into consideration. Yet, in dealing with the pediatricians, we were confronted almost daily with the justified demand for an outline of those topics to which the psychiatrist may be expected to contribute his share.

We have found it practicable to divide the personality difficulties of children into the following main groups:

1. Personality difficulties forming essential features or sequels of physical illness.

2. Personality difficulties expressing themselves in the form of in-voluntary part-dysfunctions.

3. Personality difficulties expressing themselves clearly as whole-dys-functions of the individual.

The subdivisions are those utilized in the arrangement of the second section of this book. It must, however, be emphasized that this grouping does not in any way pretend to be the equivalent of diagnostic classifica-tion or a nosological scheme. This is exactly what we wish to avoid. It is rather intended to serve as an objective, plastic, and nosologically un-biased *table of contents* of the psychopathology of childhood, based on the variety of complaints and of well recognized reaction patterns.

The main advantages of this grouping, or table of contents, lie in the fact that it includes every form of children's personality difficulties, that it does not depend on any artificial and arbitrary distinctions between neurotic and neuropathic and psychopathic and neurasthenic and psy-chasthenic, and what not, and that its freedom from nosological restric-tions makes it possible to take unbiased cognizance of the frequent occur-rence of any variety of combinations of complaints.

This attitude leads logically to a revision of the usual concept of psycho-pediatric diagnostication. Instead of subscribing to any fixed set of di-agnostic vocabulary, we come to view "diagnosis" as a reformulation of the complaint, as offered by the various informants, on the basis of the avail-able data obtained through adequate history taking and thorough examina-tion. Diagnosis thus resumes its original meaning of knowing something sufficiently well to discern it from other sets of facts; it becomes a clear statement of the problem as it presents itself in the individual case to an experienced investigator who is at the same time familiar with the manifoldness of other similar and dissimilar reaction patterns.

Finally, the complaint factor often serves as a valuable indicator of our therapeutic success or lack of success. The clearing up, or persistence, of the difficulties complained of may frequently, though not always, be used as a measure of the reasonableness and adequacy of the handling of the maladjustment under consideration.

We may briefly mention an additional feature which occasionally comes out in the sizing up of a problem. A mother brings her boy because of his stuttering; in the course of the interview one learns that the child has always been enuretic. To the parent, the speech difficulty was sufficiently alarming to assume the form of a complaint; the bedwetting, however, which the patient shares with two siblings and which had also been present in the father, has come to be viewed as a sort of family tradition, and it did not occur to the informant to even think of it as a complaint, in spite of the repeated question, "Are there any other complaints?" It was therefore not brought out spontaneously and only entered into the picture when the subsequent systematic examination broached the subject of urinary habits. A little girl has an acute cardiac illness; the prescription of complete rest causes the mother to wonder if this could be carried out satisfactorily, considering the temper tantrums which the child has had for years; it is the first time that these outbursts of anger assume the proportions of a complaint in the eyes of the family. Another child is presented as daydreaming and preoccupied and not progressing in school; reluctantly and in a round-about manner, masturbation is reported by the mother after the father has encouraged her with the words, "You better tell the doctor about that other thing." In brief, a complaint may be *leading* or *incidental*. The very fact that this is so, is sometimes of great significance in the evaluation of the whole setting, as may be easily deduced from the examples quoted,—the alarm over stuttering with complete indifference about the enuresis; the arousal of concern over temper tantrums which threaten to interfere with the prescribed rest treatment; the open discussion of daydreaming and lack of concentration combined with initial concealment of the sex problem.

It is appropriate to refer here to Adolf Meyer's[1] fundamental paper, in which the importance of the complaint factor for teaching purposes and for the practical handling of cases has been brought out very convincingly.

[1] Meyer, Adolf. The "Complaint" as the Center of Genetic-Dynamic and Nosological Teaching in Psychiatry. New England Journal of Medicine 1928, 199, 360–370.
  Also: Kanner, Leo. The Significance of the Complaint Factor in Child Psychiatry. American Journal of Psychiatry. 1933, 13, 171–181.

CHAPTER V

THE AGE FACTOR

"CHILDHOOD" is a collective term. It includes all ages between the neonatal period and the termination of puberty. It presents the individual *in statu nascendi*. It carries him from a condition of complete helplessness to the very threshold of that degree of independence and creative activity which is commensurate with his constitutional, social, and educational background. Between those two landmarks, so many, so frequent, and so conspicuous alterations occur, that in comparison the periods of adolescence, middle age, climacteric involution, and senescence, no matter how eventful they are, appear much more homogeneous and much less variable.

Socialization is the outstanding achievement at the end of this span. Therefore, its gradual development lends itself perhaps better than anything else for a subdivision of the period of childhood. Fully realizing that the lines should not be drawn too rigidly in a process of evolution, that there exist no abrupt changes, and that a good deal of overlapping will have to be expected, we may distinguish three more or less characteristic periods of childhood:

Period of elementary socialization.

Period of domestic socialization.

Period of communal socialization.

PERIOD OF ELEMENTARY SOCIALIZATION

It comprises the first fifteen to eighteen months of life, in the course of which the infant is totally dependent on the persons of his environment. Under circumstances of normal health and protection, the functions acquired at that age arise almost entirely from "within," that is, from the propensities inherent in the species. Their adequate development at the proper time may be delayed or hindered through physical illness or, in unusually rare instances (of which the famous case of Kaspar Hauser is a classical example[1]), through faulty management. Being brought up in a dark room will have a bad effect on early space orientation. Being kept constantly in a restraining crib may postpone the progress of locomotion. Being raised in a silent environment may have an influence on early auditory orientation and the time and form of linguistic achievements. As a rule, however, in the normal individual the acquisition of these and the other accomplishments takes place according to certain laws of nature, allowing but slight variations.

Very soon after birth, on the first day of life, the beginning of visual adaptation can be observed in the form of contraction and dilatation of the pupils. There is also winking upon touch of the eyelashes. At two weeks,

[1] Evans, Elizabeth E. The Story of Kaspar Hauser from Authentic Records. London. 1892.

the child fixes his eyes on objects. At four weeks, he follows moving light. At two months, he has learned to accommodate sufficiently to see large objects and to notice the approach of a person. At four months, he begins to show selective attention to faces, to blink at the approach of objects (hand, pencil), but may not yet notice an inch cube placed before him. At six months, he reaches directly for objects, begins to look for things dropped before his eyes, to express recognition, and to react to mirror images. At approximately eight months, he has developed sufficient eye-hand coordination to pick up very small objects. He has achieved a degree of space orientation which will be helpful in his first locomotive attempts.

There is also early evidence of auditory adaptation. At one week, the child is startled by loud noises. He is soon found to blink at sharp sounds. At about one month, he may attend to voice and music and be quieted by talking or singing to him. At four months, he turns his head in the direction of voices heard and, at six months, in that of a ringing bell. At nine months, or a little later, he begins to adjust to words. His audition is now complete enough to assist the infant in the acquisition of language and in the finer discrimination of sounds.

The sense of touch is well developed at birth. The child reacts markedly to temperature changes. The slightest tactile stimulus applied to the lips evokes a sucking movement. At three months, the child uses his fingers with the purpose of producing tactile sensations. The first exploratory activities are connected with the sense of touch. Pain experience, however, develops more slowly. Internal pain (colic) seems to be felt much sooner than the application of painful external stimuli. At the end of the first year the sensation of pain has reached sufficient acumen to prepare the child for future avoidance of danger, based on experience and precept.

Taste and smell have not been studied in infants satisfactorily to permit of very exact statements. They appear at a very early period, and at ten or eleven months, the children are capable of fine discriminations. It seems that quite often a child may derive pleasing gustatory or olfactory sensations from things which to the adult are unpleasant, and vice versa. This fact has often proved helpful to parents in their administration of castor oil or codliver oil, but has also made them wonder why sometimes the "flavored" drugs were accepted less willingly than the unflavored preparations.

The active motor striped-muscle performances preparatory to locomotion commence at about the end of the first week when stretching may be observed. At four months, or a little before or after, the child has learned to hold his head up and to lift it when placed in a prone position; when placed on his side, he will roll onto his back and, a little later, when put on his back, roll over to lie on his stomach. At nine months, he sits up without support. At one year, he usually stands with help, creeps, and makes stepping movements when held in a suspended position so that the feet just touch the floor. At eighteen months, the average infant has learned to walk alone. Sometimes, this final achievement may be slightly deferred by allowing the child too much dependence on "baby bins" and "walkers."

After about a week, the infant's crying assumes meaningful modulations indicative of discomfort, hunger, sleepiness, or rough handling. The next step towards linguistic expression occurs at approximately four months in the form of vocalization, coincident with the first sounding of loud laughter. At about nine months, monosyllables are coupled together to form words, such as "mama," "papa," or "dada." At one year, the vocabulary consists of at least three words, at eighteen months of about five words. It is then that the sounds, at first meaningless, are beginning to be associated with persons or objects, indicating the onset of verbal symbolization, or "language" as a means of communication.

Aside from the gradual taking in of the surroundings directly through the senses, adaptation to the environment takes at an early time the shape of active and more complex functioning. Its first manifestations are groping (first purposeless, later exploratory, and then with a goal; for instance, for the lost nipple) and manual defense movements. At six months, the relations to the outer world have been sufficiently established to permit an elementary type of observation ("regarding" things) and of physical contact (holding, reaching). Between nine and twelve months, imitative activities may be observed. At this period, we find signs of a certain degree of inventiveness (obtaining a cube from under an inverted cup or from within a paper wrap) and ability to carry out simple commissions. At one year, the child has usually learned to refrain from performing acts which are forbidden and a few months later, to inhibit them habitually.

Whether the affective responses of a newborn infant are more of an undifferentiated character, as Sherman[1] has tried to demonstrate, or whether he is capable of expressing the three "primary" emotions of love, fear, and anger, as Watson[2] has taught, is a question still open to controversy. Watson has shown that loud noises and sudden withdrawal of support arouse in the baby a reaction comparable to fear in the older child or in the adult, that anger is evoked by the hampering of his bodily movements, and that a love response is caused by stroking the skin, especially of the lips, face, breast, and the genital zone. At about two months or a little later, the average child is capable of smiling. At one year, he has already experienced embarrassment, developed preferences and dislikes with regard to objects, foods, and people, and learned to bid for attention.

The greater part of the twenty-four hours of the new-born's day is occupied by sleep. At six months, the baby still sleeps from sixteen to eighteen hours, at one year for about fourteen hours. He has therefore gained a slowly increasing amount of time for his adaptation and expansion of interests and activities.

Thus, at the end of approximately the first eighteen months of life, the normal child has acquired the necessary sensory, motor, linguistic, emotive, orientative, and adaptive equipment to make him ready for the task of domestic socialization.[3]

[1] Sherman, M., and I. C. Sherman. Sensory-Motor Responses in Infants. Journal of Comparative Psychology. 1925, 5, 53–58.

[2] Watson, John B. Behaviorism. New York. 1925.

[3] The data presented above were compiled chiefly from the following sources: 1. Personal observations; 2. Arnold Gesell. The Mental Growth of the Pre-School Child. New York. 1930; 3. Winifred Rand, Mary E. Sweeny, and E. Lee Vincent. Growth and Development of the Young Child. Philadelphia and London. 1930.

PERIOD OF DOMESTIC SOCIALIZATION

It comprises the rest of the pre-school age, from eighteen months to about four or five years. It begins at a time when the child has learned to consider himself as an integral part of the family unit. Its principal achievements consist of the elaboration and broadening of the functions evolved during the first period, training of personal habits, and the establishment of interpersonal relations between the child and the members of the household and visitors in the home. It revolves about the home as the only or main focus of interest and source of information. From it, the child emerges with a knowledge of family structure, with a primitive cosmic space and time orientation (earth, sky, sun, moon, stars; day, night, summer, winter), with a vocabulary suited for simple conversational needs, with a capacity for imaginative and competitive play, with some degree of numerical comprehension, with the realization of certain personal responsibilities, and with some appreciation of authority.

Sense perception becomes more acute and discriminative, especially with regard to the inclusion of details. Stereognostic and color vision are added. Audition, olfactation, and taste receive innumerable new impressions, and gradually a rich empirical background is established, allowing the child to correlate these impressions more and more closely and correctly with their sources. The sense of touch, in the early portion of this period, is utilized much more extensively than is usually believed for associating the "feel" of objects with their nature, purpose, and names. Casual experiences bring to the child the first judgments of weight.

Locomotion soon begins to include running, chasing, expert climbing of stairs, getting on and off a chair, mounting and skilful steering of a tricycle or kiddie car. The original uncertainty and clumsiness gives way to well-controlled and finely coördinated graceful movements which make the child capable of careful handling of his toys, drawing attempts, self-feeding, and self-dressing.

Verbal symbolization, once started, progresses with astonishing rapidity. The passive vocabulary, that is, understanding of words heard, grows even much more quickly than the number of words actively employed by the child. Economizing symbolization in the form of thinking and reasoning makes itself perceptible at about two years through planned performances, for instance, when a child goes spontaneously into the adjoining room to fetch a desired object, or when he plays hide-and-seek (even though, at that age, he will "hide" in a place where he is not really concealed from view). About a year later, he will give evidence of thinking by asking questions not only about names, in which he has already indulged for some time, but also for more complex information, showing that he "wonders" and "wants to know." Piaget, who has done pioneer work in the study of children's "philosophies," gives the following enlightening classification of questions asked during the age period which we are now discussing:

The whys of casual explanation;
the whys of motivation;
the whys of justification;
the whats;

the whens;
the hows.[1]

The knowledge, thus obtained, is of course, unsystematic and fragmentary, but slowly prepares the child for the organized mode of school information.

Submission to orders, assertion of his own will, attention to stories with rendition of their contents, and spontaneous narration are functions well performed at the end of this period. Gesell says of the child of that age level: "Indeed, before five years of age, within his limits, he becomes an entertaining raconteur, whereas four years earlier he was unable to articulate a single word."

The period of domestic socialization is the time *par excellence* for adequate and effective habit training, which is one of the most essential postulates for the acquisition of future communal adjustment. Domestication, to be sure, has in many ways set in before the eighteenth month, but now its aims consist much more clearly and consistently in guiding the child towards emancipation and conventionalization through the teaching of "manners." Habit training is at this level concerned primarily with the functions of eating, elimination, sleep, and clothing. It is now that the very essence of childhood, which De Sanctis defines as "the attitude of becoming an adult," can be developed along normal, natural lines or hindered by unwise parental management. It is now that regularity, self-dependence, and the generally accepted form of personal habits must be firmly established in order to pave the way to smooth communal socialization. Continuation of bottle feeding through a part or the whole of this period, the practices of forcing, coaxing, bribing, threatening, punishing, entertaining the child in connection with every meal and every morsel, dressing and undressing him at a time when he can be taught to perform these activities alone, failure to introduce proper urinary functioning, inability to check, persistent thumbsucking, earpulling, nosepicking, or nailbiting, may assert themselves at a later time, even though the child may "outgrow" the one or the other individual difficulty.

Training in the home will also have to give close attention to emotional habits. Watson has shown conclusively how they are formed and how they can be controlled. Whether we wish to think of them as "conditioned reflexes" or prefer to deal with them in the broader light of more complex psychobiological reactions, so much is true that emotional stability or instability in later life is based to a large extent on early training and example in the home. It is now that the foundations for fear reactions and temper tantrums and unusual attachments are often laid or removed.

The period of domestication is coincident with a mode of behavior which may be said to be almost universal and which is commonly referred to as resistiveness, or negativism, or spitefulness. After the child has learned to discern between that which is "I" and that which is not "I," he is in his

[1] Piaget, Jean. The Language and Thought of the Child. Translated from the French. New York. 1926.

Piaget, Jean. Judgment and Reasoning in the Child. Translated from the French. New York. 1928.

very nature egoistical, concerned with the satisfaction of his own wishes, with no consideration of the desires and conveniences of others. There has been no opportunity so far for him to get along with people; the people have done everything to get along with him, to protect him, to feed him, to put him to bed, to clothe him, etc. Then, at about two years, he is given tasks and slowly mounting duties. If, in any way, they interfere with his pleasure, he asserts his will by contradicting. He expects his own wants to be carried out promptly, but is apt to meet commands with "No" and "I won't," with pouting and sulking. It is one of the most important educational measures of this period to convert this egoism into socialized altruism and family solidarity, by making the child know his privileges as well as his responsibilities. Acknowledgment and respect of parental authority has to precede the later necessity of accepting (and being capable of criticizing intelligently and constructively) the authority of the school, of the law, and of ideal as well as formal conventions. Parental authority, to be respected, must be respectable. The antics of an alcoholic father and the educational inconsistencies of a moody mother may, at this time and later, undermine the child's conviction of its justification. James S. Plant has excellently demonstrated the dangers inherent in the parents' abuse of their powers by converting the "reasonable" authority to which they are entitled and morally obliged, into "unreasonable" authority, which may make a cynic or a delinquent of the youngster.

Play life is another highly significant link in the chain of features preparing the child for communal adaptation. The imitation, however naïve, of adult occupations, the contact with children from other homes, the formation of groups other than the family unit, the participation in any sort of a temporary team, the competition against another team, are most instructive and transfer for the first time a portion of the child's interests and activities to extramural scenes.

During the period of elementary socialization, the child has been weaned from the nipple and crib to become an active member of domestic life. During the period of domestic socialization, he is weaned from exclusive dependence on the home and thus made ready for the final stage of childhood, the all-momentous task of communal socialization.

THE PERIOD OF COMMUNAL SOCIALIZATION

It begins with the branching out of the child's contacts into the community texture at about four or five years of age. Single steps in this direction have occasionally been made before, in the form of visits to relatives and neighbors, being taken for walks and rides and to stores. and to church, and attending the circus or the movies. The horizon expands. The child, aside from having his well-established position in the family, enters into a number of other circles, in which he assumes certain functions, and soon, in addition to "my daddy" and "my mother" and "my brother," he tells of "our house" and "our yard" and "our dog"; he then adds "our street" and "our block" and "our neighbors," and a little later, "our class," "our school," "our teacher," "our minister," "our ball team," "our dramatic club," etc. The child has grown community-conscious. The school becomes a highly important factor in his life. The play activities are more and more organized and assume the value of recreation, of relaxation from work.

From this period, the child emerges with informations, abilities, and ambitions, which will carry him through the *Sturm und Drang* of adolescence into the midst of full-fledged life adjustments. The heterosexual pattern has been molded to a degree which makes for future family foundation, when economic independence and emotional maturity will be reached. Physical growth is approaching its termination, and intellectual growth (that is, capacity, and not actual utilization and experience) is completed at approximately sixteen years of age.

It is in this period that, more than ever before, the child must be taught and given opportunities to stand on his own feet. With the domestic habits of eating, sleeping, clothing, elimination, care of toys, and adaptation to the family established at the end of the second period, the child must now learn to go out alone, to regulate his relations to playmates, schoolmates, teachers, and people with whom he forms more casual contacts, to make decisions and take the consequences, to choose his own friends, to fight his own battles, to compete fairly, and to consider the conveniences, rights, and properties of others, without, on the other hand, being so submissive and meek as to give up too easily his own privileges and possessions. All this is made possible by the development of ever finer subtleties of abstract thinking.

Realization of the successive periods of socialization is of high educational value and indispensable in the evaluation of children's behavior disorders. The main difficulty which arises from spoiling, oversolicitude, and overprotection lies in the fact that domestication is protracted far beyond its natural boundaries. A drastic example is that of a thirteen-year old-boy brought with the complaint of childishness, whining, fear of strangers, and nailbiting. He is physically healthy and has high average intelligence. The mother has done everything that possibly could be done to keep him from growing normally into communal adjustment. She has made him sleep in her bedroom, helping him to dress and to undress; she would never let him go out alone, even accompanied him on his way to and from school, went belligerently after any boy, often younger and smaller than her son, whom he accused of beating or insulting him, and gave in to any of his wishes if he only cried persistently enough. In other instances, even domestic socialization is delayed or prevented for a long time. We see more frequently than one should like to believe children who are breast fed at two years and given the bottle at four years; who are fed, washed, clothed, and even carried about at an age when the average youngster has long learned to take care of himself in all these respects.

Children are occasionally brought to us with a great deal of consternation on the part of the parents and sometimes with the remark of the referring physician that the patient seems to have undergone "definite personality changes." We then may find a healthy, intelligent youngster of two and a half to three and a half years, whose "personality change" is described as a tendency, which had not existed before, to contradict and to disobey and to say "No." Only the knowledge of the existence of a transient period of resistance in the normal development of children will save us (after a complete examination, of course) from attaching undue importance to a mode of behavior which is as far from being pathological as is the physiological loss of weight during the first days of life.

Consideration of the age factor in child psychiatry is therefore just as essential as attention to the age factor, for instance, with regard to the height and weight of a child, and often vastly more important.

For the sake of completeness, we may be permitted to mention that attempts to subdivide the period of childhood have been made before. The most elaborate one is that by Baldwin, who gives the following classification:

1. Affective epoch: Epoch of the rudimentary sense processes, the pleasure and pain process, and simple motor adaptation.
2. Epochs of objective reference:
   a. Epoch of simple presentation, memory, imitation, defensive action, instinct.
   b. Epoch of complex presentation, complex motor coördination, of conquest, of offensive action, and rudimentary volition.
3. Epoch of subjective reference: Epoch of thought, reflection, self-assertion, social organization, union of forces, coöperation.
4. Social and ethical epoch.[1]

The usual division into infancy, pre-school age, and school age roughly corresponds to our own classification.

[1] Baldwin, James Mark. Mental Development in the Child and the Race. New York. 1911.

CHAPTER VI

THE SOMATIC FACTOR

IN THE discussion of the various factors to be considered in the psychiatric examination of a child, we wilfully and emphatically begin with a discourse on the physical condition and its significance for the final evaluation of the personality problem. We do that, aside from other reasons, as a reaction to the wrong notion prevailing among so many practitioners, that the child psychiatrist's or mental hygienist's interests and activities are relegated entirely to the patient's "psychology." It is true and practically inevitable that the present day's division of labor in the vast realm of medicine has made it impossible for the specialist in one field to do the work of all other specialities. Just as the pediatrician will leave the operative care of appendicitis or pyloric stenosis to the surgeon and the treatment of cataract to the ophthalmologist, so the psychiatrist will depend on the pediatrician for a thorough physical examination of his little patients.

In our own clinical setting, every child referred to us because of a behavior difficulty has been gone over carefully in the pediatric ward or dispensary. He is then sent to us for consultation, not because "there is nothing the matter with him physically," but because either in the absence or in the presence of positive organic findings, he has been found to present a psychiatric problem, the investigation and treatment of which appears desirable. A psychiatrist who would remain ignorant or negligent of the child's tonsillitis or rheumatic condition or mediastinal tuberculosis or any other organic ailment, would indeed fall down on his job and have to be reminded that, no matter what his specialty, he is a physician first, last, and all the time. This, however, does not mean that the discovery of an infected tonsil should be immediately looked upon as "the" cause of whatever behavior difficulty exists, or that the presence of phimosis or an occult spina bifida justifies its immediate correlation with enuresis. Besides, we can do very little, if anything, for the spina bifida. But we can do a great deal for the enuretic child.

What are the types of relation between the existence of organic ailments and the complaint of personality disorders?

In an era when physicians as well as psychologists were wont to deal with man as something like a corporal container, lodging a detachable soul, it did not seem illogical to discuss the varieties of mutual influences which mind and body exercise upon each other. It seemed, then, a comparatively simple task to ponder over the destructive results wrought upon a previously unimpeded mental working by certain diseases, mostly of a neurological or infectious character, and, on the other hand, to observe the indentations left upon the somatic host by the morbid vagaries of a deranged mind. Concurrent physical and mental symptoms of an unsound reaction were immediately translated into terms of cause and effect, the mind or the body being viewed as the primary origin or the secondary recipient of the pathological manifestations.

Today we have no desire to speculate on such a question, the very nature of which would cause us to revert to a medically impractical dualistic trend. Viewing man as a mentally integrated unit, we rather take the individual as we find him and take proper cognizance of the difficulties which we encounter, whether they are in the nature of a diseased organ or a disturbed physiogenic or psychogenic function or set of functions. We may then distinguish the following forms of relation between somatic conditions on the one hand and personality difficulties on the other hand:

Anergastic reaction forms.
Dysergastic reaction forms.
Certain oligergastic reaction forms.
Somatic manifestations of "functional" personality disorders.
Personality difficulties having direct relation to (non-neurological) physical illness.
Personality difficulties having more indirect relation to physical illness.

ANERGASTIC REACTION FORMS

Adolf Meyer, justly dissatisfied with a psychiatric classification based on the rigid nosological concept of "disease entities," prefers to deal with that with which one is confronted in psychopathology as "frequently recurring combinations of facts, which sometimes occur in pure culture and sometimes in combinations." He does not term them "disease entities" in the sense of "disease" of traditional medicine but, more modestly, "reaction types" or "reaction sets," requiring in each case specification of the etiological factors and course. "A number of these sets of facts do, however, suggest fairly definite and specific events, corresponding to the traditional 'disease entities.' We should, however, have it understood that we do not treat the group of facts as 'fixed entities,' but rather as events which we have reasons to discuss as standard samples of what makes up psychiatry, to be kept at a minimum, but to be multiplied when facts call for it and new types and combinations prove to be valuable differentiations. We take up those events which have a sufficiently definite meaning and importance —groups of facts sometimes in pure culture, sometimes incomplete or complicated by admixtures, but after all each requiring consideration in its own terms." (Meyer.)

The word *ergasia* (from the Greek *ergazomai*, to be active, to work) is used as the common denominator for all those sets of facts, denoting, if combined with different prefixes, the principal varieties of psychopathological behavior patterns.

One of these groups is the *anergastic* form of reactions, patterns of activity denoting actual loss in the sense of demonstrable focal or diffuse destruction of cerebral tissue. In the child, the standard types are the disorders attributable to juvenile paresis, brain tumor, meningitis, encephalitis, trauma, birth injuries, congenital anomalies of the central nervous system, amaurotic family idiocy, hydrocephalus, and reactions in the shape of epileptoid responses on the ground of circumscribed or more wide-spread structural alterations. The postencephalitic behavior disorders constitute an important chapter under the heading of anergastic performance pictures. The connecting link in all these reactions is a deficit, chiefly of memory and judgment, and often of intellectual capacity in children with structural defects of the central nervous system.

DYSERGASTIC REACTION FORMS

In infectious diseases, intoxications, and nutritional disturbances we may encounter psychiatric problems, usually of a more transient character, appearing mostly in the form of delirious reactions. The outstanding features are hallucinatory episodes, commonly of a fearful or worrisome type, and disorientation or at least misinterpretation of the situation due to haziness or scare. Here, we deal with disturbances which are not based on serious structural damage, but on temporary and remediable affections of the nervous tissues (usually edema) and their metabolic support in fevers or under the influence of poisons or faulty nutrition.

CERTAIN OLIGERGASTIC REACTION FORMS

The term oligergasia (from Greek *oligos*, small, scanty, and *ergasia*) refers to defective development. It is true that certain anergastic conditions, such as the pictures presented by children with hydrocephalus, tuberous sclerosis, or Tay-Sachs' disease, show a very marked developmental deficit from the very beginning; but there we have in each instance a definite "organic" cerebral structural alteration.

There is, however, a number of well-defined clinical syndromes in which mental (and physical) retardation of growth and development is a striking occurrence, but which have no known brain pathology. Many of these groups are more or less closely correlated with the organs of internal secretion. This is true of the cretin and the myxedematous child and of so-called dysgenital imbecility.

It must, on the other hand, be stated here that there is a sufficiently large group of idiotic and imbecile children in whom neither an abnormal brain condition, nor an abnormally shaped skull, nor an unusual endocrine or metabolic pathology can be found. This fact applies to a much higher degree to the vast number of children of an intelligence level lower than that of the average individual of the same age, yet not low enough to be classed as idiots or imbeciles. But before one decides that a patient's reactions are "feebleminded" in the sense of defective intelligence without anatomical substratum, it is well to do a complete neurological examination, in order to exclude anergastic or endocrine possibilities.

SOMATIC MANIFESTATIONS OF PERSONALITY DISORDERS

In the foregoing three categories, the relation between physical status and inadequate psychiatric functioning is of a sort which depends on the existence of permanent or temporary neurological disorders or of inner-secretory disturbances. The personality difficulties are of a definitely organic, or organogenic, nature; they are either cerebrogenic or endocrinogenic.

A different type of relationship is found in the numerous instances in which a mainly psychiatric "functional" disorder of the child as a whole finds its expression wholly, or more often partly, in a deviation of one form or other of physical functioning, which cannot be identified or correlated with any anatomo-pathological findings. They may appear in the shape of substitutive hysterical paralyses or contractures or anaesthesias. They may, to use a term coined by Esther L. Richards, occur as the "body protest" of a child (or adult) against unbearable emotional or environmental stress.

Everyone knows that a person may have a headache without having a sick brain. Excitement or anxiety may be accompanied by palpitations in people whose circulatory system is absolutely normal. Others may, in spite of a healthy digestive apparatus, become nauseated or even vomit at the sight of something unpleasant or disgusting.

In children, unusual strain or frustration or unhappiness may find its outward manifestation in headache, vomiting, enuresis, stuttering, or twitchings of selected muscle groups, even though the brain, the gastrointestinal system, the kidney and bladder, the larynx, and the muscles do not reveal the slightest anomalies to the most exacting examiner.

In this connection we must mention a number of findings in various organs, which represent actual demonstrable physical conditions, yet which are commonly associated with the whole-function of the personality rather than solely with the organ which is found to be at fault. Many authors like to speak of them as "neurotic" or "neuropathic" traits or as signs of a "neuropathic" disposition or constitution or diathesis. A number of them is obviously connected with a "dystonia" of the vegetative nervous system, either with vagotonic or with sympathicotonic preponderance. Some people want to include in this division the conditions in which eosinophilia is a frequent phenomenon. The same, and other investigators like to point especially to conditions arising on the basis of protein sensitization as related to general personality difficulties. In recent years, hypoglycemia has been more or less closely allied with behavior disorders; this has led Henderson and Gillespie in the latest (third, 1932) edition of their "Textbook of Psychiatry" to separate a special group of so-called "glycopenic" disorders (migraine, cyclic vomiting, crises of collapse, night terrors, etc.).

Asthma, eczema, food idiosyncrasies, mucous colitis and spasms of the colon have been proclaimed as the outstanding representatives of this group. In our present state of medical knowledge, we shall do best not to speculate too much on how "neuropathic" these conditions are. If we find them unassociated with personality problems, we shall treat the local manifestations alone; if we find in the patient thus affected any psychiatric difficulties, we shall attack the local complaint as well as the child *in toto* with all the problems that he presents.

PERSONALITY DIFFICULTIES HAVING A DIRECT RELATION TO NON-NEUROLOGICAL PHYSICAL ILLNESS

Every pediatrician has made the common observation that certain types of sickness are often associated with modes of reaction which may be derived from the somatic discomfort from which the child suffers. The child who has myocarditis or pericarditis is often found to be listless and apathetic; this reaction may not have been present before the onset of the cardiac disease and may clear up entirely after recovery. It is also well known that children with itching skin affections frequently become irritable and restless and remain so until their pruriginous condition or scabies or eczema or urticaria is relieved. The easy fatigability and general discomfort of the mouthbreather are another pertinent example.

PERSONALITY DIFFICULTIES HAVING A MORE INDIRECT RELATION TO PHYSICAL ILLNESS

It is known that conditions of ill health, though not directly responsible for personality difficulties, may imprint their marks on the general reaction of children in a more indirect manner. Without being compelled to speak immediately of an "inferiority complex," one realizes, for example, how often crippled children become extremely self-conscious and sensitive and even unnaturally seclusive. The effects on the emotional life of the "ugly duckling" of the family or of the unattractive or squint-eyed "wallflower" are equally familiar to any observer.

There is, of course, a majority of children in whose lives the usual exanthemata or other similar episodes of brief duration or even protracted bodily ailments seem to cause no change whatever in the once established behavior pattern nor to create new difficulties of any kind. It is, after all, only a small percentage of physically ill children whose faulty adjustment to their conditions makes psychiatric assistance necessary. The average child goes through a siege of bronchitis or measles, which leaves no other trace than a faint memory and perhaps an entry in the family album. There are many children with chronic otitis media or repeated upper respiratory infections, who, in spite of these conditions and the need of frequent medical manipulations, preserve their usual modes of adaptation.

As a matter of fact, it is remarkable how well children sometimes react to drastic changes arising from serious illness.

In another group of children, investigation of their behavior problems reveals a more or less definite relation of the difficulties to previous illness. We find that some of these little patients have developed satisfactorily, have average or superior intelligence, are quite well adjusted socially, and are members of stable, healthy families. There has been no complaint as to their conduct prior to the onset of reactions attributable to the illness.

George H., nine years old, was referred for psychiatric consultation because of spells of shortness of breath, which began in September, 1930. His mother first noticed the breathing difficulty at the table and thought "he was in a hurry to go out and play." The spells at first occurred at lunch only, later also at dinner time. He unfastened his belt, saying that this gave him relief. For a number of years he had presented a feeding problem, was "particular about certain foods," and his parents "had to encourage him to eat." More recently he also had Sunday morning headaches.

George was the son of a 42-year-old healthy store manager, who for several years had suffered from "nervous indigestion" which, however, did not bother him of late. The mother was an intelligent, robust woman of 40 years. George was the second of two children; his older sister, 19 years of age, had a very good school record, worked steadily as a telephone operator, and was normal in every respect. There were two miscarriages between the births of the two children. With the exception of the paternal grandfather, who died of tuberculosis, there had been no serious acute or chronic illnesses, physical or mental, nor remarkable peculiarities in any member of the family in either branch for at least three generations.

George was a full term child, born without any complication. He was breast fed for two weeks only, gained weight steadily, and offered no feeding problem for the first few years of his life. Dentition, the development of locomotion and speech occurred at the usual time. At the age of one year he had an upper respiratory infection which lasted one month. The family physician diagnosed the condition as "asthma" and warned the parents that it might return in the future. He prescribed a strict dietary régime and advised that the child be watched closely and brought back whenever they noticed the slightest sign of breathing disturbance. At 18 months, he was circumcised. At two years he had whooping cough, at three years measles, and at six years scarlet fever ("very slight"). When he was seven years old, he was admitted to the Harriet Lane Home with acute anterior poliomyelitis, which was exceedingly mild and left no traces after a quick recovery. In August, 1930, his tonsils and adenoids were removed.

He began to go to school at six years and did exceptionally well in his studies and in his contacts with the teachers and schoolmates. In September, 1930, he was transferred to another school, due to change of residence. He felt uneasy about the sudden disruption of his previous associations and resented particularly the much longer distance between his home and the new school. It was then that his breathing difficulties began.

George was a well developed, well nourished boy. Physical examination showed no abnormalities. At $9\frac{1}{2}$ years, he had a mental age of almost 12 years (intelligence quotient of 118). He was somewhat childish in his reactions, was a spoiled child, who expected (and got) everything at home and was not given sufficient opportunity to develop a sense of responsibility and personal independence.

We have here, as everywhere else where we deal with human reactions, a combination of factors which must be taken into account in sizing up the boy's difficulty. It is remarkable, and a sign of a stable personality make-up, that, in spite of maternal oversolicitude, he has done splendidly for nine years, with the exception of feeding difficulties in school age, which were found to be considerably exaggerated by the mother. During the first few years of his life he did not know that he was expected to have a recurrence of "asthma." Later, even after being told to observe himself closely and to report any evidence of its appearance, the entire home and school setting was satisfactory enough to preclude any attention to his somatic functioning. But as soon as the change of schools and the greater distance created a situation unpleasant to the boy (whose father had reacted to financial worries with gastric complaints), the "asthma" began to assert itself. Real illness of short duration at the age of one year, aided by medical prophecies and parental apprehensions, helped to pattern the behavior trends in a healthy and intelligent, but spoiled, child after a period of approximately eight years.

George and his coöperative parents were informed about the nature of his "asthma." He was given adequate recreational outlets and personal responsibilities which he had lacked before. His "asthma" disappeared promptly, together with the feeding problem and the Sunday morning headaches. He is at present a well-adjusted, normal boy.

Grace T. presented a similar history, except that in her case the hypochondriacal tendencies had been formed at a much earlier date and that the family was less coöperative. She was $10\frac{1}{2}$ years old at the time of examination, with a mental age of $12\frac{1}{2}$ years (I.Q. 117), in good health, but eight pounds underweight. After serious illness in childhood (bronchopneumonia at two years), she was made the center of family solicitudes and indulged so much that she became fully convinced that she was a sick child. The manifestations of her previous illness, reiterated hundreds of times by her elders, and observation of the symptoms of her father's gastric ulcer gave her ample material for the formation of her complaints. They were met on the part of her parents and older brother with great anxiety, indiscriminate use of tonics and sedatives, tonsillectomy, periods of rest in bed and subordination of the entire household to whims of a supposedly sick girl, whose bronchopneumonia at two years had given the family an opportunity for making an invalid of the child. She presented a feeding problem, only liked certain foods, disliked vegetables, and the mother, feeling that she must force nourishment into this "sickly" child, had for years "nagged, coaxed, cajoled, punished, made promises, prepared special dishes," etc., with most unpleasant results. Grace had it in her hand to keep the parents worried and practiced a "cough," which reminded them of her bronchopneumonia and made them her slaves. For fear that close observation during the day was not enough, she was made to share her grandmother's bed, who reported her to be a restless sleeper and to grind her teeth at night.

When examined, Grace stated that she had a pain in her stomach (pointing to the entire upper part of the abdomen), occurring mostly in school. "The harder the work is, the more pain I have. I have no appetite for candy or ice cream, only for chocolate, the good kind. Sometimes my brain goes flooie. My hands begin to shake when I write my arithmetic lesson." The school teachers, of course, were not concerned about her previous attack of bronchopneumonia and must be made to worry about her through the medium of her abdominal "pain," "cough," and "shaking."

Grace's parents learned with some effort to regard and treat her as a normal and healthy child. Her desire for attention and ostentation was directed into the more constructive channels of participation in dramatic classes. She soon gave up her hypochondriacal reactions and is now a healthy and well-adapted girl.

There is a small group of cases in which the physical illness with its symptoms, the necessity of taking the child frequently to the doctor or clinic, and the additional financial demands, may create in unsympathetic parents a slowly increasing resentment against the inconveniences arising from the need of adequate care. In some instances it comes to a point where delay of improvement is taken by the parent almost as a personal insult to their desire for comfort and the blame placed on the child's supposed "stubbornness." Thus the sick child finds himself in a hostile environment to which he may learn to react in an equally disagreeable manner.

William K. was a nine-year-old boy of superior intelligence (I.Q. 115). He was found to have allergy to feathers but to be otherwise healthy in every respect. He had had nightly attacks of breathing difficulty and "being smothered" for the past five years. Almost every night he woke up "fighting for breath."

William was the son of a clerk who had a limited income. The father had much less education than the mother who used her better schooling as a means of subduing her husband and impressing her assumed superiority upon him. She had two children, the older was a healthy, well-behaved boy of 13 years.

William developed normally and went through diphtheria, whooping cough, and mumps, without any complications during the first two years of his life. At that time the family constellation was harmonious and devoid of any frictions. But when the boy began to have his respiratory troubles, the mother (and the father who shaped his opinions after hers) found his presence in the home inconvenient and sent him off to the country to stay with his grandmother using the excuse that the fresh air would help him. During the next four years the boy got along splendidly in spite of his nocturnal attacks. He was obedient, did well in his studies and was not considered a problem child at home or in school. When his grandmother died, he was returned to his parents. Instead of having the child examined, his shortness of breath was promptly interpreted as "just stubbornness" and a "habit" by the mother, who kept nagging him, supported by the father and by the brother who was held up to him as a model child free from any such "nasty habits." It so happened that the transfer to another school, occasioned by the boy's change of residence, necessitated his being placed temporarily in a less advanced group in his classroom. This the mother took to be a proof of the child's "feeblemindedness" and it furnished her with a "cause" for what she spoke of as his "misbehavior." He was submitted to more nagging, to being referred to as the black sheep of the family and a "moron" and life was made miserable for him. Only then, under the strain of constant humiliation and scolding, he commenced to have temper tantrums, refused to get up in the morning and developed twitchings of his eyelids and nostrils.

Even after examination had revealed the rôle of the feathers, his mother was loath to accept that whole-heartedly and to deprive herself of an excuse for worrying the child. It it were not for her attitude, it is quite improbable that the asthma itself would have created the behavior difficulties; certainly it had not done so while he was with his more sympathetic grandmother. But indirectly, through the hostile home environment, it contributed to the formation of an undesirable pattern as reaction to the family's resentment of the nocturnal attacks over which the child had no control.

If otherwise normal children in a stable environment are apt to develop behavior difficulties on the basis of an old illness because of parental attitudes, certainly one may expect hypochondriacal tendencies to grow out of physical disease in emotionally handicapped children raised in an unstable environment. We again take the complaint of asthma as a paradigm.

Marie S., not quite six years old, normally intelligent, spoiled badly by her parents and an aunt, who lived with the family after having spent a number of years in a mental institution, came from a stock in which hay fever had been rife for generations. In the past two years, she had had three asthmatic attacks. The child, who had always presented a serious feeding problem, was instantly entered into the list of the asthmatic family members after the first dyspnoeic episode and given a *carte blanche* which, because of her illness, entitled her to behave as she pleased. If she had been a difficult child before, she now became very much worse making up for the rarity of the asthmatic experiences by filling the intervals with situationally determined attacks of abdominal pain and vomiting. She offered an instructive illustration during her examination. She at first was very communicative and showed considerable initiative in the conversation. She seemed alert and answered questions of the intelligence test promptly and satisfactorily. With the mounting difficulties, however, she became conspicuously pale, then gagged several times, and finally, when the test grew beyond her grasp, sat down in her chair, bent forward and vomited, being very careful not to soil her new dress. In the ward, she sometimes put her finger in her mouth to produce regurgitation in response to a disagreeable situation.

Here we have a girl whose original instability, as shown in her feeding difficulties and spoiled child reaction, became increased and assumed the form of hypochondriasis and vomiting (occasionally produced artificially) against the background of a few asthmatic attacks, giving her the privileged position of an invalid child.

The child was found to be sensitive to orris and feathers. A few asthmatic wheezes and whistles were heard particularly over the upper pulmonary lobes anteriorly. She had a sinus arhythmia.

The intelligent mother learned to overcome her desire to pamper the child and to avoid unnecessary manifestations of alarm in her presence, with the result that her difficulties lessened. The psychopathic aunt in the home, with her emotional outbursts, still presents a difficult problem.

Ben H., eight years old, never had asthma. But he was a member of a family which was subject to breathing difficulties. The paternal grandmother, the maternal grandfather, an aunt, a cousin, had histories of "asthma" or "hay fever." Mental disturbances and suicides had occurred rather frequently in both branches of the family. The child displayed behavior deviations in the form of food capriciousness, twitchings of the hands and face, temper tantrums, blinking, etc. He was badly spoiled. Three years ago, he had pneumonia, leaving him with a cough which soon was "diagnosed" as asthma by his parents. The cough did not differ at first from the common variety, but when the child grew older he realized that he was expected to have "attacks" of shortness of breath, with the result that he began to have paroxysms, much to the family's alarm. During visits with friends and during his stay at the Harriet Lane Home, the cough, the feeding difficulties, and the twitchings were totally absent. The mother's appearance in the ward, however, immediately produced a paroxysm of coughing.

The physical examination proved the child to be entirely normal. He was placed in the neutral environment of a private boarding school where nobody expected him to have asthma or any other illness. He adjusted well there within a short time and was rid of all his behavior difficulties, including his cough.

It has thus been demonstrated in a number of illustrative cases that physical illness or discomfort may either alone or, more often, in a variety of combinations with additional factors (originally unstable personality, unwarranted prognoses or prophecies, undesirable parental attitudes, etc.) tend to establish or exaggerate behavior difficulties in children of varying degrees of intelligence and forms of emotional responsiveness. It must be realized at the outset that the sort of illness discussed here may leave the child's personality unscathed in a large majority of instances, just as other more or less eventful occurrences in the course of early development may not leave any mark on the individual's attitudes and performances in most cases, and in a number of others enter quite conspicuously into the formation of certain inconvenient and, in a sense, "abnormal" reaction tendencies.[1]

---

[1] Kanner, L., and S. E. Lachman. The Contribution of Physical Illness to the Development of Behavior Disorders in Children. Mental Hygiene. 1933, 17, 605–617.

CHAPTER VII

THE INTELLIGENCE FACTOR

THE HUMAN individual is endowed with a body which is capable of growing and developing along lines determined by the species, from embryonic ontogenesis, through the processes of early maturation and puberty, to climacteric and senile involution and the final termination of the life cycle. He is further equipped with certain urges and drives which take care of the need for preservation of the self and the race. He shares these qualities (in a form of his own, to be sure) with the lower animals, which also have their somatic characteristics and their "instincts" and drives. His adaptive possibilities, however, are enormously increased and his creative faculties aroused and maintained by another function or combination of functions which represents the highest peak of evolution and which is commonly designated as intelligence. The nature of this function is so complex that it has defied any attempts at too rigid a definition. In one of the standard dictionaries (Winston) it is interpreted as:

1. The ability to learn, to profit by experience, or to acquire knowledge;
2. The ability for reasoning and abstract thinking;
3. The ability to meet a new situation, to solve a problem, or direct one's conduct or thinking effectively.

It must be stated that the ability to profit by trial and error has been found to some extent to be present in animals as low as chickens. Köhler's famous experiments have proved the capacity of anthropoids for a certain degree of inventiveness.[1] Yet such performances are tied up too closely with immediate sense-experiences, and even in the ape, where there is a slight trend to delayed reactions, this has its natural limitations in the inherent action-tendencies of the species.

Bühler, basing his work on phylogenetic considerations and on direct observation of children, has advanced the theory that the mental development of the infant passes through three stages:

1. Instinct. "A ready-for-use inheritance of modes of behavior set going in a definite way according to a preformed natural plan. . . . Instincts have an extremely conservative character; they function with extraordinary certainty and precision where everything remains unaltered, and fail when the individual enters upon new conditions of existence. Naturally they once had come into being too, and were not exempt from change, but this only came about in the course of and at the cost of many generations."
2. Training. It is built up on the capital stock of instinctive modes of behavior and makes use of "associative memory," by suppressing some instincts, accentuating others, and forming new combinations. "The human

[1] Köhler, Wolfgang. The Mentality of Apes. Translated by Ella Winter. New York. 1925.

49

trainer deals in reward and punishment and thereby merely imitates what nature shows him, for in its wild state the animal also learns by success and failure." Play is one of the practices of the child's training.

3. Intellect. Its main characteristic is inventiveness "by means of insight and reflection." It works from within and with a certain amount of independence. It grasps entire situations with their peculiarities and adapts itself to them by discovering ways and means which can be arrived at through cognition only. It depends on adaptive and inventive plasticity.[1]

Regardless of whether or not this theory of three successive stages of mental development might be open to controversy, so much is certainly true that the child, at the age of about ten or eleven months, coincidental with the first acquisition of language, emerges with orientative-discriminative abilities, which from then on show a steady increase. They are as much a part of the genus as is the specific configuration of the body and the capacity for tissue growth. They may be fostered or hindered in their transformation into performance by a variety of factors, just as the capacity for bone development may be fostered or hindered.

During the past few decades, methods have been devised, by which the child's intelligence can be measured objectively. The test most commonly employed is that worked out by Binet and Simon in France and adapted for English speaking persons by Terman (the Stanford Revision of the Binet-Simon Intelligence Scale).[2]

The scale begins at the three-year level and is followed up for each year successively until the age of ten years, when the interval is increased to two years, until the level of the "superior adult" at eighteen years. The following table, compiled by Dr. Meyer and quoted here with slight alterations, gives a picture of the psychobiological reactions used in the tests:

Naming:[3]   *Year*

Key, penny, knife, watch, pencil (three of five)............Three
Colors: red, yellow, blue, green..........................Five
Coins: nickel, penny, quarter, dime.......................Six
     nickel, penny, quarter, dime, dollar, half-dollar.....Eight
Days of the week...Seven
Months...Nine

Carrying Out Spoken Requests:

Points to parts of body: nose, eyes, mouth, hair (three of
    four)..Three
Performs three commissions given at once: put key on chair;
    open door; bring box.................................Five

[1] Bühler, Karl. The Mental Development of the Child. Translated by Oscar Oeser. London and New York. 1930.

[2] Terman, Lewis M. The Measurement of Intelligence. Boston, New York, Chicago. 1916.

[3] Terman wants it clearly understood that naming colors is not a test for color discrimination but for the "verbalization of color perception." To test color vision, we use the excellent tables devised by Dr. Shinobu Ishihara, which may be obtained from the C. H. Stoelting Company in Chicago. As regards the identification of coins, it has been found that children from poor homes do slightly better with it than those from families of wealth and culture.

Personal Data:

Gives last name...Three
Gives sex..Three
Gives age..Five
Discriminates between right and left......................Six
Gives number of fingers without counting; on one hand, on
  the other hand, on both hands together..................Seven

Discriminations:

Of length: two lines with difference of one centimeter.......Four
Of forms: finding of shown geometrical figures (circle, tri-
  angle, square, rectangle, etc.) on an identical chart.......Four
  Readjusting two halves of cut triangle...................Five
Of weights: 3 and 15 grams...............................Five
  arranging blocks of 3, 6, 9, 12, and 15 grams............Nine
Of beauty: Three sets of pretty and ugly faces...........Five
Of completeness: omission of eye, nose, mouth, arms.......Six
Of time of day: morning or afternoon.....................Six
Of date: year, month, date (within three days), and day of
  week...Nine

Reaction to pictures:

Enumeration of at least three objects.....................Three
Description...Seven
Interpretation..Twelve

Repetition of Sentences:

Six syllables...Three
Twelve to thirteen syllables..............................Four
Sixteen to eighteen syllables.............................Six
Twenty to twenty-two syllables............................Ten
Twenty-eight syllables....................................Sixteen

Repetition of Numerals:
Forwards:

Three digits..Three
Four digits...Four
Five digits...Seven
Six digits..Ten
Seven digits..Fourteen
Eight digits..Eighteen

Backwards:

Three digits..Seven
Four digits...Nine
Five digits...Twelve
Six digits..Sixteen
Seven digits..Eighteen

Counting:

Four pennies..Four
Thirteen pennies..Six
Counting backwards from 20 to 1 in 40 seconds............Eight

Calculation:

   Adding value of three 2-cent and three 1-cent stamps......Nine
   Problems involving simple subtraction....................Nine
   Arithmetical reasoning...................................Fourteen

Reading and Writing:

   Writing from dictation: See the little boy..................Eight
   Reading of fire story with reporting of at least eight items....Ten

Drawing:[1]

   Copies square with pencil...............................Four
   Copies diamond with pen and ink........................Seven
   Copies designs after ten seconds' exposure................Ten

Word Resources:

   Using three given words in one sentence...................Nine
   Giving three words rhyming with day, mill, spring.........Nine
   Naming sixty words in three minutes.....................Ten
   Arranging sets of eight shuffled words....................Twelve

Definitions:

   By use: chair, horse, fork, doll, table, pencil...............Five
   Superior to use: balloon, tiger, football, soldier............Eight
   Abstract terms: pity, revenge, charity, envy, justice........Twelve
   Differences: fly and butterfly; stone and egg; wood and glass
      ....Seven
      idleness and laziness; evolution and revolution; poverty and
      misery; character and reputation.....................Sixteen
      king and president...................................Fourteen
   Similarities: wood and coal; apple and peach; iron and silver;
      ship and automobile..................................Eight
      snake, cow and sparrow; book, teacher, and newspaper; wool,
      cotton, and leather; knife blade, penny, and piece of wire;
      rose, potato, and tree...............................Twelve
   Central thought of a paragraph.........................Eighteen
   Meaning of words (list of one hundred):
      Twenty words......................................Eight
      Thirty words......................................Ten
      Forty words.......................................Twelve
      Fifty words.......................................Fourteen
      Sixty-five words...................................Sixteen
      Seventy-five words.................................Eighteen

Judgment:

   Comprehension: First degree............................Four
                  Second degree..........................Six
                  Third degree...........................Eight
                  Fourth degree..........................Ten
   Detecting absurdities in four of five statements...........Ten

[1] These are not tests of "drawing ability" but more of form perception and reproduction. In the third, the main factors involved in success are "attention, visual memory, and a little analysis" (Binet).

Inference from circumstances.........................Fourteen
Moral of fables: Four points.........................Twelve
                 Eight points.........................Sixteen

Imagination:

Inversion of clock hands.............................Fourteen
Writing "Come quickly" in code.......................Sixteen
Physical relations: path of cannon ball; weight of fish in
    water; hitting distant mark with rifle..............Sixteen

Induction:

Rule for holes in folded paper.......................Fourteen
Problem of enclosed boxes............................Sixteen

Ingenuity:

Tying bow knot around stick..........................Seven
Finding lost ball in circular field: inferior plan...........Eight
                                      superior plan...........Twelve
Measuring seven pints with 3 and 5 pint vessels; eight pints
    with 5 and 7 pint vessels; seven pints with 4 and 9 pint
    vessels...Eighteen

From this list, it becomes evident that a considerable number of assets is included in the evaluation of a child's "intelligence": comprehension of language heard or read; ability to repeat words and sentences mechanically; the use of language as a means of communication; the range of the vocabulary; form perception and reproduction; memory and immediate recall; reasoning, resourcefulness, and imagination; inventiveness; logical thinking; adaptation to new situations; judgment; ethical attitudes (in some of the comprehension tests); critical powers (detection of absurdities); arithmetical abilities; organizing facilities (arrangements of weights; forming a sentence of shuffled words); minimal ability of aesthetic judgment; observation; discriminative and orientative functions; and many more items. Both the questions and the answers have been sufficiently standardized to enable the experienced examiner to be as certain about his conclusions as is, for instance, the cardiologist about the result of his examination of the heart.

For statistical reasons and for the purpose of an abbreviated terminology, the result of the intelligence test has been condensed into the so-called intelligence quotient, or I.Q., which is obtained by dividing the actual, chronological age of the child into his mental age. According to the I.Q., one may roughly group the children into a number of categories, realizing all the time that children belonging in the same class with regard to their I.Q. may differ widely in many other respects, such as emotional maturity and stability, habit training, constitutional factors, physical condition, and environmental features.

I.Q.	*Classification*
Above 140......................	Near genius or genius.
120–140.......................	Very superior intelligence.
110–120.......................	Superior intelligence.
90–110.......................	Normal, or average intelligence.

80–90 . . . . , ... Dullness.
70–80 . . . . Border-line deficiency.
50–70 . . . . Moron.
25–50 . . . . Imbecile.
Below 25 . . . . Idiot.

Aside from the standardized rating, a great many things of considerable importance may, and should, be learned during the performance of the test. It is essential to note the child's general attitude and behavior. One will gain insight into the degree of his responsiveness; whether he is alert or listless; whether he reacts spontaneously or needs much urging and encouragement; whether he is attentive, or easily distracted, or preoccupied; whether he is composed or uncomfortable; at ease or tense; quick or slow; or hesitant; or embarrassed; o r unusually shy; or "smart-alecky"; whether he is persistent in his efforts or gives up easily; whether he is interested or indifferent; serious or playful. One child was very suspicious, fearing that the questions might be just a design to divert his attention from an impending operation or injection. Another reacted soon after the beginning of the test with the remark, "Think you can catch me, do you?" A little girl coöperated excellently, until the question was asked (Year VI), "What's the thing to do if it is raining when you start to school?" She then became mute and tense; the mention of school had touched upon her outstanding difficulty. In restless and stuttering children it is often interesting to note how at first the hyperactivity or speech difficulty is absent or almost absent for some time during the examination and then reappears or becomes more pronounced when the tasks become too difficult. The procedure also gives one an opportunity to observe the degree of the child's fatigability.

The type of answer, whether correct or incorrect, is often very telling and offers valuable leads. There is the five-year-old girl who is brought in as presenting a serious feeding problem. The mother impatiently interrupts any advice with regard to regulation of the child's feeding habits with the statement that that is exactly what she has always done. But when the girl is asked, "What ought you to do when you are hungry?" she replies promptly, "My mother gives me candy." An excitable boy of twelve years with night terrors, when expected to name sixty words in three minutes, enumerates a long list of terms, in which murder, weapons, kidnapping, and robberies play a predominant part. He lives in a neighborhood full of rowdies and is sent to moving picture theaters almost every day. It has been his ambition to become a gangster. One negro boy's frequent truancy, kept secret both by the patient and his parents, came out when he innocently stated that the thing to do when he was on his way to school and noticed that he was in danger of being late (Year VIII) was to "play around in the streets."

It is essential, in the scoring, to differentiate between complete failure and close approximation of the correct answer. Thus, an eleven-and-a-half-year-old boy with lipodystrophy and concomitant, largely environmentally determined personality difficulties had an intelligence rating of ten years, giving him an I.Q. of 85. But he came so near to the right solution of the twelve year problems and even some of the fourteen year problems that the registration of the I.Q. alone, without proper credit for his additional achievements, would decidedly give a wrong picture of the boy's intellectual capacity, on which advice with regard to school adjustment and educational expectations depends to a considerable extent.

The I.Q. in itself does not tell of the distribution of the plus and minus scores over the different years. One boy, aged nine years and ten months, has an I.Q. of 100. His chronological and mental age coincide exactly. But the highest level at which he has no failures is the seventh year. From then on he "scatters" up to the twelfth year. This shows that, at almost eleven, he misses some of the eight, nine, and ten year requirements, making up for the deficit by solving some of the twelve year problems. The highest age at which all requirements are fulfilled is called the "base line." An unusually low base line with a very high degree of scattering is occasionally significant and should make one think of actual deterioration. We find such pictures sometimes in adult schizophrenic patients and in children whose intelligence has suffered in the course of life as a result of an organic process, such as encephalitis or brain tumor or juvenile paresis.

The outstanding advantage of the standardization of intelligence is that one no longer has to "guess" at a child's endowment. Personal impressions may often be misleading and occasionally even deceive the most experienced examiner. There is the quiet and shy child with a very poor school record, who was referred for psychiatric consultation with the remark that she was "obviously feebleminded." She was found to be of high average intelligence. Her school difficulties were the result of frequent changes of residences and schools, of being kept at home for weeks at a time, of having no recreational outlets and no privacy for her homework. She was given an opportunity to make up for lost time, to attend the same school regularly, to play outdoors sufficiently, and to have a corner of her own. The child not only progresses well in her studies now, but has become alert and self-confident and happy and given up the hypochondriacal complaints which were the reason of her being taken to the dispensary. At another time, a pediatrician returned a Mongolian dwarf to me with a certain amount of indignation. The child had been found to be seriously retarded by my assistant. The referring physician thought the boy so "cute" and "cunning" that he was convinced my assistant must have made a grave mistake. The child was restandardized in his presence, with the same result as before. Shyness is often mistaken for "backwardness," and shrewdness or loquacity for "intelligence" not only by parents, but often also by teachers and physicians.

Another advantage of the rating is the fact that it gives us a dependable means of comparing a child's intellectual capacity at different times with the same method. This is especially helpful in determining the result of thyroid medication in cretins. One of these patients advanced within eighteen months from an I.Q. of 65 to one of 89. In another case, the quotient dropped from normal to below 70 within less than two years. The enormous loss indicated an organic process; it was one of the first symptoms of juvenile paresis.

This is the place to correct the wrong notion, prevailing among so many physicians and laymen and helping to discredit psychiatry, that the mental examination consists solely of the determination of the I.Q. Children are often referred to the psychiatrist "for standardization," with the idea that the quotient will in every instance give the clue for the existing problem. It is important to realize that the possession of intelligence gains or loses in value according to whether or not it is properly utilized or taught to be properly utilized. Even in the adult, a high I.Q. is by no means a safeguard against bizarre superstitions or fraudulence or instability. Furthermore, the child's experience and general stock of information must be included in the final evaluation of his intelligence. Just as the presence of a chronic tonsillitis alone does not satisfactorily "explain" enuresis, even though it may have something to do with it, so any degree of mental retardation alone should not be made responsible for a psychiatric problem, without investigating into the other factors dealt with in this volume.

This is also the place to touch briefly upon a question with which the psychiatrist is often confronted and which was most drastically put to me by a judge in a Criminal Court. Can a boy of, let us say, fifteen years with a mental age of eight years be compared in every respect to a normal eight-year old? Decidedly not. The one is seriously handicapped but perhaps physically stronger, perhaps sexually mature, whereas the other is essentially "normal" and has a capacity for further average development. On the other hand, a slight degree of retardation is not always a liability, nor is superior intelligence always an asset, if the total personality is considered. A stable, but somewhat retarded garbage collector, who has found his place in life and aptly raises and supports a family, is far superior to the highly intelligent lad who forges checks and plunges from one trouble into another. In short, an attitude of sound relativity is necessary in evaluating the significance of the results of the Binet-Simon and other tests. Very grave deficits in the sense of idiocy and imbecility are, of course, always serious handicaps.

Page 57 contains a survey of the intelligence quotients of 1000 children who were referred for psychiatric consultation.

The arithmetical average lies at 84, the median at 86.2. It would even be much higher if it were not for the fact that practically every idiotic and imbecile child has been referred for standardization. It is evident that the vast majority of the children fall in the groups of morons, borderline deficiency, dull, average, and slightly superior intelligence. The table shows plainly that the common behavior disorders are only in a comparatively small number of cases closely associated with low grade feeblemindedness.

What are the possible correlations between the intelligence factor and personality difficulties of children?

The *idiot* or *imbecile* or *low grade moron* grows up with a severe handicap, arising from his total or almost total inability to learn to adapt himself even to the simplest demands of his complex environment, calling for ever new adjustments to a multitude of changeable and changing situations. He is not capable of thinking in abstracts, of independent planning, and of assuming duties and responsibilities. He cannot elaborate his experiences to the point of self-protection, avoidance of danger, and respecting the integrity of objects as well as of persons, especially of the baby brother or baby sister. If he is not sufficiently protected, he is liable, particularly in

I.Q.	Number	Per cent
Below 30	22	2.2
31–35	5	0.5
36–40	6	0.6
41–45	11	1.1
46–50	18	1.8
51–55	32	3.2
56–60	32	3.2
61–65	35	3.5
66–70	63	6.3
71–75	59	5.9
76–80	102	10.2
81–85	112	11.2
86–90	105	10.5
91–95	85	8.5
96–100	100	10.0
101–105	76	7.6
106–110	53	5.3
111–115	36	3.6
116–120	22	2.2
121–125	12	1.2
126–130	5	0.5
131–135	7	0.7
136–140	2	0.2
Total	1000	100

the early years of life, to do great damage to himself and to others. The impulsive mode of acting, not guided by any well-directed goals, may induce him to wander away from home aimlessly, without being able to find the way back. Being uninformed and uncritical, some of the girls of this type have fallen prey to the persuasions and cheap bribes of somewhat less retarded people who have abused them sexually. Venereal infection or the birth of mostly feebleminded offspring of very young mothers are often the sinister results. Every juvenile court knows how frequently children of this sort, because of their easy suggestibility due to lack of criticism, have been used as tools for delinquencies planned by others, either by being frightened or flattered or promised handsome rewards. "Pica," or "perverted appetite" is sometimes reported in these children at an earlier age, not so much because of a real anomaly of appetence as because of lack of discrimination.

Frederick K., 3 years and 10 months old, was the feebleminded son of an alcoholic father who was morbidly jealous, beat his wife, and left the family whenever he pleased, often returning unexpectedly in the middle of the night with a great deal of cursing and clatter, and of an unintelligent "nervous," and hypochondriacal mother. He had gone through rickets, a series of sore throats, and measles, and had phimosis. The child had been taken to the dispensary on various occasions because he drank ink, spirit of niter, and ammonia. One time he grabbed a butcher knife and cut his baby brother's face with it. The mother also complained that he ran out in the street and "defied the automobiles." He talked and walked in his sleep. His enunciation was very indistinct. His sister, Emily, was also seriously retarded (I.Q. 63), had temper tantrums, and diurnal enuresis was destructive, bit her finger nails, and was deaf "in school only."

Irene L. had a mental age of 5 years at 10 years and ten months. She soiled and wet herself constantly both at night and in the day time. She often wandered away from home, taking up with strangers, and had been picked up and returned by the police a number of times. There was occasional vomiting after eating sweets. She had been breast fed for two years. At the age of eighteen months, she was taken to the Clinic because she had swallowed a small Christmas tree ball (in June!). She had a right alternating lateral strabismus, leucoderma, and dental caries. Her father was an alcoholic, "drunk and cursing and jealous all the time," and had deserted the family three years ago. The mother, a Polish immigrant, was illiterate. A sister, 19, had had enuresis until twelve years of age.

Albert J. was 4 years and 10 months old. His mental age was barely three years. The mother brought him with this complaint: "I can't do anything with him. He defies you in punishment or anything else. If he does anything and I wish to punish him, he will just defy me. I won't beat him but just spank him or slap. He has awful crying spells." This parentally mismanaged and ill-understood child, at the age of three years, while "husking corn," "accidentally" got into the kitchen table drawer, took out a paring knife and ran it into his right eye, which later had to be completely enucleated.

These are a few examples of the perils which surround the ill-protected and ill-supervised feebleminded child. It must, however, be stated that destructiveness is sometimes also encountered in children of normal or even superior intelligence with faulty habit training and poor emotional control. The backward child destroys his toys because he does not comprehend their real meaning and purpose. The intelligent child destroys them either because of curiosity (to know "what is inside," or "how it is made," or "what makes the doll close her eyes or say, ma-ma"), or in a temper tantrum, or in order to get attention, or to terrorize his environment.

In the *dull* and *borderline children* the personality difficulties more or less closely associated with the intelligence factor often do not start until school age. The educational curriculum is necessarily adapted to the grasp and achievements of the average child. The youngster who cannot keep pace with the well-outlined requirements will have the choice between a number of alternatives. If he is ambitious, he will try to make up for his poverty of natural endowment by means of increased effort, reducing or eliminating the time for recreation and relaxation through play. He will overwork himself and be under a constant strain which, particularly if it is accompanied by frustration, may result in personality difficulties. The situation may become aggravated by parents or teachers who do not realize the real nature of the child's handicap and are too prone to identify failure with "laziness" or "lack of ambition" and to contrast the child with brother Jack or sister Jane, who do so splendidly in their studies. The retarded pupil, who is less eager to conform to the prescribed standards to which he simply cannot conform, not being able to comprehend the things that are being taught and discussed, may become preoccupied with other matters more easily accessible to his imagination and indulge in daydreaming. He then will be branded as suffering from "lack of concentration." Or he may become restless, "hyperkinetic," and even "mischievous," taxing the teacher's patience and attempting to acquire in this mode the respect of his classmates or even the semblance of a hero or of a martyr. Another child, who has not hit upon any of these forms of reaction, may develop a hatred of the school, where he is bored and perhaps teased by the schoolmates, and play truant. Or he may discover that illness will give the parents the most plausible cause for keeping him at home. When there is no actual discomfort, he may fabricate headaches or stomachaches and in the course of time develop hypochondriacal habits.

The child, of course, does not, and cannot (and should not), know that he is "backward," that he lacks the required capacity for the class work standardized for the average child of his age. His apathy, restlessness, mischievousness, truancy, hypochondriasis, or irritability are the outward manifestations of his realization of failure and frustration for which he is blamed and the source of which he does not understand. These difficulties usually disappear when the strain is removed from the child by means of proper school adjustment.

William P., a nine-year-old boy with an I.Q. of 86, was referred because of enuresis, nailbiting, irritability, occasional temper tantrums, headaches, and fatigability. He was in the low fourth grade in a country school headed by an energetic teacher who had the ambition to raise her pupils' scholastic performances to the level of the work done in the city schools; as a matter of fact, she wanted them to excel their urban contemporaries. Correction of his refractive error did away with the headache, but the other difficulties persisted. While in the second grade, the boy had formed an intense dislike of his teacher and the school. He was put back a half grade, remaining in the same classroom. This had the result that, according to his mother, "he sees younger children going ahead of him and that makes it very hard for him." The following letter was written to the school teacher: "We are writing you, with the mother's consent, concerning William P., who attends your school and is now in the fourth grade. The boy has come to our Clinic with several complaints. His headaches disappeared after his poor eyesight had been corrected with glasses. We have found the child to be slightly below the average intellectually and feel that he will improve if he is dealt with leniently in school. If he lived in B., we would send him to an ungraded class for a time; but since this is not possible in your community, we feel that the boy would do much better if he were not pushed beyond his capacity." Through the mother, a personal interview with the teacher was arranged, in which the details of the problem were discussed. As a result, the child became much happier, his irritability and temper outbursts left him, and he ceased to bite his nails and to wet the bed. Owing to improvement of the total situation, his school work was of better quality and carried out with greater enthusiasm and with admiration for the once hated teacher.

A similar type of school adjustment helped to relieve June C., aged eight years, I.Q. 81, of her various tics (blinking began when she entered the first grade; six months later, wrinkling of the forehead and frowning were added; when she was promoted to the second grade, the habit of nodding her head made its first appearance). The family physician, treating the "symptom" rather than the child, told the mother to call June's attention to the twitching every time it occurred and was surprised when informed that "this had made her worse"; he was at the end of his resources. The child was transferred to the slow-moving group of her class and her tics ceased to be the family topic of conversation, and the fear that they "might develop into St. Vitus's dance" was eliminated. Two weeks later the social worker could report that the tics had vanished and that the child had given up her crying spells. Her difficulties have not returned since then (more than two years ago).

The child of *average intelligence* may also have his reactions to an over-estimation of his endowment. This is especially the case when overambitious parents create in their offspring an artificial clash between their unlimited expectations and the child's normal, and normally limited, capacity. As a result, we see children with behavior disorders arising from the strenuous effort to compete with the prodigy of a cousin who has "skipped" so many grades or to attain perfection in every subject, so that the parents may proudly display the school reports to an admiring assembly of uncles and aunts and neighbors.

If it were true that a low I.Q. is at the bottom of every personality difficulty of a child, then we should not expect to see psychiatric problems in the *intellectually superior* youngster. Our table shows that of 1000 children not less than eighty-four with quotients above 110 presented behavior problems. In only a small number of those, it is true, is the problem in any way associated with the intelligence factor. In our cases, we had an opportunity to observe the following types of relationship:

Undue emphasis, on the part of the environment, of the child's accomplishments in recitation, music, chess or checkers, solving arithmetical problems, or the production of "bright sayings," may get the child into the habit of considering himself, and demanding to be considered, the center of attention. If he becomes insatiable in this respect, he may learn to substitute foul means for fair in order to attain his goal.

We have pointed out that the retarded child may suffer from being expected to do more than he can do in school. The superior child often is harmed by not having enough to do. Being a year or more ahead in mental age, he will find the class requirements extremely easy. He will be through with his prescribed tasks so early that he will have a surplus of unoccupied time on hand. If this is not filled with organized activity, the child may drift into restlessness, "michievousness," or daydreaming. Even though the mechanism is altogether different, the outcome, therefore, may resemble the disorders growing out of lack of grasp in the backward child.

In another group, the intellectual superiority is linked with intellectual curiosity to such an extent that the child is in danger of becoming too one-sided in his interests and activities. Here we have the typical "book-worm" who may so lose himself in a fantastic world of fiction that he may push aside the normal need for actual life experiences and for the necessary play association with other children.

Thomas G., seven years old, came of a stable family. He was an only child. He was brought with the complaint of restlessness and "going from one habit into another" (twisting his face, touching his nose and ears, biting his nails). He was found to have large tonsils and an inconsistent functional systolic murmur at the apex. He had a nine-year intelligence, I.Q. 124. In addition, he approximated most of the ten and twelve year tests very closely. During the interview he was hyperactive and ostentatious, "but a model of good behavior so long as his attention and interest were occupied with the test questions. He regretted that he was not asked more questions." The boy's difficulties had begun at the time when he entered kindergarten. At home, he had been taught to read and to write and to draw and, with his excellent endowment, learned very well. His achievements had made him stand out as the child prodigy of the family and neighbors, who showered upon him attention, praise, nickels, and candy. The school had nothing new to offer; he knew everything that was taught. He was treated just like any of the other children. He therefore invented new ways of forcing the attention of his environment upon himself. He first wiggled about in his seat, then kept talking and giggling, then developed his "twitchings" and "twistings" and "jerkings," which a physician did not fail to "diagnose" as incipient chorea. He became the *enfant terrible* of his classroom and later on at home and in Sunday school. He became outright impudent. His school work suffered from his fidgetiness and carelessness. The treatment consisted in directing his activities into more constructive channels and occupying his energies sufficiently, having him promoted to a higher grade more commensurate with his actual capacity, having him take piano lessons (he had shown interest in music), arranging for organized recreation, and discouraging over-indulgence and open admiration at home. The child now is the leader in the higher class, receives the best marks in conduct, effort, and progress, has learned to assume and carry out responsibilities, and the alleged "incipient chorea" has vanished entirely. His tonsils, of course, were removed.

Melvin E., eleven years old, combined with his I.Q. of 118 an insatiable intellectual curiosity. In addition to being very conscientious about his school work, he went to Hebrew School every afternoon for two hours, read three newspapers daily, spent hours in libraries, read while riding in the street car, read during meals, read in bed, read everything everywhere and always. The complaint was blinking, grimacing, and twisting of the lips. His constant reading was a reaction to an incident in a lower grade. He had worn glasses for years, and on one occasion the gymnastics teacher excluded him on that account from some exercises, referring to him as "goggles," much to other boys' amusement. Melvin decided that, if his glasses prevented him from athletic equality with his classmates, he would show them what he could do "spiritually." The boy had a most remarkable stock of information. But he had obtained it for the price of isolation, one-sidedness, dissatisfaction with himself, and tics. His reading and studying schedule was curtailed and he was advised to join the Y.M.H.A. and to participate in their sports program. He now associates much more freely and his tics have left him.

There exists still another mode of relationship between good intelligence and personality difficulties, in that it can be used constructively in the child's proper adjustment.

Peggy W., thirteen years old, had a congenital double athetosis of a mild degree. She was the daughter of a former professor of physics at a leading university, now employed by the Government, and an intelligent mother who, however, described herself as "nervous, quick-tempered, impatient, and intolerant" and who "can see nothing good in the child" because of "those movements." The girl's sensitiveness, evoked by her clumsiness, had been kept alive and increased by constant (undeserved) criticism and nagging. She had an I.Q. of 115. This was held up to the mother as a decided asset, commanding parental pride and aid. The knowledge changed the mother's attitude towards the child. Peggy had compensated for her physical defect by "thinking up" stories and dramatic plots which, considering her age, had decided merits. In the small community in which the family lived a small "literary club" was organized, in which, among other things, Peggy's productions were read or enacted. With her extreme sensitiveness diminished, her school work improved to such a degree that now she is among the first in her class in her academic work. She has found her place in the sun, after the detection of an asset of which neither she nor the family had known before.

In children under three years of age, the Binet-Simon test cannot be applied. Whenever a determination of the child's endowment seems indicated, we made use of the very helpful scheme devised by Gesell.[1]

It is at that early stage, of course, not exactly an "intelligence" test, but rather a not too rigid measurement of the child's developmental progress, as compared with the observed and statistically gaged "norms of development" with regard to motor, linguistic, adaptive, and personal-social behavior. All four modes of performance may uniformly advance beyond the "norm," or may fall behind uniformly. But there may be a dissociation in the sense that, for instance, the motor development of a two-year-old has reached the minimal requirements of the eighteen-months level (walking alone; climbing stairs), whereas linguistically he has not proceeded beyond vocalization (four months), and in his adaptive and personal-social behavior, he may conform to the achievements expected of the average infant of twelve months.   •

[1] Gesell, Arnold. The Mental Growth of the Preschool Child. New York. 1930.

CHAPTER VIII

THE EMOTIONAL FACTOR

ONE MAY recognize in the mentally integrated individual three sufficiently distinguishable types of whole-functioning:

The *cognitive* or *intellectual* functions, which include comprehension, capacity for learning and reproducing, thinking, reasoning, judgment, inventiveness, skill, information, and utilization of past experiences.

The *conative features*, manifesting themselves in the urges, drives, desires, appetites, action-tendencies, habit formations, degree of initiative and aggressiveness, manner of persistence in striving for a goal, and the speed of performance.

The *emotional responses* to life situations.

There has been a good deal of theoretical controversy among philosophers and academic psychologists as to how many emotions there are, as to which are primary or elementary and which are secondary or composite, and as to how they should be classified. Descartes had six primary emotions (admiration, love, hate, desire, joy, sadness), Spinoza had three (joy, sadness, desire), Shand has seven (fear, anger, joy, sorrow, curiosity, repugnance, and disgust). According to McDougall, there are six primary emotions or preparation reactions (fear, disgust, wonder, anger, subjection, elation, tenderness), to which are related the instincts or end reactions of flight, repulsion, curiosity, pugnacity, self-abasement, self-assertion, and parental care. Others have attempted to divide emotions into objective (love, hate) and subjective (joy, sorrow), or into retrospective (regret, satisfaction) and prospective (hope, dread, anxiety), or into weak and strong ones. The distinction between those "passions" in which pleasure predominates (love, courage, benevolence) and those in which pain predominates (rage, hate, pity, fear, indignation, envy, shame, jealousy), reaches back to Aristotle and has ever since then played an important part in the discussion of affective reactions; to these Stratton has recently added excitement as an hedonically undifferentiated emotion (either standing alone, or as the precursor, or as the successor of other emotions).

There has been considerable airing of the question which of the emotional responses are inherited and which are acquired. In general, one may say, that the individual, by virtue of his being a human specimen, brings with him potentialities for certain forms of responses to certain types of life situations involving danger, facilitation of, or interference with, his goals and wishes (success or frustration), praise or lack of recognition, and different other sorts of welcome or unwelcome experiences or anticipations.

Watson[1] was the first to study experimentally the emotional responses of infants during the first months of life. He found that from the very day

---

[1] Watson, John B. Psychology from the Standpoint of a Behaviorist. Philadelphia and London. 1919, pp. 198–206.

63

of birth they reacted to a group of situations in a mode which impressed the observer as an indication of "fear": sudden catching of the breath, clutching randomly with the hands, sudden closing of the eye-lids, puckering of the lips, then crying. The principal settings which called out such behavior were: 1. Loud sounds. 2. Sudden removal from the infant of all means of support, such as dropping it from the hands to be caught by an assistant or sudden pulling of the blanket upon which it is lying when it is just falling asleep. Hampering of the baby's movements was answered in a manner which may be looked upon as "rage": "If the face or head is held, crying results, quickly followed by screaming. The body stiffens and fairly well-coördinated slashing or striking movements of the hands and arms result; the feet and legs are drawn up and down; the breath is held until the child's face is flushed. In older children the slashing movements of the arms and legs are better coördinated, and appear as kicking, slapping, pushing, etc. These reactions continue until the irritating situation is relieved, and sometimes do not cease then. Almost any child from birth can be thrown into a rage if its arms are held tightly to its sides; sometimes even if the elbow joint is clasped tightly between the fingers the response appears; at times just the placing of the head between cotton pads will produce it." An observable "love" response was produced by stroking some "erogenous zone," tickling, shaking, gentle rocking, patting, and turning upon the stomach across the attendant's knee: "The response varies. If the infant is crying, crying ceases, a smile may appear, attempts at gurgling, cooing, and finally, in slightly older children, the extension of the arms, which we should class as the forerunner of the embrace of the adult." Watson concluded that fear, rage, and love (or, as he was willing to call them, X, Y, and Z) are the three emotional reactions "belonging to the original and fundamental nature of man."

The negative results of Watson's experiments are as instructive as his positive findings. Three babies from the Harriet Lane Home were exposed to the nearness of animals (black cat, rabbit, pigeon, various beasts at the Baltimore Zoo), to the presence of strangers, to the sight of fire, and taken into a dark room, without exhibiting the slightest sign of fear. A little baby boy, Albert, whose response to animals (rabbits, dogs, white rats, and inhabitants of the Zoo) had been one of calm curiosity and interest, was presented in the laboratory with a white rat, for which he instantly reached in an exploratory fashion. When he almost touched the animal, a loud noise was produced with a metal bar, resulting in a reaction of shrinking and withdrawal. When the child, after a time, again reached for the animal, the procedure was repeated, and the withdrawal response became more pronounced. After the seventh experiment, Albert showed definite signs of strong fear at the mere sight of the rat.[1]

Several things can be learned from Watson's early work with infants. It shows first that there are certain relatively simple life situations (noise, loss of support, restriction of movement, stroking), which from the very beginning of life evoke characteristic reaction patterns pictured in the child's body posture, motility, facial expression, and the quality of his

[1] Watson, John B., and R. Rayner. Conditioned Emotional Reactions. Journal of Experimental Psychology. 1920, 3, 1–14.

cry. We learn secondly that other settings which are believed by the laity to be natural producers of fear in children (animals, darkness, strangers, fire) failed to elicit any such response in babies who had spent their first few weeks in a hospital ward and had not had an opportunity to be taught at home to fear those situations. The experiments with little Albert demonstrate thirdly the fact that affective responses can be taught or "conditioned," that is, that some events which have previously been accepted neutrally may, through repeated associations with simultaneous pleasant or unpleasant experiences, come to evoke affect-loaded attitudes. We see furthermore that just as all other human potentialities need time and gradual maturation to assume a more and more complex actuality, so the emotional life evolves slowly and its expansion and amplification depend on age, grasp, and previous experiences. It would hardly be correct to say that X, Y, and Z, or fear, rage, and love are the only emotions constituting the fundamental equipment of man, Watson's assertion to the contrary notwithstanding. It takes, for instance, a greater degree of general ripening than that existing within the first two hundred days (the ages of Watson's babies) to be at all capable of feeling or displaying jealousy; yet we know from numerous examples that jealousy need not be taught and that the response is as much of a pattern and, in a way, as "fundamental" as that of fear or of rage.

The question regarding the number of emotions, a pet preoccupation of earlier psychology, has become futile in the light of a broader psychobiological attitude. We have come to know that the names of emotional expressions, emotional attitudes, emotional reactions in general are not names for any existing entities. They are snapshots from the linguistic camera, conveying an impression of the sum total of facts involved in a special type of human behavior. The meaning of the term "fear" implies the idea of existing or anticipated danger as well as the individual's attitude in the face of this danger. There are other sets of facts which, in spite of their resemblance to the combination alluded to as fear, show sufficient dissimilarity to have warranted the creation of other names, such as apprehension, dread, fright, terror, horror, alarm, consternation, etc. The same is true of anger, worry, joy, love, hate, pity, and their numerous verbal nuances. These are not "different" or "similar" emotional entities but brief designations of certain broad constellations involving a situation, a person's response to it, and his more or less conventionalized manifestation of the response. Furthermore, such responses may be exaggerated or concealed, they may be pretended or "acted" (not only on the stage), and they may be controlled and intellectualized, just as, on the other hand, cognitive activities may assume a highly affective coloring. Over and above, it seems to us essential to realize that the emotional life of a person is not merely a series of sudden, situationally determined bumps and upheavals with completely neutral intervals, but that it is a continuously diffuse and regulative whole-function, more or less intense, differing more or less in its character and its mode of expression and in the individual's degree of awareness of it, more or less proportionate to the character of the situation, more or less directly dependent on some specific event. In other words, in occupying ourselves with the affective functioning of children (and of

adults), we are interested not only in its episodic and dramatic culminations but also in the temporarily or permanently immanent emotional tension states and moods and attitudes and personality traits, in such features
as the general feeling of satisfaction or unhappiness, the sense of security,
a condition of sensitiveness or of suspiciousness, etc.

For practical clinical purposes (and for these purposes only), it may be
well to distinguish between several types of emotional functioning:

"Normal," natural, serviceable emotional reactions. We are so
constituted that certain types of situations do certain things to most of
us. Realization of danger is almost invariably connected with fearful avoidance or shrinking. What specific form the fear reaction will assume under
the specific circumstances, depends on the degree of nearness and intensity of the perilous situation, on the individual's personality and training, on his experience or lack of experience with similar events, and on any
number of other factors. The fundamental constellation of danger plus
some sort or another of fear is to be considered as a normal, natural human
phenomenon. Education of children will have to make use of it, in order
to adapt them to the complexities of their environment. They must be
taught to know the dangers inherent in venomous snakes or poisonous
mushrooms, in playing with matches, in the handling of a loaded pistol, or
in crossing a street during heavy traffic. Thus the innate potentiality of
fear is intellectualized, rationalized, made serviceable, turned into a necessary means of self-protection, converted into life-preserving caution; it
may even, under certain conditions, be transformed into an attitude of
facing and braving, instead of evading, the danger and assume the shape
of courage. Jealousy, through training, may be purged of the element of
hostility and become highly useful as creative competition. Anger, controlled and led into reasonable channels, serves as a powerful cultural agent
as righteous indignation and resentment of obvious injustice. The absence
of caution, competitive interests, and justified resentment is a problem
not less serious than complete abandon to strong emotional impulses.

Strong emotional reactions commensurate with the situation.
There are events in human life which make affective upheavals understandable and more or less normal. Profound grief after the loss of a parent
may well be expected to lift a child out for some time from the regular
routine, interfere with his attention in school, with his interest in play activities, with his appetite and his sleep. The preparations for a birthday
party or the Christmas Eve anticipations may well create an excitement
in which the child's behavior differs markedly from his usual mode of
performance. From the youngster's point of view, certain seemingly unreasonable responses may also be included in this category. If a child has
been made to believe that the ragman puts naughty children into his bag
and does all sorts of cruel things to them, abducting them from their homes
forever, it is highly comprehensible that the sight of the ragman may produce an intense fear; it is not the child's response that is abnormal but the
type of training that has paved the way for it.

*Strong emotional upheavals not reasonably commensurate
with the situation.* In the first two groups we have dealt with normal or
near-normal affective reactions. The third group leads us straight into psycho-

pathology. Emotional immaturity and instability and faulty training may result in sweeping, highly dramatic, uncontrolled outbursts entirely out of proportion to the responsible setting. Temper tantrums are a classical example. A stormy scene with kicking, screaming, destructiveness may follow nothing more than the mother's refusal to produce a penny. Sometimes, in comparatively rare instances, a logical connection between the reaction and the situation cannot be directly discovered and the behavior can be understood only after a painstaking analysis of the child's personality. This is, for example, true of the phobias. A setting which to the observer (and even in the patient's own judgment) seems completely neutral may produce a veritably paralyzing terror: being in a closed room, finding oneself in the midst of a crowd. In most cases, however, it is either a mildly disturbing immediate occurrence that is reacted to very vigorously or a more general and protracted discomfort which leads to emotional tempests (e.g., anxiety attacks) Very infrequently, in children who are so disposed, there is a most violent acute affective sequel to a frightful or resented happening, lasting for from a few hours to a few weeks, which remains a single event in the child's life (Ziehen's ecnoia). Usually, however, the paroxysms repeat themselves and assume the proportions of emotional habits.

Emotional habits. Breathholding spells, temper tantrums, crying spells, fear of the dark or of animals may be corrected at their inception by judicious management. Otherwise they tend to recur as often as the slightest opportunity arises. The child becomes, if you wish, "conditioned" to a certain type of response to a number of similar situations. The response becomes a habit. It is this form of children's emotional reactions with which the parents, the teachers, and the physicians are most frequently confronted.

Wholly incongruous emotional responses. In a small number of children, especially in the odd, peculiar youngster, in the imbecile, and in the schizophrenic, one may observe reactions which are altogether contrary to one's usual expectations. There are outbursts of laughter or weeping or rage or hilariousness which seem to come out of a clear sky and to have no foundation whatever in the external situation. On the other hand, events of first magnitude which other people would naturally meet with more or less strong emotional reactions, may be regarded with utmost indifference which impresses one as bizarre and incomprehensible if one considers the importance of the event (for example, deprivation of liberty by being confined in an institution, death of a near relative).

Transient emotional attitudes. We have so far dwelt on adequate or inadequate, reasonable or unreasonable, commensurate or not commensurate responses which are limited in time and may be termed more or less acute and more or less obviously connected with a concrete situation. There exist, however, also emotional reactions which are spread over a much longer period, are as a rule not dramatized and are less dependent on the stimulation by specific happenings. They are protracted attitudes, moods, affective tones, sometimes alluded to as dysphorias, governing all activity rather than being circumscribed episodic performances standing out as momentary outbursts from an otherwise inconspicuous behavior. Without ever having temper tantrums, a child may go through a period of general irritability, poutiness, sulkiness, crossness, surliness, grouchiness. Without necessarily having any definite objects of fear, there may be a general attitude of shyness, timidity, suspiciousness. Marked self-consciousness or sensitiveness may underly all of the youngster's contacts with his surroundings. There may be a mood of mild elation, merriment, mirth, gaiety, or, on the other hand, of sadness, downheartedness, gloominess, pessimism. It is, or course, easily understood that in the course of such moods the child may at times burst out with stronger and more drastic ventilations of his feelings, except that it is exceedingly uncommon to see at so early an age the manic-depressive culminations which one finds in the adult. The relation of these transient attitudes and moods to life situations are often not evident at first glance and may be very subtle. But after it has been learned and after the difficulties have been improved, the child's disposition may be favorably influenced.

More permanent emotional traits. It is well known that people differ more or less essentially in their receptiveness to various types of situations, in the manner and intensity of emotional elaboration and expression, in the occurrence, quality, and duration of moods, in other words, in their "temperaments." As among adults, so we find among children the calm youngster whose reactions are usually quite commensurate with his experiences, the excitable person whom the least event (a shopping trip, a stranger at the door, a dog across the street) is apt to work up to a height of responsiveness, and the phlegmatic boy or girl who seems to be left unmoved by the very same trip or stranger or dog and even by happenings in which he or she is much more directly and significantly involved; the compassionate child who responds with sympathy to the suffering of others, who is highly considerate of the feelings of the parents, siblings and playmates; the cold individual who does not seem affected by what happens to others; the cruel child who even enjoys the minor or major miseries of those with whom he lives.

Emotional reactions are perhaps suited better than any other form of human functioning to serve as a demonstration of psychobiological and sociobiological integration. It is utterly impossible to think of them detached from the individual's total personality and from the situational features. They are both responses to environmental influences and indicators or signs of what goes on in the responding person. The "meaning" and understanding of any sort of emotional behavior are determined fundamentally by the setting in which it occurs, by the manner in which the individual is involved and in which he feels himself involved, by his previous experiences with similar situations, by his previous reactions to similar situations, by social conventions, by his temperament, and by many other factors. At the same time, the response manifests itself to the observer in a fashion from which he usually can infer the nature of the individual's experience and what takes place within him. This is accomplished by means of a complexity of physiological happenings which vary according to the general emotional pattern and according to its intensity. We have learned from Watson's work that even infants in the first weeks of life, when affected in the sense of X, Y, or Z (fear, rage, or love), assume certain postures with involvement of changes in the muscular tone, in the physiognomy, in the respiration, in the general activity; the picture displayed in X is different from that shown in Y and Z, but sufficiently typical for the same emotion. It is, as a matter of fact, this behavior of the infant's body which made it possible for Watson to conclude that there was an emotional re-action at all present. The bodily surface manifestation of the emotions, which comprises posture, tonicity, motility, facial expression, complexion, and visible respiratory changes, has for many centuries been made the sub-ject of more or less scientific interest and within the past one hundred years been studied from the anatomical, physiological, phylogenetic, and interpretative angles.[1] The less conspicuous visceral participation has been made accessible to fruitful research in the more recent past and has been shown clinically and experimentally to be an integral component of the emotional whole-functioning, involving the vegetative nervous system, metabolism, the endocrines, digestion, breathing, circulation, and even the electrical skin resistance in a more or less specific manner.

One may roughly distinguish three degrees of somatic participation in emotional reactions:

Physiological participation as a normal, natural part of the psycho-biological emotional reaction. Its intensity is usually, though not always, proportionate to the intensity of the response. Since man, incessantly con-fronted with various needs of adaptation and with all sorts of factors help-ing him or interfering with his goals, it is to be expected that he is hardly ever, not even in his sleep, absolutely neutral emotionally and that, there-fore, there are more or less subtle visceral tensions present at any time. At the occasion of stronger feelings, they naturally become more readily demonstrable and have been found to show some degree of specificity in accordance with the different emotional reaction-patterns.

Near-physiological participation. It does happen, even in healthy and stable individuals, that one or another of the somatic components may step out of the frame of the total reaction in a disproportionately con-spicuous and usually unpleasant manner. Strong grief or disappointment may be accompanied by a more or less severe headache or by lack of ap-petite with or without measurable alteration of gastric motility or secre-tion. It is known that sudden fright may result in a hardly resistible urge to defecate as a part of the fear response. The examination diarrheas of some students are an almost proverbial example of what apprehensive tension may occasionally do to an individual. The mild nausea that often goes with disgust may at times be increased to the point of vomiting. Though no longer strictly physiological, these intensifications of certain features of visceral participation may be termed near-normal or near-physiological reactions in contra-distinction to the third group of out-spokenly morbid somatic dysfunctions on an emotional basis.

Pathological participation. A noticeable portion of the psychopa-thology of childhood is made up of complaints in which abnormalities in the somatic participation have come to play an essential rôle. Breathholding, palpitations, pallor, syncopes, anorexia, constipation, diarrhea, colospasms, nausea, vomiting and headaches are some of the outstanding manifesta-

[1] A representative bibliography will be found in: Kanner, Leo. Judging Emotions from Facial Expressions. Psychological Monograph, No. 186. Princeton. 1931.

tions. They may derive their origin from and owe their repetition to one or several of the following features:

Unusual intensification. There are children in whom the personality makeup, training, and sometimes observation of similar reaction forms in the elders create a greater readiness for extraordinarily strong bodily responses in the presence of any emotional setting. These are, for instance, the youngsters whose worry about promotion in school is accompanied for days or weeks by loss of appetite or by vomiting.

Habitual intensification of a specific type of somatic reaction. The quantitative increase is often resorted to with sufficient frequency to make one speak of it as a habit. It may be elicited by the recurrence of single concrete situations or it may be a repeated response to some protracted and less obvious discomfort.

Intentional utilization. A child has learned that either some of the responses which we have designated as near-physiological or some similar symptom due to real physical illness has caused parental alarm, has placed him in the center of attention at home or in school, and has given him advantages and privileges not otherwise obtained. Or he has noticed that someone else in the family has derived such benefits from the symptom. He may make use of this experience more or less intentionally by fighting unpleasantness or seeming neglect by means of the symptom (headache, or vomiting, or constipation). This mode of behavior is often a factor in the development of hypochondriacal trends in children.

Diversification. Sometimes, a near-physiological somatic reaction, which has primarily been expressive of a very definite emotional setting, may come to lose its specificity and be diverted to other dissimilar situations. A baby suddenly falls from his highchair; in his fright, he catches his breath. Watson has demonstrated that catching of the breath is a part expression of fear as well as of anger in infants. It does, indeed, happen not infrequently that, after the breathholding effect of a fright, the same pattern is later used by the child to express anger. The somatic response, first experienced in a fear situation is taken over to indicate displeasure in the same child. Similarly, vomiting may at first have been a signal of disgust or an answer to overstuffing; once the vomiting type of response has been learned, it may be diverted to situations of fearful anticipation, of jealousy, and of various forms of excitement.

Automatization. The bodily concomitants may in some instances become so frequent and gradually so dominating and so detached from the original emotions that they may cease to function as specific signals in response to circumscribed affective settings. To the casual observer, they may seem to lead an independent existence with no obvious or even suggestive situational connections. This is the reason why so many physicians find it exceedingly difficult to attach psychobiological significance to some of the reactions belonging in this category. Yet there are numerous examples of psychogenic headaches or constipation or colospasms which in the course of time have become automatized. Since Brissaud, we know that many tics are in the main psychogenic reactions which have become detached from their former meaning as expressive or defensive responses.

Our pluralistic approach to the study of the mentally integrated personality contains in itself an invitation to view the emotional factor from the angle of its close interrelations with the other factors entering into the formation of personality. In order to prevent misunderstanding, we hasten to emphasize that the term interrelations is not in the least intended to imply the notion of different functional entities working side by side or influencing each other in the sense of one function doing something to another. What we propose to consider is the interesting and practically important question as to how the younger or the older child, the well endowed and the poorly endowed, the healthy and the sick, the intelligent and the unintelligent, the well trained and the poorly trained youngster is known to react emotionally, in other words, in what manner age, constitution, the physical condition, the degree of intelligence, and the environment chime with the child's affective reactivity. It is hardly necessary to state that sharp lines cannot be drawn, since all of these features are held together as the qualities, more or less fixed or changeable, of a developing individual.

The age factor. We know that infants soon after birth are capable of reactions, which impress one as fear, rage, and love. It is especially in the range of the first two emotions that abnormally strong responses may occur, usually not before the end of the first half year of life. Breathholding spells are reserved for the following two years, after which they are very rare. The expressions of fear and anger then become more differentiated, the latter appearing in their extreme form as temper tantrums. In the course of time, with the increasing participation in the environment with its complexities, the child acquires a capacity for additional emotional reactions, such as sympathy and jealousy, and for displaying different shades of the same emotional response. The richer the experiential background and the comprehension of situations, the more variegated and complex and capable of fine differentiations becomes the emotional life of the growing child. There comes a time in the pre-school development of most youngsters when they go through a period of resistiveness or negativism, on the handling of which a great deal of his future affective adaptations will depend. Again, sooner or later in the years of pre-puberty, there is a transient stage of crossness and irritability and increased sensitiveness in a large proportion of children.

The constitutional factor. Aside from racial and climatically determined differences, there are within the same national group and geographic region noticeable individual variations of emotional responsiveness. Though it is futile and unwise to raise the question as to exactly how much is due to ingrained personality traits and how much has been engrafted by environmental influences, one would expect a certain range of variations, knowing that such differences exist also in the physical configuration, in the intellectual endowment, and in other respects. One cannot get away from the common observation that there are children and adults who are from the beginning emotionally unstable, just as there are people who are from the beginning handicapped physically or intellectually. In such children's biographies we usually find a continuous string of emotional difficulties manifesting themselves at home and in school and in their relation to playmates. The fact that they are to a greater or lesser extent constitutionally determined does not at all imply that they cannot and should not be made accessible to proper modification.

The physical factor. Somatic discomfort, due to illness or fatigue or lack of adequate recreational outlets, may, as any other discomfort, serve as an unpleasant situation in response to which the child may develop emotional difficulties. The itching sensation experienced in eczema may create in the youngster a condition of marked irritability. A neglected toothache may have a similar effect. The weakness of a child with acute cardiac illness may result in general apathy and listlessness. A crippled youngster may react to his disfigurement with excessive sensitiveness or with a general attitude of despair or with compensatory boastfulness. Much will depend on the degree of physical suffering, on the attitude of the environment, on the patient's own make-up, on the presence and utilization of assets, and on other things. Besides, there are diseases which may alter very perceptibly a child's total personality and with it, of course, his emotional responsiveness, as is the case in epidemic encephalitis or in juvenile paresis.

The intellectual factor. High intelligence does not always necessarily go with emotional stability, nor does low intelligence always coincide with emotional instability. It is undoubtedly easier to teach a bright child to conventionalize his emotional reactions than it is to train a retarded child in this or in any other respect. But we have had an opportunity in the preceding chapter to point to the finding of emotional immaturity in youngsters with average and even superior intelligence quotients and, on the other hand, the occurrence of splendid adjustment in stable and well handled feebleminded individuals.

The environmental factors. Their bearing on the emotional life of the child will be treated in detail in a subsequent chapter, in preparation for which we only wish to remark here that the study of a child's emotional reactions and emotional difficulties cannot be considered complete or useful from a therapeutic point of view without the knowledge of the emotional atmosphere prevailing in his immediate environment.

CHAPTER IX

THE SEX FACTOR

SEX DIFFERENTIATION takes place at a very early period, if not at the moment of the union of the spermatozoon with the ovule. In the course of intrauterine growth and post-natal life until and after the time of pubescence, it becomes more and more marked and complicated. After many centuries of reluctance to deal with the subtect at all and of prejudices dictated in part by ecclesiastic dogmatism, it has, within a brief era of scientific approach, become almost a truism that procreative maturation does not enter suddenly into the life of an individual some time during the second decade but that it is the culmination of a continuous evolution beginning at conception. It does not differ in this respect from the general laws of somatic development and, after birth, from the successive ripening and unfolding of the mental functions. Both the sexual and psychic potentialities are brought into existence as integral constituents of the human being and have a natural tendency to evolve gradually and to show manifold individual variations within or without the limits of the average, on the basis of ingrained constitutional factors and of later nosological and environmental influences.

Any consideration of the distinguishing features of the male and female sexes will best begin with the realization that there are three outstanding types of differences: generic, personal, and those determined by social convention.

Generic differences can, of course, be studied on a statistical basis only. They include the distribution of birth rate (the ratio being 104 to 106 boys to 100 girls), mortality (being greater in the male), and the often peculiar and unexplained apportionment of morbidity. It is, for instance, well known that approximately seventy-five to eighty per cent of all cases of hypertrophic stenosis of the pylorus are found in boys, who also show a great preponderance in the incidence of color-blindness and specific reading disability (congenital word-blindness). The prevalence of hemophilia in the male and its transmission through the unaffected mother is also a matter of common knowledge. Similar experiences have been made with regard to so eminently a psychopathological reaction as hysteria which is from seven to nine times as frequent in the adolescent and adult female as in the male. In how many ways, even in matters of habit formation, generic inequalities may make themselves perceptible, is shown by the example of toenail biting, in which little girls indulge much more frequently than boys.

Personal differences exist on the anatomo-physiological and on the psychobiological levels. The first have been divided into three groups:

Primary sex characteristics, largely of a morphological nature, present at birth and capable of further development. They comprise mainly the organs of reproduction.

Secondary sex characteristics, becoming apparent at a later period of childhood. They show themselves in the general structure of the body, the form of the skeleton, especially the pelvis, the growth of the hair, the development of the breasts, the configuration of the larynx and the differentiation of the quality of voice. They include the differences in the type of respiration (abdominal in the male, costal in the female), the typical distribution of adipose tissue, etc.

Tertiary sex characteristics (Havelock Ellis), referring to those distinguishing features which are obtained not so much from inspection of the individual as from measurements of large numbers, such as the rate of linear growth, the shape of the skull, the weight of the brain, the functioning of the glands of internal secretion, and the number of the red blood corpuscles.

As to the *psychobiological distinctions,* Moll states: "Without further discussing the question, to what extent in earlier generations there has been any cultivation of psychical differences, I believe that we are justified in asserting that at the present time the sexual differentiation manifested in respect to quite a number of psychical qualities is the result of direct inheritance."[1] By "inheritance" he undoubtedly means in this connection not the transmission of parental reaction-tendencies but qualities dependent on being a member of one of the two sexes. Bucura, who has devoted a special monograph to the subject of sex differences, unfortunately paying but scant attention to their gradual evolution, stresses the stronger emotionalism, the greater tendency towards concreteness, the more vivid imaginativeness, the weaker power of volition, the greater inclination towards conservatism, the lower degree of aggressiveness, the higher and purer altruism and readiness for self-sacrifice in women.[2] The advent of exact methods of mental standardization has tended to do away with the notion, long maintained and most consistently advocated by Möbius, that women are as a rule intellectually inferior to men.[3] Certain inherent differences, however, cannot possibly be disregarded. It is a fact, which cannot be disputed and which has been established by Kerschensteiner through painstaking investigations, that boys have a superior ability to draw in comparison to girls of the same age. It is further a matter of common observation that, given equal intelligence, training, and social status, girls as a rule reach a higher degree of tactfulness, formal behavior, and ability to deal with people than boys of the same age.

Educational and conventional influences begin to work upon the child at a very early period, long before the acquisition of the secondary sex characteristics. As soon as the baby is old enough to observe, the differences in clothing and in the coiffure cannot fail to impress themselves upon his mind and to be accepted as a given part of the reality of his environment leading later on to an understandable curiosity. When, at about

[1] Moll, Albert. The Sexual Life of the Child. Translated by Eden Paul. New York. 1924, p. 42.

[2] Bucura, Constantin J. Geschlechtsunterschiede beim Menschen. Wien und Leipzig. 1913. (Chapter on "Psychische Geschlechtsunterschiede," pp. 57–83).

[3] Möbius, P. J. Über den physiologischen Schwachsinn des Weibes. Fourth edition. Halle. 1902.

the end of the second year, sentence formation, plural suffixes, and pronouns are added to the linguistic equipment, the child learns in many
languages to use different articles distinguishing between two or three
genders and, in all languages, to employ different pronouns when referring
to men and women. By virtue of equality or similarity of the garments and
of parental guidance, little girls feel that they belong together and little
boys feel that they belong together in their play interests and activities.
The other group is felt dimly as something different and is caused by the
educators to be felt as something diametrically opposite. The sexual nature
of the difference is sometimes discovered incidentally, sometimes actively
through questioning and other forms of satisfying the inevitable curiosity,
sometimes passively through information obtained from the elders or in a
less desirable form from playmates, and occasionally through actual exploration or even seduction.

It is essential to emphasize the fact that the primary and secondary sex
characteristics and the psychical as well as sociological differences evolve
gradually in the course of childhood, that the awakening of sex urge and
sex attraction undergoes a slow and subtle evolution directed by biological
processes as well as outside forces. It is unquestionably true and a matter of
common sense that the newborn is, according to his degree of intellectual
development and the absence of an adequate experiential background, acquainted with nobody and nothing but his own body, and that only very
vaguely and indistinctly. It is true that in his first gropings he comes upon
parts of his body, prominences or cavities, which he can handle and with
which he can play and which are capable of sensations which he does not
have when he touches or strokes his nipple or a toy. It is further true that
for a time, as long as he has no or little outside contacts, the family members
are the only or main persons with whom he establishes close personal relations. It is finally true that before he has advanced enough to realize the
significance of heterosexual goals he does not discriminate between the sexes
more than knowledge, education, and opportunity permit him to do.

These facts are so obvious that they would hardly deserve mention, had
not the psychoanalytic school based upon them a momentous hypothetical
structure which partly works with a translation of them into an elaborate
terminology and partly has "sexualized" them into a fascinating but unproven dramatic meshwork of happenings, beginning in utero (with an
overture taking place in the "racial unconscious"), carried through life,
and terminating at the moment of death. The fact that the infant is thrown
on his own resources with regard to his first manual occupations is interpreted as autoeroticism or "narcissism" (a term borrowed from Greek
mythology); the accessible prominences and cavities become "erogenous
zones" and their manipulations are viewed as indulgences of a libidinous
character. Thumbsucking, earpulling, interest displayed in defecation and
in urination are translated into terms of larvated masturbation. Their undisputed pleasurable effect is taken for sexual gratification. We must, to be
fair, admit that the designations sex and libido are claimed to be used in a
much broader sense than that commonly employed. But if the childhood
pleasures derived from thumbsucking are "libidinous" only in that they
are hedonic sensations, then it is difficult to see why one should so stub-

bornly insist on calling them libidinous; the whole issue then becomes mainly one of preferred nomenclature. As a matter of fact, the many assertions to the contrary notwithstanding, it is the psychoanalysts themselves who again and again in their publications draw analogies between the infant's activities and gross sexual behavior of the adult.

The child's family relations have been depicted by Freud in the light of what he called the Oedipus complex (another loan from Greek mythology). After a period of objectless, narcissistic eroticism, the boy's first love object is his mother. He is jealous of his father who shares the mother's affection, and he wishes the father out of the picture. The unfolding and solution of this "family drama" of the boy's mother-love and father-hatred (in the girl the situation is reversed accordingly) is said to play an enormous rôle in determining his future destiny, his choice of occupation, his selection of a mate, and many features of his character and relations to people.

The fact that the youngster is indifferent in his relations to members of the two sexes, (though convention sees to it that he is not altogether indifferent), makes the psychoanalysts speak of a period of bisexuality preceding the heterosexual adjustment. He goes through a time when he is "polymorphously perverse," when the aberrations which in the adult are morbid are natural steps in his development.

The conventions of civilization cause the child to "repress" his narcissism, the Oedipus stage, the homosexual inclinations, all of which are lodged in the "unconscious." They remain repressed throughout the life of the well-adjusted individual who has the ability to "sublimate" them in the form of moral attitudes, artistic productions, social connections, etc. They may appear in disguised form in dreams, mispronunciations, lapses of the pen, forgetting, and the like. Or they may fail of complete repression; they may be "fixated" or the individual may "regress" to their level. This results in abnormal or peculiar characters (anal-erotic, urethral-erotic) or in psychotic reactions. Thus schizophrenia is considered as a regression to the narcissistic stage, paranoia as a homosexual psychosis, and hysteria is viewed as based mainly on an unsatisfactory solution of the Oedipus complex.

We have merely given the skeleton of the Freudian theory of infantile sexuality. Our presentation is avowedly incomplete. To go into details would require much more space than we can afford. The popularization of the theory[1] has had two beneficial results. It has raised the tabooed subject of sex to the dignity of scientific research and it has called attention to the fact that sexual maturation, before reaching the nubile stage, is a process of long and gradual development in the course of childhood. It did, however, swing the pendulum to the opposite extreme of ascribing all human behavior too one-sidedly to the influence of sex, making the mistake of yielding all too willingly to the lure of unbridled speculation and of forgetting all the other factors which we have learned to value in the study of psychobiology.

In dealing with the sex problem, we have so far approached the subject

---

[1] Freud, Sigmund. Drei Abhandlungen zur Sexual-theorie. (I. Die sexuellen Abirrungen. II. Die Umgestaltungen der Pubertät). Dritte, vermehrte Auflage. Leipzig und Wien. 1915.

from the point of view of sex differentiation along physical, psychical, and educational lines. In the practical dealings with the everyday child, the first opportunity to consider the topic as being in any way a problem is given by the youngster himself either in the form of masturbation, which we shall take up in detail in a later section, or more frequently and almost inevitably in the form of questions. Curiosity with regard to matters which have a bearing on sex is displayed by children at an earlier age than is usually believed. Miss Hattendorf has collected a considerable number (1763) of children's questions concerning sex; those asking them (of their parents) ranged between two and fourteen years in age. The questions could be classified into eight groups: Origin of babies (40.9%); coming of another baby (14.5%); physical sex differences (12.7%); organs and functions of the body (11.9%); process of birth (10.4%); relation of the father to reproduction (5.2%); intrauterine growth (2.4%); marriage (2.0%). Pre-school children asked 49.1% of the questions, those from six to ten years asked 40.1%, and those above ten years of age asked 10.8% of all the questions. Miss Hattendorf concludes her enlightening study by saying: "The relatively large number of questions for children of pre-school age, as compared with other ages, indicates that children are manifesting interest in sex through their questions in these very early years. The subject-matter of the questions indicates what children are wanting to know in reference to sex. Interest is shown to develop from simple inquiries concerning the origin of babies, through the more intricate physiological processes of conception and birth, to the deeper sociological and psychological interpretations of customs and attitudes. The ages at which the questions occur substantiate the feeling expressed by so many writers that sex instruction should be given in the early years. The questions, in showing the trend of children's interest in sex, seem to indicate a developing interest in the subject which points to the need of a graded program in sex education for children."[1]

It is obvious that this curiosity finds at first an incentive in concrete events and observations, such as the arrival of a younger brother or sister; the first view of the genitalia of a child of the opposite sex; sometimes the incidental witnessing of parental cohabitation with puzzled wonderment as to the meaning of the act; often the overhearing of the discussion of the playmates anent the subject of sex or ridicule on the part of the playmates because of display of ignorance and naïveté. Later, when abstract thinking is added to the youngster's equipment, when adolescent romanticism and cruder preoccupations are gradually prepared through vague stirrings and the fascinating mixture of show-offishness, shy approaches, and brisk evasions, the intelligent youngster experiences as part of his early philosophical problems a growing inquisitiveness about the intrinsic significance of the existence of two sexes, about the hows and whys of matrimony, about the whence of human development. At the time of puberty, when the stirrings and urges become more circumscribed, when conventional education has managed to drive home more or less subtly and comprehensively

[1] Hattendorf, Katherine W. A Study of the Questions of Young Children Concerning Sex: A Phase of an Experimental Approach to Parent Education. The Journal of Social Psychology. 1932, 3, 37–65.

the connection between sex differentiation and the aim of family formation, when accumulated perplexities, observations, previous fragments of information, and perhaps actual experiences of some sort or another have knit a loose meshwork of knowledge, there is a desire for greater coherence and a readiness for a more complete understanding. At the beginning, the sex curiosity hardly differs from the same child's eagerness to know what causes thunder and lightning or what it is that makes the doll say, "Mamma." It then assumes a different form, due largely to the facts that the youngster begins to feel himself personally involved and that the secrecy surrounding the subject gives it a more specific aspect in his eyes.

The capacity for curiosity and the wish to satisfy it is one of the main characteristics of good intelligence. Once it is aroused, it is bent upon adequate gratification and does not suffer itself to be squelched by impatient subterfuges. Parental unwillingness to help the child may have a number of harmful and certainly not intended results. The repudiated curiosity, which the youngster cannot cast off at will and which has been discouraged as something "ugly," "dirty," "naughty," is forced into illegitimate, sneaky, secretive activities. The information is apt to come from improper sources and to be either incorrect, or obscene, or both. Ocular and manual exploration may take the place of verbal explanation. The whole question, rebuffed as indecent by the elders, assumes in the mind of the child a magnitude which may lead to preoccupations unhealthy because of their exclusiveness. The very idea of indecency and filthiness, unwisely injected into the matter, may be appropriated and carried into adult life, especially by women, interfering with normal adaptation to the heterosexual goal.

It is one of the real merits of the psychoanalytic school that it has paved the way to a saner attitude towards the discussion of sex, unencumbered by unscientific and obscuring taboos. This has led to an increasing insight into the desirability of including in the child's education the instruction in so natural and vital a topic, beyond the mere warning against the dangers of acquiring venereal infection and against existing or assumed perils resulting from masturbation. Such a realization, however, has often tended to develop peculiar slip-shod methods confusing rather than helping the youngster and, on the other hand, to go to the extreme of blurting out all and everything regardless of his preparedness and degree of comprehension, replacing the stork story at an early date by a crude description of the details of intercourse. Experience has taught that it is wisest to answer the questions when they come truthfully in the sense and spirit of the questions and to wait patiently until the next question comes.

A very intelligent girl of five approached the problem in this manner: "Daddy, when they want bread, they must have dough, don't they?" "Yes." "And when they want dough, they must have flour, don't they?" "Yes." "And when they want flour, they must have wheat?" "Yes." "Well, everything comes from everything else, does it not? Well, then, what do people come from?" She was told that people are born, that they come from their mothers. Her curiosity was fully satisfied until about a year later, when she wanted to know just what happened within the mother. It was explained that it takes nine months for the baby to grow within the mother from a tiny cell until it is big enough and capable of living without under the necessary care and protection and that the development goes on for many years to come. Two years afterwards, the question came: "Just where does the child grow in the mother?" She learned that a special organ was provided for that in the lower portion of the abdomen. When she saw a pregnant woman after that, she understood. When a little brother arrived, she was neither invited to inspect him nor prohibited from entering when he was bathed. When she noticed the genitals and made a remark about it, she was told that that is how boys are built. It was neither a shock to her nor did she seem to develop a "castration complex"; it merely was an addition to her knowledge which satisfied her intellectual curiosity aroused by the sight. At ten years, she wondered: "Mother, they say sometimes that a child looks like his father. I can well see how he can look like his mother because that is where he came from. But how is it that he can look like his father?" Her mother told her that people marry in order to found a family; that they unite in a way that would permit the "seed" to enter the mother's special organ in which the child was conceived and borne. By that time, she had acquired in school sufficient botanical knowledge which could serve as an illustration. Again, she was satisfied. Sooner or later, she will want to know more and her questions will be answered correctly, with due consideration of her grasp and of the type of question. One day her mother was not well. She was solicitous and desired to know what was the matter. She was told frankly that her mother was menstruating. The mechanism was explained to her (in an understandable manner) and she was instructed that in about two or three years she will have the same experience. It never occurred to her that there should be anything indecent about the subject. She considered it as a part of the things that children learn from their parents, just as they try, for instance, to answer frankly her questions with reference to the economic structure of her country and to her problems of cosmic orientation. She has no reason for gathering her impressions from uncontrollable sources.

Familiarity with the facts, willingness, the overcoming of harmful prudishness, truthfulness, a dosage adapted to the child's developmental and intellectual preparedness as evidenced by the type of questions, and good common sense are the parents' best requirements for efficient and sensible sex education. Direct answers of this sort mean more to the youngster than the confused and confusing "demonstrations" of the propagation of lilies to a group of children. Sex curiosity should be met as and when it arises; it is a natural phenomenon and does not have to be injected artificially.

Much has been written, and oftentimes well written, about the *specific features of puberty*. It is undoubtedly a period of vague and vacillating strivings, of peculiar fermentations, in which the attainment of the nubile stage cannot be denied a leading part. It must, however, not be forgotten that those years at the same time also mark a progressive domestic emancipation, a gradual reaching out into participation in communal life and activities, and a demand for vocational decisions and adjustments. The young individual begins to learn how to handle his own steering wheel which so far has been directed for him by his parents and teachers. He begins to include in his thinking something which has evolved just as gradually as all his other notions, that is, the thought of his future. An untamed and as yet unregulated and insufficiently utilized energy, a feeling of growing strength finds its outlets in competitive games, sports, and athletics. Simultaneously, a vast new realm is opened by the groping excursions into the fields of abstract ideation. Traditional concepts are inquired into, examined and, according to the child's make-up and background, accepted, criticized, or temporarily or permanently modified or rejected. The age-old struggle between father and son, between the older and younger generation, between settled conservatism and a hazy, militant progressivism takes place, introducing a second period of resistance, more subtle, more difficult to handle than the first period of negativism in pre-school age. It goes without saying that all this is accompanied by physiological happenings of first magnitude, the advent of menstruation in girls and of potency in boys, the final shaping of the secondary sex characteristics, and frequently evidence of transient hyperthyroidism and basedowoid characteristics; the type of eidetic imagery changes or, at any rate, becomes definitely established. Juvenile acne may make its appearance and be quite bothersome.

A few ambitious attempts have been made to discern a number of different characteristic phases of the age of pubescence. We quote briefly those elaborated by Ruppert and by Hildegard Hetzer.

Ruppert distinguishes (in the observation of the boy, A.):

1. Late childhood: years 10 to 12;4. The boy fits in nicely with the other members of the household. His parents are satisfied with him. He does his home work carefully. He plays well with his younger brother.

2. Phase of "feverish wishing" (*Wunschfieber*): years 12;4 to 13;8. He begins to quarrel and to fight with his brother and is punished by his father. Almost every day he comes with a new wish. He first asks politely for, and then impatiently demands clothes and objects (fountain pen, pen-knife, etc.) which will make him appear more grown-up. He has a strong desire to earn money and discusses different schemes. He trades postage stamps (and, in this country, sells magazines or newspapers).

3. Phase of active spite: years 13;9 to 15;1. He openly rejects his brothers and his father. He is spiteful and often disobedient. He forms a friendship with an older boy who drastically "enlightens" him about sex. He criticizes and caricatures his teachers. He wishes to acquire a bicycle without having to ask his father for it. He wants to go away to his grandparents' farm in order to be rid of the "oppression" at home and in school. He likes to read mystery and detective stories. He contradicts his parents and sometimes revolts openly.

4. Phase of spite directed towards himself: years 15;2 to 15;7. This is a period of meditation and self-observation. The own limitations are recognized. He goes alone for long walks. He is rather shy and clumsy. He begins to accept and to adjust himself to the social standards of his environment. In contrast to the preceding feeling of strength and grown-upness, he now suffers from a sad realization of powerlessness.

5. The crisis: year 15;8 to 15;9. It is characterized by a certain instability and helplessness and inner conflicts. There is a poverty of expression; he does his home work well, yet in school he has difficulty in displaying his knowledge. He complains of poor memory. He has phantastic daydreams.

There is an unwillingness to make decisions. He has headaches. There is a good deal of motor restlessness and absentmindedness.

6. Phase of relaxation and of determined ideal formation: year 16. He becomes calmer and works much in the garden. He comes to terms much easier. He is very sensitive, though. He has a definite vocational goal. He feels "like newborn" and thinks of the preceding months as of a period of illness. He is less self-critical. He gets along better with his brothers and assumes the rôle of a mentor with them. He tries earnestly to understand people and ideas. He forms his first attachment to a girl.

It is, of course, understood, and Ruppert emphasizes the point clearly enough, that in different individuals those phases begin at different times and have a different duration. Personality and outside influences naturally play a significant part.

Hildegard Hetzer found in the boy whom she observed the following phases:

1. Period of quiet gathering of forces (*Kräftesammeln*): year 13;4–13;7.
2. Period of exaggerated feeling of power: years 13;7 to 14;6.
3. Negative phase: years 14;6 to 15;1.
4. Period of boy friendships: year 15.[1]

Clinically, the sex factor is important for several reasons. We know the child who comes to us with his psychiatric problems only incompletely if we do not try to become acquainted with all the functions and factors which contribute to the making of his personality. We wish to be informed about the rôle which devious sex information plays in the evolution of the specific difficulty for which we are consulted. We aim to verify or discard, on the basis of the individual case history, the general claims of the psycho-analytic school regarding the significance of sexual trauma in the etiology of hysterical and other psychopathological reactions. We are frequently enough confronted with the problem of masturbation. We are often called upon to deal with sex precocity in children. We must handle, in private practice, in child guidance clinics, and in juvenile courts, the cases of overt heterosexual and homosexual activities, of fellatio, exhibitionism, fetishism, etc., occurring before, during, and after the age of puberty.

[1] Ruppert, Hann. Aufbau der Welt des Jugendlichen. Leipzig. 1931. Die Phasen der Reifezeit, pp. 36–73.—Hetzer, Hildegard. Systematische Dauerbeobachtung über den Verlauf der negativen Phase. Zeitschrift für pädagogische Psychologie. 1927, 28, 80–96.

CHAPTER X

THE CONSTITUTIONAL FACTOR

THE PAST few decades have witnessed a heated controversy with regard to the question whether mental "disease" is due to *heredity* or to *environment*. Definite sides were taken, with corresponding battle cries on each side.

The war, as many other wars, was waged around a non-existent or rather artificially construed cause. In the first place, we have learned that a temper tantrum, stuttering, a paranoid delusion, or a depression is not necessarily and not usually the "symptom" of a "disease entity" in the traditional sense. Secondly, we know from common sense experience that every individual's personality, whether he is healthy or ill, whether he reacts normally or abnormally, is constantly molded and influenced in its trends and performances by constitutional, endogenic, and exogenic factors, all of which must be taken into consideration. To elevate the one on the throne, simultaneously forgetting the existence of the others, would be one-sided and unscientific.

What are the relationships between a child's psychiatric problems and his constitutional make-up? And a much more important question: What are the criteria that would tell us even approximately whether and in what way in a given case the constitutional factor enters into the picture? In the handling of a clinical problem no attempt, however learned, at a definition of what constitutes constitution will be of practical help. If, for our present purpose of studying and treating children's behavior disorders, we approach the question at all, it is not with the idea of entering into theoretical discussions, but avowedly with the aim of realizing liabilities and utilizing assets that may be constitutionally determined in the child with whom we happen to deal.

Under these circumstances, we shall confine our interests to the factual material obtained from the history and direct examination of the child. We then note a few points that instantly command our attention.

Jane M. had been treated at the Harriet Lane Home for rumination which began at the age of eight months. The application of a ruminating cap improved her condition noticeably, but she occasionally indulged in the practice until her fourth year, when it disappeared entirely. She was seen again at the age of twelve years. She had always been a healthy child, developed normally in every respect, done well in school, and was a happy, sociable girl. Rumination was the only difficulty she had ever had. Her parents were stable, healthy, and intelligent people with good educational background; the father was a dependable railroad conductor, who was well thought of by his employers and associates. Jane was the fifth of seven children, one of whom died soon after birth (premature). The others were all well developed, stable and normally intelligent. Jane's I.Q. was 106.

A different picture obtains in the case of Alfred R., also twelve years old. At the same age when Jane began to ruminate, Alfred had his first breathholding spells. He had nocturnal and diurnal enuresis until ten years old. He had temper tantrums. For the last few months, frequent masturbation had been observed. He disobeyed and threatened his mother. He had a ravenous appetite. He progressed very poorly in school; he had failed three times in the fourth grade. He did not get along well with other children, always wanted to be the "big guy." He had an intelligence quotient of 76 (a retardation of three years). The father, an alcoholic garbage collector, was divorced by his wife because of abuse and non-support; he treated the children brutally. The mother was "nervous, shaking inside, can't eat or read or sew, awfully easy upset, can't sit in one place, constipated all the time"; she had lived with the father for several years and had three children before she decided to marry him. In 1924, she temporarily deserted the children. Soon after the divorce, she married a lunch-room keeper with a "terrible temper," who had just been divorced by his wife. Alfred's brother had enuresis at 16 years. His sister, 14, had enuresis and "shook." The maternal grandfather, the maternal grandmother's brother, and two maternal uncles were inmates of State Hospitals for the Insane. The maternal grandmother suffered from "smothering spells" all her life. One maternal aunt was peculiar and "acted queerly."

Jane has had no other difficulty besides her rumination, which has remained an incident in her life. Alfred has had a long string of disorders, from which he has never been entirely free; he comes of a family in which a large number of people have failed more or less completely in the task of life adjustment. In his case, we may be justified in feeling that, aside from (and in addition to) the environmental anomalies apt to arise in such surroundings, there is ingrained in the individual a certain degree of inadequacy to adapt himself to demands to which a constitutionally better endowed child would find less difficulty to adapt himself.

We shall expect such a constitutional inadequacy to be present under the following circumstances, which may serve as concrete and objective criteria:

1. An unusual accumulation of disorders of a somatic or psychobiological nature (or both), the latter spread over practically the entire span of life. The combination, for example, of congenital strabismus, undescended testicles, mental retardation, faulty enunciation, temper tantrums, and enuresis, or the concurrence of asthma, urticaria, irritability, restlessness, and stuttering will make one think of some constitutional weakness.

2. This impression will be strengthened by the finding of an unusual number of other cases of serious maladaptation in the child's ascendancy.

3. We shall be supported in our assumption by the observation (made frequently) that of several siblings one or two may show the string of disorders referred to above, whereas three or four others, grown up in the same environment and under the same type of management and having the same antecedents, develop normally. We then must be ready to assume that there must be something particular in the original endowment of that one child or those two children making them more apt to develop the difficulties which they have.

We may quote a few examples from our case material:

Gordon H., 12 years. External strabismus; partial ptosis of upper lids; marked visual defect; undescended testicles; bilateral hydrocele; peculiarly shaped ears; mental retardation (I.Q. 52); temper tantrums; feeding problem; psychogenic vomiting; truancy; stealing. Mother peculiar, Christian Scientist; maternal grandfather faith healer; brother unusually retiring, enuretic, extremely fearful, retarded in school. An older sister was well adjusted.

Benjamin M., 11 years. Enuresis; blinking; nailbiting; disobedience; hypochondriacal pain in left side of abdomen. Father psychopath, gambler, alcoholic, bootlegger, had served several jail sentences, did not support the family; mother unintelligent, illiterate, easily excited; sister, 13, "cranky," had "hollering spells," was asthmatic, complained of frequent urination; paternal uncle wet the bed until 18 years old; maternal cousin had enuresis "even while he was a soldier." Two younger sisters were normal.

Albert H., 5 years. Adenoid facies; hypertrichosis; mental retardation (I.Q. 70); defective speech; temper tantrums; feeding problem; stealing; fatigability. Father paranoid (imagined "the Catholics were against him, the foreigners plotted to keep him from holding his jobs"), morbidly jealous, deserted the family; mother had been in School for the Blind, feebleminded, had enuresis and temper tantrums in childhood, married her husband "to spite her parents," had "dizzy spells" and "the blues," complained of "gas on her stomach"; maternal grandfather died of alcoholism; maternal grandmother immoral, had two illegitimate children; maternal uncle was arrested for burglary; maternal aunt had congenital lues; two maternal aunts once disappeared from home for a whole week. A younger brother, 3, was well developed.

Charles R., 12 years. Lifelong enuresis; since age of six years, shaking spells, headaches, headshaking, temper tantrums; faulty enunciation; mental retardation (I.Q. 74). Father alcoholic, was arrested for non-support; mother was treated for "nerves"; sister had an illegitimate child after a "fake marriage"; brother had enuresis until 18 years of age; brother, 6, had night terrors. Two sisters well adjusted.

Allan M., 7 years. Constipation in early infancy; frequent colds; feeding problem; cruelty to other children; destructiveness; cried easily, emotional immaturity. Normally intelligent. Father had an "easily excited disposition"; mother easily excited; sister, 6, feeding problem, restless; paternal grandfather spent nine years in psychopathic hospital; paternal uncle and two aunts very unstable and hot-tempered; maternal uncle had record of forging checks, embezzlement, gambling, and drinking; two paternal great-uncles had depressions.

Margaret H., 11 years. Right internal strabismus; lefthanded; functional systolic murmur; mucous colitis; some mental retardation; odd behavior; reversed syllables when talking (cil-pen for pencil, etc.); negativistic; temper tantrums, screaming spells; feeding problem; nailbiting; nightmares; fear of the dark; headaches. Stubbornness a "family characteristic" on mother's side; father very peculiar, stuttered occasionally, "nervous," "likes to be the center of the stage," not truthful, came from a "nervous family"; maternal grandmother spent eight years in psychopathic hospital; maternal grandfather died of pernicious anemia; maternal uncle shot himself recently; paternal cousin an idiot; carcinoma rife in father's family; brother, 16, stuttered. A sister, 15, and a brother, 10, were well adjusted.

William H., 10 years. Congenital nystagmus; refractive error; rhythmic shaking of the head; frequent colds; chronic constipation; excitable, restless; afraid of the dark; mentally retarded (I.Q. 79). Father had convulsions in infancy; paternal grandmother had asthmatic attacks; brother, 4, had congenital nystagmus, shook his head, had several convulsions, restless, had temper tantrums and strong fear reactions, fecal incontinence. Another brother, 9, was well adjusted and healthy.

It has probably not escaped the reader's attention that, in our enumeration of objective criteria, we have failed to include the recent studies on the correlation between the *configuration of the body* and the personality make-up of an individual. These studies have been introduced into psychiatry and carried out most consistently by Kretschmer.[1] He distinguishes three types of physique: the thin, lanky, visceroptotic, oval-faced "asthenic" type with a narrow intercostal angle; the short, stocky, round-faced thick-necked "pyknic" type with a wide epigastric angle; and the strong-boned, long-limbed, muscular "athletic" type of body build. He finds that these constitutional "types" are closely associated with certain general "character" traits: the asthenic group with a cold, chilling, reserved, ingrowing, dreaming, sensitive, highly ambitious, "schizothymic" or "schizoid" (Bleuler) make-up; the pyknic with a warm, inviting, communicative, outgoing, practical, good-natured, easily elated or easily depressed, "cyclothymic" or "syntonic" (Bleuler) personality; the athletic standing somewhere between the two, perhaps closer to the asthenic than to the pyknic.

As far as the clinical work with children's psychiatric problems is concerned, we can, at least for the time being, derive no practical aid from any such classification even if it does seem to open up a fruitful field for academic curiosity. Regardless of the width of the intercostal angle or of any other measurements, there is such a variety and manifoldness of the pictures presented, that only a pluralistic examination of the constitutional, physical, intellectual, emotional and environmental factors will lead to a satisfactory diagnosis in the individual case, as a basis for an adequate therapeutic program. We must, for the same reason, especially guard ourselves against any sort of formulation calling for an exact statement, expressed in percentages, as to how much of a child's behavior disorder is constitutional and how much environmentally determined. It is not our desire to separate things which are so thoroughly fused and integrated that they cannot be separated, or to draw lines which cannot be drawn even approximately or artificially. The actual facts in each case and the concrete criteria outlined above will serve as sufficient guides. The value of including the constitutional factor (in the sense of our delineation of the concept) in the evaluation of the problem consists largely in helping us to know better just what kind of human material we are dealing with in the child and his family and to plan our therapeutic program accordingly.

[1] Kretschmer, E. Physique and Character. Translated by W. J. H. Sprott. New York. 1926

CHAPTER XI

THE ENVIRONMENTAL FACTORS

WE HAVE, so far, discussed the essentially endogenic factors to be considered in the study of a child's personality difficulty. We have tried to demonstrate the fact, forcing itself upon one's attention in every individual instance, that it is impractical, unwise, and really impossible to base child psychiatry on the arbitrary emphasis on any one of these factors exclusively. No matter how significant the sex problem, the intelligence quotient, a condition of ill health, or the constitutional element may turn out to be in the final evaluation of the underlying complaint, we must always take in the patient's entire personality make-up. In doing so, we have seen again and again that, just as we cannot afford to separate the somatogenic and intellectual and emotional and hereditary features, it is inconceivable to deal with them apart from the consideration, examination, and utilization of the environmental setting.

Non-psychiatric medicine, when dealing with exogenic sources of illness, is interested chiefly in their influences on the infrapsychobiological functioning; it therefore limits itself usually to climatic and atmospheric conditions and to bacterial, nutritional, chemical, and mechanical insults and their effects. It is, because of the very nature of its principal concerns, not mindful of the problems of interpersonal relations. Yet it is these relations which are active not less constantly and consistently and are certainly not less complex and variable and life-shaping than the weather and the food and the infectious germs. They are—and this is a point not always properly appreciated by the average physician—not less accessible to exact and objective study. It is true that they cannot be reached by any measurements comparable to barometric or caloric determinations nor by anything similar to X-ray or autopsy or the microscope. But they can be observed and registered just as accurately, and measured by performance, of which verbal expression is an essential part. The factors of intelligence and of emotion have a practical meaning only if viewed in the light of interpersonal relationship; they have no significance *per se*, not even for most purely theoretical academic purposes.

The term "environment" comprises not only the immediate surroundings of a child. We have recently had two examples which most vividly demonstrated the inroads which events of communal or national importance may make on the contents of a psychiatric office hour. One was the Lindbergh tragedy. Fear of kidnapping was instilled in some of the children by anxious parents, with the result that general timidity, nightmares, and panic-like reactions called definitely for energetic readjustment. On the other hand, there were mothers who for the first time, for fear of abduction, began to pay serious attention to the aimless wanderings of their retarded or epileptic children, who until then had remained untreated. The second instance was the much-discussed case of an adolescent psychopath with a long record of behavior problems and parental mismanagement, who, together with a feebleminded youth, committed a murder, was captured after a dramatic escapade, and sentenced to death. Numerous parents, incited by the newspaper headlines and minute accounts of his early difficulties, brought their offspring to the clinic, eager to have them examined and to be advised as to the proper method of handling them. Often the parental alarm proved to be unwarranted or greatly exaggerated; in other cases, the event had a beneficial effect, in that it thus made possible the planning of an organized attempt at straightening out at an early date personality disorders which, if neglected or misdirected, may indeed lead to serious maladaptations in later life.

THE HOME

It is only natural that the home looms first and foremost among the situational factors which contribute to the molding of the child's personality.

We have pointed out that the first fundamental period of childhood, that of elementary socialization, takes place entirely in the home and that the second period is essentially one of progressive domestication, ushering the child into the ultimate task of communal adjustment. The specific form which this gradual maturation assumes in the individual child will therefore depend not only on his own constitutional endowment but also to a large extent on the influences, examples, and standards of the "milieu" in which he spends the years of his greatest plasticity and impressionability. Realization of this fact will guard us against the total neglect of that which the individual brings with him, his inherent capacities and limitations of a physical, intellectual, or adaptive nature; it will cause us to accept Stern's "theory of convergence," stating that both predisposition and environmental factors must work together in order to establish a particular mode of reaction tendency.

If we speak of home influences, a vast complexity and manifoldness of factors forces itself upon our attention. For the sake of a clear organization of our material, we may, however, single out a number of features which were found empirically to be of especial significance for the formation of the child's personality. They are:

Interpersonal relations between the parents and among other members of the family.
Effect of broken homes.
Parent-child relations.
Relation to brothers and sisters and place in the family.
Economic conditions.
Moral and social standards.
Superstitions and other notions of the parents.
The problems of the step-child and the foster-child.

Interpersonal relations in the family. One of the great advances in nineteenth century civilization was the growing realization of the importance of proper feeding, ventilation, and light for the physical development of children. If one considers that bathing was an unusual event in the lives of the wealthy noblemen of Louis Quatorze, and that the tooth-pick was an exceedingly rare implement in their time, we have indeed progressed far. But it was reserved for our own age to put on a scientific basis the recognition, utilized long before by clever biographers, auto-biographers, and novelists, that the early home influences contribute a great deal towards the mental development of the individual. Harmonious family life is one of the best guarantees for the smooth adjustment of a normal child and for the optimal adjustment of one handicapped physically, emotionally, or intellectually. The study of the home conditions of patients presenting behavior disorders reveals in a vast majority of cases the existence of domestic frictions. It is most frequently due to an "incompati-bility" of the parents, resulting in quarrels and unhappiness which is re-flected in the entire home atmosphere. Paternal alcoholism and in-law interference figure prominently in our material as the exciting causes.

In not less than 26 per cent of our cases the father's excessive drinking has contributed to the disorganization of the family life. Where there was no separation or desertion, there has in most instances been a change in the child's attitude from the healthy respect of reasonable paternal authority to the dread or contempt of the drunkard's unreasonable authority, en-forced by brutality. Chronic alcoholism is often allied with morbid jealousy, which leads to distasteful scenes of wife-beating and vile accusations in the presence of the children.

There was the man who, in his drunkenness, terrorized his wife by dragging his sleeping son out of bed in the middle of the night and beating him cruelly, because he knew that this would hurt the mother more than if he would beat her; as a result, the boy developed a strong fear reaction, night terrors, and tics.

There was the man who kept a loaded gun under his bed, lying for hours in ambush for the "men" whom he suspected of having relations with his wife; their son, a boy of superior intelligence and in good physical health, became worried over the situation, "brooded" a great deal, cried most of the time, and his preoccupations finally interfered seriously with his progress in school; it was possible, in this case, to dissuade the father from imbibing; the gun was removed from the home; the mother became less fearful and excitable and asked the social worker just what the doctor had done to the man to effect such a change in him; the child, relieved of his terror and anxiety, now does much better in his studies. Unfortunately, it is not always possible to obtain such satisfactory results through working with alcoholics.

There was the orphan who lived with her grandparents; the grandfather, in his alcoholic fury, made life miserable for his wife and for the child, and the grandmother made up for it by overspoiling the girl who was brought to the clinic as a timid, whining, enuretic youngster of ten years, who shook like a leaf at the sight of any man.

There was the drunkard who dragged his child every day to the movies to spite his wife; the boy soon also learned to worry his mother and to defy her educational attempts by means of temper tantrums; the father, "annoyed" by the scenes, said that he could not blame his son for disliking her ways and took him with him to his speakeasy, often returning after midnight.

It is easily seen that any clinical work with behavior disorders of children that does not appreciate the etiological value of parental alcoholism with its excrescences and does not consider it in the therapeutic plan, fails to do justice to the problem and is, in most instances, not even of a palliative character.

Drastic examples of parental dissensions on the basis of in-law interference are furnished by the following cases.

Doris D., twelve years old, was referred to us because of her general restlessness, crying spells, shyness, despondency, nailbiting, lipbiting, pavor nocturnus, and sleepwalking. The child had a congenital malformation of the heart with complete auriculo-ventricular dissociation and was hard of hearing as a result of bilateral otitis media at eight years. (Auditory difficulties were rife in the family; the father had been treated for "bilateral nerve deafness"; the paternal grandfather was totally deaf; a brother had been hard of hearing since an automobile accident two years ago; another brother had chronic otitis media). The mother came of a wealthy family, which very strongly opposed her marriage to a street car conductor. After the father's progressive deafness had caused him to lose his job, they were destitute. The mother's parents offered to care for her and the five children on the condition that she divorce her husband. This she did not want to do. They moved to the paternal grandparents' poverty-stricken home, which had no bathtub and no electricity and was located in a poor, noisy neighborhood. The in-laws, unintelligent and temperamental people, not only made the mother feel her dependence most keenly, but also instilled into the father suspicions and caused incessant frictions and quarrels with, at times, manual accompaniments. The children were encouraged and often forced to take sides. The offers from the maternal family's quarters were repeated, producing in the mother indecision and increasing her irritability. It was in this setting that the girl's difficulties developed. The other children also suffered severely from the domestic situation, responding to it in a similar manner.

Mary B., ten years old, was brought with the complaint of being "nervous and scary"; she talked in her sleep, had night terrors, fainting spells, and temper tantrums; she bit her finger nails. The parents got along nicely until they moved near the paternal grandparents. Then things began to happen. The grandmother took a hand in the situation and poisoned the home atmosphere by means of unfounded accusations against the mother, which the father, a dull Italian laborer, took for supreme revelations. His jealousy aroused, he kept scolding and, after a time, beating his wife. The child became desperately afraid of him and displayed the reactions which formed the contents of the complaint.

Parental dissensions may arise from many other sources. They may be based on differences of religious attitudes and affiliations, creating a grave problem with regard to the children's religious education. They are often due to divergent ideas with regard to child training generally, each of the parents pulling in the opposite directions of extreme leniency and despotic strictness. Or definite psychopathic trends of one of the parents may seriously disturb the peace of the home. An overindulgent aunt or grandmother or the presence of an unsympathetic, impatient grandfather, on whom the family is financially dependent, have proved to interfere with the consistent rearing of children and, directly or indirectly, to precipitate behavior difficulties in them.

Sidney K.'s parents were hard working, stable, responsible people who, if interviewed separately, spoke intelligently about the proper ways of raising children, especially their only son, eight years old. But when their correct theories were to be translated into practice, they failed to work. If the father refused to give him a nickel, the mother gave it to him. If the father insisted upon having him go without food between meals, the mother stealthily loaded him with candy and cake, "because he asks for it so cute and promises that he will be a good boy." There was constant discussion between the parents, resulting in loud arguments in his presence. Sydney was brought to the clinic as a "feeding problem," which promptly disappeared when the parents had learned to agree with regard to his management.

Broken homes. Thirty per cent of the children referred to us because of personality difficulties came from broken homes. The sudden disruption or slow disintegration of the family unit may take different shapes and be due to a number of reasons, the most frequent of which are:

Death of one parent or of both parents.
Illness, necessitating protracted hospitalization.
Desertion.
Separation.
Legal divorce.
Nomadism.
Carelessness.
Extreme poverty.

In the cases of desertion, separation with or without legal procedure, and carelessness, a long period of domestic unpleasantness has usually preceded the breaking up of the home. The final disintegration was the outcome of many years of non-integration. Lack of support on the part of the father often complicated the picture.

Robert F. was thirteen years old. His father had at one time built up a very profitable business, owned a large home, had servants and chauffeurs and a considerable bank account. His wife, making up for the meagre years of her childhood and adolescence, developed an uncanny talent for spending much more money than was available. She made expensive trips to Europe, entertained luxuriously, especially at a time when growing competition made itself sorely perceptible. Her two children were raised almost entirely by the servants. Her husband's pleas and admonitions were met with crying spells and had the result that she spitefully turned away from him and roused his anger by frequent flirtations with other men. When finally, after much domestic unhappiness, the man lost his business and had to give up his residence and his automobiles and many other conveniences, she left him, taking her two children with her. The father secured a position in a tailoring establishment and earned enough to support a family of modest tastes. The relatives tried to effect a reconciliation, which could not be established because of stubbornness on both sides. It was, however, decided that the father should keep the boy and the mother should keep the girl. While Robert could see his mother and her relations whenever he wanted, his sister was not permitted to visit her father. The children's emotions had been played upon a great deal long before the separation, until they had become callous and lost their interest in the whole affair. The paternal grandmother, with whom the father and son had made their home, expected, after each visit to the boy's mother, to hear from him tales of her misbehavior, while the maternal relatives were eager to obtain information about anything that might incriminate the father. Since facts were not available and the boy soon found out that he could gain favors by inventing stories, he made a regular sport of using his imagination, and soon lies were carried back and forth. He also began to prevaricate about other matters and played truant in school, giving the most fantastic excuses, until he took to stealing and landed at the Juvenile Court.

Pauline M. was only eighteen months old, and yet she already showed the effects of a disruption of the home. Both parents were very temperamental young people of Hibernian stock. After a few months of "fussing and fighting," the mother went to live with her parents, who spoiled the child badly. Pauline learned to gain attention by refusing to eat and by means of breathholding spells. Everyone pitied her plight of being left without a father. Both parents, when interviewed separately, told tearfully how much they would like to get together again, but one waited for the other to come with apologies.

Louis S., now twelve years old, was brought up by his mother and aunt with the idea that his father had died of pneumonia. Several months ago, while he was supposed to be sleeping, he overheard a conversation between the two, during which his father's name was mentioned and they expressed curiosity as to what had become of him. Louis did not have the courage to ask them about what he had heard, but a few days later he began to tease his paternal grandparents until they told him that his parents had separated when he was three months old and that the father had disappeared and never been heard of. They made him promise that he would never let on at home that they had mentioned the fact to him because there was an agreement that he should remain ignorant of it. Louis became preoccupied, pictured his father in all kinds of situations and dangers, imagined scenes in which he suddenly met his father, saving him from perils or being rescued by him; the idea occurred to him that he might be the son of a millionaire who would turn up some day, or he was suspicious of the secrecy and felt that his father might be in prison for some crime. He had, in spite of slight intellectual retardation, done well in school before, but his daydreaming interfered seriously with his studies, and he developed a tic of his shoulders. After he had been given an opportunity to get acquainted with all the known facts and the secrecy had been definitely eliminated, the tic faded away and his school work improved.

These instances have been selected at random from our case material. It is, of course, rarely the fact of family disintegration alone that creates personality difficulties in children. It is usually only one of the contributing factors, but a factor which cannot be disregarded if we wish to do full justice to the individual problem.

Personality disorders occasionally arise from the interruption of the normal home life through death of the father, or of the mother, or of both, or from the fact that a parent has been sent away to a tuberculosis sanitarium or to a psychopathic hospital. In other cases, families are broken up through carelessness of the parents, who bring offspring into the world and then scatter them among their relatives. Especially at the present era of general economic distress, we have had the experience that well-meaning, but destitute mothers brought their children to welfare agencies, to the clinic, or to the Juvenile Court, with some invented complaint, in the hope that the children will be placed in an institution for feebleminded children or in reformatories, where they at least would get proper food and clothes. In one instance, the parents who had always been anxious that their children receive a good education kept them away from school, calculating that, because of their truancy, they would be committed to the so-called Parental School, to which truants are sometimes sent in this community.

We have had a small group of children whose difficulties were largely due to the frequent breaking up of their homes, with the preservation of the family structure. For all practical reasons, we may speak of the background as of nomadism. Not few of these children come from intelligent and well adjusted families. The many and often unexpected changes of residence, with the need of giving up again and again friendships and acquaintances and playmates, were determined by the father's occupation. This was especially true of several children of army officers who had been transferred in short intervals from one post to another and who had taken their families with them.

We have especially in mind the case of an intellectually superior girl who each time the family moved made remarkably good adjustments at first but gradually became very unhappy because she formed attachments which were suddenly disrupted; she kept writing to her former friends and even sent them gifts, but after an occasional first reply the children did not keep up their correspondence with her. She soon began to abstain from forming new associations with a feeling of "What is the use?" and to withdraw into herself. She was brought to us with the complaint of downheartedness, daydreaming, reading all the time, poor progress in school (or, better, in the schools which she successively attended), lack of attention and concentration, irritability, and masturbation. To make things more complicated, she was sent to live with different relatives for a few weeks any time when a new order to move arrived. The father, caused to realize the principal difficulty, made it possible to persuade his superiors to obtain for him a more permanent location. For the past fifteen months they have lived in one place. The child has again become happy and contented, does splendidly in her studies, has many friends, and has ceased to present any personality difficulties.

It is, of course, needless to assert that there are many children who come from broken homes without ever presenting particular behavior disorders. Much will depend on the child's own make-up and on the circumstances preceding, accompanying, and following the fragmentation of the family. It is also true that in some instances the breaking up of the home has a beneficial effect on the personality development of children. We have, as a matter of fact, to resort to it sometimes for therapeutic purposes, in order to free a child from harmful mismanagement, cruelty, neglect, or from the devastating influences of immorality in the home.

Parent-child relations. If, as we have seen, strained relations between members of the family may, directly or indirectly, so affect a child as to create personality disorders, it is obvious that the specific form of association between the parents and the child himself must be of particular significance in the formation of his character and habits. It is especially the management of his domestic socialization and the preparation for faultless communal adjustment that may seriously deviate from sound and sane standards. Most parents do their job well, with the use of common sense and the knowledge that a child must be given a chance to grow into healthy manhood and womanhood, to receive protection when and where it is needed, to be fed and clothed and educated properly, and to develop responsibilities of his own in due time. Behavior disorders usually arise from the following main types of parental aberration from this normal standard of child rearing:

Parental oversolicitude, overindulgence, and overprotection.
Parental indifference and neglect.
Parental hostility and rejection.
Excessive parental ambitions for the child.
Loading excessive responsibilities on the child.

The oversolicitous parent keeps the child from growing up. The result is prolonged immaturity and dependence, which may be carried over into adult life if not remedied at a sufficiently early date. The features of elementary socialization may become stationary for an additional year or two or three years, and communal adaptation may be delayed or even hindered beyond the age of puberty. The children are kept permanently "babified," the boys become "sissified." They are spoiled in every direction. They are given to eat whenever and whatever they please. No routine of feeding or sleeping is established. At ten or more years, they are taken into their parents' beds any time they ask for it. They obtain everything they want through the medium of whining, crying spells, screaming, or kicking. They are dressed and undressed many years after the average child has learned to perform these functions unaided. They are kept away from school when they express the slightest complaint, or when a cloud shows up in the sky. They are made to wear extra sweaters and galoshes and heavy underwear on days when other children are out playing happily and healthily in light clothes. When they do play outside, their mothers stand at the window watching everyone of their moves, ready to run out any time they feel that a playmate has treated them too roughly. The parents fight their children's battles, often with tots much smaller than the supposedly injured offspring. The parents blame the teachers or the educational system in general for their children's failure in school. The slightest cough, stomachache, headache, scratch, or bruise is seriously considered as the possible symptom of some grave disease. Admonitions are showered upon these children from the minute they open their eyes in the morning until they go to sleep at night.

As a result, these children never learn the value or even the meaning of regularity, self-care, responsibility, or independence. They have the experience that whining or temper tantrums make them rule the household and gain their ends; therefore, they make a habit of whining and of having tantrums. They remain infantile in their behavior; they talk baby talk; or they wet or even soil themselves; they do not know how to play with other children or how to act in the presence of adults. They may become cowards, not having learned how to protect themselves; or they may grow up to be deceitful and sneaky, hitting their playmates and running instantly to hide behind the mother's skirt. They present feeding problems. They may develop hypochondriacal tendencies, knowing that a complaint of headache or stomachache will add to the attention they receive and help them to get more hugs and more nickels and more toys.

No treatment of feeding difficulties or temper outbursts or enuresis will have the desired success, if the underlying parental overprotection with all its implications is not remedied. It is the ideal of medical therapy to remove the etiological factors rather than to alleviate single symptoms; in psychiatric problems, symptomatic treatment will mostly be wasted effort, if the total personality and the total situation are disregarded.

Martin R. was examined on his eighth birthday. He was rushed to the hospital by an agitated mother because "he is thin, he is going down so." He was found to be in perfect health and of high average intelligence. He had an older sister of eleven years, who had the good fortune that her mother was ill after her birth and she was raised adequately by her grandparents and by a colored mammy. She was a resolute girl, who had energetically withstood later maternal spoiling and was therefore *persona non grata* with the mother, who concentrated all her efforts on Martin. According to Mrs. R.'s story, he had at five months a "mysterious disease," the chief symptom of which consisted of sucking two fingers and for which "specialists" were consulted; against their advice, all kinds of mechanical restraint were applied. At two years, he "nearly died" of uncomplicated pertussis. Mild chicken-pox at seven years "drove her frantic." She had constantly "changed diets, doctors, and teachers on him." She did not let him play with other children "because they were too rough"; even his play with his sister was supervised "because she is so strong and he is such a delicate child." To make him fatter, she gave him two glasses of milk and a pint of cream with each meal, the single dishes being buttered and greased *ad nauseam*. She dragged him to physicians, osteopaths, and chiropractors. She brought him to the clinic, determined to get a "diagnosis," because she was convinced that Johns Hopkins would discover the serious disease from which he suffered (Hopkins did; it was the maternal attitude), and if she would receive no diagnosis, she was going to take him to the Mayos at Rochester and, if necessary, to other clinics (all except those in New England, because "she did not trust the Yankees," being a Virginian). Only through work with the intelligent and sensible father was it possible to save this child from further mismanagement.

Bernard H., seven years old, with a mental age of nine years and in good health, had an excellent stock of information and a splendid vocabulary. An emotionally unstable father, who had an "artistic temperament," and an overindulgent mother had done everything in their power to deprive him of childhood's pleasures. He was an only child for four years; his birth was followed by three miscarriages, making the parents feel that he would remain the only heir. He was to become a perfect human specimen and a "genius." He was permitted not a second of privacy; at night, he slept with an aunt, who was to report each morning how he rested; since he was to take a nap for two hours each day, he did not always promptly fall asleep in the evening. This was interpreted as "insomnia," and doctors were consulted. His stools were counted, and if the number did not come up to the mother's expectations, she resorted to cathartics. At six years he was sent to a "private school" in which he was the only pupil; the "teacher" was to submit to everyone of the mother's peculiar educational whims; he was kept out of "school" for two to three weeks at a time whenever the parents decided that he needed a rest. He was not allowed to associate with other children because the families in the neighborhood were "socially inferior" and some of their boys, much to Mrs. H.'s horror, "disgraced themselves by wearing overalls." This seemed below the dignity of a future genius. The child had no recreational outlets. He was irritable, responded with understandable nausea to the large volume of food which he was forced to consume, and healthily rebelled against the parental mismanagement. In a more sensible environment, he would undoubtedly have offered no personality problem whatsoever. The parents, disappointed that he did not turn out to be the perfect boy of their vague conception, told themselves and the child that he "bordered on hysteria" and nagged him unmercifully, aside from causing him to take patent medicines, tonics, and sedatives.

It is interesting to observe that most overindulgent parents, anxious to warn and protect their children against imaginary perils, are at the same time nagging, scolding, perpetually admonishing parents. Thus an inconsistency in the handling is created, which cannot fail to have its damaging effect on the children.

Parental carelessness and neglect often results in inadequate habit training or total lack of habit training.

This was especially apparent in a three-and-a-half-year-old, somewhat retarded girl, whose mother categorically declared her unwillingness (which she sometimes, perhaps not incorrectly, called inability) to bother with the details of child rearing. Helen was an unwanted child in the first place. When first seen, she was still bottle fed and had no control of her excretions. In a boarding school, within less than two months, she could be taught to feed herself with fork and spoon, acquired good bowel control, and ceased wetting herself during the day; her nocturnal enuresis became less frequent; the bottle was dispensed with entirely; her temper tantrums disappeared.

Hostility of a parent against all children or, more often, against one particular child, is fortunately not very frequent. Where it exists, it is apt to create serious personality difficulties in the victim. It is usually the unwanted child that is rejected by the father, or by the mother, or by both. Sometimes matrimonial disappointment is the underlying factor. Hatred of the marital partner may be transmitted to the child or the children bearing resemblance to him, or to her, as the case may be.[1]

Carl R., eleven years old, was the oldest of three children. Dorothy, 9, was backward in school. Gloria, 7, had skipped a grade, was very intelligent, but wet the bed every night. Neither of the two sisters was con-

[1] Newell, H. W.: The Psychodynamics of Maternal Rejection. American Journal of Orthopsychiatry. 1934, 4, 387-401.

sidered a problem at home. Carl, however, was brought to the Clinic by the mother, who felt that he should be committed to a boys' reformatory because of "meanness and badness." She was at a loss and very vague when asked to give specific examples. She reported that the school had complained about his behavior; "he has to be sent down to the principal, he just carries on, is very annoying to the teacher, and very sassy." Compare this with the school report which was received a few days later: "The principal knows Carl and has not found him a school problem at all. She heard the conversation that the mother had with the teacher, in which the mother asked the teacher if Carl was a problem. The teacher told her he was not. She is sure the mother has not succeeded in giving the child a bad reputation. He does well in his work, and his conduct is excellent." The mother told a story that neighbors accused her boy of masturbatory and homosexual practices on a vacant lot; this story could not be substantiated. The boy had an I.Q. of 103; he had an old mediastinal tuberculosis. During the interview and following contacts, he was found to be coöperative and truthful, intellectually, emotionally, and morally superior to his mother, who had managed to convince him that he was ripe for a correctional institution and that there was something wrong with his head. He seemed hungry for a word of encouragement. It was the mother who needed correction and who had a great deal wrong with her.

In another instance, a somewhat retarded boy, when asked about his difficulties, stated that he had sawdust in his brain and that all he needed was to be hit with a hammer over his head good and hard. His mother had told him that. When an attempt was made to correct her notion, she became enraged at her son for misquoting her; she had said "mallet" and not "hammer!"

Eugene D., nine years old, was brought with an almost unending list of complaints by his mother who stated that she had been "nervous since I have been married and have had children." She was disappointed in her marriage. Her husband, a bacteriologist, was rather pedantic and irritable and very strict in money matters. She could never forget that Eugene's arrival deprived her of the pleasures of playing golf and of swimming in which she had indulged before. She could not find anything good in the child. When she took him to the clinic, she told him that he would probably be retained and that it would take at least a whole month to get him straightened out. She played with the possibility of sending him to a reformatory. She persuaded him that he had St. Vitus' dance and diabetes. She insisted that he was an "unusual type, a freak, and a dual personality," and that living with him was harming her own health and giving her a "nervous indigestion." Eugene was a well built, attractive, normally intelligent boy. His main difficulty was a severe degree of reading and writing disability, which called for specific training and sympathetic understanding on the part of those about him.

Some parents are extremely ambitious for their children, pushing them beyond their capacity, stuffing them with music lessons and religious education, when even the school work is too much for their grasp. The result is that conscientious children, trying to live up to the expectations, are under a constant strain and have no time nor opportunity left for healthy relaxation and recreation. Others rebel against the enforced heavy program mapped out for them and resort to hypochondriasis or to spiteful reactions, in order to get away from tasks which they simply cannot perform. In others, again, the parents' disappointment that they did not carry out the order to become geniuses may create more or less serious behavior problems.

Quite frequently parental ambitions and pride express themselves in the form of showing their offspring off to visitors and neighbors. At any given occasion, the child is requested to sing songs, to show the school report, to recite poems, to solve conundrums, etc., etc. As a reward for his performances, he receives praise and hugs and nickels and candy. His "cuteness" and "cleverness" is discussed in his presence. In this manner he is taught to consider himself, and to expect to be considered by everyone else, the center of attention. If there is no logical chance for displaying himself, he soon begins to make himself seen and heard by other means, such as grimacing, noisy behavior, or teasing the parents or siblings.

Just as overprotection, with delayed development of responsibilities, often leads to personality problems, so do difficulties sometimes arise from burdening a child with too many duties at a time when he is not ripe for them.

Sleepwalking and night terrors and anxiety attacks developed in a pale, undernourished, eight-year-old girl of low average intelligence, when she was given practically full charge of the household duties (in addition to her school work). The mother had undergone a gynecological operation and was too weak to do anything. The father had been twice in a psychopathic hospital with suicidal depressions. He had "spells" similar to the child's anxiety attacks and evidently supplied her with this form of reaction pattern. The frail little girl was suddenly confronted with the care, including laundry and scrubbing of floors, of the entire family, consisting of the parents, herself, a brother, two sisters, a sister-in-law, who did not help her at all but "just sat around," and a nephew. After being sent to a convalescent home, she did not walk in her sleep and did not have a single attack.

A healthy boy of eleven years, with an I.Q. of 96, with a history of eczema, had always been well adjusted. He was brought to the clinic with the complaint of fear reactions. About three to four times a week, the parents went out at night to movies or on visits and did not return until quite late. He was left alone with a two-year old sister. He did not mind that for some time. Once he went out for a few minutes and locked himself out. This frightened him considerably. Since then he had been afraid to remain alone at home.

The unnatural and pathological proportions which parental mismanagement may sometimes assume are best demonstrated by the following instance:

Virginia L. was a six-and-a-half-year-old girl in good health and of superior intelligence. Her father, a bigoted, boisterous psychopath, 62 years old, saw in her a future occupant of the State Penitentiary and tried to "reform" her with a razor strap, by keeping her imprisoned at home, and by reading passages from the Bible to her. He "diagnosed" her case as an "hysterical Christly frame of mind." He once noticed that she "moved" under her covers and decided that she must be masturbating; he thought that painting her clitoris with iodine would be the most appropriate remedy. Once she picked up a peanut from the street; aside from lecturing to her about this being an early manifestation of a criminal tendency, he forced her to eat a pound of peanuts, which he bought; it made her very sick, and while she suffered he pointed out to her the high educational value of his procedure. They lived on a farm and for the first six years of her life she had absolutely no contact with other children. After moving to a small town she was never permitted to leave the house and backyard lest she might be contaminated by talking to colored children who lived two blocks away. Her mother, 28 years old, afraid of her husband, was ordered to accompany her on her way to and from school. Virginia was to wash and wipe the dishes three times a day. Once she said she would not wash more than ten dishes at a time; this her father took for unheard of disobedience and punished her severely. To mark the distinction between weekdays and the Sabbath, she was to sit still all during Sunday. She was an only child. She slept in the parents' bedroom, so that the father might "catch her" when she masturbated. When she fell asleep while he, read the Bible to her late in the evening, he took that for a sign of an irreligious attitude. She once remarked that she would like to have curly hair; he scolded her for not being satisfied with what she had. He described himself as an "expert of man's body" and had always doctored her himself. When he stated that she was decidedly a potential criminal, the mother remarked, "Either that or a genius." It was, indeed, a sign of the child's unusual stability that, in this peculiar setting, she developed no other difficulties than "occasional" lack of appetite and temper tantrums (always in the father's absence). She was sent to a boarding school, where she behaved normally in every respect.

Relations to siblings. Sometimes the specific type of association with the brothers and sisters may contribute its share to the development of personality problems. The only boy among several girls or the only girl among several boys is apt to be spoiled by the others or, on the other hand, may feel, and actually be, isolated. Resentment and friction has, in a number of our patients, been created by the parents' attitude of preferring one child to another or of contrasting them openly. Occasionally, both the child praised and the one blamed may be harmed; in the former, conceit and an unjustified feeling of superiority may be the result; the latter may react with lack of self-confidence and of self-assertion, or with spite, or with jealousy of the rival. Not a few instances of hatred between siblings in later life date back to unequal treatment during the period of childhood.

The child, who is given charge of a younger sibling and who is expected to devote much of his time to the new arrival, may in one case form a strong attachment, but in another feel that he is done an injustice by curtailing his time of recreation and play. The baby may be considered a burden and an annoyance.

The youngster who for several years has been an only child may strongly resent the new addition to the family, if he is given less affection and less attention than he has previously received. In some cases the onset of behavior disorders coincides exactly with the birth of a younger brother or sister.

The child's place in the family, in order of birth, may at times be of significance in the evaluation of the psychiatric problem for which examination and treatment is requested. Much has been written about the *only child*. It is, of course, not at all true that, as has been claimed, being an only child is a disease in itself. Many only children develop normally if they are well endowed and wisely managed. The literature contains conflicting statements as to the frequency of behavior disorders due to a child's "onliness." It is true that an only child is apt to be more exposed to parental oversolicitude and overindulgence than others. This is especially the case if he derives his solitary position from the loss through miscarriage or death of one or more siblings, making the parents feel that they should all the more protect their surviving offspring. It must also be remembered that, in some instances, a child remains "only" because of the death of one of the parents, precluding the birth of other children.[1] It was in our material hardly ever the fact of the "onliness" alone that gave rise to the existing difficulties. It is also not irrelevant to know that sometimes the real trouble may begin at the time when a child's position in the family ceases to be solitary; jealousy and bids for attention may manifest themselves for the first time upon the coming of a second child.

We sometimes deal with "artificial" only children that is, those coming from a larger family, whose care has been taken over by fond grandparents.

A certain amount of "scrapping" among brothers and sisters is a common occurrence. There are, however, children who, because of their dullness, or sensitiveness, or because of some specific peculiarities, are selected by the rest for continuous "teasing," with sometimes very unpleasant accompaniments and results.

There was the enuretic boy whose sisters "shamed" him every morning and dominated him with the threat of telling his playmates about his wetting; the boy became irritable and vindictive and retaliated by throwing objects at them and coming to his mother with complaints about them, which were mostly products of his imagination.

There was the somewhat retarded boy whose brother called him "goofy" and managed to make the surname popular in the neighborhood; the brother himself was, by the way, equally retarded and not less of a behavior problem.

There was the fourteen-year-old boy who came with the complaint of staying out late; he was desperately afraid of his brother, aged 24 years, who, assuming the disciplinary functions of the dead father, beat him cruelly; the boy had, unsuccessfully, tried to sneak into the house at a time when he expected his brother to be in bed.

There was Harold B., 15 years old, who had a history of tuberculosis and acute anterior poliomyelitis with impairment of the use of the right arm, with an I.Q. of 75, and mild stuttering; his older brother and younger sister had bestowed upon him the title of "dumbbell," would not permit him to whistle or sing while they themselves indulged in these pleasures, and bossed and angered him to such an extent that he threw stones at them and once landed a knife in his sister's leg; he was placed in a boarding home, where he showed no sign of irritability and where his speech difficulty improved considerably.

[1] Of the abundant literature on the only child, we quote a few publications which are especially instructive: Hooker, Mary Ferris. A Study of the Only Child in School. Journal of Genetic Psychology. 1931, 39, 122. Machacek, J., and F. Fremel. Studien über einzige Kinder. Zeitschrift für Kinderforschung. 1926, 32, 340.

Goodenough and Leahy, in conclusion of an interesting study, state that "there is probably no position in the family circle which does not involve, as a consequence of its own peculiar nature, certain special problems of adjustment."[1]

Economic situation. Problem children come from all social and economic strata. Parental overindulgence, ingrained mental retardation, epileptic or postencephalitic personality changes, paternal alcoholism, family dissensions, or emotional disturbances are apt to occur among the rich as well as the poor. Yet there are difficulties which are more or less closely associated with the family's financial status. They may be due to a general home atmosphere of worry over existing or threatening poverty and, especially in an era of growing unemployment, over the fact or the dread that the father might lose his position or be "laid off." Impoverishment may call for new adjustments which create personality problems in the child (less comfort, change of residence, loss of friends, cheaper clothes, etc.). On the other hand, climbing upon the economic ladder may lead to problems of its own (change from public to private school, cold reception, if not exclusion, of the "newly rich" by those whose acquaintance is sought, snobbishness, the parents' exaggerated ambitions to "refine" themselves and their children). The type of neighborhood and playmates will be dictated by the family's income. Inadequate means will result in crowded quarters with insanitary living conditions, unhealthy sleeping arrangements, and lack of privacy. Extreme, but by no means rare, examples are the children who are kept away from school on winter days because there is no money to repair their shoes, or the development of enuresis in unheated homes with the toilet in the back yard.

This is the place to mention one of the features of poverty-stricken homes, which deserves a great deal of consideration in connection with children's behavior problems and character formation. Due to crowded quarters, various members of the family share at night not only a room, but also the same bed. It is astonishing that not less than 22 per cent of our patients of over four years of age come from homes with unsatisfactory sleeping arrangements, in the sense that they occupy the same room or the same bed with a parent or sibling of the opposite sex. It should, however, be emphasized that this is often due to reasons other than financial inadequacy. As a matter of fact, we have observed that older boys of well situated families, who sleep with their mothers or aunts or sisters, often presented more serious personality difficulties than those whose improper sleeping situation has been enforced by the inability to pay rent for another room or to purchase another cot.

The most outstanding results of such arrangements and of the causes and attitudes connected with them are general immaturity, protracted dependence, childishness, and spoiled child reactions. Masturbation is often a problem in these children because of the constant sexual stimulation which, in three of our cases, has given rise to incestuous practices.

We have seen a group of boys between six and fourteen years of age

[1] Goodenough, F. L., and A. M. Leahy. The Effect of Certain Family Relationships Upon the Development of Personality. Journal of Genetic Psychology. 1927, 34, 45-71.

who had been made to sleep with their mothers after the father's death or desertion.

One woman even boasted of the fact that, after her husband's departure, she had taken her two younger boys, aged eleven and seven years, into her bed and that they were unusually attached to her. Neither she nor John, the eleven-year old, wanted to hear anything about being separated at night. John, healthy, normally intelligent, had remained infantile in his reactions and especially immature in judgment and in sizing up situations.

Kenneth, ten years old, was the youngest of three brothers; the other two were twenty-four and twenty-two years old. Because of the discrepancy in age, he had always remained the baby. "Baby" and "honey" were the only names he heard at home. His father died eight years ago of pneumonia, and since then he had always slept with his mother. He presented a feeding problem, blinked his eyes, cried easily, and had an aërophagic tic ("makes such funny noises with his throat"), for which he had been given tonics for years and prescribed "rest cures" in bed for weeks at a time. His I.Q. was exactly 100, but his behavior was that of a child of less than five years. His schoolmates called him "Mary" because of his effeminate appearance and conduct.

One mother brought in great alarm her eight-year-old boy with the complaint of "smothering spells," which he got only when she "pressed him too hard" while hugging him in bed at night; the boy masturbated frequently, while the mother looked on and "hollered at him."

Roland's father was killed in an automobile accident one year ago; his mother took him (he was eleven years old) and his five year old brother into her bed; she was hypochondriacal, constipated, felt a "knot" in the epigastric region, "could never lie on her back," vomited often, and had backache "in the end of her spine and in her neck." The two boys developed similar complaints; they were all on "diets." In bed, they "massaged" each other, and all three, including the mother, derived sexual pleasure from the manipulations. Roland was a masturbator.

Moral and social standards. It is at home that children receive their first instructions of what is right and what is wrong. Not knowing of any other standards, the parental attitudes and activities are the pattern *par excellence* until they grow old enough to compare it with others. But by that time the impressionable child has already taken over a good deal of that which had served as the only observed model of social behavior.

We have discussed the possible effects of parental alcoholism on the development of a child's personality. A home atmosphere of chronic dependency and begging is hardly beneficial for the establishment of civic interests and responsibilities. Open conflicts with the law and sexual immorality of the parents or older siblings will not fail to leave their marks on the child, either in the form of imitation, or in that of shame, worry, resentment, and (justified) disrespect of parental authority. Illegitimacy is not in itself a problem; but it may become a serious difficulty because of the attitude society often takes towards the illegitimate child, aside from the fact that these children are more apt to come of poor stock than those born of married couples.

We cite a few case histories which demonstrate the influence upon children of undesirable moral and civic standards in the family:

Josephine B., a girl of 6½ years, was an illegitimate child. Nothing was known of the father except that he was a chronic alcoholic with a "violent temper." The mother was alcoholic, immoral, untrustworthy, and uncoöperative. Her husband, whom she married at the age of 14 years, an illiterate fruit vendor, deserted her several times. The oldest son, 24, was in jail for stealing an automobile and for larceny of jewelry "for his wife"; he was syphilitic. A daughter, 20, was a prostitute. Another son, 14, was feebleminded and a truant. He and two younger twin brothers had a Juvenile Court record of burglary. Of the twins, one had internal strabismus, and the other compound hyperopic astigmatism. The family was chronically dependent and known to the Family Welfare Association, the Prisoners' Aid Association, the Bureau of Catholic Charities, the Juvenile Court, the Criminal Court, and the School Attendance Department. There had been innumerable evictions. Josephine was found to be utterly neglected, dirty, without the slightest trace of habit training. She had an I.Q. of 91. She was sent to a boarding school where, under wise management, she is doing splendidly.

Rita T., 12 years old, was sent for consultation because of the mother's complaint that she was slow and nervous and that she stuttered. She had a mild myopia, slight hyperthyroidism, was lefthanded, and had an I.Q. of 73. There was both a history and actual evidence of masturbation (large and red labia majora; chafing between legs). Her sister, Ruth, 9 years old, was normally intelligent, had mediastinal tuberculosis, was very irritable and afraid of the dark. The father, a heavy drinker, had deserted the family three years ago. The mother was feebleminded, hypochondriacal, and immoral. She deserted the children nine times in four years. She had been taking Ruth with her as "decoy" when she went to room with strange men. At one time, police found her, a drunken stranger, and Ruth in bed together in a disorderly house. There were two other children in the family: Carl, 16, feebleminded, had internal strabismus. Dorothy, 14, had been a chronic truant and sex delinquent since the age of eight years. Carl and Dorothy had had incestuous relations for a long time. Carl beat the children brutally.

Doris L., at 12 years, had a record of smoking, drinking, sex promiscuity, forging a check for $25.00 and staying out at night; she had gonorrhea. She was intellectually retarded. Her brother, Andrew, eight years old, I.Q. of 79, had enuresis and fecal incontinence. The father was a chronic alcoholic. The mother had seven illegitimate children from four different men. One was killed while driving an automobile after being discharged from the Training School for the Feebleminded. Another, 21, was schizophrenic and an inmate of a New York State Hospital. The mother had had numerous miscarriages. In 1930, she served thirty days in jail for running a disorderly house. The paternal grandfather died of an alcoholic psychosis in a psychopathic ward. There was justified suspicion that it was the mother who initiated Doris in her alcoholism and sex practices.

Peculiar medical notions in the family. In taking a psychiatric case history, it is of interest to know not only what the actual difficulties are but also what they mean to the child and to the family. The patient whose enuresis is explained on the basis of a "weak bladder" or "kidney trouble" will react differently to attempts at establishing normal urinary habits than the youngster who is made to feel that the wetting is a personality problem which can be remedied rather than dependent on the moods of a bladder which plays tricks on him. And yet, the weak bladder and kidney still figure strongly in the "etiology" given out to parents by physicians, who do not seem to realize that they are imparting notions which, aside from being incorrect, may become outright harmful.

One of the most frequent fallacies that we were called on to correct was the dread of "heredity." It is, in many instances, not hereditary influence itself, but the apprehensive expectations based on the existence of something or other in the family that may give rise to serious behavior disorders.

The aunt of a six-year-old girl was epileptic. Since the child was born the whole family watched for signs of epilepsy in her, especially since the aunt had a few convulsions in the presence of the pregnant mother, making everyone fear that the baby might have been "marked." Betty was never left alone for a second, so that the anticipated convulsions should not be overlooked. Someone remarked, when Betty was about two years old, that she had a "funny look under her eyes, just like the aunt." This was sufficient to increase the vigilance and the dread. Any time she failed to answer a question immediately, this was interpreted as an epileptic "absence." She was dragged from one doctor to another, and at one time luminal was prescribed. Habit training was completely neglected. She always slept with the parents. The child remained enuretic, could not dress nor undress herself, had temper tantrums, crying spells, and feeding difficulties with frequent gagging and vomiting. She was not epileptic and had low average intelligence.

Irene L., twelve years old, offered an extreme example of parental fear of hereditary recurrence of "insanity." Her father was an irritable man, had neuritis in his shoulder, complained of sleeplessness; he was a timid man who had little to say at home or anywhere else; it was his greatest desire to be let alone and to escape the nagging of his wife. Her mother, the main provider, ran a grocery store and managed to pay the rent and to feed and clothe the family adequately; she was easily excited and, having a keen sense of responsibility, worried over every little thing that happened or might happen, and suffered from insomnia. There was a grandmother in the picture, who was shaking her head for thirty years prior to her recent death. Irene had gone to see her every Sunday. A few months ago, a cousin, Dave, in a depression with obsessive trends, escaped from a State Hospital and committed suicide. Since then the memory of Cousin Dave haunted the mother who began to watch her two younger children, Irene and Morton, very closely for manifestations similar to those Dave had shown at the very beginning of his mental derangement. Irene, made apprehensive and feeling that she was doomed to become insane (the term "heredity" had become a household word in her surroundings), began to shake her head like her grandmother, to complain about her shoulders like her father, to suffer from sleeplessness like both parents, and having heard of hallucinations occurring occasionally in Dave, every noise and every flash of light scared her terribly. Her brother, Morton, eleven years old, reacted to the same situation with grimaces, night terrors, and rapidly increasing irritability. Before the death of Cousin Dave, both children, who were physically healthy and normally intelligent, had presented no personality problems. Marked improvement set in promptly after the dissipation of the mother's dread of "heredity."

The request for an operation is often expressed in connection with all kinds of psychiatric problems. Some parents come fully determined to have the child's tongue clipped because of his stuttering or other speech disorders, or to have a circumcision performed to cure enuresis, or to remove feeble-mindedness by means of brain surgery. The latter demand is quite frequent and enhanced by overenthusiastic newspaper reports of the miraculous deeds of brain surgeons. One mother insisted on an operation for un-descended testicles to cure the poor eyesight of her imbecile son.

The laymen (and some physicians, for that matter) have a peculiar idea about "nervousness." They take it to be the expression of "weakness or irritability of the nerves" which, therefore, must be "strengthened" by tonics or "calmed" by sedatives. If the one does not work, it is often supplanted by the other, or else the tonics are "changed on the child." The pharmaceutical firms supply a sufficient variety to suit every taste and every pocketbook. We have seen children, who were raised for many years on prescribed (!) medicines of all sorts for such problems as bedwetting, feeding difficulties (which are called "anorexia"), or restlessness. Hypo-chondriacal trends are thus made almost inevitable.

"Worms" are a popular etiology for all forms of behavior problems, and their presence should indeed be excluded in the routine physical examina-tion. Many are the youngsters who are tortured with daily cathartics or even enemas, without it ever occurring to the parents to find out for a day or two if they are really needed. A twelve-year-old girl was slightly con-stipated at the age of two years; since then she had been given castoria and enemas for eight years, only to "switch over" to senna leaves.

Many are the children who are branded with "diagnoses," which range from "mean" or "lazy" to "hysterical" or "crazy." They are made to believe that they are just that, and their self-confidence is severely shaken. One mother persuaded her child that he was a "freak" and a "dual person-ality," and another that he had "sawdust in his head."

What prophecies can do to a child is best seen in the case of the mas-turbating girl who, in elaboration of parental predictions, came to fear that she would have to be operated on soon, that she would have to have her face lifted, and that her children would be feebleminded. A boy became desperately afraid when his father, himself a hypochondriacal person, explained that his failure to button his coat upon leaving the movie theater would result in pneumonia, and then proceeded to describe pneumonia in the direst terms.

The problems of the stepchild and the foster child. There are instances where the arrival in the house of a step-parent or placement of a child in a foster home is the best thing that can happen to a child and indeed may act as the most appropriate remedy of an existing personality difficulty. It may do away with the ill results of a broken home and restore successfully the disrupted family unit. In other cases the new arrangement may create more or less grave problems. It will depend to a great extent on the personalities of the adults and their attitude towards the child. Rejection of the stranger, who may be looked upon as an unwelcome in-truder, jealousy, unwillingness to accept him or her as an authority may aggravate the situation. A stepmother or foster mother may be as overindulgent, or as negligent, or as hostile as an own mother, creating similar difficulties. According to Charlotte Bühler, the characteristic social attitude of the foster child is his uncertainty, which appears to result from the uncertain life conditions.[1] Kühn found that, in his material, eighteen per cent of neglected girls and ten per cent of neglected boys were stepchildren and their specific traits were a tendency to brood, distrust, self-assertion, and sensitiveness.[2]

Alice G., eight years old, had internal strabismus, was lefthanded and intellectually retarded. Her mother died soon after her birth. She was tossed about among unsympathetic relatives, until her father remarried when she was three years old. The stepmother, a conscientious woman, treated her as well as a good-natured and thoughtful mother would treat her own child. About a year ago the stepmother became pregnant. She was told by superstitious neighbors that the appearance and actions of an older child may influence the looks and behavior of other children in the home. In order to provide an optimal setting for the newborn, she spoke of having Alice's eyes operated on, started to "break" her from the use of the left hand, and tutored her with the intention of "brightening her up." Alice, fearing the operation, under the strain of the change of handedness and expected to acquire knowledge which she could not grasp, became irritable, extremely unhappy, had crying spells, and for the first time in her life resented her stepmother as a stepmother, telling her that her own mother would have been much better to her.

THE NEIGHBORHOOD

Neighborhood contact is usually the child's first lesson on extra-domestic social structure. It supplies him for the first time with means of comparing his own status with that of other children. It provides the earliest opportunities for comradeship, formation of play groups with, however loose and primitive, common interests, and for intercourse with adults other than the members of his own household. It remains, for a time, the child's entire universe, with a vague notion of something beyond, a notion which expands and becomes gradually clearer, as the vicinity begins to include more and more blocks and the church and a few stores and walks and automobile or street car excursions. To the rural child the world for the first few years looks altogether different than to the urban child; it looks, at least in preschool age, different to the child raised in a quiet suburban section than to the one reared in a noisy business district or brought up in the slums. The parents' relation to the neighbors will have its influences on the type of association among their offspring. It will make a difference whether the family lives in a congenial environment or whether the parents and the child are rejected or ignored because of economic or religious or racial inequality. Frequent changes of location with the need of ever new adjustments may leave their marks on the personality development of some children. Absence of coëval playmates may create in a child a pathetic feeling of solitude.

[1] Bühler, Charlotte. The Social Behavior of the Child. Handbook of Child Psychology. Edited by Carl Murchison. Worcester. 1931, p. 420.

[2] Kühn, H. Psychologische Untersuchungen über das Stiefmutterproblem. Beihefte zur Zeitschrift für angewandte Psychologie. 1929, No. 45.

Jean was a highly intelligent girl of not quite six years who was an only child; her parents lived in a small colony amidst retired business people. The youngest other child in the community was fourteen years old. Jean stood for hours at the window, hoping against hope that some child might pass by the house. If this ever happened, she became excited and beckoned to the child to come near. If her attempts were unsuccessful, she flew into a rage and then wept for hours. She kept begging her parents to move into another section. She criticized them for "keeping her a prisoner all her life." When, on rare occasions, she did have an opportunity to be with other children, she did not know what to do with them, having lived among adults only, and was even more unhappy with them than without them.

Melrose was a healthy and intelligent six-year-old girl who had always presented a feeding problem. Her parents had a little confectionery store with adjoining living quarters. They were eager to carry out instructions given them at the clinic, but were constantly interfered with by old customers, who were in the habit of walking into the dining room and kitchen and of taking a hand in the management of Melrose's feeding. The parents, for fear of losing some of their best customers, were helpless and finally decided to send the child away for a time.

In view of such occurrences, it is necessary, in the psychiatric examination of individual cases, to inquire carefully into the type and possible influences of the neighborhood. It is there that healthy associations are formed and outdoor recreations take place, but it is also there that unsound reactions may be established and, especially in the slums, foundations for antisocial trends and gangdom activities may be laid.

THE SCHOOL

In our civilization, every child, unless too severely handicapped physically or intellectually, spends at least eight years in school. They stand out as major experiences in a person's life history, not only because of the knowledge received there but also because several hours are spent there each day together with a group of coëvals and with one or several teachers with whom at least temporary relations are established. The school may be an altogether pleasant experience, helping to give to the child sufficient information, ability to participate in group activities, and conventional skill to assure a smooth communal adjustment in the future. But it may also be a breeding place of unhappiness, fears, daydreaming, resentment and behavior disorders of all sorts, if serious difficulties arise and are maintained within its walls or are carried into school from the outside. There are several features which are especially apt to call forth personality problems in school children:

Unhealthy relations to the teacher.
Unhealthy relations to the classmates.
Physical illness.
Lack of recreational outlets.
Being in the wrong grade.
Frequent changes of schools.
Long absences from school.
Late registration.
Experience of failure.
Parental interference with the school regulations.

Relation to the teacher. Teachers are human beings, subject to physical and emotional difficulties like the rest of us. To the child, however, they are (and should be) persons with supreme authority, and regarded by him with awe. The average pupil covets the teacher's approval as much as he desires to be praised by the parents. She is usually thought to be more powerful than the father or mother, because her criticism is expressed in the more respected and, therefore, more potent form of the written monthly or quarterly report. If she uses her position wisely, the normal child will do well under her care and the difficult youngster will profit from the contact. There exists nowadays a tendency to blame always the teacher for the ill-conduct of a school child, just as some people indulge in wholesale condemnation of modern parenthood. The sincerity and good will of the average teacher are just as much above reproach as are the intentions of the average parent.

But the average teacher is often in a very difficult position. She is expected to teach certain subjects to a certain, usually quite large, number of pupils who either live up to the grade requirements and are promoted or fail to do their work satisfactorily and must repeat the grade. This would be a very easy task if she were confronted with a physically, intellectually, and emotionally homogeneous group. Yet this is never the case. Her skill and patience are tested severely by the youngsters who are unusually shy, who tremble or stutter or cry when called upon to recite or to read, or by those who are consistently late, very slow, restless, mischievous, spiteful, openly antagonistic, ostentatious, or who ask to be excused every few minutes because of a frequent urge to urinate. There, it is no longer a question of merely imparting the knowledge of spelling or long division or the rivers of Spain; it becomes an equally, or even more, important problem of the individual handling of these children with the definite aim of finding the reasons for their devious behavior and socializing them sufficiently to conform to the conventional standards of conduct as well as to the postulated class achievements.

In order to be able to handle the individual difficulties of her pupils, she herself is in need of adequate preparation, experience, and guidance. Patry enumerated "certain forms of personality difficulty, habit reactions and emotional and social maladjustments, or mismanagement of functions and opportunities, which occur in an average or normal professional group of women," reported to him by several school superintendents in the course of one single week: self-centeredness (person who lacks the ability or willingness to see things, dispassionately, objectively, from the other person's point of view. Everything is interpreted from her own angle); self-satisfaction (person who lacks a desire to improve herself professionally or socially, who feels self-sufficient and displays a bumptious attitude); unnaturalness (teacher who is too self-conscious of her position in life and who feels that, to be respected, one must hold himself aloof); mental dishonesty with herself and others (unwillingness to face present facts of reality; a lack of desire to accept her limitations and an attempt to overcompensate for them to the extent of trying to give the impression that she knows more than she does; a tendency to evade or smooth over difficulties and procrastinate rather than deal squarely with the now and here);

lack of sympathetic and friendly attitude and manner in dealing with others; taking herself too seriously; tendency to inhibit others rather than to draw them out in a positive manner (instead of shaping opportunities for her contacts to flower out and develop and express her pupils' personalities, such a person wipes out confidence or belief in herself because her approach is negative rather than positive); inability to discuss matters frankly from an impersonal point of view; unwillingness to take criticism; shut-in or withdrawal type of reaction (the person who is too introspective, lacks cordiality, and finds difficulty in socializing herself); moodiness; sarcasm; being group centered in her own profession only, with lack of participation with other professional and social groups; working with one eye on the clock and merely complying with the letter of prescribed requirements; failure to establish healthy habits of work, play, rest, and sleep; "schoolmarmitis" (magnified self-awareness of herself in the rôle of dispenser of knowledge and wisdom to children and, on occasion, to their parents; a tendency to "lord it over" and a patronizing attitude towards others).[1]

It is from such attitudes and traits that undesirable relations may arise between teachers and their pupils, in whom fear reactions, meekness, disrespect of authority, vindictiveness, hatred, and even contempt may develop. On the other hand, the well-balanced, sympathetic, and understanding teacher will inspire trust, respect, love, and admiration of her person as well as enthusiasm for the work which she requires.

In recent years, the nation-wide establishment of parent-teacher associations, the spread of mental hygiene information, and the creation of the position of visiting teachers, who form a valuable link between the school and the home, have tended to introduce sound and helpful relations between the teacher, the pupil, and the parents.

Relation to classmates. At the time of entrance into school life, children come with different personalities and varying degrees of socialization. The only child, who has had little or no opportunity to associate with coëvals, may find it more difficult to fit into a crowd than the youngster who comes from a large family and who has been permitted to play with children in the neighborhood. The aggressive child is more apt to assume the functions of leadership, while the shy or meek child will more likely be among those led. Schneersohn conducted original and illuminating observations of the spontaneous formation and dissolution of play groups during the recess period, permitting an insight into the social tendencies of the individual pupil; he paid especial attention to the type of children entering into a group, the type of game played, the rôle of each member within the group (leader, rival, follower), the interest in the game, etc. There is the boy or girl who instantly attracts a number of others and directs their activities; there is the child who faithfully remains in the circle once it has formed itself; there is the child who remains at the periphery as an onlooker; there is the drifter who, within a few minutes, changes his participation a number of times; there is, finally, the lonely child who remains unattached during the entire period. It is the drifter

---

[1] Patry, Frederick L. The Rôle of Psychiatry in the Personal Hygiene of Professional Women. Hospital Social Service. 1932, 25, 481–488.

and the solitary child and the bully who call for particular study and adjustment.[1]

Every adult knows from his own experience how during school life lasting friendships are formed, but also how envy and jealousy, cruelty, denunciation, or revengefulness may at an early date mar the character of a child and also cause a good deal of suffering in the victims. Many classes have their "teacher's pets" who with their privileges often combine the disadvantage of being teased by the others. Many classes have their permanent clowns who make up for their personality difficulties by constantly attracting the teacher's and classmates' attention, by becoming martyrs when punished, and heroes when they can "get by" without being discovered or disciplined.

It is the parents who domesticate the child, who feed and clothe him, teach him proper habits, and prepare him for communal socialization. It is the teacher who imparts to him knowledge and supervises his first type of communal group contact. It is among the classmates that he must acquire a "group spirit," which is so essential in later life.

Physical illness. The ill child cannot work as efficiently nor play as vigorously as the healthy child. Depending on the type of his discomfort, he may appear irritable, languid, or easily fatigued. It is, therefore, necessary that school children undergo periodic physical examinations and are immediately seen by the school or family physician as soon as any disorder is suspected. Mouthbreathing due to chronically infected tonsils and adenoids, general weakness because of undernutrition, and errors of refraction are responsible for a good many poor marks. Children whose left-handedness is "broken" by the teacher (now fortunately a relatively rare practice), may react with more or less apparent personality difficulties. In the more progressive communities, the school system provides satisfactory facilities for the physically handicapped child; it has special classes for the cardiac child, so that he may not climb stairs, or at least has elevators for his use; it has open air classes, rest hours and lunches for those who are in need of those arrangements; it has special schools for crippled children, where they receive individual attention and medical, particularly orthopedic, treatment; it has special classes for the conservation of sight and of hearing. Handicapped pupils whose schools have no such provisions are indeed at a severe disadvantage, which may show itself psychobiologically as well as physically.

Lack of recreational outlets. "All work and no play," is a bad policy for children. If the youngster is to have adequate recreational facilities, he needs time, a place, and playmates. The time may be curtailed by an over-ambitious teacher who loads her pupils with an excessive amount of home work, in order that her class should excel, or by parents who fill all their offspring's spare time not occupied by school activities with music lessons and music practice, with religious education, and with errands or money earning jobs, or by the child himself whose pedantic or obsessive character causes him to spend hours and hours on the slow writing and

[1] Schneersohn, F. Sociability of Abnormal Children and Social Child Psychology American Journal of Psychiatry. 1933, 12, 1307–1337.

rewriting of his home work. Other children again develop the habit of voracious reading to the extent of refusing to go out and play. One often sees parents who declare that they "do not believe" in leaving their children "unoccupied"; they prefer to have them help in their stores, or with the laundry, or scrubbing the floors.

In order to play, a child needs not only time, but also a place. In the tenement districts, this is a very serious problem. Sufficient parks and playgrounds must be provided within easy reach. So many a boy has suffered himself to be received in a gang and indulged in its activities because he could find no other mode of satisfying his recreational needs. It is the slums that need the most, and have the fewest, branches of organized boys' and girls' clubs and other recreation centers. It is here that adult loafers and delinquents and prostitutes are in abundance and apt to initiate unsupervised and uncritical children into the practices of begging, stealing, and sex activities.

Insufficient recreation because of lack of playmates is found chiefly in the diametrically opposite stratum of society. Here, the child is surrounded lavishly with costly toys; he is taken on vacation trips, led through museums and galleries, and has his tutor or governess. But he may nevertheless be lonesome and lack the thrilling experience of group play. We think, for example, of the mother who would not let her "sugarplum" play with other boys because their parents permit them to wear overalls. Or we think of the highly intelligent girl of fourteen years whose mother, herself of a solitary nature, would not allow her to associate with other girls, not even with her private school classmates, because "you can never tell what kind of families they come from."

Lack of adequate recreational outlets through healthy play association with coëval children may revenge itself severely. It may make the child less fit and less eager to do his work, due to fatigue or to monotony. It may create in him envy of those who are more fortunate in this respect. It may cause him to seek in truant wanderings the adventures denied him in the form of organized games. It may induce him to look for satisfaction in daydreaming or in the development of hypochondriacal complaints.

Being in the wrong grade. A child who has been pushed up the grades beyond his innate capacity and grasp, or a child who is far too intelligent for the grade in which he finds himself, may be led to fill the time, unoccupied by the one because he cannot participate and by the other because he comprehends too quickly, with motor restlessness, mischievousness, or daydreaming, or even cause him to resort to truancy.

Frequent changes of schools are mostly due to equally frequent changes of residences. Let alone the harmful and humiliating practice, employed in so many schools, of putting the child back a grade or a half grade automatically whenever he comes from elsewhere, the need of repeated readjustments may soon not be fulfilled if the youngster develops the feeling of "What is the use? I shall probably have to move again anyway." There will be an element of uncertainty in the child, lack of a feeling of belonging somewhere, and absence of loyalty and group spirit.

Long absences from school may be the result of sickness, of "rest cures" prescribed erroneously for the treatment of "nervousness," of lack of proper clothing in poverty-stricken families, or of the habit of taking the child along on the parents' more or less extensive travels or visits to distant relatives. The child loses time and, upon his return, finds himself in the same grade with younger children and sees his former classmates ahead of himself.

Some parents, especially immigrants from Eastern and Southern Europe and overprotective mothers, feel that a child at six years is too young and immature to be sent to school. Often, if there is a brother or a sister one or two or even three years younger, they wait until both are good and ready and enter them in the first grade together. Thus the child finds himself with children much younger and smaller than he is and is kept back not only in his studies but also in his general development and maturation.

It is not difficult to see that the child who has experienced failure both in every day school activities and in the final day of reckoning at the end of the semester, is exposed to all kinds of problematic situations, arising from within as well as from without. The very occurrence of failure has, of course, its causes which must be studied in every instance: physical illness, lack of intellectual capacity, unhappy home conditions, etc. The child who, for any reason, is not promoted may develop a feeling of excessive shame; if he has worked hard without success, he may be prompted to give up his efforts in the face of failure. He may learn to look for excuses and find a scapegoat in the teacher's supposed "meanness" or prejudices or in his own somatic functioning, thus beginning to complain of headaches and stomachaches of a hypochondriacal nature. It is also important to know how the child's failure is met by the others. Teachers, classmates, and parents are too liberal with terms, such as "stupid" or "lazy," and the parents try often to avert failure through nagging, punishment, or "tutoring" (usually by themselves in an inexperienced, impatient, and even hostile manner). If the child is retarded, no force in the world can make him comprehend or do things which are beyond his capacity; force will be a waste of effort, its lack of results will irritate the "tutors," and intensify in the child the feeling of failure. If the child is "lazy," the reason must be found. It is not natural for a healthy, normal child to be apathetic, listless, indifferent, disinterested, inactive; if he presents these traits, he may be ill; or he may not be able intellectually to take part in the grade work; or he may know the work so well that he is bored; or he may be preoccupied; behind his "absentmindedness" there may be hidden a wealth of highly dramatized and prolific fantasies.

Parental interference with the school regulations. There are parents who are jealous of the school. They feel that the educators alienate the child from them. They therefore watch suspiciously for any occasion to "rub it in," mostly in the child's presence. The overprotective mother gets worked up if her offspring is placed too near the window or too near the radiator or too far from the window or from the radiator. To her, every poor mark instantly spells prejudice or "meanness" on the part of the teacher; she does not fail to persuade the child that this is so. We have known parents dishonest enough to make corrections in the child's arithmetic or spelling tests and then bring them back to the teacher with the impudent accusation that the paper had not been marked right. The possible effects on the child's character of such practices are obvious. There is the attitude, not at all uncommon, that public education is a one-sided duty of the community; the school has its obligations, the performance of which is criticized with a sharp tongue, and the parent sends her child to school as a special favor to the authorities and wishes that to be known and appreciated by everyone. Instead of coöperating with the school, it becomes a constant issue of home versus school. On the other hand, we have seen hostile mothers who made every attempt possible, fortunately without success, to prejudice the teacher against the child.

The oversolicitous and impulsive mother of a healthy boy once took a notion to run into the classroom in an agitated condition to curse the teacher because she gave the pupils too much home work to do (an unfounded accusation), and to drag her son away from the school in order to teach him herself. The boy's sufferings from the whole affair can hardly be described. He liked school and this really was the origin of the mother's action; she was jealous that anyone or anything should share the child's affections with her.

Another boy stated that he disliked (and on several occasions "hooked") school because "the teachers are mean to children when they expect them to work too hard"; his mother had told him so; she had written notes excusing his truant absences on the grounds of sickness.

A father was in the habit of accusing the teacher of his only, badly spoiled son of ignorance in the elements of arithmetic (because his own child had told him so). He worked himself and the boy into a paranoid attitude. Once when he came to fetch the boy home from school he saw an example on the blackboard and precipitated a scene, claiming that the teacher had made a mistake. It took several teachers and the principal a long time to convince him that it was he who was mistaken about the result of the problem. He nevertheless continued to criticize the school and threatened to bring the matter before the school superintendent. He instructed the boy to look for an occasion to "get even with the lot."

The hateful mother of an intellectually superior boy, who stubbornly tried to convince his physician that his asthma was a "bad habit," ran almost daily to his teacher insisting that the boy was "feebleminded" and should be placed in a special class for retarded children.

CHAPTER XII

DIAGNOSTIC SYNTHESIS

Psychiatric examination is an analytical procedure. It begins with a biographical analysis of all events which seem to have mattered in the patient's life and a reconstruction of the situational frames within which those events have taken place. The biography leads logically to an analysis of the patients assets and liabilities as they appear at the time of the investigation. Here we are concerned with all those features which have entered into the formation and integration of the child's individuality. Even though, for the sake of systematic organization of the material, the single factors must be taken up successively, they are, not even for the moment, dealt with as detached or separable entities. From the very beginning, there is a unifying starting point in the form of the complaint and a unifying goal in the form of the determination of the total personality of the child about whom the complaint has been made. The child's anatomy and physiology and physiopathology and intellectual capacity and emotive responses and ambitions and action tendencies do not exist or function apart from each other. In registering the presence of facial acne, it makes a difference and must be stated what the acne means to the patient and those associating with him; it may have no psychobiological significance whatever; the child may be very sensitive about it and become preoccupied with its possible effect on others; an anxious mother may be unduly alarmed about it and drag her offspring from one doctor to another; the playmates may have teased the child about it and caused unhappiness; a physician's incidental remark anent its probable duration may have made a lasting impression; superstitious lore with regard to its assumed connection with sexual intercourse may have influenced the pubescent or adolescent boy's thinking and activities. The same is true of any other item which is brought out in the course of the investigation. To quote just one more example, we find that a slight degree of mental retardation may never come to light if nothing unusual is expected of the child and, on the other hand, give rise to serious emotional strain if overambitious parents want him to go through college and university or, again, may make the child stand out as an intellectual giant in a feebleminded family. All such possibilities make one appreciate the value of a relativistic attitude as well as the fact that, in the course of the analysis, we do not merely cite unrelated addenda but consistently work towards a well-rounded knowledge of the specific mode of fusion of the available data in the integrated personality in whom we are interested.

Psychiatric diagnosis is a synthetic procedure. All medical diagnosis is based on synthesis, as is indicated in the original meaning of the terms "symptom" (things which "fall together"') and "syndrome" (that which "runs together"). In non-psychiatric medicine, however, the main aim consists in piecing together a number of "symptoms" which concur often enough to have them stand out as a definite disease picture. This is a justified method, and experience has taught that, with the progressing subtlety of our clinical and laboratory means of examination, the establishment and recognition of these pictures has become more certain and clearcut, even though we have to allow for more or less conspicuous variations. This is also true of a number of psychiatric conditions, except that they offer a much wider range of individual differences. In the anergastic, dysergastic, and certain oligergastic reaction groups, we have before us constellations of symptoms permitting of a diagnostic terminology in the traditional sense: encephalitis, juvenile paresis, typhoid delirium, Mongolism, or cretinism. The "name" gives us a fair idea of the clinical manifestations common to practically all instances of the illness designated, even though, in approaching the individual problem, we cannot afford to disregard the total personality of the affected child (as, indeed, we must not overlook it under any circumstances, psychiatric or not psychiatric).

But if we come to deal with the rank and file of children's behavior disorders, we look in vain for any single word or words that would at once convey the entire situation in which we are interested diagnostically and therapeutically. "Enuresis" is certainly not a diagnosis in the same sense as is, for example, "Hirschsprung's disease" or "aortic insufficiency"; nor is the I.Q.; nor is "nailbiting," nor "fear of the dark." There have been attempts to unite certain of these personality problems under collective headings. We are thus burdened with concepts, such as "neuroses" and "neuropathies," and "constitutional psychopathic inferiorities," and plain "nervousness." The various authorities operating with these terms have, of course, very precise personal notions of what they mean when they use them. But in the first place, very few, if any, agree with each other. Besides, perusal of the literature leaves one with the somewhat disturbing impression that the very same behavior disorder, let us say, enuresis, is called a "neurosis" by one, a "neuropathic trait" by another, and an "hysterical symptom" by still another. Some authors make unconvincing distinctions between neuropathic and psychopathic manifestations, which, at best, are artificial and can be accepted in good faith only. The issue becomes even more confusing if one is confronted with a child who presents several complaints; we have pointed out in the preceding chapters that this is a rather frequent occurrence. In such a case, we may find that the same patient is neurotic and neuropathic and psychopathic simultaneously. It is difficult to see what one can do with this sort of diagnostication, which is based on opinion rather than on the statement of concrete facts. Furthermore, if we do accept these designations, it must be conceded that almost every child referred because of a psychiatric problem (if he is not anergastic or delirious or feebleminded) is a "neurotic" or "neuropathic" child, and these terms assume the rôle of generalizations instead of telling us precisely what is wrong with the patient.

Far be it from us to want to give the semblance of iconoclastic heresy. But, in working practically with children and having to send to the referring pediatrician a clear report of each patient's difficulty, we found it best to refrain from any generalized terminology, for the reasons enumerated above. Neurosis and neuropathy (aside from the misleading etymology which would point in the direction of involvement of nervous tissue) are not diagnoses in the original and accepted meaning of this word. They do not lead anyone to "know" what the problem is and to distinguish it from other problems. The term "malaria" does that sufficiently, but the term "neurosis" does not and cannot do it.

We must therefore return to the statement that psychiatric diagnosis is a synthetic precedure. It differs from non-psychiatric diagnosis by virtue of the greater complexity and manifoldness of the "symptoms." It must, in each individual instance, go back to the factors obtained in the complaint and in the course of the examination. Any one word cannot do justice to it. It is a reformulation of the complaint on the basis of the available data.

A few concrete examples may serve to illustrate the point:

Lifelong feeding problem and frequent diurnal enuresis in a healthy six-year-old boy of high average intelligence, youngest in a family of four, badly spoiled by an invalid father and a hypochondriacal mother.

Stubbornness, temper tantrums and crying spells in a healthy, normally intelligent three-year-old girl with internal strabismus and signs of old rickets, beaten and nagged by an unintelligent, deaf mother, who is disappointed in her married life.

Masturbation and school difficulties in a pale, undernourished, feeble-minded eleven-year-old boy with dental caries, whose brother, 19, has a history of masturbation and enuresis; alcoholic, brutal father, died eight years ago; stepfather resents his behavior.

Hypochondriasis, crying spells, and truancy in a slightly undernourished, somewhat retarded twelve-year-old girl with visceroptosis and vasomotor instability; complaints began after promotion and transfer to another school; the child does not feel equal to the task and wishes to repeat the grade.

Irritability, daydreaming, nailbiting, and belching in a twelve-year-old girl of superior intelligence, with spastic colon, who finds it difficult to adjust herself to the family's recent financial disaster, forcing them to move into a socially inferior neighborhood.

A physically and mentally healthy, well adjusted seven-year-old boy, handicapped by a moody, emotionally unstable mother who has branded him as a "feeding problem" and changes schools, doctors, and "diets" almost every week.

A physically healthy seven-year old boy of superior intelligence, somewhat restless, who, because of parental snobbishness and misapplied social standards, was kept from any associations with other children, sent to a "private school" of which he is the only pupil, and stuffed with piano and violin lessons and chess studies; the victim of an excitable father who works with "hands, hair brush, and razor strap" and of an obese, untruthful, moody, self-righteous mother.

Stubbornness, daydreaming, feeding problem, thumbsucking, masturbation, and specific reading disability ("congenital wordblindness") in a normally intelligent seven-year-old boy with dental caries, mediastinal tuberculosis, and a history of many illnesses (among them diphtheria, otitis media, and mild poliomyelitis), badly spoiled; sleeps with eight-year-old sister who has crying spells, sucks her thumb, and offers the same feeding problem.

Anxiety attacks, enuresis, and nailbiting in a parentally and medically mismanaged, physically healthy, normally intelligent ten-year-old girl, whose attacks have been treated as "leaky heart" with digitalis, protracted rest in bed, prohibition of school attendance and of play, and general over-indulgence.

Feeding difficulties, psychogenic vomiting, and occasional stuttering in an alert six-year-old boy of high average intelligence, with infected tonsils. Broken home. Spoiled by grandmother. Stuttering began during presence in the home of a stuttering relative. Family fears serious physical illness as the cause of his difficulties.

It can hardly be doubted that this type of diagnostic formulation tells us much more about the individual problem and serves far better as a basis for therapeutic planning than the non-descript term "neurosis" or "neuropathic constitution." It takes in the whole situation with its genetic-dynamic aspects, speaking of the child rather than of his "disease."

THIRD SECTION

THE PRINCIPLES AND AIMS OF
PSYCHIATRIC TREATMENT

CHAPTER XIII

GENERAL THERAPEUTIC CONSIDERATIONS

PSYCHIATRIC treatment does not and cannot limit itself to a more or less isolated concentration on the complaint itself. The behavior difficulty brought to the physician's attention is an indicator of a general maladjustment in which various factors may be involved in different combinations and degrees. The very fact, which cannot be emphasized often and strongly enough, that so-called monosymptomatic behavior disorders are so rare as to be the exception rather than the rule, ought to make one sensitive to the complexity of the problems of a psychiatric nature. The unreasonableness of "treating" separately the bladder, the larynx, or the stomach of a child who is enuretic, stutters, or has "anorexia" with gagging and vomiting is very obvious and needs no further comment.

In every medical approach, history taking, examination, and recognition of the type of illness are already steps directed towards adequate therapeutic planning. This is even more true in the case of psychiatric management. Any remedial program will depend on the knowledge of that which is to be relieved, namely the patient rather than a detached organ or habit, with all the influences of a physical, constitutional, intellectual, emotional, and situational character which have entered into the formation, development, and course of the difficulty. Such information is indispensable; it is the *conditio sine qua non* for successful relief. It furthermore prepares the soil for confidence and coöperation on the part of the patient and his family.

It is often surprising to notice how well pleased children and parents are if they realize that one actually makes a serious effort to understand the situation, instead of automatically reaching for the prescription pad. A slipshod, haphazard questioning may sometimes have the result of irritating the mother who may feel that the physician unnecessarily pries into her private affairs. But we have yet to meet the parent who would fail to appreciate the advantages of a tactful, sympathetic, interested, and well-conducted systematic investigation, unless feeblemindedness or a paranoid attitude interferes intellectually or emotionally with the required rapport. In such a case, this very discovery is a point which will have a decided effect on the therapeutic arrangements. The physician's skill in the handling of people and in making the desire to overcome the difficulties a mutual concern of himself, the child, and the family is a factor as significant as his knowledge of the problem and of the best method of its treatment. This is especially true of the manner in which the diagnosis

117

is communicated to the parents. The formulation should avoid alarming terminologies. A mother may well accept the explanation that her offspring's present level of intellectual capacity makes it difficult for him to fulfil the requirements of the grade in which he is and that the strain from which he suffers will be relieved by his being placed in an ungraded class; she may, however, be hurt and indignant if the term "feebleminded" is flung at her; she will leave the office in an unhappy and dissatisfied mood, and the adjustment will more than likely not be made. This does not at all imply that anything should be withheld from the parents. They should be told all the pertinent facts, but in a form which would assure the maintenance of peaceable contacts.

It is unfortunately true that we are sometimes confronted with situations which are more or less unmodifiable. We may be living in the best or, at any rate, one of the best of existing civilizations. But the facilities for children's care are far from being perfect. Financial inadequacy, political meddlings, the indifference and ignorance of legislators, and the lack of progressivism and vision on the part of some of our courts are facts which cannot be disregarded. The present state of psychiatric knowledge and abilities may not be ideal, but it is far abreast of the social structure of our day. It is a good thing to realize this state of affairs and include in one's calculations the limitations which it implies. Such a sober realization has its definite advantages. It inspires one to work for better opportunities; at the same time, it saves one from the disappointment of aspiring to the unobtainable. It discourages Pollyannish attitudes and illusions. But some of our commonwealths are more progressive and considerate and better equipped economically than others and are leading the way to improvement. Besides, the open-minded physician will not permit himself to be stunned by these difficulties. He will assume a melioristic viewpoint, which will cause him to do the next best thing, if the best thing is beyond his reach.

The modifiability of the situation may also be impaired by the type of people with whom one deals. Parental convenience, indifference, or outright unwillingness or even total lack of grasp are factors which cannot be left out of the account. It is true, at the same time, that "lack of coöperation" should never be used as an ever-ready excuse. This is the place to insist tenaciously on the fact that it is an essential part of the treatment to assure coöperation. The relative number of "uncoöperative parents" is, in a way, a measure of the physician's efforts and abilities in this direction. No practical worker, it is true, will go on squandering his time and endeavor on "human material that is fundamentally unadjustable, and unadjustable by virtue of a chronic habit-formation as fatal to its victims and as demoralizing in its influence as the addiction to narcotics or alcohol."[1] But it takes a penetrating study of personalities and family groups and a great deal of experience before such a verdict can be reached. And even then, one should maintain a melioristic attitude.

The need of a melioristic viewpoint in medicine, and more especially in

[1] Richards, Esther Loring. Conservation of Social Energy. Hospital Social Service. 1924, 9, 278–288

psychiatry, cannot be advocated vigorously enough. It keeps one from being ensnared in the super-optimistic elation of those who, once they have found some formula, announce that they have a cure-all, whether this be endocrine gland extracts, or getting at the repressed sexuality, or what not. But it also does away with undue pessimism, which is ready to throw up the arms in despair if perfection cannot be obtained or if a "cure" is not accomplished. Nothing does more harm in medicine than thinking in the two extremes of cure and failure. To illustrate: We certainly are not in a position to "cure" feeblemindedness as such; but we do have it in our power to help the feebleminded child to find his way in life. We can protect him from evil associations which may abuse his suggestibility and poverty of judgment; we can protect him from the burden placed on his shoulders by overambitious parents or teachers; we can find for him a type of occupation and setting in which he will be proficient, useful, satisfied, and happy. On the other hand, one may "cure" a child of disobedience by beating him into frightened submission; but it would be an Eisenbarth cure indeed, creating problems much more serious than the disobedience.

Nor are we capable of commanding the course of human events. If we have helped a stuttering child through general adjustment and specific measures, we have no guarantee that with new situational difficulties at a later period he will not react again with stuttering, or tics, or something else. But the patient and the parents will now have confidence enough to come back and to ask for assistance at an early date.

Good psychiatric treatment is not satisfied with temporary contacts; it institutes a follow-up system which makes it possible to guide the child and his family for a protracted stretch of time, so that any new problem may be reached and straightened out at its inception.

The complaint, of course, is the guiding line all through the treatment. Its cessation may usually be considered a safe measure of therapeutic success.

If we consider the limitations and utilize the assets existing in the child, the family, and the total setting, we are doing the best that we can, without having to look for perfectionism and without being bothered about "permanent" one hundred per cent cures. The ancient Romans were a practical people; they coined a proverb which might serve as a motto to every conscientious physician. It says: *Ultra posse nemo obligatur*.

The treatment itself consists of several steps, which must be undertaken simultaneously or successively, wholly or in part, depending on the individual case and on the type of the complaint. They are:

Work with the child.
Work with the family.
Work with the community.
Specific therapeutic aids.
Follow-up work.

We shall, in the following chapters discuss each of these points separately.

Hartwell has summarized in an interesting way the main concerns involved in the psychiatric treatment of children. He advises:

1. To think *about* the child by understanding his mental life.
2. To think *for* the child and lay plans to help him.
3. To think *with* the child and thus seek to cure him.[1]

It is a good policy not to make one's recommendations in a dictatorial manner. It is much more helpful to develop the therapeutic program before the parents as an understandable, logical, and acceptable conclusion of the history and examination. One must also make sure that the measures advised can really be accomplished. Otherwise one might make the same mistake as did a certain European medical celebrity, one of whose patients, a poor laborer, had saved for months to get together the rather high consultation fee and at the end of the interview was told that what he needed was a long ocean trip. One must also not be too rigid and self-righteous to consider reasonable and more convenient alternatives which may suggest themselves in the course of the treatment. Sometimes new and unexpected circumstances may arise in the situation calling for alterations or even for a revision of the original plan.

In order to be fully prepared for an authoritative presentation of the program, it is advisable to have answered to oneself the following questions:

To what extent is the child modifiable?
To what extent are the parents and their attitudes modifiable?
To what extent is the total situation modifiable?
What are the difficulties that call for modification?
What are the best methods of their modification?
What are the obstacles most likely to interfere with such a plan?
How can these obstacles be overcome?
What are the assets that can be used constructively?
How can we best assure optimal coöperation and confidence?
If the ideal plan cannot be carried out, what would be the next best procedure?

When all these questions have been decided upon, we are ready to begin with the actual treatment.

[1] Hartwell, Samuel W. Fifty-Five Bad Boys. New York. 1931.

CHAPTER XIV

WORK WITH THE CHILD

REGARDLESS of the number of people and types of situations which must be taken into account in the management of children's personality disorders, one should never lose sight of the fact that the therapeutic aim is directed primarily towards the youngster who is our patient. This statement may sound trivial and superfluous. But it is based on the observation, made more than occasionally, that some workers, in their efforts to obtain the family's coöperation and to make the necessary communal adjustments, sometimes leave the child himself out of their direct contacts and work "over his head," permitting him to remain uninformed and passive. Things begin to happen which, under the circumstances, seem unexplained, mysterious, and not necessarily connected with the complaint in the youngster's thinking. Tonsils are removed, glasses are prescribed, arrangements with the school are made, placement in a boarding home is decreed, while the principal and central figure in the plot is not confronted with the whats and whys and purposes of all these activities. No matter how correct and useful they are, the patient's unpreparedness and lack of active and understanding participation in the entire scheme may have a decided effect on the intended modification. It is thus that at times a fundamentally wrong approach (for instance, the unwarranted prescription of a drug for a child to whom its object has been clearly explained) may have better results than a fundamentally correct plan carried out without his knowledge and collaboration. Common sense, of course, will exclude from such direct contact any child who, because of his age or low intelligence, lacks the capacity for personal concern with his psychiatric difficulty and with the therapeutic program.

The first postulate in every case is the correction of all physical ills detected in the course of the examination. It is, from a practical point of view, quite immaterial whether or not the existing malnutrition, anemia, myopia, dental caries, adenoid vegetations, or mediastinal tuberculosis has anything to do with the temper tantrums, fear reactions, feeding difficulties, or any other behavior disorder. In a child who offers no personality problem whatever the recommendations with regard to the restoration of bodily health will be the same. Realizing that we deal with the person as a whole and not with an isolated complaint, we cannot fail to set up in the patient an optimal condition of comfort and well-being as an ideal opportunity for successful adjustment. We may be able to relieve a child of his bedwetting even though his teeth continue to decay; but we certainly have not, in this case, solved all of his difficulties; our job has not been a complete one. Besides, no matter how futile and speculative it may often be to tie up all psychiatric problems with existing physical illness in the sense of causal relationship, it is doubtless true that the old idea of *Mens sana in corpore sano* is much more than a time-worn adage. Behavior being a set of functions mentally integrated in the total personality, its smooth working depends to a large extent on an optimal integration in every respect.

It must, however, be stated that we definitely limit our activities to the physical disorders that have been actually demonstrated. We abstain from "treating" or advising to "treat" hypothetical, not really observable dysfunctions which are postulated by this or that author or by this or that school as the one and only cause of the complaint with which we are concerned. If, in a child with migraine or convulsions or vomiting, we find a hypoglycemic condition, we feel that its very existence calls for specific treatment. But we cannot take seriously the rule laid down by some investigators who advocate the feeding of sweets to all children who have night terrors on the basis of the unproven assumption that pavor nocturnus is the expression of a glycopenic state, even if the blood sugar happens to be absolutely normal. The same holds true especially of the theories about pluriglandular disturbances and their claimed but not commonly evinced relation to behavior disorders. Wherever they can be brought out by clinical or laboratory examination, they unquestionably need attention. But wherever this is not the case, we do not succumb to the lure of abstract speculation and are more interested in rational therapy than in the increase of the sales record of pharmaceutical firms.

Just as in history taking and during the investigation, so also in the discussion of therapeutic arrangements it is best to interview the patient and his parents separately. Thus the child is spared the father's or the mother's I-told-you-so comments, and it is much easier for the physician to find a suitable formulation and approach in the absence of parental interference. The preceding exploratory contact with the youngster has already given ample opportunity for the establishment of a satisfactory rapport with the physician, which, of course, is indispensable. As long as the child is apprehensive, sullen, indifferent, or spiteful, little, if any, collaboration can be expected. The psychoanalysts have fitted the relation between patient and physician into their general scheme by giving the physician the rôle of a "phantom of the original libido object," a situation, in which "the oldest, repressed, forgotten, unconscious relations of childhood appear in new form." This so-called "transference" is considered a highly important factor in the treatment; resistance, or negative transference, must be broken, postive transference must be achieved, maintained, kept from going too far, and finally resolved, sublimated and transmitted to other, more desirable libido objects. It would not be fair to deny anyone the privilege to call coöperation a positive transference and lack of it a negative one. The same may be said (and really has been said) to be the case in the relations between defendant and judge, prisoner and warden, pupil and teacher, employee and boss, congregation and minister, subject and king, or even man and God. But it seems in order to wonder whether the physician's rôle as a "libido object" exists in the child's "unconscious" or whether it is mainly the product of the analyst's conscious speculations. For our own purposes and for anyone trained to deal soberly with the concrete facts in the matter, it seems sufficient to know that the patient listens to us attentively, understands what we have to say to him, is capable of accepting facts which have been furnished by himself, by his parents, and by an objective examination, and is willing to participate in an arrangement which promises to relieve him of his difficulties.

A significant step in the treatment is the correction of faulty attitudes and notions which the child has formed with regard to his personality disorder under the influence of his environment. In working with an enuretic child, it is necessary to do away with his idea that it is a "weak bladder" or a "weak kidney" which is responsible and that, therefore, the condition simply cannot be helped. The youngster with a tic will have to be freed from the false label of St. Vitus's dance which has been pinned on him. One boy went about with the self-conceived notion that his problems were caused by some mysterious force in him to which he kept referring as "It": "It makes me blink my eyes when I am tired." "Sometimes It suddenly makes me jerk my arms. I do not want to do it, I don't even know that I am going to do it. It just takes my arm and jerks it." "It makes my head ache." Physicians, teachers, and relatives often use the term "nervousness" as an explanation offered to the child or to each other in his presence for his behavior difficulties. They do not realize that this word, which they consider rather harmless and frequently with a feeling of relief that there is not "something worse," may set up some strange ideas in the child. We have made it a point to study the meaning which the term had in the thinking of the patients who used it. Here are some typical examples of the statements which were made:

"Nerves are in your hands. Nervousness is when you put your hand on anything it shakes like."

"Nervousness is when you wiggle and cannot sit still. Nerves are in the teeth. When they don't work right, they make you wiggle."

"Nervousness means that you are shaking all the time. That is all I know. Nerves? I think they are part of the bones. I think they are in the back of my neck." (This boy had been treated by a chiropractor.)

"Nervousness is due to the condition of your nerves. They are somewhere inside the body. I do not know just where they are."

"Nervousness is when you shake all over or something like that. (Demonstrates.) It is something like St. Vitus's dance, that is what my mother says." Question: "What are nerves?" Answer: "I don't even know whether we have any or not."

"Nerves is in your head. They look something like snakes. It makes you talk in your sleep and walk in your sleep. If you are scared or upset, it is because your nerves is bad."

Nervousness, at all events, in the thinking of a child does not signify the reaction of the total personality but the action of the "nerves" of which he has a very vague notion. He therefore looks upon it as an organic condition which is believed to be the "cause" of his restlessness, shaking, stuttering, temper outbursts, or any other behavior disorder. As long as we permit the patient to reason in this manner, it would be illogical to convince him of the need and of the reasonableness of his personal efforts. It is not enough that we know ourselves that the difficulty which we wish to remedy is a whole function of the patient's personality; we must formulate our information to the child who is old and intelligent enough in an intelligible and constructive manner. The frequent summing up of the problem as being one of "nervousness" may do more harm than good.

In dealing with the child, we must create in him confidence in ourselves as well as self-confidence in his ability to overcome the difficulty. The patient must learn that we are personally interested in him, that we do everything we can to understand him, to determine his physical health, and to learn of his attitudes and of his home and school relations, that we take him and his statements seriously, that we are sympathetic and wish to help him, that we think well enough of him to "let him in" on the program, which is worked out together with him as well as for him, and that we expect him to take an active part in its materialization.

This method of consensus as the main therapeutic prerequisite has been found to be superior to two other procedures, one of which has been quite popular in Germany since its introduction by Bruns,[1] while the other, though practiced rather widely, has fortunately never been awarded the dignity of a "scientific" measure. We refer to the *methods of surprise and of deception*. The surprise method is a modification of the old custom of firing a pistol shot unawares behind the patient to cure him of his delusions, tics, or stuttering. The hypochondriacal child is outwitted by some sudden trick which is to prove that the stomachache complained of really does not exist. More or less ingenious apparatuses have been devised, which work with light flashes and unexpected noises and electric shocks to surprise the child into moving an hysterically paralyzed limb. In this country it is still quite customary in medical circles to grab in haste for a pitcher of cold water which is poured over the child who has a breathholding spell or a temper tantrum. If it were our sole purpose to "cure" the hypochondriacal stomachache, the hysterical paralysis of the arm, or the temper tantrum, such a drastic surprise measure would perhaps be in order, though it does not even guarantee the maintenance of free motion of the arm after the child has left the physician's torture-chamber. And if the "surprise" does not happen to succeed at once, not even a temporary "'cure" is achieved. If we wish to treat the child as an individual, we shall certainly not be satisfied with these tricks, but prefer to proceed more slowly on the basis of personality adjustment and consensus.

The deception method, much more widely employed, has been kept out of the textbooks. But the number and variety of its uses at home and in the practitioner's office is legion. This method is not interested in the child himself nor in his environment nor in the dynamics of the difficulty. It knowingly deceives the child into thinking that his enuresis is really based on a weak bladder and that the medicine prescribed will strengthen the organ, so that "it" (i.e., the bladder) will not wet the bed. It works with the notions underlying the placebos of dubious fame, which help the drug stores more than the patients. It is, after all, a fraud if one deliberately leaves the child under the wrong impression that his hypochondriacal pain has its origin in a sick organ and then prescribes some bitter medicine, the bad taste of which is intended to discourage the patient from further complaining. The analysis of a representative number of prescriptions of

[1] Bruns, L. Die Hysterie im Kindesalter. Halle. 1906.

asafetida would reveal facts which may not speak too well of the psychiatric resourcefulness of the medical profession.

Adjusting the child to the reasonable demands of a suitable environment is one of the principal objects of psychiatric treatment. It includes proper sanitation and physical care, adequate feeding and clothing, regular hours, sufficient recreational outlets, frank and sensible information, good example, and that degree of socialization which is commensurate with the child's age. To secure all this, we must add to the direct contact with the patient himself the therapeutic work with his family.

CHAPTER XV

WORK WITH THE FAMILY

PSYCHOBIOLOGY deals with interpersonal relationships. These relationships play a powerful rôle in the evolution of normal and abnormal behavior. Sociobiology is an essential feature of psychobiology. If we speak of the individual as a whole, we understand the "whole" to include the situational dynamics of his reaction patterns. Just as we have found it impractical to treat an organ or a complaint without the consideration of its being an integral part of the personality, so it is impossible to deal with the patient detached from his environment. Hence, our therapeutic efforts, to be successful, cannot afford to abandon the approach to those people whose activities we have learned to be linked most intimately with the patient's habits and the molding of his character.

We shall naturally first concentrate our endeavors on the persons with whom the child is in constant and close contact, who have the logical and legal authority over him, and whose coöperation or lack of coöperation spells success or frustration of any therapeutic program, psychiatric or not psychiatric. In conformity with our plans, we shall expect the parents to do something directly for their offspring and more indirectly to work on themselves in his behalf.

No matter what we wish to do directly to the child, we need the family's mediation and consent. It is to them that we must leave the administration of drugs or dietary measures. They are the only ones in a position to carry out the physician's recommendations with regard to the proper methods of training. It is from them that we must obtain the permission for any major step in the examination and treatment, from the puncture of a vein for a blood specimen to the arrangements for a tonsillectomy or the desired school adjustment.

Most of these recommendations would be almost futile and at times even create additional problems if we fail to establish parental coöperation. We have seen how parental overprotection, overindulgence, oversolicitude, overambition, indifference, carelessness, rejection, etc., are highly important factors in the development of behavior disorders. The need of a correction of any unhealthy parent-child relation is therefore imperative. Such a change can take place only if the necessity and practical application has been demonstrated to the parents intelligibly, convincingly, and concretely.

"Educating the educator," to quote a term coined by Hanselmann,[1] is very often a highly important part of our therapeutic task. "Education" is derived etymologically from Latin *e*, out, and *ducere*, to lead or to pull. "Training" has its origin in Latin *trahere*, to draw, to pull, to drag. "Rear-

[1] Hanselmann, Heinrich. Einführung in die Heilpädagogik. Erlenbach-Zürich und Leipzig. 1930, p. 461f.

ing" and "raising," of Anglo-Saxon source, mean to elevate, to lift up, to "bring up" a child. Child training, in other words, has from time immemorial been looked upon as the task of pulling, drawing, or lifting the young individual up to the state or level of the adult educator. If this state or level is satisfactory, we have good reasons to expect desirable results from the elders' educational activities. If it is not, the educators themselves are in need of guidance, and it is the physician (and, upon his initiative, the social worker, or some trusted and interested member of the family, or the minister or priest) who must provide it if he wishes to relieve the child of his personality difficulties. We cannot hope to attain a good readjustment of a maladjusted youngster, as long as the etiologically active environmental maladjustment persists unabated.

It would, of course, be impossible to enumerate all the items which one may have an opportunity to present to the parents. The interview devoted to a discussion of the treatment will shape itself according to the type of complaint, the intelligence and emotional attitudes of the parents, and the degree of their willingness, or suspicion, or outright resistance. There are, however, a few points which one must always keep in mind in working with the family:

The existing problem must be formulated to the parents frankly but tactfully, in simple and understandable everyday language, devoid of professional terminologies, in an inoffensive manner which would assure acceptance. The strength of the formulation rests to a considerable extent on the ability to go back to the statements which were offered by them in the presentation of the complaint and to the additional facts obtained in the course of the examination. The mother may frown at sweeping generalizations, but she will listen attentively to any explanation which is introduced by remarks, such as, "You have said yourself that. . . ," "Your own observations have led you to believe that. . . ," or, "Our painstaking examination has very carefully considered your assumption that the child may have St. Vitus's dance, but we are in a position now to relieve you of this fear." The mother realizes that she is taken seriously, that her own observations and interpretations and apprehensions have not been brushed aside, and that the "diagnosis," instead of being handed to her in the form of some Latin term or medical slogan, is brought clearly to her understanding. She knows exactly, or at least as much as the physician does, what is wrong and why it is wrong.

Biochemical tests, BMRs, microscopical slides, roentgenograms, and I.Q.s are most valuable guides to the physician, who has the physiopathological and psychological background for their proper evaluation. It is a grave error to present them to the uninformed or to the insufficiently or wrongly informed layman who in nine cases out of ten will not understand the pictures or figures and sometimes make improper use of them. The physician, laboratory technician, social worker, or psychologist who hands them out confuses rather than impresses the patient or the parent.

The treatment should be planned with the parents and not dictated to them. They are entitled to know why certain recommendations are made. Advice must be concrete and palpable, given best in the form of a program for the twenty-four hours of the day. Every step must be made to appear logical, reasonable, and helpful.

One mother went to a dispensary with her lisping and enuretic boy. The interne had good reasons for wanting a Wassermann test. He took the child to a room without saying anything, stuck a needle into his arm, and obtained the blood. The mother fainted. She indignantly left the dispensary. Anxious to help her child, she took him to our clinic. She reported that at the other place the doctors had pumped the child's blood for a transfusion (she said "transflusion"). Had she been told before, she stated, that blood was needed, she would have gladly given her own instead of her boy's "who is so anemic." It was explained to her that the blood was not needed for a transfusion but for an important test of the child's condition. She immediately realized the justification of the procedure and would have acquiesced had we asked her to give her consent to any other manipulation. It would have been so easy, with just a few explanatory words, to gain the confidence of this really coöperative woman.

Conviction is never obtained through argumentation. "Constructive composure," to use Meyer's word, is the physician's most forceful armamentarium in dealing with patients and their relatives and with people in general. The therapeutist who loses his patience is at a great disadvantage. Constructive composure must be cultivated as much as the knowledge of physiology or pathology.

It is unwise to blame parents for what they have done or omitted. It is far better to speak calmly of the complaint as a result of these actions or omissions and to offer alternatives which will yield better results and do away with the difficulties under consideration.

Faulty notions must be corrected in the parents as well as in the intelligent child. They may be of a superstitious nature, they may consist of wrong ideas about heredity, they may be due to the pseudo-scientific or ill-digested popular literature with which the book and magazine market is flooded, or they may have an iatrogenic origin in wrong or misunderstood diagnostication and prognostication.

It is often necessary to discuss the problem and its adjustment with both parents, either together or separately, as the case may be. It is, however, unwise to play one parent against the other.

Work with the family must often include the direct or indirect dealing with members of the household other than the parents. It will sometimes be necessary to check the detrimental influence of a teasing brother or a spoiling grandmother or a superstitious maid.

One must be careful not to demand of the parents anything that they really cannot do for financial or other reasons. One must also keep in mind the degree of the modifiability of the individual family members as well as of the total situation.

Wherever it is found that other members of the family or of the household present similar, or other personality difficulties, efforts should be made to arrange for their examination and treatment.

CHAPTER XVI

WORK WITH THE COMMUNITY

THERE ARE innumerable instances in medical practice in which treatment and prophylaxis are limited strictly to the contact between the physician on the one hand and the patient and his near relatives on the other hand. But frequently the horizon of therapeutic resources must be broadened to include the druggist and, more indirectly, the pharmaceutical factories, the hospital facilities of the community, and the aid of a consulting specialist and perhaps of a trained nurse. The modern physician fully realizes that the advances made along the lines of public hygiene have placed on him obligations going beyond a mere restriction to office interviews and bedside activities. He understands the soundness of reporting infectious diseases. He has learned to accept as essential necessities the appointment of medical public health officers and school physicians. He has become interested in all matters of legislation touching upon the physical welfare of the populace and upon the privileges and duties of his profession. In other words, he has become community-minded.

In the psychiatric work with children's personality disorders the knowledge, utilization and creation of adequate community facilities often becomes an important part of the therapeutic program. Dealing with the patient and his family alone may not suffice for the attainment of a satisfactory adjustment. In behalf of the child, contact with one or another or several communal agencies may be needed.

The school. The average child spends at least eight of his formative and most impressionable years in school. We have, in a previous chapter, tried to explain the various difficulties which may arise, alone or together with other sources, from faulty adaptation to the educational and socializing requirements of the school. The educators have learned to appreciate the advantages of considering each child as an individual with specific abilities and limitations as against the old-time method of teaching a certain amount of scholastic wisdom to a "class" regardless of the personality make-up of its constituents. In spite of all talk of a feeling of rivalry and of a delimitation of competencies, the interested teacher is not only willing to give to the physician an idea of his pedagogical system and aims but is grateful for any help which he can receive from the medical profession in making easier his task of coping effectively with the handicapped pupil. Before asking for and accepting advice he has, of course, the right to expect that the adviser is well-informed about that which the school can or cannot offer. He is a poor psychiatrist indeed who would wish to dictate radical changes for which neither the school nor the community are adequately prepared. But he can help his patient considerably if he calmly discusses with the teacher his personal needs and the best mode of their gratification. This is true not only of the crippled, deaf, blind, stuttering, mentally retarded, or intellectually superior child but of any pupil who presents behavior difficulties in the classroom. The physician will be useful in explaining and remedying so many complaints of lack of attention and concentration, daydreaming, restlessness, mischievousness, listlessness, poor progress in spite of good intelligence, and persistent truancy. He will be helpful in steering pupils into the special classes for hearing and sight conservation and speech training and for dull or feebleminded children. He will assist the school authorities in the difficult task of vocational guidance. Close contact with our educational institutions will increase the efficiency both of the educator and of the psychiatrist or psychiatrically intelligent physician in their attempts to alleviate the personality disorders of pupils with whose adjustment they are both concerned in equal measure.

Psychiatric institutions. It may often seem advisable to commit cretins, Mongolian, the congenitally amaurotic, and other idiots, imbeciles, or low grade morons to training schools for the feebleminded. Hospital placement may be required for epileptic, postencephalitic, or schizophrenic children, or juvenile paretics. The physician must, therefore, through personal visits, familiarize himself with the location and therapeutic standards of such institutions and keep in constant touch with them if he wishes to learn of the progress of his patients after they have been committed. He will render inestimable service to his city or county or state if he educates the public and its legislators sufficiently to have them build such hospitals where they do not exist in spite of urgent need and to improve those which have not kept pace with the advancement of pediatric and psychiatric knowledge.

The courts. It has been only within the last two or three decades that children's delinquencies have come to be looked upon as expressions of personality maladjustments which are in need of medical, and more especially psychiatric, investigation and treatment. Young thieves and burglars and sex delinquents are not immediately fined or sent to prison. The establishment and development of our juvenile courts is one of the outstanding achievements of the early part of the twentieth century, as far as scientific attempts at prevention of crime are concerned. One does not have to be unduly optimistic to feel that here a significant step has been made in the right direction. The juvenile court of our own community, supplied with a broadminded judge, an efficient staff of probation officers, a pediatrician, and a psychiatrist is an excellent example of the eminent rôle which these institutions have come to play in the field of mental hygiene. No modern physician dealing with children can afford to ignore them. Nor should he remain uninformed about the progressive efforts of our correctional reformatories for boys and girls, both communal and private.

Boarding homes. The disruption of the family unit through death, hospitalization, separation, desertion, or penalization of one or both parents, or a home environment disastrous to the child's development may necessitate his placement in a suitable boarding home. This is the place to state and to restate vigorously and emphatically that the psychiatrist and juvenile court judge appreciate as much as anyone else, if not more, the desirability of preserving the family structure as often and as long as is reasonably possible. There are demagogues who delight in accusing them of breaking up homes to the right and to the left, indiscriminately and unnecessarily, and of tearing children away brutally from the loving care of their parents. This is a deliberate falsehood. But if a child has become delinquent or developed other equally serious personality disorders in a setting of alcoholic or sexual orgies, psychotic entanglements, habitual and apparently incorrigible thievery or other flagrant conflicts with the law, or criminal neglect and cruelty, then both the patient and the community are served and tragic catastrophes are, and must by all means be, prevented by removing the child from his unfortunate and unhealthy environment. It is not the psychiatrist's job to change the social structure of the day. He is too busy doing psychiatry. But it is his job to help the individual youngster brought to him because of behavior disorders, and if this help cannot be accomplished without removing him from a maladjusted home (and only then), his therapeutic efforts will be based on the patient's removal from his home. He will have to see to it that suitable, stable, understanding, coöperative, and intelligent people should be selected for the purpose of taking over the child's reëducation and further training along the lines prescribed by him. Since there are agencies which, as Richards says, "go about placing dependent and semidependent children with less intelligence than a forestry department displays in reforesting neglected areas," it is up to the physician or to his social worker to make sure that the placement is really a curative measure, instead of creating new difficulties in place of, or in addition to, the old ones.

Welfare agencies. The charitable agencies will often have to be called upon to aid in the financing of boarding home placement. Where it is found that hunger, lack of clothing, and improper housing conditions are a part of the difficulty, the agencies will be approached to render first aid and give relief in the form of financial assistance and of providing work for the unemployed members of the family.

Other community contacts may occasionally be indicated, such as work with the church, with the child labor bureau, with the societies for prevention of cruelty to children, with special agencies interested in crippled or deaf or blind children, with summer camps, recreation centers, etc., as the case may be.

The psychiatrically intelligent physician will soon perceive that the contact is a mutual one. If he has displayed sufficient knowledge, understanding, practical ability, and tact, the agencies not only will try to coöperate when approached by him but will also come to him with their own patients and problems of which there are many. They will only too gratefully give him many opportunities to impart his insight to larger groups of people, educators, nurses, parent-teacher associations, and others, and it will even happen that his own colleagues will invite him to speak to them of these matters, which they slowly begin to look upon as indispensable tools of their medical equipment.

CHAPTER XVII

SPECIFIC THERAPEUTIC AIDS

THE PRINCIPAL aim in dealing with the rank and file of psychiatric disorders of children consists of readjustment of the maladjusted patient through work with himself, with his family and, whenever indicated, with one or another communal agency. This is the guiding line in the treatment of every type of personality difficulty. Depending on the nature of the complaint, however, the necessity may arise for employing measures which serve as valuable and sometimes indispensable supplements. They are not "the" treatment; they are aids in the treatment.

Some time ago a psychiatrically interested young pediatrician came to us with the expression of puzzlement over the fact that there had been no improvement of the tics of a fourteen-year-old boy in spite of the advice to ignore them, which had been given to the mother two years before and carried out religiously. The advice to ignore the tics apparently had been considered as exhausting the therapeutic needs of the case. It was regarded as "the" treatment. And it was not successful. It failed because it overlooked completely the main issue of studying the patient's personality and adjusting the basic problems underlying the development and maintenance of the tics. The boy was somewhat retarded intellectually but very conscientious and, with extreme effort, had managed to go through the grades until the age of twelve years when for the first time he was not promoted. At the same time, undeserved unemployment befell his father. The boy, due to the ensuing economic stress, had to forego pleasures and privileges which he had previously enjoyed. He later solved his own problem. He left school at fourteen and was given a newspaper route. The knowledge that he helped to support the family, however meagerly, gave him an unprecedented feeling of self-confidence. He no longer had to cope with the fact, which he naturally could not comprehend, that despite hard work his scholastic attainments were unsatisfactory to the teachers and to himself. His tics disappeared within a short time. The advice to ignore them may have been correct as a therapeutic accessory, but as the only measure regardless of the more fundamental factors at play it was bound to fail.

For this reason, if we speak of specific therapeutic aids, or supplements, or accessories, we presuppose that, however important they may be and however unsatisfactory effects their omission may prove to have, they are secondary to the work discussed in the preceding chapters. An occasional hypnotic may be indicated in a case of persistent insomnia, yet its administration is not even patchwork nor a justifiable "palliative" if the basis of the sleeplessness is not ascertained and attacked, with all the physical, emotional, and environmental factors that may be involved.

The specific aids may be pharmaceutical, educational, and suggestive. The *mechanical devices of restraint* which were (and still are?) quite popular in dealing with thumbsucking, nailbiting, and masturbation should be discarded. They are of the same order as is the recourse to whipping used by parents who do not know how otherwise to assert their authority. They accentuate, instead of attenuating, the difficulty. They may, in a minority of cases, relieve thumbsucking or masturbation, but they do not help the thumbsucker or the masturbator.

Pharmacological aids are indicated in demonstrable endocrine disorders, in lues, in the epilepsies, in migraine and other severe headaches, and in a number of other conditions. The indiscriminate use of tonics and sedatives as "placebos" cannot be discouraged emphatically enough.

Among the *educational measures*, adequate habit training and the establishment of habit regularity are issues of the utmost importance, which fall in the category of therapeutic essentials in the task of readjustment; they are a major part of the treatment and not accessories. Of the more specific educational aids, we like to mention the so-called *star chart*, which is sometimes helpful (as a supplement) in cases of enuresis, feeding difficulties, and temper tantrums. The days of the week are written on a sheet of paper, which is given to the child. With the help of lines, provisions can be made for two or three or more weeks. The patient is to paste a gold-colored paper star in the corresponding space at the end of each twenty-four hour period during which he has remained dry or eaten well or displayed no tantrums. If he has wet himself or has not eaten well or has had an outburst, the space remains blank. When there is reason to doubt his truthfulness, the more reliable of the parents is given, unbeknown to the child, an identical chart which is to be treated in the same manner and brought back together with the youngster's chart. The child is promised a toy or a book or a party or anything else that he has been wishing eagerly at the end of the first week or two weeks in which there would be no blank spaces. Care must be taken that the promise is really kept. It is, to judge from our experience, not useless to repeat that the star chart should be employed only as an accessory, after all necessary attempts at personality adjustment have been made. It should be applied only to children old and intelligent enough to understand and be interested in the procedure.

The following is a reproduction of the star chart of a ten-year old boy who all his life had wet his bed every night. It was made out after certain features of faulty training had been corrected and undesirable sleeping arrangements changed and a needed school adjustment made. We may add that his enuresis has not recurred within the period of more than a year which has elapsed since he returned the star chart.

	First week	Second week	Third week	Fourth week
Sunday	Star	Star	Star	Star
Monday	Star	Star	Star	Star
Tuesday		Star	Star	Star
Wednesday		Star	Star	Star
Thursday	Star		Star	Star
Friday		Star	Star	Star
Saturday	Star	Star	Star	Star

It is only fair to state that the results are not always so prompt as in the child whose chart we have reproduced. But the incentive of the prize and particularly the feeling of achievement which even a solitary star may give to a child who has wet his bed every night may be of considerable value.

Suggestive methods are usually divided into waking suggestion and hypnotism. There are people who erroneously believe that psychotherapy is identical with suggestion. Psychotherapy is the sum total of efforts which we make in behalf of the adjustment of a person with personality difficulties. It includes education and habit training and improvement of environmental disturbances; it may involve the treatment of physical disorder; it may have to concern itself with vocational guidance. It is made up of all that with which we have dealt as work with the child, with the family, and with the community, as specific therapeutic aids, and as follow-up work. "Suggestion" is only a part of psychotherapy. The more we can do for the adjustment of a child, the less we shall have to suggest.

It is, of course, legitimate to speak, if one wishes to do so, of waking suggestion if one tries to instil greater self-confidence into the patient and to make him feel that he can overcome his difficulty. One may, however, look at the matter from a different angle. The child either is or is not capable of overcoming his difficulty. If he is, any assurance given out to that effect is a statement of the truth rather than a suggestion. If he is not, no amount of suggestion will help, and other methods will have to be employed.

We have, on another occasion, had an opportunity to demonstrate the fallacies of the "suggestive" surprise and deception methods. Pototzky[1] reports good results with what he calls *Milieusuggestionsmethode*. It consists of talking the patient into believing himself transplanted into a pleasant environment. After painting a poetical picture of the calm beauties of the sea shore or of the mountains, he proceeds to tell the child, "You feel so rested, so delightfully calm, that you cannot comprehend how you ever could be so unbridled and swept away by anger," or, "In this sweet quietude you have finally won the feeling that you will sleep quietly also at night," or, "You now feel so strong, that you have the feeling that you are able to move again your paralyzed leg."

The method of *hypnotism* in the treatment of children's behavior disorders has been used especially in Germany. The results are not too encouraging and do not invite indiscriminate imitation. Its indications are so restricted as to be almost negligible. It may be considered in obstinate cases of stuttering or enuresis after the ordinary steps have failed and no other method is available. Even then one must make sure that the child has the proper understanding of the nature of the procedure and that his family does not share the popular superstitions anent its supposed mysteriousness. The hypnotizer must have had ample experience not only with adults but especially with children. It is better not to hypnotize enough or at all than to hypnotize too often.

We may again restate as a result of our experience that the better we are oriented in the genetic-dynamic factors of the individual problem, the

[1] Pototzky, C. Zur Methodik der Psychotherapie im Kindesalter, mit besonderer Berücksichtigung der "Milieusuggestionsmethode." Zeitschrift für Kinderheilkunde. 1919, 21, 104–112.

more we know of the child's liabilities and assets, and the more systematically we go about the task of adjustment, the less frequently we shall have to work with any mode of suggestion.

We cannot close the chapter on specific therapeutic aids without a brief reference to the assistance of a competent *social worker* who can do a great deal helping the family to carry out the physician's recommendations and who can save much of his time by working out a direct contact with the child himself. The psychiatric social worker is not only an "investigator" but a valuable therapeutic agent. Adequate training, common sense, and experience must, of course, be expected of her. One must be careful not to select the type of worker, fortunately diminishing in number, who goes beyond the physician's arrangements and feels called upon to lecture to the parents on the castration and Oedipus complexes and on the significance of their offspring's high or low I.Q., or who feels that her duty is performed if she brings in a detailed description of the pattern on the living room carpet and an enumeration of the book and magazine titles seen in the patient's home. A good social worker is a decided asset, and no child psychiatrist can afford to be without one.

CHAPTER XVIII

FOLLOW-UP WORK

OPINIONS are divided as to whether a physician has fulfilled his duty if he has prescribed proper medication and a suitable daily routine or whether he should go out of his way to make sure that his recommendations are actually carried out. It certainly is to the credit of the profession that the much spoken of "fear of losing a patient" entails much more than mere monetary considerations. It is based on the desire for continued confidence and on the scientific curiosity to watch and direct the course of the illness and the period of convalescence.

In dealing with children's psychiatric problems, the initial program is not the treatment, but the beginning of the treatment, which is kept up by means of a well planned follow-up routine. Its intensity, its duration, and the frequency of direct contacts depend on the nature of the individual problem. Its aims are manifold:

Follow-up work is the best and perhaps the only way of testing one's own therapeutic skill as well as the validity of the methods adopted. It gives one an opportunity to recognize and correct diagnostic and remedial errors, from which no one is exempt.

It helps one to control the situation in the sense of ascertaining coöperation on the part of the child, the family, and, wherever indicated, the child-caring agencies of the community.

It makes it possible to appraise and treat the obstacles which may arise in the arranged readjustment of the patient and his environment.

It serves to check one's unwarranted optimism or pessimism with regard to the degree of modifiability of the people and situations with which one deals.

It makes one aware of relapses or new difficulties at their very beginning and helps one to straighten them out before they become more firmly intrenched.

It keeps the physician informed about accomplished or anticipated major alterations in the environment, about sickness, deaths, changes of residence, financial reverses or gains in the family, promotion or failure in school, etc., and about their influences on the patient.

Most of our knowledge of the dynamics of adult behavior and its deviations has, until recently, been based on retrospection. It was mainly through adequate history taking that the early personality difficulties of a psychotic or otherwise maladjusted patient came to light. His biography had to be written backwards, as it were.

This method of retrospective analysis has its decided advantages and is indispensable in psychiatry. It is, however, highly desirable to study life histories from the beginning as well as looking back from the height of a famous person's great achievements or from the depths of a stranded individual's entanglements. It is one thing (and an important one at that) to ask, "What were the childhood reactions of this depressed, or schizophrenic, or epileptic man or woman?" and another thing to ask, "What is going to become of the child who presents this or that behavior disorder?" It is from this type of investigation that psychiatry may be expected to derive momentous gains in the next generation or two. The more complete the original case records and the closer and longer the follow-up work, the better are the chances for gaining insight into the evolution of personalities and of personality disorders.[1]

[1] The high informative value of adequate follow-up work has been recently demonstrated by Ruth E. Fairbank, whose excellent paper, The Subnormal Child —Seventeen Years After. Mental Hygiene, 1933, 17, 177–208, presents a study of the material which had been previously worked up by C. Macfie Campbell (The Subnormal Child—A Survey of the School Population in the Locust Point District of Baltimore. Mental Hygiene. 1917. 1, 96–147).

PART TWO

FIRST SECTION

PERSONALITY DIFFICULTIES FORMING ESSENTIAL
FEATURES OR SEQUELS OF PHYSICAL ILLNESS

CHAPTER XIX

ANERGASTIC REACTION FORMS

THE ANERGASTIC reaction groups are composed of those mental disorders which are intimately connected with histo-pathological alterations of cerebral substance. They are therefore always combined with clinical neurological changes which are of primary diagnostic importance. The psychiatric involvements are essential components of the morbid conditions and may clear up after recovery from the disease of the central nervous system with which they are associated, or they may leave the personality damaged for the rest of the patient's life. This is not the place to go into the details of the somatic symptomatology, for a study of which we must refer to the pertinent textbooks and monographic presentations. Here we are largely interested in a discussion of the psychopathological features. One may say as a general rule that the tissue alteration or destruction is mostly allied with a loss, a deficit, or an arrest of the mental functions. The *congenital* malformations of the brain result in a more or less severe retardation of intellectual development and in those personality disorders which go with feeblemindedness and with the bodily handicaps (paralyses, contractures, choreiform or athetoid movements, ataxia, blindness, deafness) arising from the disease. The *acquired* cerebral lesions may affect the child in the sense of a complete or partial standstill of mental growth, of a dropping out of functions already possessed, or of a general change of the emotional, adaptive, and social reactivity ("change of personality") with or without intellectual impairment. In acute illnesses, there may be a varying degree of reduction of consciousness, ranging from mild drowsiness to profound coma, and delirious reactions. In the more chronic disturbances, memory, judgment, comprehension, and the capacity for verbal communication may suffer. The functions of speech may never be acquired, or they may be learned incompletely or at a late period, or, if already developed before the onset of the illness, may be wholly or partially abolished; there may be motor or sensory aphasia, or paraphasia, or perseveration (constant repetition, independent of external stimuli, of a word or a phrase), sometimes associated with various forms and degrees of alexia, agraphia, and apraxia. Headache is one of the most common symptoms of cerebral disease and of especial diagnostic significance if linked with projectile vomiting or with vertigo. Convulsions may occur in any of the conditions which make up the anergastic group. Sleep is often disturbed, most characteristically in epidemic encephalitis.

Among the psychopathological *sequels* of brain diseases are intellectual inadequacy, epileptiform conditions, faulty utilization of experience, especially in the sense of inability to realize and to avoid danger, and antisocial trends. Confusional states may cause the children to wander away from home aimlessly. Institutional custody must frequently be resorted to and vocational adjustment is often impossible and always a very difficult problem.

MALFORMATIONS OF THE BRAIN

Cerebral malformations, both congenital and acquired, are practically always associated with varying degrees of intellectual defect, most frequently with idiocy or imbecility, and in the majority of cases require institutional care. Children with gross deformities, such as acephaly (absence of the entire central nervous system), anencephaly (absence of the hemispheres with cerebellar atrophy), and cyclops (lack of symmetrical arrangement of the brain and one-eyedness) are fortunately not viable and are either born dead or die within the first few hours after birth. Some of the other anomalies are of greater psychiatric importance and are therefore briefly discussed.

Porencephaly. The name porencephaly roughly indicates the presence of a "hole in the brain." There is a lack of cerebral substance, either unilateral or bilateral, located mostly in the anterior or middle parts of the brain and sometimes permitting a communication between the surface of the cortex and the lateral ventricle. True or congenital porencephaly is said by some to be due to intrauterine anemic necrosis (Kundrat) or traumatic encephalitis, and by others to be a developmental anomaly. False or acquired porencephaly originates in local atrophy with the formation of a cystic cavity as a result of hemorrhagic or inflammatory lesions. Aside from spastic paralysis (hemiplegia or diplegia), the main symptoms are convulsions, defective speech, and varying degrees of feeblemindedness. Of Kundrat's eighteen cases, only three survived the period of infancy. Tredgold states that "several cases have been described in which a large cavity existed in one hemisphere, and yet there was little or no appreciable mental change."[1]

Microcephaly. Microcephaly is an unusual smallness of the brain with a corresponding smallness of the skull, out of proportion to the other measurements of the body. True microcephaly, which is considered a developmental anomaly, has been distinguished by some from so-called pseudo-microcephaly, which is said to be the result of intrauterine cerebral diseases. The brain is not only small but may also present various deformities, such as macrogyria, simplification of the convolutional pattern, heterotopia (islands of gray substance within the white matter), absence of the corpus callosum, and differences in the extent of the reduction in size of the various parts of the brain. Nor is the skull merely a miniature of the normal cranium; the head is cone-shaped (oxycephalic), the occiput is often flattened, and the forehead receding. Many microcephalics are helpless, mute, untidy idiots. Others may learn to speak, to perform simple tasks, and to keep themselves reasonably clean. Vision and hearing are not impaired, but there is often a marked insensibility to pain. Some of the children attain intelligence quotients of between fifty and sixty or even slightly higher; these are vivacious, usually restless, imitative, and may learn to read and write, to do simple arithmetic, and to perform easy duties or even earn a living under supervision. Convulsions are said to occur in approximately one-half of all cases. Growth is often stunted. The duration

[1] Kundrat, H. Die Porencephalie, eine anatomische Studie. Graz. 1882.—Tredgold, A. F. Mental Deficiency (Amentia). New York. 1916, p. 74.

of life is less than that of the average population but approximately the same as that of other types of idiots and imbeciles. Many die of tuberculosis. It has been justly pointed out that the shape of the head is of greater diagnostic significance than its size; as a matter of fact, there are many normally intelligent dwarfs with small skulls which, however, are well formed and the measurements of which are well in proportion to those of the rest of the body.

Hydrocephalus. Hydrocephalus is an accumulation of an abnormal amount of cerebrospinal fluid in the ventricles (internal hydrocephalus) or in the subarachnoid space (external hydrocephalus). It is either present at birth, when it is mostly intraventricular, or acquired during life. It is due to obstruction in the cerebrospinal pathways leading to the cerebral subarachnoid space (Dandy). Among the various factors which have been made responsible are traumatic insults, infectious diseases, and psychoses affecting the mother during pregnancy, parental lues, alcoholism, and tuberculosis, intrauterine vascular anomalies of the embryonic brain, inflammation of the ventricular ependyma, and occlusion or displacement of the communicating orifices between the ventricles. Hereditary and familial occurrence has been reported. The amount of fluid averages about one quart, but as many as five quarts have sometimes been found. Its excessive quantity results in an impairment of the development of the cerebral substance. There is often a flattening or even an obliteration of the convolutions and sulci and a pressure atrophy of the tissues. The skull is greatly distended, the cranial bones are thinned and widely separated, and the fontanelles may not close for many years. The shape of the head is marked by prominence of the frontal and parietal protuberances. There is a noticeable disproportion between the sizes of the head and of the face. The veins of the scalp and of the forehead stand out prominently. The orbital roof is pushed downward. Congenital hydrocephalus is often associated with other developmental anomalies, such as dwarfism, harelip, spina bifida, clubfoot, and encephalocele. Sometimes there is nystagmus, strabismus, or optic nerve atrophy. Those children who do not die at birth mostly have serious mental defects. Although there are very mild cases which show only slight intellectual impairment or even normal intelligence, the majority is found in the idiotic or imbecile class. Those patients are usually good-natured, affectionate, and cheerful, though clumsy and awkward in their movements, and they often have difficulty in holding up and fixating their heads. Convulsions are not uncommon.

Acquired hydrocephalus may be due to cerebral tumor, obstruction of the aqueduct of Sylvius, cicatricial occlusion of the fourth ventricle, lues, meningitis, encephalitis, or it may be "idiopathic."[1]

AMAUROTIC FAMILY IDIOCY

Amaurotic family idiocy, or the Tay-Sachs disease, was first described by Warren Tay (*Symmetrical Changes in the region of the Yellow Spot in Each Eye of an Infant. Transactions of the Ophthalmological Society. London. 1881, 1, 55*) and later studied systematically and established as a clinical

---

[1] Consult Walter Dandy. Chapter on Hydrocephalus, in "The Brain." Practice of Surgery, edited by Dean Lewis. Vol. XII, pp. 213–255. Hagerstown. 1933.

entity by B. Sachs (*A Family Form of Idiocy, Generally Fatal, Associated with Early Blindness [Amaurotic Family Idiocy]. Journal of Nervous and Mental Disease. 1896, 21, 475*). These two titles contain the essential symptomatology and prognosis of the condition. They refer to the frequent familial occurrence, as many as three and four affected siblings having been reported. The mental defect does not appear until the onset of the clinical manifestations of the illness, usually between the fourth and tenth months of life; before that time, the development may have been normal along motor, linguistic, and adaptive lines. Then follows an arrest and progressive deterioration to the point of idiocy and an increasing general weakness. The ocular changes are pathognomonic for the disease; they appear as the well-known *cherry-red spot* in the region of the macula lutea and atrophy of the optic nerve with rapid impairment of vision until absolute blindness is reached. Death occurs before the termination of the third year. The reflexes may remain unaltered, or they are increased or diminished. Spastic or flaccid paralyses are a frequent finding; often the helplessness and inability to lift the head or perform any sort of movement is due chiefly to the child's extreme prostration. Bulbar symptoms have been observed, especially disturbances of deglutition. Nystagmus and strabismus have been noted in some cases. Hyperaesthesias and vasomotor disorders have been recorded. A peculiar feature is an unusual sensitiveness to sound (hyperacusis). Another characteristic peculiarity is the predilection of the disease for the Jewish race; it was, as a matter of fact, believed that other races are spared entirely, but a sufficient number of affected Gentile patients has been reported to correct this opinion.

The *pathology* has been studied extensively by a number of investigators, especially by Schaffer, Globus, and Hassin. Sachs has spoken of an "agenesis corticalis" or "a defect in the development of the highest nerve elements of the cortex." Further studies led him to conclude that the condition was due to a degeneration of the ganglion cells throughout the entire central nervous system. Hassin, who speaks of the changes as "developmental and degenerative phenomena," has found the thalamus to be particularly affected. Schaffer and Globus (quoted from Sachs) give the following characteristics: "1. A widespread cytopathological process; an unusual swelling of the cell protoplasm and of the dendrites; a swelling of the hyaloplasm, which causes a mechanical destruction of the cell fibrils and reduces the cell body to a mass of detritus. The axis-cylinder does not appear to be involved in this general swelling. 2. Every cell of the entire central gray matter and of the spinal ganglia is similarly affected."

Various *etiological theories* have been advanced, in addition to the factors of heredity and racial preference. An "inherent biochemical property" of the protoplasm cells has been accused. The endocrines have been made responsible, but glandular therapy has had no effect. Bielschowsky believes that the disease should be traced to the absence of some ferment essential to normal cell metabolism, as evidenced by the deposit of a lipoid substance.

Of twenty-three families tabulated by Sachs, five of the parent groups were more or less closely related. It is interesting that of a pair of twins of the same sex one was affected while the other was spared.

The diagnosis is easily made with the aid of an ophthalmoscope. The prognosis is bad. All that can be done therapeutically is to make the remaining few months as comfortable as possible for the patient.

Spielmeyer and H. Vogt have described a *juvenile form* of the Tay-Sachs disease, beginning between the ages of four and sixteen years, progressing much more slowly, and differing from the classical infantile form in that the typical cherry-red spot is absent and there is no predilection for the Jewish race. Both forms are fortunately very rare.[1]

TUBEROUS SCLEROSIS

Tuberous sclerosis, or Bourneville's disease, is extraordinarily rare. It was first described in 1880. It is characterized by multiple small sclerotic areas of the cortex, adenoma sebaceum of the skin, especially of the face and back, and congenital tumors of various internal organs (kidney, heart, stomach, uterus). Convulsions and progressive mental deterioration are the outstanding clinical symptoms. The anatomical changes begin in intrauterine life, the seizures appear during the first weeks or months after birth, rarely later than the end of the first year. The patients usually die young from the growth of the tumors, intercurrent disease, or status epilepticus.[2]

MONGOLISM

Mongolism, Mongoloidism, Mongolian idiocy or imbecility, or Kalmuck idiocy, owes its name and its separation as a distinct group to Langdon-Down's attempt in 1866 to work out a classification of idiocy on an ethnological basis. It is characterized by a marked defect in the mental development and specific somatic anomalies affecting chiefly the configuration of the head, the eyes, the tongue, and the extremities. The head is mostly small, brachycephalic, rounded, showing hardly any protuberances, and flattened out in the back so that the occiput and the neck almost form a continual straight line. The eyes have oblique palpebral fissures; there is an epicanthal fold of the skin at the medial angle; the two eyes are very near each other, although the flat bridge of the nose sometimes gives the opposite impression and has caused some observers to claim that the eyes are normally or widely placed. The limbs are soft, thin-boned, and relatively short, the hands thick and stubby, the fingers are tapering, and especially the little fingers are sometimes disproportionately small. The thumbs and big toes are abducted and at a considerable distance from the rest of the digits. The lines of the palms show no definite pattern; there is "a confusion of lines like those on a piece of crumpled paper which has been unfolded" (Wyllie and Shrubsall).

Besides these pathognomonic features, there exist in varying number of

[1] For a more detailed information we refer the reader to the following communications: Sachs, B., and Louis Hausman. Section on Amaurotic Family Idiocy. In Nervous and Mental Disorders From Birth Through Adolescence. New York. 1926, pp. 306–320. Bibliography on pp. 324–327.—Provotelle. De l'idiotie amaurotique familiale. Paris. 1906.

[2] Bourneville, D. M. Recherches sur l'Épilepsie et l' Idiotie. Paris. 1890.—Freeman, W. Tuberous Sclerosis. Archives of Neurology and Psychiatry. 1922, 8, 614.

cases many other bodily deviations from the normal; absence or hypoplasia of the nasal bones; all sorts of deformities of the external ear; occult spina bifida; umbilical and abdominal herniations; diastasis of the recti muscles; undescended testicles; prognathism; malformations of the heart (in about 10% of all cases; especially patent interventricular septum); strabismus; nystagmus. Considerable muscular hypotonia is a common and outstanding symptom.

To these congenital anomalies are added others which appear sooner or later after birth, such as dryness, inelasticity, and loss of the normal lustre of the skin; delayed, irregular, and faulty dentition; retarded body growth and sex development; a peculiar spotted form of bilateral lamellar cataract (rarely before the ninth year); formation of deep transverse fissures on the dorsum of the tongue which are practically always present after the fifth year and which John Thomson ascribed to persistent and forcible sucking of the tongue. These furrows and lingual protrusion from a small and narrow-palated mouth are counted among the typical symptoms of the condition.

As the name "Mongolian idiocy" indicates, the mental picture is dominated by a more or less extreme degree of feeblemindedness. The patients rarely reach an intellectual level exceeding four years; a seven-year capacity is about the highest attainment ever reported. Contrary to many other idiots and imbeciles, the Mongols are known to be quiet, good-natured, well-behaved, and affectionate. Sutherland (*The Mongolian Imbecile. British Medical Journal. 1909, 1, 1121*) once said that these patients seem to be blessed with "the possession of a secret source of joy." In spite of the defect and the resulting parental indulgence, temper tantrums or other outbursts are almost never observed. Masturbation is rarely practiced by Mongols. They usually do not lie nor steal, nor are they willingly destructive. They appear placid rather than torpid. As infants, they lie peacefully in the crib playing with their hands and feet, without paying attention to their surroundings or trying to attract attention. Due to the general hypotonicity of the muscles, they are limp and late in sitting up. Locomotion is not acquired until the third year. Words are not formed until very late, and the patients hardly ever learn to express themselves by means of other than the simplest sentences. There is no spontaneity or initiative in their actions. Simple orders are carried out obediently. Even the most primitive form of reasoning is wanting. The children eat and sleep well. They know no fear nor caution nor excitement. An interesting feature commonly observed is a tendency to imitate other people's performances and gestures. This is often done with a good deal of pleasure, the expression of which imparts to the child, with his slanting eyes and protruded tongue, a somewhat clownish appearance. Van der Scheer mentions the Mongols' love of rhythm and music.

The patients' resemblance to members of the Mongol race is certainly only incidental. For a long time, it was believed that the condition occurs in Caucasians only, or even exclusively among Aryans. Tumpeer, in 1922, reported an unquestionable case in a Chinese boy and Bleyer, in 1925, published two cases (in a third, admixture of white ancestry could not be excluded with certainty) in negro children. Of 292 Mongols seen at the

Harriet Lane Home, 267 were white and not less than 25 were negroes. Crookshank speculated on an atavistic basis of the disease and found that the lines of the palm and the posture are similar in the Mongolian idiot, the real Mongol, and the orang-utan.[1] Even though there are some undeniable resemblances in certain somatic features and in some cerebral details (open operculum, increased curvature of the corpus callosum), there are enough differences to outweigh the similarities. Besides, the Mongolian idiot is an idiot, whereas the millions of Chinese and Japanese with their highly developed civilizations give no evidence of being phylogenetically or otherwise inferior to any other race.

It may be mentioned that young Mongolian idiots look very much like each other to the point that mothers in clinics have mistaken strange children for their own. As they grow older, however, they begin to show more individual features.

Of the many etiological theories, the one most widely accepted is the assumption that Mongolian idiots are "exhaustion products," that is, according to Shuttleworth, "dependent upon conditions adversely affecting the maternal reproductive powers; the advanced age of the mothers, and frequent childbearing being the most noticeable causative factors. . . . Exhaustion, illness of whatever kind during the period of gestation may produce imperfection in the evolution of the foetus and its tissues, which we know as Mongolism." It is true that from fifty to sixty per cent of all patients are the last born of their families and another twenty-five to thirty per cent are among the youngest. But there is still a fair number of children left who are among the first born and approximately five to ten per cent are oldest. It is also true that from thirty to fifty per cent of the mothers (Shuttleworth: 33%; Turner: 42%; Van der Scheer: 45%) were older than forty years at the birth of the Mongol child. Approximately thirty per cent of the last born were "late arrivals," that is, they were born more than five years after the birth of the preceding sibling. Abortions and stillbirths are comparatively frequent in the families in which there are Mongol children. It is interesting that higher degrees of mental retardation are uncommon among their brothers and sisters in whom, on the other hand, congenital physical anomalies are often encountered. Syphilis, tuberculosis, alcoholism, and psychoses of the parents are believed by some investigators to cause or contribute to the "exhaustion." Also worry, emotional shock, and illness during pregnancy were considered essential; if this were so, one would expect to see many more Mongols than really exist.

Others accused abnormalities of endocrine functioning as responsible for the condition. Especially the thyroid, the thymus, and the anterior lobe of the pituitary (Timme) have been blamed. Positive evidence for any of these claims has not been produced. Glandular therapy has had no satisfactory results.

[1] Tumpeer, H. Mongolian Idiocy in a Chinese Boy. Journal of the American Medical Association. 1922, 19, 74.

Bleyer, A. The Occurrence of Mongolism in Ethiopians. Journal of the American Medical Association. 1925, 84, 1041.

Crookshank, F. G. The Mongol in Our Midst. A Study of Man and His Three Faces. Third Edition. London. 1931.

Lutrovnick, in his thesis, suggested that Mongolism consists of a developmental arrest of the organs in the median line of the body. Van der Scheer added, on the basis of eighteen autopsy findings, that there is a hypoplasia of the median structures of the forebrain. He ascribes Mongolism to increased intrauterine pressure due to narrowness of the amniotic cavity, resulting from faulty implantation of the ovum in an abnormal mucous membrane of the maternal uterus.

Institutional training is the best available form of treatment. It is often exceedingly difficult to persuade the parents to send these patients away from home because, more than any other backward children, they endear themselves in the hearts of those about them, being calm and appearing always contented and affectionate. They require good physical care, the more so since they have a low resistance against intercurrent illness and their mortality rate is quite high. If they are not too retarded, they are trainable to a limited extent and can acquire sufficient skill to take care of their daily needs and even to do some simple work under proper direction and supervision.

Mongols rarely reach the age of maturity. The average age at death is said to be between fourteen and fifteen years. According to Brousseau, those Mongols who survive the years of adolescence begin to age very rapidly and appear much older than they really are.

The occurrence of two or more Mongols in one family is very unusual. It is interesting that 32 cases of Mongol twins have been reported in the literature, whose twin siblings were normal (dizygotic in all instances where the type of twinning was specified). Five instances have become known, in which both twins (always of the same sex) were Mongolian idiots.[1]

BRAIN TUMOR

Cerebral tumors are about five times less frequent in children than in adults. The commonest forms are gliomata and tuberculomata. The relation of cerebellar location to site in the cerebrum, according to Cushing, is two to one, while in adults it is one to five. The symptoms are usually divided into general and focal or localizing ones. The *general* signs are mostly referable to intracranial pressure; they consist of headache, nausea, and sudden, projectile vomiting not necessarily associated with the ingestion of food, vertigo, slow pulse, papilledema, stupor, and generalized convulsions. The *focal* symptoms depend on the site and extent of the neoplasm. This is not the place to discuss them, we must refer to the textbooks of neurology and pediatrics. We may only state summarily that they arise either directly from the destruction of cerebral substance at the place of the tumor or from pressure on, and displacement of, the neighboring tissues. Paralyses and Jacksonian epilepsy in tumors of the motor zone;

---

[1] There are a few excellent monographs on Mongolism: Still, G. F. Mongolian Imbecility. Kings College Hospital Reports. VI. 1898–1899.—Lutrovnick. Sur les manifestations mongoloides chez les enfants européens. Thèse de Paris. 1908.— Suchsland, O. Die mongoloide Idiotie. Dissertation. Halle. 1909.—Van der Scheer, W. M. Beiträge zur Kenntnis der mongoloiden Missbildung. Berlin. 1927.—Brousseau, Kate. Mongolism. A Study of the Physical and Mental Characteristics of Mongolian Imbeciles. Revised by G. Brainerd. Baltimore. 1928.

motor aphasia, often preceded by bradylalia in growths in the region of Broca's area; word-deafness, paraphasia, auditory aura in convulsions, disorders of smell and taste in temporal lobe tumors; disturbances of stereognosis and of the sense of position, alexia, agraphia in parietal location; hemianopsia and visual hallucinations in affections of the occipital lobe and the optic pathways; ataxia, vertigo, and prominence of pressure symptoms, especially choked disc, in cerebellar tumors are some of the leading indicators in an attempt at localizing orientation.

Psychic abnormalities are said to exist in from sixty to eighty-five per cent of all cases. It must, however, be mentioned that these figures were obtained from adults only or from mixed adult and infantile material. The mental symptoms reported are not specific for cerebral tumors in general nor for the type of growth nor for the site of the neoplasm in particular. It is usually said that frontal lobe tumors are associated with peculiar personality changes attended by a varying degree of intellectual deterioration, poverty of judgment, mild euphoria, and more especially facetiousness and a tendency to punning (*"moria"*: Jastrowitz, or *"Witzelsucht"*: Oppenheim). Most of the psychopathological features are indeterminate and consist largely of dullness, somnolence, listlessness, apathy, indifference, irritability, mild depression, sometimes confusion, disorientation, and stupor. The speech disturbances and hallucinatory experiences have been mentioned in the preceding paragraph as being of help in localizing efforts, though it is well known that they cannot be relied upon very strictly in that respect. The best aid in diagnosis is furnished by the method of air-injection (ventriculography, cerebral pneumography).

BRAIN ABSCESS

The commonest cause of localized collections of pus in the brain is acute or chronic otitis media or mastoiditis. The abscess is then mostly situated in the temporal lobe or in the cerebellar hemisphere on the side of the ear affection. In a small group of cases the origin is traumatic or rhinogenic or metastatic from bronchiectasis, pulmonary gangrene or abscess, ulcerative endocarditis, and actinomycosis. The symptoms of acute cerebral abscess and of the terminal stage of chronic abscess are those determined by its site plus signs of intracranial pressure (headache, projectile vomiting, slow pulse), fever, drowsiness increasing to the point of deep coma, slow respiration, and convulsions. Delirious reactions may be present. Chronic abscesses are usually divided into four stages: initial, latent, manifest, and terminal. In the period of latency the symptoms are very vague and mostly slight; there may be mild headaches or rises of temperature, loss of weight, apathy, slight confusion or depression or transient hilariousness, and sometimes convulsions. Abscesses located in the left temporal lobe are often associated with word-deafness with or without alexia and agraphia.

MENINGITIS

In all forms of meningitis, there is clouding of consciousness which may vary from drowsiness and apathy to profound coma at the height of the disease or in the terminal stages. Delirious reactions may be mild, or associated with intense fear and hallucinations, or reach the proportions of violent manic-like excitement. In the surviving cases, deafness may become a permanent difficulty, especially in the epidemic form, and low degrees of feeblemindedness may be the result. Ziehen states that "meningitis is one of the main causes of imbecility." We saw recently an unusual onset of tuberculous meningitis in a two-year-old boy; following two convulsive seizures, he presented for several days prior to the manifestation of the characteristic symptoms the feature of perseveration. His consciousness remained clear and he answered questions relevantly and promptly, but as soon as he was left to himself, he kept repeating, "Machine has got lights" (reference to his toy automobile), and "I have a bridge in there" (pointing to his mouth and alluding to an episode which occurred the day before he had the convulsions; his older brother who had lost many of his deciduous teeth spoke of having a "bridge"—the toothless gums—in his mouth, whereupon the patient insisted that he also had a bridge). Both phrases had been some of his last statements before his seizures and were muttered automatically again and again until the final coma set in.

PARA-INFECTIOUS AND POST-VACCINAL ENCEPHALITIS

Symptoms indicating an involvement of the central nervous system during the course of measles had been described now and then for the past two hundred years. But it was not until the middle of the second decade of this century that the attention of pediatricians began to center about conditions which clinically resembled the features observed in epidemic encephalitis. Boenheim found among 5940 cases of measles eleven with convulsions of unclear origin, eight with serous meningitis, and six with encephalitis. The incidence has, however, markedly increased in the last few years. The cerebral complications usually begin from five to eight days after the appearance of the exanthema. Aside from different neurological signs (tremors, tonic and clonic spasms, myoclonus, paralyses, choreic-athetotic motility disorders, cerebellar symptoms, transient blindness, abnormal reflexes, changes in the spinal fluid), the same variety of psychopathological manifestations as in the lethargic form has been noted. There may be drowsiness, somnolence, or the reversal of the sleep curve characteristic of epidemic encephalitis. Sometimes delirious reactions occur, which may assume the proportions of manic-like violent excitement. In a case of a seven-year-old girl reported by Eckstein, definite personality changes were complained of by the parents at the end of six months.

Scarlet fever is most rarely associated with encephalitis. Boenheim found only one such instance among 2240 cases, and Eckstein saw none in 2059 children.

The nervous complications of varicella were divided by Glanzmann into the following groups:

Meningitis varicellosa (fever, headache, opisthotonus, somnolence, delirium, agitation, mild paresis); good prognosis.

Encephalitis.

Ophthalmoplegia externa.

Chorea.

Acute cerebral tremor.

Cerebellar ataxia.

Myelitis.

Isolated cases of optic neuritis, polyneuritis, and multiple sclerosis.

Encephalitic symptoms were also observed in mumps.

The convulsions of whooping cough, which are fatal in the majority of cases, were thought for a long time to be based on hemorrhages only, but more recent histological studies have favored the assumption of "grave necrobiotic alterations" of the brain substance.

Eckstein, in 1929, collected from the literature and from his own material ninety-two cases of post-vaccinal (para-vaccinal) encephalitis. The incubation period between the date of vaccination and the onset of cerebral symptoms ranged between two and twenty-six days, in the majority of cases its duration was between ten and thirteen days. In the acute stage, there was fever, somnolence, frequently convulsions, often paralyses, visual disturbances, sometimes meningitic features, and in the different cases all sorts of other neurological disturbances. The outcome was as follows:

Died	33
Completely recovered	25
Improved	7
Unimproved	2
Undetermined	8
Serious mental defect	7
Character changes	2
Residual paralyses	8
Total	92

According to Flexner, recovery from post-vaccinal encephalitis, if it takes place, tends to be complete. "This outcome is independent of the stormy course and alarming character of the disease at the outset, and is in striking contrast with the end-result in cases of epidemic encephalitis of all grades of severity."[1]

EPIDEMIC ENCEPHALITIS

Jelliffe says in the introduction to his monograph on "Postencephalitic Respiratory Disorders" (New York and Washington, 1927): "In the monumental strides made by neuropsychiatry during the past ten years no single advance has approached in importance that made through the study of epidemic encephalitis. No individual group of diseased reactions has been as widely reported upon, as intensively studied, nor as far reaching

---

[1] Eckstein, A. Encephalitis im Kindesalter. Berlin. 1929.—See also: Boenheim, C. Über nervöse Komplikationen bei spezifisch kindlichen Infektionskrankheiten. Ergebnisse der inneren Medizin und Kinderheilkunde. 1925, 28, 598.—Glanzmann, E. Die nervösen Komplikationen der Varicellen, Variola und Vaccine. Schweizerische medizinische Wochenschrift. 1927, 57, 145.—Wilson, H. E., and F. R. Ford. The Nervous Complications of Variola, Vaccinia, and Varicella with Report of Cases. Bulletin of the Johns Hopkins Hospital. 1927, 40, 337.—Flexner, S. Postvaccinal Encephalitis and Allied Conditions. Journal of the American Medical Association. 1930, 94, 305-311.

in modifying the entire foundations of neuropsychiatry in general." No other condition, indeed, has stirred the medical world to such an extent, increased our insight, confirmed knowledge that had been gained previously and discarded errors that had been made before, and contributed to the abolition of the superannuated hyphen separating, rather than connecting, the "neuro"-prefix and "psychiatry." No other illness has at the same time precipitated such an unprecedented cloudburst of hypotheses as has epidemic encephalitis, emerging in the wake of the pernicious grippe epidemic during the latter part of the World War.

Constantin von Economo, in the spring of 1917, described as *encephalitis lethargica* an acute inflammatory cerebral affection, tending to appear in epidemic form, characterized by protracted somnolence and general prostration, accompanied by cranial nerve palsies and a variety of other neurological symptoms, and (as was later discovered) followed usually by serious personality changes with or without outspoken intellectual defect. Kinnier Wilson, in 1918, suggested the term *epidemic encephalitis*. Because of the frequent involvement of the basal ganglia, Sachs recommended the designation of *central or basilar encephalitis*. The disease is popularly referred to as "sleeping sickness."

Epidemic encephalitis may occur at any age, from earliest infancy to latest senescence; there is a predilection for mature and robust individuals. The male sex seems to be preferred in a slight degree.

The bacteriological agent is not known. Rosenow's findings of a coccus have not been corroborated. Other investigations point in the direction of a specific filtrable virus bearing close resemblance to that of herpetic keratitis. The manner in which the infection spreads is also still open to discussion. Only very few instances of familial occurrence have been observed, and only on surprisingly rare occasions physicians and nurses have been victimized by their contact with encephalitic patients. The agent is most likely lodged in the oral cavity and in the nasopharynx and transmitted to the brain through lymphatic pathways. It has not been satisfactorily determined whether the relation to influenza is more than just one of chronological coincidence.

Identical or at least similar epidemics and sporadic cases have in all probability occurred before the great pandemic of 1916 and the following years. Those best known and most frequently cited are the sleeping sickness of Tübingen in Germany in 1712, reported by Rudolf Jakob Camerer (Camerarius), with delirium, somnolence, ptosis, and ocular symptoms, and "Nona," coincident with a wave of influenza in northern Italy in 1890 and manifesting itself in the form of mostly fatal states of sleepiness combined with ocular palsies. Some authors felt that they could trace the disease back to the days of Hippocrates, Livy, and Aretaeus of Cappadocia.

With regard to the pathological anatomy, there are certain characteristic features, the most outstanding of which is the preference for involvement of the midbrain and basal ganglia, although there is no part of the central nervous system which may not be affected in the individual case. Another striking phenomenon consists in the fact that in this serious and often very diffuse cerebral disease gross macroscopical alterations are either absent or very mild and not at all characteristic. The ventricles and the cerebrospinal fluid show no changes. The brain surface appears from pink to dark red and congested, the meninges are usually slightly edematous. Microscopically, there is a marked congestion of all the blood vessels with perivascular degeneration of white matter. Small hemorrhages are often found.

Any attempt to discuss the clinical manifestations of epidemic encephalitis must be preceded by a reference to the polymorphous, protean, almost unlimited variety of its symptomatology which defies any rigid grouping. Not unlike syphilis and hysteria, the condition or certain of its features may resemble a good many other things. Barker rightly speaks of "the great diversity of syndromes met with, the apparent absence of any constant chronology in the development of the syndromes, and the aping by this malady of almost every well-known and well-defined neurological symptom-complex." The most ambitious classificatory effort was undertaken by Tilney and Howe, who distinguished between "eight fairly well-defined subgroups or clinical types," the lethargic, cataleptic, paralysis agitans, polioencephalitic, anterior poliomyelitic, posterior poliomyelitic, epilepto-maniacal, and acute psychotic types; to these they added an infantile form, encephalitis neonatorum, "the recognition of which depends rather upon the extremely early age of incidence than upon any particular clinical feature." Barker, in a report to the Association for Research in Nervous and Mental Diseases in 1920, submitted the following grouping:

1. The somnolent ophthalmoplegic type (febrile or afebrile).
2. The paralytic (akinetic or hypokinetic) type.
3. The amyostatic type (Parkinson-like and cataleptic syndromes).
4. The hyperkinetic type (myoclonic forms, choreatic forms, epileptic forms).
5. The psychotic type (delirious forms, depressive forms).
6. The hyperalgetic type (painful forms).
7. The tabetic type (Argyll-Robertson pupils with loss of deep reflexes and, sometimes, with lancinating pains).
8. The ataxic type.
9. The abortive type (formes frustes; imperfect, rudimentary, and ambulatory forms).
10. The aberrant type (intestinal forms, cutaneous forms, vagal forms, etc.).

For our own purpose, it seems convenient to adopt Felix Stern's division into acute encephalitis on the one hand and postencephalitic manifestations on the other hand.

Stern subdivided the acute forms into three groups

1. The hypersomnic-ophthalmoplegic form.
2. The irritative-hyperkinetic form.
3. The atypical forms.

The disease may begin abruptly or be ushered in by prodromal signs, such as headache, abdominal pain, aches in the extremities, easy fatigability, increased irritability, upper respiratory infections, and mild meningeal symptoms. The nature of these symptoms makes it quite understandable that they are encountered in older children much oftener than in small infants who are incapable of expressing themselves. Eckstein reports a four-week-old baby who suddenly failed to nurse well; on the next day, it refused the breast altogether, would not take milk from the bottle and did not respond to spoonfeeding; the tongue was pushed convulsively against the palate; in the following days it slept incessantly and developed a typical encephalitic picture.

The *hypersomnic (lethargic)-ophthalmoplegic form* is characterized by somnolence and ocular palsies. The children sleep for several days or weeks, being roused with difficulty and unable to stay awake for any length of time. The depth of sleep varies in the individual cases from drowsiness and sleepiness over natural sleep to lethargy and coma and has no relation to the presence or absence of fever or to the height of the temperature. In most instances sleep is normal; pulse rate, respiration, electrical skin resistance, and the general appearance do not differ from the conditions found in the nocturnal sleep or diurnal naps of healthy individuals. Even the dream life is similar. If has been noted that youngsters who have had nightmares or pavor nocturnus attacks previously may also have them in the encephalitic sleep. The patients may be roused sufficiently to answer a question intelligibly or to take nourishment but may doze off again instantly in the midst of conversation or of a meal. In the brief intervals of waking there may be a good deal of yawning.

Sometimes *delirious reactions* are observed. Stern differentiates between "initial deliria" preceding the lethargic stage, deliria accompanying the somnolence, and deliria associated with the hyperkinetic form. Those occurring in the interruptions from sleep are usually mild, fleeting, superficial, and uncharacteristic, the hallucinations simple and non-dramatic; the whole picture resembles that of vivid and somewhat fearful dream reactions. Occupational deliria are not common in children; occasionally the patients during sleep pull at the bedspread, mumble, or jerk the arms about as if in defense or in response to some dream situation.

The lethargic condition is frequently associated with *ocular disturbances*. Older children who are able to relate their experiences often complain of seeing double. Whether or not diplopia occurs in early infancy can, of course, not be ascertained. Ptosis, various forms of strabismus, and spontaneous nystagmus are not unusual. The statistical data, as compiled by various authors, with regard to ocular symptoms vary from fifty to as high as ninety per cent. Seventh nerve palsies are next in reported frequency. It is interesting to note, that, aside from the more general involvement of the oculomotor nuclei, there are definite geographical differences in the distribution of the affection of the cranial nerves.

Though in most instances the lethargic state remains a single episode at the very onset of the malady, relapses may occur. One boy of thirteen years had encephalitis in January, 1925, when he spent two weeks in bed; he slept continually for ten days, had fever up to 103°, saw double, and had twitchings of his face, legs, and arms; after two months, there was again an elevation of temperature and he slept for three days. Since then, for over a year, he had periods of somnolence, lasting from a few hours to several days.

The *irritative-hyperkinetic form* may develop as the only initial feature of encephalitis or emerge in the course of the lethargic state. The abnormal muscular contractions may range from tic-like twitchings and jerkings to choreiform movements, athetoses, and convulsive seizures. The motility disturbances may be restricted to individual muscles or muscle groups, involve one extremity only, affect one entire side of the body, or be generalized. Hohman, quoting Goodhart and Kraus and citing examples from his own case material, describes as "dystonias" movements which involve certain larger muscle groups, are simpler and less bizarre than athetotic performances and have a more purposive appearance. One of his patients displayed a constant slow rhythmic raising of the shoulder and abduction of the arm, with flexion of the elbow and partial supination of the hand; another showed frequent rhythmic repeated movements of flexion at the knee. The relative monotony of the choreiform picture in encephalitis as compared to Sydenham's chorea, is also emphasized by Eckstein.

The *atypical forms* may show all sorts of deviations from the more classical disease patterns. Often the acute stage is so mild and uncharacteristic, that a diagnosis cannot be established until later when the appearance of typical sequelae retrospectively shed light on the real nature of a seemingly insignificant and transient febrile stupor, an unexplained convulsion, or ptosis. This is also true of the forms which during the acute phase do not essentially differ from an ordinary upper respiratory infection. At times the onset is linked up with some mild infectious disease, though it may be evident from the after-effects that a lethargic encephalitis must have taken place and not an encephalitis associated with mumps or pertussis or whatever the illness might have been which has later been made responsible by the parents for the ensuing changes.

The acute stage is often followed in children immediately by what has been termed a *post-acute period* (*nachakutes Stadium:* Stern). It is then, if not already at an earlier date, that extreme *overtalkativeness* makes itself perceptible. It was Hohman who called attention to this peculiar phenomenon. He states: "Words pour out in veritable torrents and often this overtalkativeness is not accompanied by an oddity of thinking, expression, or activity. In some cases there may be great overactivity as well and the child presents then a typical hypomanic picture. In some cases the overtalkativeness and overactivity may persist for years."

Especially interesting and pathognomonic for the post-acute stage is the peculiar *reversal of the sleep curve* which was first described by Von Pfaundler and later by Hofstadt under the name of agrypnia. The reader will find it discussed in the chapter dealing with the sleep disturbances of children. For the sake of completeness, it may be mentioned in this connection that also during the acute onset persistent insomnia may be a disturbing symptom which, according to Hohman, is of ominous prognostic significance.

Lethargic encephalitis resembles syphilis in this respect that after an apparent recovery from the primary insult a variety of pathological symptoms may develop at a later time on the basis of the original damage. Sometimes there may be a direct continuation of neurological, metabolic, and mental disorders. The initial restlessness, reversal of sleep, or tic-like movements may be sustained for long periods, the original strabismus or epileptiform seizures may last a lifetime. Again, there may be an interval of from several months to as many as five years in which there is no outward evidence of any disturbance, physical or mental, and following which, without the slightest noticeable provocation or in the wake of some seemingly insignificant discomfort, one or more typical sequelae may make their appearance. Some of them may have been present in a rudimentary or more conspicuous form during the acute or post-acute stages; others enter into the clinical picture as something new and foreign to the individual. The outstanding syndromes were enumerated by Hohman as follows:

1. Behavior and mental disorders.
2. Sleep disorders.
3. Parkinson-like syndrome.
4. Tics, chorea, athetoses.
5. Paralytic and convulsive residuals.
6. Endocrine syndromes and vasomotor disorders.

The first two types of disturbances may be grouped together as psychobiological disorders, the next three as neurological sequelae, and the last item may be classed as vaso-vegetative dysfunctions.

Of the *neurological* group, the *amyostatic*, or *akinetic-hypertonic*, or *Parkinsonian symptom* complex, which is observed in about fifty per cent of adult cases, is less frequent in children. Already in the acute stage, a mask-like expression of the face with marked reduction of mimetic activity and a certain degree of general rigidity is a common observation. These features, however, give way to a restoration of the normal muscle tone, and the face resumes its usual physiognomy. It is not until some time later that the paralysis agitans type of symptoms gradually assumes characteristic and easily recognizable proportions. There is a progressive slowing of motility and of the mental activities. Speech becomes monotonous. The arms are held in flexed position and do not swing in walking. There is constant drooling, with the saliva flowing over the chin down on the clothes, forming a thin pane between the half-open lips, or hanging down from the mouth like a thick rope. The body is bent forward, and there may exist the typical Parkinsonian propulsion or retropulsion and speeding up of the gait. The cog-wheel phenomenon may be elicited. This development is rarely seen in children younger than ten years of age. The prognosis is not favorable.

Among the hyperkinetic sequelae, *choreiform and athetoid movements* have been observed. *Tic-like performances* are not infrequent. These are a few complaints gathered from the material at the Harriet Lane Home for Invalid Children and the Henry Phipps Psychiatric Clinic of the Johns Hopkins Hospital: "Twitching of shoulders and face; marked grimacing." "Sniffing." "Nose blowing, more especially at bedtime." "Habit of hitching his coat over his abdomen." "Spitting, which began three years after onset, not present in school nor at night; at home she keeps going to the bathroom or to the coal scuttle and spitting into it." "Snapping the fingers all the time and picking the nose." "Blowing the nose in a peculiar fashion; drawing the mouth to the side 'as if he were going to have a fit'." "Stuttering." "Putting her fingers in her mouth and then rubbing her hair with the wet fingers; a good deal of respiratory activity in the form of sighing and puffing."

Respiratory disorders are not uncommon in postencephalitic states; Jelliffe devoted a special monograph to these phenomena. He quotes Gabrielle Levy's classification which (with slight modifications) is as follows:

1. Disorders of respiratory rate (tachypnea and bradypnea).
2. Dysrhythmias or disorders of respiratory rhythm (Cheyne-Stokes, breathholding spells, forced or noisy expiration, inversion of the inspiration-expiration ratio).
3. Respiratory tics (yawning, hiccough, spasmodic cough, sniffing).

In addition to the tics, Hohman mentions the occurrence of *obsessive-compulsive features*, such as rubbing the cheek and ear after wetting the fingers, crossing oneself in rhythms of three, nine, or twenty-seven, and similar modes of behavior. It may also be stated in this connection that Hohman was one of the first investigators in this country to report "forced conjugate upward movements of the eyes" which have become known as *oculogyric crises;* they are seen chiefly in Parkinsonian patients. Hohman thinks that the eye muscle spasms are "evidence of a persisting inflammatory focus in the midbrain." His four patients were all adults. We have seen this condition in a fifteen-year-old boy who had acute encephalitis at five years and whose crises ("His eyes go up in the air") were followed by headaches.

The *paralytic residuals* are most frequently concerned with ocular and facial palsies. In many instances, the ptosis and strabismus of the acute stage are transitory but sometimes they may persist. Hemiplegias, diplegias, or paraplegias are relatively rare. *Convulsions* may continue long beyond the onset, and in some infrequent instances they may not appear until a few years after the acute encephalitis.

With regard to *metabolic* after-effects, the most outstanding feature is the rapid gain of weight of some of the children. One of our patients gained eighteen pounds within two months. The clinical picture of dystrophia adiposo-genitalis has been reported. Diabetes insipidus has been observed. Sexual precocity is sometimes noticed. Single cases of severe hypertrichosis have been described.

The postencephalitic sequelae which are especially difficult to handle, which are often not recognized as such by the parents, the school authorities, and the general practitioner, and which may pass for a long time as "plain meanness" and be treated with unsuccessful punishments, are the *behavior disorders* which are not at all uncommon in these children. A few of the complaints may serve as eloquent examples:

A boy of twelve years, an only child, who had "always screamed louder than other children," had an attack of fever, vomiting, and delirium, which was diagnosed as "influenza," in March, 1926. He was in bed for three weeks. About two weeks after getting up, he again had vomiting spells with pain in the right side of the head and neck, lasting two days. Since then, there was a marked change in his general behavior. He kept barking and growling like a dog and shaking his head, at which time he seemed fully absorbed by his actions. He developed a voracious appetite and gained weight rapidly. He complained constantly of rightsided headaches. He became very restless, quarrelsome, and threw himself about at home and in school. He had temper tantrums. He spoke of being weak in his knees and fell occasionally. He had a small pet dog of whom he had been very fond and whom he had guarded and protected previously; after the change of character had taken place, he cruelly mistreated the animal. There was a coarse tremor of his hands and he held his jaw rather rigidly when talking. At twelve, he had a mental age of a little more than thirteen years.

A boy had for two weeks, at the age of five years, a "stupor with some features of delirium," after which he was awake and restless at night and wanted to sleep all the time during the day for a whole year. In the delirium he had been heard to say "Take that radiator off my chest." For several months following the "stupor," he had unaccountable flights of temperature, up to 105°, with vomiting and drowsiness about twice to three times a week. Since then, according to his parents, he never was the same; he was "like a different child." He became progressively more difficult to manage. After stuttering for about two months soon after the onset, he developed the habit of sniffing. He was afraid of the dark, of dogs, of being hurt, and of traveling in trains "for fear of a railroad wreck" (no one of his acquaintance had ever been in one, nor had he ever witnessed a traffic accident). Since the age of eight years, he grew gradually more and more irritable and had violent temper tantrums, sometimes without any evident provocation. When reading a book, he would suddenly throw it on the floor; afterwards he would cry and feel sorry, saying that "there was something in him, he just could not help it." He would dig scissors into anyone who crossed him; once he chased his grandmother with a carving knife; another time he held his brother, four years his junior, under the water in the bathtub. He had a fierce hatred of his brother (the only other child in the family) since he had wanted a sister and had been promised he would get one. He had talked of getting rid of his brother and of killing him. He hit him over his head when the little boy was three years old; the child "never was without bruises somewhere" inflicted upon him by the senior sibling. When taken to a restaurant and apparently engaged in eating, he suddenly stopped, screamed at the top of his voice, threw the dishes on the floor, cursed his mother, and attempted to run away. He professed to be very religious, prayed a good deal, said that he "does not want to sin." He had become very childish in his play, would not associate with other children, had a battered doll to which he clung all the time; he took it everywhere, dressed it, talked to it, fed it, tried to sew for it, and slept with it. He had a peculiar way of playing with his hands; he pretended that they were dinosaurs, moved them toward one another and made them fight, walked them up imaginary cliffs and acted as if they fell off. His affections varied from demonstrativeness to cold indifference. When observed for some time, he appeared extremely restless, got up, sat down, walked about the room, made constant movements with his fingers and hands, pulled at his sleeves, rubbed the thumb of one hand over the finger tips of the other, twitched his face, etc. When put to bed at night, he would lie and stare at the ceiling and talk to himself for three or four hours, sometimes till three o'clock in the morning; his mother would find him breathing through his teeth and working his hands like claws on either side of the face. In his sleep, he had fright reactions of the pavor nocturnus type. He wet the bed every night. His intelligence remained normal. He was in the course of several years examined by several physicians who declared him to be a "spoiled child." His parents separated on his account; his father said he could not live in the house with such a child, claiming the whole behavior picture was due to the mother's indulgence, as the doctors had said. No school would keep him. Upon the recommendation of Dr. Esther L. Richards, he was placed in a suitable boarding home in the country where, under consistent discipline, he showed steady improvement. He slept ten hours during the night, attended school regularly, and behaved well. A certain amount of overtalkativeness and the respiratory tic of sniffing were kept up for some time.

In the following, we abstract briefly a few further behavior pictures from the case records of postencephalitic children:

Complete change of personality with restlessness, irritability, inability to concentrate enough to stick to school work or the simplest job. Violent temper tantrums when crossed. Later open stealing. A reformatory refused to keep the boy because of excessive masturbation and homosexual activities. Frequent changes of positions, stealing from employers; wandering about the streets for the rest of the day when sent on an errand in the morning. At fourteen, when sent to deliver goods, he would be found in the servants' quarters trying to make illicit advances to the maids. In the juvenile court for stealing a bicycle.

Abrupt change of character following a one-week-period of droopiness, sluggishness, and diplopia. The girl developed attacks of yawning and of dyspnea, after a typical post-acute stage with reversal of the sleep curve. Explosive outbursts in which she would strike people; combativeness and screaming spells in school. Tic of blowing the nose. Fine tremors of the tongue and fibrillary twitchings of the lips on showing her teeth. Extremely hyperactive deep reflexes, the slightest touch with the fingers eliciting a tremendous response. Intelligence remained normal.

"Sleeping sickness" at seven years, with somnolence for three weeks ("Sometimes it was hard to tell whether he was living or dead"), double vision, and delirium ("He saw things, he saw people passing his bed in the daytime"). Then his whole disposition changed. He used to be a quiet, contented, well-behaved boy. After his illness, he always wanted to be on the go, visiting everybody in his village, telling invented stories; careless about his appearance, would not sit still at the table, dropped food, was easily excited, cried a good deal, had temper outbursts. He developed the habit of spitting and drooling. He had headaches, divergent bilateral strabismus, and exophthalmos. At ten, he had a mental age of eight years.

Change of personality with restlessness and peculiar activities. Tendency to rhythmical movements of the hands, such as wiping them across his lips. The boy roamed about the streets, gazed at the stars and threw kisses at them. Often gave irrelevant and disconnected answers. (What city is this?—"Baltimore, Maryland. The Indians were the only real Americans.") Slight ptosis of right eyelid; the right side of the face somewhat smoother than the left. Mental retardation of about eighteen months at seven and a half years.

The striking feature in all of these examples consists in every single instance in an alteration of the patient's personality sooner or later after the acute stage of epidemic encephalitis. Children who have been quiet, manageable, obedient, well-trained, become generally restless, overactive, intractable, disobedient, and manifest asocial and antisocial tendencies which have been alien to them before. There is a constant but ill-regulated push of motor activity, expressing itself in the inability to stick to one thing for any length of time, running about, changing the goal or even lack of any apparent goal, jumping, shouting, laughing, crying, overtalkativeness, explosiveness, destructiveness. Routine becomes practically impossible. In school, the patients are inattentive and cannot concentrate on their studies; scholastic progress, therefore, suffers even in those pupils whose intelligence has not been impaired. They become wilful, stubborn, are given to temper tantrums, lose any feeling of sympathy, become cruel, hit their playmates, teachers, and parents, use obscenity, lie, steal, wander away from home, and drive their environment to exasperation. Threats, punishments, rewards, admonitions have only very temporary results. The children do for moments regret their misbehavior, they may apologize and promise improvement and be sincere in their promises. They often feel that they "could not help it," as if some irresistible force has driven them to act as they did. Any regret, however, is only transient, and they immediately go back to the same mode of behavior. There is a marked lability of affect, moodiness, periods of indifference and lack of consideration for others alternating with touching tenderness. As the picture progresses, the children may become dangerous to their surroundings, mistreat brutally smaller siblings and playmates, are liberal with the use of their fists and teeth and fingernails, with weapons of all sorts from a stick or stone to knives and pieces of furniture. One seven-year-old boy nearly shot his uncle to death with a loaded revolver which he had removed from the pocket of an automobile and threw lighted matches into a haystack. Sexual delinquencies are not infrequent, from forcing other children to practise mutual masturbation to exhibitionism, homosexuality, and rape. Occasionally paranoid trends exist; the children complain that people are talking about them and have it in for them. The symptomatology varies in the individual cases. The behavior bears no appreciable relation to the physical condition, except that the slow Parkinsonian is less apt to display so drastic and violent a reaction as the postencephalitic non-Parkinsonian. Nor is there any necessary relation to the type of home environment; children from stable and well-adjusted families may show the same form of disturbance as those coming from less desirable homes.

Thiele, in his excellent presentation of the psychiatric residuals of encephalitic children and adolescents, distinguishes three principal foundations of the behavior disorders:

1. Pathogenic, process-determined character changes.

2. Reaction tendencies which had been a part of the patient's original personality make-up, made dormant by adequate training, and becoming manifest ("activated") under the influence of the disease.

3. Reactive misbehavior arising from a response to being ill and the closely associated changes in the living conditions and in the attitudes of the environment. It is these "secondary" features that, according to Thiele, can be used as the most promising lever and starting point for a therapeutic approach.

It is most remarkable that the personality change may sometimes run in exactly the opposite direction. Grossman reports the case of a ten-year-old boy who before his illness had been wilful, quarrelsome, difficult to manage, and always up to some mischief; following a mild attack of encephalitis, he became docile, obedient, and amiable, and stopped fighting with his brothers and sisters.

In some cases, the *intellectual abilities* suffer no losses. In the majority, there may be two distinct types of mental deterioration. The mental growth of a child who is hit at an early stage of development, during the first two or three years of life, may come to a complete standstill. The achievements acquired prior to the illness may remain or be damaged only to a slight degree, but nothing new is learned afterwards. Thus, when seen at school age, those patients have the typical characteristics of idiots or low grade imbeciles. If the encephalitis occurs during school age, there is often only a partial development of further attainments, with a gradual dropping out of previous acquisitions. This results in a Binet-Simon performance which is typical of various forms of organic illness, the anergastic picture with a low baseline and considerable scattering below and above the age at which the encephalitic attack had occurred. It does, of course, also happen that lethargic encephalitis is engrafted upon a constitutionally feebleminded child.

The postencephalitic *sleep disturbances* may be a continuation of the post-acute reversal of the sleep curve. Occasionally, this "agrypnia" does not make its appearance until a few years after the onset of the illness, but this is a rather rare occurrence. Sometimes one finds in the later life of these patients a condition which closely resembles narcoleptic attacks, except that the cataplectic component is usually absent.

Considering the polymorphous nature of the disease, it is easily understood that, save in times of an epidemic, the *diagnosis* may offer considerable difficulties. Barker has enumerated the conditions with which the acute stage is most likely to be confused. They are: meningitis; influenza and grippe infections; Heine-Medin disease; the infectious form of multiple neuritis; typhoid fever; mumps; infectious arthritis or myositis; tetanus; hydrophobia; forms of encephalitis, myelitis, or encephalomyelitis other than those due to the specific virus responsible for the lethargic form; uremia; acidosis; cholemia; drug intoxication (veronal, cocain, alcohol, etc); botulism; cerebral hemorrhage, cerebral thrombosis; cerebral embolism; sinus thrombosis; cerebral atherosclerosis; cerebral, cerebellar, pontine, or cerebello-pontine angle tumor. The classical syndrome of fever, somnolence, diplopia and other ocular disturbances offers the least diagnostic difficulties, especially if followed by the typical and pathognomonic post-acute reversal of the sleep curve.

The postencephalitic sequelae, especially the psychobiological alterations, are easily recognized if they can be traced back to an acute encephalitic attack. Once one has become acquainted with the abrupt personality change, it is difficult not to think of it if a similar history is presented. Otherwise the mistake is not infrequently made that the patients are treated for a long time as "bad" and "mischievous" or as "psychopathic personalities" or sometimes as "hysterical." In one of the cases quoted above, the child had for a long period been termed "spoiled," with the result that his father indignantly left his wife, who, so he had been advised, had through her overindulgence brought about the patient's unbearable behavior disturbance. The absence of cataplectic seizures and a history of double vision or other symptoms of the acute encephalitic stage will serve as criteria distinguishing postencephalitic sleep disorders from true narcolepsy.

There exists no specific *treatment* of acute lethargic encephalitis. "Not only," says Hohman, "do we have no reliable or even promising therapy for the disease itself, but since we know nothing about its mode of contagion we are powerless to suggest measures for the control of the spread of the disease. Isolation is to no point, because we know of no contact infection." Convalescent serum is reported to have had beneficial results in some few cases, especially of sporadic encephalitis; yet in a disease with such a varied course and unpredictable prognosis it is possible that the casual improvement may not have been due to the serum, after all. Lumbar puncture has been recommended. It is useless to recite the many drugs and other remedies that have been attempted, since none of them has had a noteworthy effect. The illness takes its course, an unforeseen, capricious course, regardless of the initial symptoms, differing geographically, differing individually, with no definite chronology in the sequence of stages (Achard has called encephalitis a polymorphous and "acyclic" disease).

Of the sequelae, the Parkinsonian syndrome offers the best therapeutic possibilities. Hyoscin hydrobromide, in initial doses of $1/150$ gr. in older children and $1/1000$ gr. in patients under three years of age, increasing slowly to larger units, four times per day, helps to relax the rigidity and to improve the mental slowing.

With regard to the postencephalitic behavior disorders, all investigators agree that little can be done to resocialize the patients. Bond and Appel have recently sounded a more optimistic note in their monograph in which they describe the good results of their intramural methods of personality readjustment. Of the forty-eight cases which they tabulate, there were twenty-nine "good" boys and girls made "bad" by the disease, six "bad" boys made "worse," and thirteen boys who had been in trouble since infancy. Of the total number, six made an "excellent" adjustment, in twenty-one the results of treatment were "good," in four "fair," nine were "improved," there was a "slight gain" in six, and "no gain" in two patients while managed within the walls of a hospital school (Department for Mental and Nervous Diseases of the Pennsylvania Hospital in Philadelphia). Twenty-six children followed after being discharged, have the following behavior record at home: "Excellent," three; "good," three; "fair," one; "doubtful," seven; "poor," twelve. It therefore seems that protracted institutional training or, at any rate, reëducation away from the home environment offers a better outlook than ambulatory treatment or a too early return to the family.[1]

[1] It is impossible to give, within the frame of a text-book, a complete bibliography of epidemis encephalitic. A vast literature has accumulated within the past fifteen years, since Von Economo's first communication. The following publications have been selected on the basis of guiding the reader toward a good orientation rather than on that of originality or importance exclusively: Acute Epidemic Encephalitis

LEAD ENCEPHALOPATHY

Lead intoxication is more frequent in children than is stated in most textbooks, both pediatric and psychiatric. Not less than eighty cases were seen at the Harriet Lane Home. Forty of these came to the attention of the clinic within a few days; they were all negro children, coming from the same neighborhood, and the source of the lead poisoning could be traced to the inhalation of fumes from the burning of old battery casings, on sale in a small store in the vicinity.[1] All other instances but one were referable to the habit of chewing the paint off toys, furniture, and wall plaster. In one case, the family lived in a dilapidated house; the plaster kept falling from the kitchen ceiling into the cooking utensils and right into the food. Of the forty cases which did not result from the use of storage batteries for fueling purposes, nineteen were colored and twenty-one were white children. Twenty-three of the patients showed no clinical symptoms whatever, the lead line of the gums or laboratory findings being the only evidence. All others had varying degrees of bodily involvement, the mildest manifesting themselves in the forms of obstinate constipation, occasional headaches, fretfulness, occasional abdominal pain with or without vomiting. In a number of instances definite cerebral participation becomes apparent sooner or later, often resulting in signs of intracranial pressure. After days or weeks of irritability, restlessness, drowsiness, or apathy, and sometimes without such prodromal changes, sudden projectile vomiting, convulsions, visual disturbances, delirium, coma, paralysis, ataxia, or any combinations of these symptoms announce the presence of an encephalopathy. The younger the patient is, the longer the poisoning continues, the greater the intensity of exposure, and the more the children have been weakened by coëxisting diseases, the less favorable is the prognosis with regard to future development. Ten of the children died, four at the age of two years, three at three years, and one each at one, four, and five years; of these several were rachitic, one had congenital syphilis, and one had luetic parents. Intellectual arrest, often to the point of idiocy, is a frequent outcome. It must, however, be remembered that the pica habit is itself often, though by no means always, an indication of mental retardation. On the other hand, our experience justifies the plea for thinking of the possibility

---

(Lethargic Encephalitis). An Investigation by The Association for Research in Nervous and Mental Diseases. New York. 1921. (It is from this volume that Barker and Grossman have been quoted.)—Stern, Felix. Die epidemishe Encephalitis. Berlin. 1922.—Tilney, Frederick, and Hubert S. Howe. Epidemic Encephalitis. (Encephalitis Lethargica). New York. 1920.—Eckstein, A. Encephalitis im Kindesalter. Berlin. 1929.—Hohman, Leslie B. Encephalitis. In Abt's Pediatrics. Vol. VII, pp. 866–911. Post-Encephalitic Behavior Disorders in Children. Johns Hopkins Hospital Bulletin. 1922, 33, 372.—Thiele, Rudolf. Zur Kenntnis der psychischen Residuärzustände nach Encephalitis epidemica bei Kindern und Jugendlichen. Berlin. 1926.—Bond, Earl D., and Kenneth E. Appel. The Treatment of Behavior Disorders Following Encephalitis. New York. 1931.

[1] Williams, Huntington, Wilmer H. Schultze, H. B. Rothchild, A. S. Brown, and Frank R. Smith. Lead Poisoning from the Burning of Battery Casings. Journal of the American Medical Association. 1933, 100, 1485–1489. (Contains a good bibliography on lead intoxication in children.)

of saturnism in all cases of low degrees of feeblemindedness; the question as to whether the child was in the habit of gnawing paint should always be included in the history taking. In the absence of a typical lead line, the diagnosis can be made by the examination of the blood for achromia and basophilic stippling of the red blood cells and for spectroscopic evidence of lead,[1] of the spinal fluid for increase in cells, globulin, and in pressure, and roentgenologically by lead deposits at the end of the long bones bordering on the epiphysis.[2] The treatment consists of immediate removal of the source of the intoxication and the administration of phosphates.

JUVENILE PARESIS

The occurrence of general paresis, or dementia paralytica, in the young was first observed in 1877 by Clouston,[3] whose patient, a sixteen-year-old boy, presented clinical features similar to those seen in adult paretics. Since then, hundreds of cases have been reported and smaller or larger series collected and analyzed. By 1903, approximately one hundred and forty instances had been published. At the present time, the case descriptions contained in the literature are almost innumerable.[4]

[1] Shipley, P. G., F. McN. Scott, and H. Blumberg. The Spectrographic Detection of Lead in the Blood as an Aid to the Clinical Diagnosis of Plumbism. Bulletin of the Johns Hopkins Hospital. 1932, 51, 327.

[2] Park, E. A., D. Jackson, T. C. Goodwin, and L. Kajdi. X-Ray Shadows in Growing Bones Produced by Lead; Their Characteristics, Cause, Anatomical Counterpart in the Bone and Differentiation. Journal of Pediatrics. 1933, 3, 265.

[3] Clouston, T. S. A case of General Paralysis at the Age of Sixteen. British Journal of Mental Science. 1877, 23, 419–420.

[4] The outstanding monographic presentations based on a thorough study of larger groups gathered from the literature or from the investigators' own material are listed below:

Gudden, H. Zur Ätiologie und Symptomatologie der progressiven Paralyse mit besonderer Berücksichtigung des Traumas und der im jugendlichen Alter vorkommenden Fälle von Paralyse. Archiv für Psychiatrie. 1894, 26, 430–471.

Alzheimer, A. Die Frühform der allgemeinen progressiven Paralyse. Allgemeine Zeitschrift für Psychiatrie. 1895, 52, 533–594. Forty-one cases (thirty-eight from literature and three of his own).

Thiry, C. La paralysie générale progressive dans le jeune âge. Thèse de Nancy. 1898. Sixty-nine, all from literature.

Mott, F. W. Notes on Twenty-two Cases of Juvenile General Paralysis with Sixteen Postmortem Examinations. Archives of Neurology. 1899, 1, 250–327.

Hirschl, J. A. Die juvenile Form der progressiven Paralyse. Wiener klinische Wochenschrift. 1901, 14, 515–518. Twenty cases, observed within a period of ten years.

Frölich, W. Über allgemeine progressive Paralyse der Irren vor Abschluss der körperlichen Entwicklung. Inaugural-Dissertation. Leipzig. 1901. Forty-seven cases.

Wollburg, G. Über Dementia paralytica im jugendlichen Lebensalter. Inaugural-Dissertation. Kiel. 1906. Thirty-three cases.

Fairbanks, A. W. General Paresis in Childhood. Journal of the American Medical Association. 1908, 51, 1946–1954. Thirty-eight cases.

Dahl, W. Über jugendliche progressive Paralyse. Inaugural-Dissertation. Würzburg. 1909. Seventy-one cases.

Upon Klieneberger's suggestion offered in 1908, it has become customary to limit the designation of juvenile paresis to the cases arising from congenital lues and to speak of those rare conditions which develop on the basis of early acquired syphilis as "early forms of progressive paralysis" (*Frühformen der progressiven Paralyse*).[1]

Whereas in adult paretics the male sex predominates at a ratio of approximately two to one or three to one, the distribution is about equal among boys and girls (Alzheimer, Ziehen, Bleuler), with perhaps a small preponderance of the incidence in boys (1.6:1.0 in Menninger's group; 1.4:1.0 in that studied by Schmidt-Kraepelin; 1.3:1.0 in Frölich's cases; 1.2:1.0 in Wollburg's material). A few authors (Régis, John Thompson, Wigglesworth) report a slight predilection for the female sex.

The age at *onset* was previously believed to coincide with the inception of puberty. Statistical compilations of a more recent date have tended to call for a revision of this opinion. The greatest frequency of the first manifestations of the condition has been found to lie between the ages of eight and ten years in boys, and between ten and twelve years in girls. In exceptional instances, the diagnosis was established before the sixth year of life (never earlier than during the fourth year). It seems worthwhile to quote a statement made by Menninger with regard to the beginning of juvenile paresis: "There are two very distinct types of onset: the vague and indefinite development of the disease in a mentally and often physically inferior child which may be apparent at birth or soon afterward; second, a more or less acute break, after some years of normal development of the child. In a later stage of the disease, these two groups are not distinguishable clinically and at any stage they are identical serologically." Similarly, John Thomson states: "The disease may set in in children who had previously seemed quite normal; but, in most cases indications of mental defect have been present from early infancy."

Since juvenile paresis always depends on a *hereditary transmission of syphilis*, two lines of investigation have suggested themselves: a study of the offspring of adult paretics and an examination of the antecedents of juvenile paretics. The classical communications of Junius and Arndt are of especial informative value.[2] They found that, while the average fertility of the total population of Berlin amounted to three children for each mar-

---

Huguet, J. F. J. Observations et réflexions sur la paralysie générale dans le jeune âge et la syphilis héréditaire. Thèse de Paris. 1913. Seven cases.

Schlicht, J. Kasuistische Beiträge zur Lehre von der juvenilen Paralyse. Inaugural-Dissertation. München. 1905. Fourteen cases.

Schmidt-Kraepelin, T. Über die juvenile Paralyse. Berlin. 1920. Forty cases.

Klauder, J. V., and H. C. Solomon. Juvenile Paresis with a Presentation of Twenty-Three Cases. American Journal of the Medical Sciences. 1923, 166, 545–559.

Menninger, W. C. Juvenile Dementia Paralytica. A Study of Forty Cases. Journal of the American Medical Association. 1930, 95, 1499–1502.

[1] Klieneberger, O. L. Über juvenile Paralyse. Allgemeine Zeitschrift für Psychiatrie und psychiatrisch-gerichtliche Medizin. 1908, 65, 936.

[2] Junius, P., and M. Arndt. Über die Deszendenz der Paralytiker. Zeitschrift für die gesamte Neurologie und Psychiatrie. 1913, 17, 303.

ried couple, that of 1869 paretics (1312 men and 557 women) did not exceed 1.5 births; of these, 1.4 were still living at the time of the onset of the father's illness, and only 0.7 (for each married couple) when the mother broke down; the number of stillbirths was twice as high as that of stillbirths in the whole populace. Thirty-six per cent of all pregnancies terminated in abortions, miscarriages, or stillbirths. Including these cases, the mortality of the children of paretics was seventy-one per cent. It did not differ essentially from the mortality of the offspring of tabetic parents and of luetic parents with no neurosyphilitic symptoms. These figures fully explain why juvenile paresis is so much less frequent than dementia paralytica in the adult; a considerable proportion of the children die before they have an opportunity to develop the clinical features of the condition. (The relation between juvenile and adult paretics admitted to the psychiatric clinic in Munich was, according to Schmidt-Kraepelin, 40:2184, or 1.83%; the expectancy of paresis in children with congenital lues is given as 1.7%, that of paresis in 4134 syphilitic Austrian army officers was calculated by Mattauschek and Pilcz[1] to be 4.8%.)

Similar research on a much smaller material was carried out by F. Plaut and M. K. Göring (*Untersuchungen an Kindern und Ehegatten von Paralytikern. Münchener medizinische Wochenschrift. 1911, 58, 1959*). Of 244 pregnancies in a total of 54 families with one paretic parent, one hundred and thirty children survived. Of the one hundred studied, forty-five had suffered physical or mental damage. Eighteen of these had a positive, four a doubtful, and twenty-three a negative blood Wassermann. Seventeen were retarded intellectually.

As regards the ascendency of paretic children, the most comprehensive data were furnished by Schmidt-Kraepelin. 17.5% of the fathers only and 10% of the mothers only admitted luetic infection. The Wassermann reaction was positive in 22.5% of the parents. Neurosyphilis was present in 25% of the parents of the juvenile paretics. The syphilitic origin could be determined in 65% of the patients, either through statements obtained anamnestically, through the examination of the blood of the parents or siblings, or through the history of the mother's many abortions and miscarriages. Paresis in the near relatives of these patients is not infrequent. As a matter of fact, H. A. Bunker, Jr., and S. B. Meyers (*An Anthropometric Study of General Paralysis. American Journal of Psychiatry. 1928, 7, 1027*) quote H. C. Solomon as saying that "he has never seen a patient with juvenile paresis whose father or mother did not present either symptomatic or serologic evidence of neurosyphilis." Of ninety cases reported by Frölich and Klieneberger, fifteen (ten boys and five girls) had a paretic parent; not less than eight of the ten boys had paretic fathers, and not less than four of the five girls had paretic mothers. The relatively frequent combination of paresis in father and son or in mother and daughter is indeed remarkable and has been noticed also by several other authors (e.g., Pilcz). The occurrence in siblings is exceedingly rare; it has been reported

---

[1] Mattauschek, E., and A. Pilcz. Zweite Mitteilung über 4134 katamnestisch verfolgte Fälle von luetischer Infektion. Zeitschrift für die gesamte Neurologie und Psychiatrie. 1913, 15, 608.

by A. Hoch (*General Paralysis in Two Sisters, Commencing at the Age of Ten and Fifteen, Respectively. Autopsy in One Case. Journal of Nervous and Mental Disease. 1897,24,67*) and Klauder and Solomon (two sisters). Familial concurrence of juvenile paresis and tabes or other forms of neurosyphilis has been observed by H. J. Smith (*Presentation of a Tabetic Child and Paretic Parents and Brother. Journal of Nervous and Mental Disease. 1916, 44, 66*), M. Nonne (paresis and tabes in a brother and sister. *Über die Bedeutung der Syphilis in der Ätiologie der Tabes. Fortschritte der Medizin. 1903, 21, 977*), J. Grinker (mother and first son tabetic, second son paretic, third child, a girl, had cerebral syphilis of the vascular type. *A Case of Juvenile Tabes in a Family of Neurosyphilitics. Journal of Nervous and Mental Disease. 1904, 31, 753*), and others. It is remarkable that, while paresis is seen in certainly not more than from one to three per cent of the offspring of paretic parents, neurosyphilis, and particularly general paralysis, is found to be much more frequent in the antecedents of children with juvenile paresis.

The syphilitic etiology of juvenile (as well as adult) paresis has been established beyond any trace of uncertainty. We are, however, not sufficiently informed about the problem why it is that certain congenitally luetic children develop the condition, while others are spared. The theory of the existence of a neurotropic virus has not been definitely proven. The literature abounds with controversial claims; one faction makes the nature of the spirochete responsible, whereas another group looks for an explanation in the patient's personality make-up.

Often *traumatism* is brought into etiological connection with the onset of the condition by the parents or other informants. Frequently a careful investigation reveals the insignificance of the injury, which in retrospect appears magnified in the eyes of the family. In other cases one may find that the time interval between the reported fall or similar accident and the first signs of paresis has been much too long to permit of any thought of causal relationship. In a number of instances, finally, the trauma is a result rather than the cause of the illness, in that the child's deteriorated mental condition and especially his loss of judgment makes him less aware of the presence of danger and of the need of self-preservation and thus deprives him of the necessary caution.

We precede the discussion of the clinical picture by the presentation of a typical case:

Howard B. came of an unstable family. His father died in 1929 at the age of forty-three years of alcoholism. He was a lithographer by trade but never held a position for any length of time. He had been a drunkard since adolescence and often stayed away from home for several days at a time. He sat around the house "thinking" for hours when sober. The mother died in 1919 of influenza, when Howard was three years old; she had two miscarriages before the birth of the patient, who remained an only child. She was an obese (she weighed 204 pounds), unintelligent woman. The father's brother, Charles, a saloon keeper, divorced after considerable matrimonial difficulties, died in 1928 of alcoholism and pulmonary tuberculosis. Another paternal uncle, Milton, divided his time between jails, a State Hospital for the Insane ("paranoid condition with alcoholism"), and a State Tuberculosis Sanatorium; when on parole or after escaping from any of these places, he threatened to kill his wife, his sister, and other people and sometimes actually assaulted them. He and his family had been supported by charitable agencies since 1898. The father's third brother, Joseph, "drank himself to death" fifteen years ago; he was syphilitic. Another brother, George, was sober and more stable than the rest; one of his daughters, mentally deficient, had been treated for gonorrhea and had an illegitimate child; one son, twelve years old, I.Q. of 58, had a record of habitual truancy, nailbiting, and frequent masturbation; another son was brought to the Juvenile Court at fourteen years because of larceny.

Howard was born on March 31, 1915. He had pneumonia at six weeks. At three months, he began having convulsions, starting in the left leg "until he shook all over"; they recurred "off and on" for one year. When three months old, he was taken to a dispensary, where the diagnosis of congenital lues was made on the basis of a positive blood Wassermann. His parents did not bring him back for treatment, nor did they submit to the recommended examination of their own blood. He began to walk "weakly" at eighteen months; he did not talk until a little over two years of age. After that he developed well and was considered a "strong, active boy."

Since three years of age, after his mother's death, he was raised by his maternal grandparents. He entered school at six years but missed nearly all of the first two semesters because of measles and bronchitis. He then did very well in his studies for two years. He had always presented a feeding problem and "had to be humored to eat." He was enuretic until about ten years of age. He was spoiled considerably; his grandmother would not let him play with other children, she was afraid "he would be run over or something would happen to him."

He reached the fourth grade at nine years, without any noticeable difficulties. At that time, there developed a marked decline in his scholastic achievements and a deterioration in his general behavior at home and in school. He repeated the fourth grade and, at ten years, he was placed in an ungraded class until his grasp became so defective that the teacher advised that he be taken out of school entirely and kept at home.

During the same period, he became more and more irritable and very restless. He began to cry at the slightest occasion. His speech, which had been clear before, was careless and indistinct. When eating, he got food on his face and hands and clothes.

At the age of twelve years, he had a mental age of seven years and two months (I.Q. 59). At fourteen and a half years, his mental age was five years and two months with a baseline of four and scattering up to seven years (I.Q. 35). During these two and one half years, he deteriorated considerably in every respect. His physical examination showed that his pupils were unequal in size (left much larger than right), irregular in shape, and did not react to light. His speech was inarticulate and indistinct. There were Hutchinsonian incisors and poor development of the dental enamel. The tongue deviated slightly to the right. Genitalia were underdeveloped and pubic hair was sparse. Ophthalmoscopically, a central macular degeneration was noted in the right eye, and in the left eye there was a large patch of atrophic choroiditis just above and to the temporal side of the nerve head. His vision was impaired as evidenced by groping. He had a prominent Olympian brow. Blood and spinal fluid Wassermann reactions were strongly positive. There was a two plus Pandy and a cell count of 5. The colloidal mastic test was 3321000000.

His behavior, at fourteen and a half years, was that of a child hardly older than three years. He had wet and soiled himself for the past few months. His vocabulary was narrowed down substantially. He mostly occupied himself with a picture book, pointing to objects and talking in a baby-like manner in simple words and phrases, such as "See the dog," or "There is a horse," repeating them over and over. He did not reply to questions but responded to simple requests. There were occasional short-lived crying spells and episodes of screaming and destructiveness.

A few months later, he was reported to put everything he picked up into the stove and to play with fire. He became unable to dress himself. On several occasions he wandered away from home aimlessly. He spoke of hearing and seeing things.

He was committed to a State Hospital in March, 1930. He was inoculated with malaria and later given sulpharsphenamine intravenously and intramuscularly. In September, 1930, he was reinoculated; after that he received bismuth salicylate and arsenicals. He began to have numerous convulsions, sometimes a whole series lasting for a full hour. His gait became unnatural and awkward. His vocabulary was limited to the one word, "pussy cat." He was utterly untidy. A third malaria treatment in March, 1932, and mercury inunction did not halt the progress of his deterioration. Blood and spinal fluid Wassermann remained positive throughout, the cell count rose to 24, the colloidal gold curve in February, 1932, was 5544332100.

At present, the boy is utterly helpless, completely demented, and merely vegetates.

The *physical symptoms* of juvenile paresis are in many ways similar to those of adult patients. The *pupillary changes* are the most frequent and most striking findings. In the following table, we give some of the figures which K. Weiler (*Untersuchungen der Pupille und der Irisbewegung beim Menschen. Zeitschrift für die gesamte Neurologie und Psychiatrie. 1910, 2, 101*) observed in adult paretics, as contrasted with those which W. Stöcker (*Über eigenartige Unterschiede im Pupillenbefund bei progressiver Paralyse der Erwachsenen und der juvenilen Form. Zeitschrift für die gesamte Neurologie und Psychiatrie. 1914, 26, 564*) and Schmidt-Kraepelin obtained from their studies of juvenile patients (all numbers are given in percentages):

Pupillary changes	Adults (Weiler)	Children	
		Stöcker	Schmidt-Kraepelin
Anisocoria	27	67	60
Reflex rigidity	57	17	12.5
Absolute rigidity	34	67	82.5
No changes	9	11	5
Optic atrophy	4–12 (Gudden, Kraepelin, Mendel)	33	17.5
Irregular outline		39	35

It appears from this table that difference in the size of the pupils, absolute rigidity (that is, failure to respond to both light and accommodation), and optic nerve atrophy are more common in juvenile paresis and that reflex rigidity (that is, lack of reaction to light with preservation of the contraction upon convergence) is more frequent in adults.

In the juvenile form, hyperactivity of the *tendon reflexes* is more common than their decrease or total absence. Ankle clonus and the Babinski phenomenon are also more apt to be elicited. All this speaks for a preference of the illness for the affection of the pyramidal tracts to the degeneration of the posterior columns (Homburger).

There is also a greater frequency in the occurrence of all sorts of *tremors, spasms, convulsions,* and *contractures.* In the case history quoted above there were "spasms" between the ages of three months and one year and then again rather severe convulsions during the last two years. Toward the end, shortly before death, as many as a hundred and more convulsive seizures may happen in one day. The attacks may be epileptiform in character or resemble more the Jacksonian type. The different forms of episodes which may take place in the course of the illness range from mild headaches and migraine-like conditions with nausea and vomiting, fainting spells with general tremors, attacks of dizziness with grinding of the teeth, to outspoken convulsions.

The *speech disturbances* resemble more closely those of the adult form; in paretic children one often hears a sort of articulation which is similar to "baby talk" and later slowly deteriorates into indistinct and unintelligible mumbling. The test phrases devised for older people ("Third riding artillery brigade"; "Methodist Episcopal"; "Around the rough and rugged rocks the ragged rascal ran"; "She sells seashells at the seashore;" etc.) are hardly applicable, mainly because some of the words contained in them are not known to the little patients. The speech difficulties come out noticeably enough in conversation or when the child is requested to count quickly. The speech usually is clumsy, thick, monotonous, and not well articulated; at the beginning, or in milder degrees, it is merely halting and hesitating; in others it is more hasty, precipitated, and abrupt, and after a good beginning, soon ends in indistinct mumbling. Slurring is frequently observed. A good deal depends on the progression of the illness and the state of general deterioration. In the case which we have quoted it is seen how within a few years a boy with normal phonation gradually lost the ability to pronounce words and to express himself, until his vocabulary contained the only remaining word, "pussy cat." There is a short step left from this condition to absolute mutism. In the earlier stages, faulty sentence formation (agrammatism) and the substitution of wrong words for the ones intended (paraphasia) may be noted. Or syllables may be omitted, or reduplicated, or transposed, or sometimes there may be a seemingly compulsive "logoclonic" repetition of the same word or word fragment. Towards the end, in cases of extreme dementia, shouting and screaming may become the only form of vocal activity.

The *handwriting* may also be impaired in the sense of tremulous characters, omissions, repetitions, and transposition of letters or words, failure to write in straight lines, orthographic errors, and substitutions (paragraphia). The ability to write may finally be totally lost, or the script becomes meaningless and cannot be deciphered.

The *gait* equally depends on the patient's general condition. It may be well preserved for a long time. There may be a tendency to stumbling as the first indication of a motility disorder. Spastic gait is more frequent than ataxic gait in juvenile paretics.

Romberg's sign seems to be less common than in adults. Coarse tremors of the tongue and lips, however, are a not unusual condition, as are circumscribed paralyses which mostly occur as residuals after convulsive seizures.

It may be said that the majority of the patients are undersized and generally underdeveloped. Hypogenitalism is quite common. In the girls, menstruation begins late or never.

Sensibility is usually not affected in the earlier stages, and later it can hardly be determined because of the child's inability to coöperate intelligently.

Serologically, the Wassermann reaction of the blood is almost always positive; the spinal fluid presents pleocytosis, increased globulin, positive Wassermann reaction, and the characteristic paretic colloidal gold curve.

The principal feature of the *mental disturbance* consists in a *progressive intellectual deterioration*, involving chiefly comprehension, memory, and judgment. The native endowment, as measured by the Binet-Simon test, may have been average or below normal. In both events, we usually are informed by the parents or by the teacher that after a year or two or three years of smooth progress in school there has been a noticeable slump with ever declining capacity. This is not a temporary standstill as in the non-paretic dull or moron child, who has to wait until he slowly reaches another year of mental age within a chronologically much longer period of time, but a definite and rapid retrogression or rather loss of something that has already been achieved. The deficit is not an even one at the beginning; there is a dropping out of some functions, while others are still preserved. While in the feebleminded person the intelligence quotient remains stationary within the limits of a few points upward or downward, it sinks incessantly in the juvenile paretic. Furthermore, the unevenness of the downfall manifests itself in a considerable scattering in the test. A patient who at the age of eight years, before the onset of the illness, had an I.Q. of 100, may at ten have one of only 70, with a baseline of six years, and at twelve one of about 50, with a base of not more than four years, doing perhaps a number of five, six, seven, and eight year tests but none of those normally performed by a nine-year-old child. In other words, we have a type of intellectual deterioration which is quite characteristic of all progressive anergastic reactions in children of school age. The result is that the patient at first fails in his grade and then, where there are no ungraded classes, keeps being demoted to an ever lower grade until finally the parents are advised to remove him altogether from the school.

The *impairment of comprehension* is slow and gradual. At first, it is the more complicated new things that the child has difficulty to grasp, such as introduction of long divisions, decimals, fractions, or grammatical rules. Later on, simpler explanations are not understood. In severe cases, when the dementia has far progressed, verbal communications may no longer have any meaning to the child, who not only has lost his own capacity for oral expression but also the conception of remarks, however trivial, that are made in his presence. Ultimately, attentive fixation and looking about may be the only signs that the patient takes any notice whatever of what goes on in his environment.

It is remarkable that, as long as orderly conversation can be maintained, the *impairment of memory* and of immediate recall is much less pronounced in children than in adult paretics. Korsakoff pictures with confabulations hardly ever occur in the juveniles.

Judgment is most gravely affected. There is no realization of illness. Criticism and self-criticism are abolished. In spite of poor marks and constant demotion, the patients are mostly satisfied with their school achievements. Only occasionally do they complain of lack of concentration. They make contradictory statements without in the least sensing the discrepancies. Knowledge of the difference between right and wrong, beautiful and ugly, harmless and dangerous becomes sooner or later abolished.

Simultaneously with all this, there is a steady decline in the child's *formal behavior*. After maintaining good habits of conduct and cleanliness for a number of years, he becomes slovenly in his table manners, spills food on his clothes, eats voraciously and indiscriminately (just "gobbles"), loses his bowel and bladder control, is subject to ever changing moods, cries easily, has temper outbursts, mumbles to himself, appears absentminded and is generally childish in all his performances.

Very often, the general deterioration of intelligence and conduct remain the outstanding clinical feature. We then speak of the *simple form* of paretic dementia. In a small number of patients, the picture takes on a more *euphoric* and slightly *expansive form*. Delusions of grandeur hardly ever reach the grotesque and limitless dimensions which they assume in the adult. The child may brag about his ability, his beautiful clothes, his pretty singing voice, or his brilliant future, but he does not own and dispense millions of dollars and does not possess all the banks and railroads of the United States or of the world, as do the older paretics. Even these *small delusions of grandeur*, as they have been called (by Babonneix), are mostly of a transient nature. The *depressive form* of paresis is still less common in children. Here again the mood is not so outspoken as in the adult. The patient is shy, slightly hypochondriacal, and easily frightened.

The *pathology* of the illness does not differ essentially from that of adult general paresis. Autopsy reports stress the presence of chronic leptomeningitis, cortical atrophy, a large amount of fluid in the pia-arachnoid spaces and in the ventricles, changes in the pyramidal tract and in the posterior columns, and small weight of the brain.

The *prognosis* has been absolutely bad until the introduction of the malaria treatment, and even now is far from inspiring great optimism.

The *diagnosis* is comparatively easy if one considers the character changes, the speech alterations, the pupillary symptoms, the decline in intelligence with the scattering in the Binet-Simon test, and the typical laboratory findings.

Inoculation with malaria or relapsing fever, which may be combined with the administration of mercurials or arsenicals or bismuth, holds out some hope, however slight. Schmidt-Kraepelin, in her monograph, has given a review of the various modes of treatment employed in juvenile paresis (malaria is not included), which we quote below:

A. Symptomatic remedies:
   Narcotics. Hypnotics. Antispasmodics.

B. Etiological remedies:
  a. Antisyphilitic drugs: Mercury. Potassium iodide. Salvarsan (intravenous) and salvarsan-serum (intraspinal). Fowler's solution.
  b. Fever producing remedies: Sodium nucleinicum. Tuberculin.
  c. Antitoxin producing remedies: Dead streptococcus cultures. Typhoid fever. Cholera. Relapsing fever.
  d. Organotherapy: Lipoid emulsions (subdural). Lymph gland extracts. Tela choroidea. Bone marrow preparations.

Institutional care in a well conducted hospital is advisable from the beginning of the illness and indispensable in later stages.

CEREBRAL TRAUMA

Any physician has had the experience that parents are prone to explain behavior difficulties of their children on the basis of some early fall or automobile or other accident, assuming that the impact has permanently damaged the brain. Often the physician is called upon to give his own opinion in individual cases on the connection between bodily insults and later psychopathological developments; the question comes up in many court litigations.

One may roughly divide cerebral traumatism in childhood into three groups:

1. Antenatal injuries, due to a fall of the gravid mother or to a direct and violent insult to the pregnant uterus.
2. Birth injuries.
3. Postnatal head trauma.

Not enough is known about those antenatal injuries which did not lead to abortions, miscarriages, or stillbirths or to early death. The differentiation post partum between intrauterine and natal insults is often exceedingly difficult.

Birth injuries have been made the subject of valuable anatomical and clinical studies for the past seventy years, since the publication of W. J. Little's classical paper, *On the Influence of Abnormal Parturition, Difficult Labor, Premature Birth and Asphyxia Neonatorum, on the Mental and Physical Condition of the Child, Especially in Relation to Deformities (Transactions of the Obstetrical Society, London, 1862, 3, 203).* Important investigations are linked permanently with the names of Sigmund Freud (*Cerebrale Diplegien. Wien. 1892*), Sir William Osler (*The Cerebral Palsies of Children. A Clinical Study from the Infirmary for Nervous Diseases. Philadelphia. 1889*), Gowers, Sarah J. McNutt, B. Sachs, G. S. Collier, Bronson Crothers, Ylppö, Dollinger, Ph. Schwartz (*Erkrankungen des Zentralnervensystems nach traumatischer Geburtsschädigung. Berlin. 1924*), F. R. Ford (*Cerebral Birth Injuries and Their Results. Medicine. Baltimore. 1926, 5, 121-194*), and many others. Ford came to the conclusion that "cerebral birth injuries are rather rare than common, and the great mass of infantile palsies can no longer be lightly attributed to faulty obstetrical procedures." He felt that "the true cerebral birth palsies are represented by the congenital hemiplegias, the monoplegias and the asymmetrical and unequal bilateral spastic paralyses." On the other hand, he stated that "very convincing

(the parts — both arms or legs —)

evidence has been gathered that the congenital diplegias which constitute by far the largest group of infantile spastic palsies as seen in the pediatric department (235 out of 280 in all) are not attributed to meningeal hemorrhage at birth, but are the result of various pathological processes of intrauterine origin." The outstanding causes of cerebral birth injury are direct insults to the head while it passes through the birth canal, due to difficult or protracted labor, damage done through instrumental delivery or breech extraction, precipitate labor, and prematurity; reduced coagulability of the blood, giving rise to hemorrhagic disease of the new-born, has also been claimed as an etiological factor which, however, has not been accepted by many investigators.

We are here interested mainly in the problem of the *psychopathological consequences* of birth injuries. According to Ford, most of the infants with congenital diplegia (which he does not consider a result of birth injuries) fail to reach the second year of life; "mental defect obviously could not be estimated accurately, but was almost invariably present." On the other hand, he finds that "intelligence is comparatively unaffected" in the congenital monoplegias, hemiplegias, and double hemiplegias of a definitely traumatic origin. "Severe grades of mental defect," he states, "are probably not related to birth injury with the exception of that type which develops in association with frequent convulsions." Ford's studies confirm the statement of Weygandt who, in his monograph on idiocy and imbecility of children in Aschaffenburg's *Handbuch der Psychiatrie*, warns against too ready a connection of faulty intellectual development with difficult birth or labor. Whereas many authors attribute from five to twenty per cent of serious mental defects to birth injuries (Piper: 9% Potts: 12%; Wulff: 14%; Beach and Shuttleworth: 17.5%), Tredgold does not feel that more than 1.5 per cent of all cases of idiocy can be traced to birth trauma as an etiological factor and that those children are invariably epileptic.

On the other hand, Groves B. Smith reported recently that of fifty children with histories of birth injuries, 22 per cent were normal intellectually, 16 per cent were morons, and not less than 62 per cent belonged to the group of "uneducable" defectives (40 per cent imbeciles and 22 per cent idiots). He concluded that "the existence of associated epilepsy, athetoid movements, and speech defects tends to cause personality deviations and 'scattering' in intelligence tests, which renders the intelligence as being somewhat unreliable both in evaluation of the present mental level and as a prognostic indicator of future development." He found antisocial tendencies in the group with the least mental retardation, the behavior being characterized by irritability and lack of concentration. Cameron pointed out that palsied children, because of their poor control over their bodies, miss in their infancy the information that healthy babies derive from crawling and later walking all over the house and from various sorts of manual exploration; due to the lack of such experience they often seem to be less intelligent than they afterwards turn out to be, and their chances for ultimate improvement under education should not be underrated.[1]

[1] Cameron, H. C. Intracranial Birth Injury. Lancet. 1923, 2, 1292—Cameron, H. C., and A. A. Osman. Late Results of Meningeal Hemorrhage in the New-Born. British Medical Journal. 1923, 1, 363.

Schroeder, from whose article we quoted the data pertaining to Smith's study, made an investigation of 146 behavior problem children referred to the Institute for Juvenile Research in Chicago and classified as having infantile cerebral palsy; in addition, he studied 79 children showing signs of cerebral injury at birth without developing palsies. He found that difficult labor tends to determine behavior problems which, however, are chiefly the result of mental retardation. Distractibility and hyperactivity are characteristic traits in the birth traumas but no behavior difficulty is specific. Children with cerebral birth injuries who do not develop palsies show the behavior characteristics and mental retardation common to those with cerebral birth palsies; differences in behavior that occur in this group are largely explained by the absence of orthopedic handicap. Schroeder feels that children with cerebral injury at birth who show distractibility and hyperactivity, although free from birth palsies, should be included in the classification of the results of birth trauma. It must be mentioned that Schroeder's material is made up mainly of children who have been brought for examination *a priori* because of retardation, delinquency and "nervousness," so that birth injured and birth palsied children not having any of those difficulties did not come to his attention.[1]

The results of *postnatal injuries* have been studied mainly in adults. It is, from this point of view, highly significant that so thorough and excellent a book as *Nervous and Mental Disorders from Birth Through Adolescence* by Sachs and Hausman devotes barely one page to the discussion of *Injuries to the Brain and Its Coverings*, giving a brief description of concussion and dealing just as briefly with fractures of the skull. The best classification of the psychopathological sequels of cerebral trauma comes from Adolf Meyer. He distinguishes:

1. Direct post-traumatic deliria.
   a. Delirium accompanying febrile conditions.
   b. "Delirium nervosum" of Dupuytren, not differing from deliria after operations, etc.
   c. Delirium as a phase in the slow emergence from coma following trauma.
   d. Protracted deliria, usually with numerous confabulations.

2. The Post-traumatic Constitution.
   a. Mere facilitation of reaction to alcohol, grippe, etc.
   b. "Vasomotor neurosis," headaches (especially on stooping or sudden changes of position), dizziness, attacks of meningismus, increased fatigability, irritability, intolerance to alcohol. (This form has been described by Friedmann and attributed by him entirely to vasomotor irritability.)
   c. "Explosive diathesis" (Kaplan). Great irritability, especially after the use of alcohol, sometimes leading to acts of violence often quite unmotivated or even to an epileptic seizure.
   d. "Hysteroid" or "epileptoid" episodes (in the form of "absences") with or without convulsions.
   e. Types of paranoic development.

[1] Schroeder, Paul L. Behavior Difficulties in Children Associated With the Results of Birth Trauma. Journal of the American Medical Association, 1929, 92, 100–104.

3. Traumatic defect conditions.
    a. Primary defects allied to aphasia.
    b. Secondary deterioration in connection with epilepsy.
    c. Terminal deterioration due to progressive alteration of the primarily injured parts, with or without arteriosclerosis.

4. Psychoses in which trauma is merely a contributing factor: General paralysis, manic-depressive and other transitory psychoses, catatonic deterioration and paranoic conditions.

5. Traumatic psychoses from injury not directly affecting the head.[1]

In children, it is especially disorders of the second category that are met with as the result of cerebral trauma. Where intellectual defects occur, they are mostly connected with convulsive phenomena. The term *dementia traumatica*, as used among others by Ziehen, should be employed with the greatest caution. Sometimes mental retardation has been present but not recognized by the family before the injury. We have, as a matter of fact, seen cases where the head injuries were the result rather than cause of feeblemindedness. A retarded boy who had not learned how to avoid danger ran with all his might with his head against a stone post, sustaining a severe injury; the same child once turned on the gas jets and crawled into the baking oven, calmly awaiting further developments. Weygandt says rightly: "It is difficult to answer the question with regard to traumatic idiocy; undoubtedly there exist single indisputable cases. Generally, however, the accident is often overrated as an etiological factor." We have seen one child, a girl now twelve years of age, who would fit into Meyer's group 3a; after a fall down the cellar steps at the age of two and a half years, she lost her speech entirely and has never been able to learn to speak or to comprehend spoken or written language, while she is well capable of communicating through signs and gestures.

Pierce Bailey, in 1903, reported irritability, temper tantrums, boisterousness, fighting, and unmanageableness as the main behavior problems of several children who had sustained cerebral injuries. An eight-year-old boy showed marked personality changes after being run over by a heavy wagon. His parents could no longer control him, he was extremely irritable, fought his playmates constantly, went into "violent passions," got out of bed at night and moved about the house. It is this type of post-traumatic character alterations which has caused several authors (for example Osnato) to draw analogies between the results of head trauma and the sequels of encephalitis. Kasanin, who studied the personality changes in children following cerebral trauma, finds that there are certain resemblances, especially as to extreme emotional instability, temper tantrums, egocentricity, and inability to follow a definite goal in life. He continues: "The parallel stops when we come to the question of ultimate prognosis. As seen from our cases, there is, in spite of a long period of various conduct disorders, a tendency toward adjustment on a somewhat lower level, while the cases suffering from sequelae of epidemic encephalitis show, as followed to the

[1] Meyer, Adolf. The Anatomical Facts and Clinical Varieties of Traumatic Insanity. Proceedings of the American Medico-Psychological Association. Washington, May, 1903.

present time, a grave prognosis." In all but one of Kasanin's fifteen cases (all boys) there is evidence of marked emotional instability and antisocial trends. Stealing figures in the complaints about eleven of the boys, temper tantrums in eight, marked irritability, truancy, and staying away from home in six each, restlessness is a feature in several of the cases, less common difficulties were masturbation, homosexuality, attempted intercourse with the sister and other girls (in one instance), lying, disobedience, cruelty, destructiveness, depressive features, vasomotor instability, fatigability, enuresis, and grimacing. In eight cases, the accident was followed by severe headaches, and marked vertigo figured in three of the boys. Kasanin emphasizes the diagnostic importance of the frequent inability to stand heat or closed-in places; Healy has also laid stress on this particular characteristic. It is of interest to note the great frequency of psychoses, alcoholism, convulsions, and serious other difficulties and maladjustments in the families of the majority of the patients.[1]

In the cases of forensic complications, the testifying physician will do well to familiarize himself with the following facts:

1. The exact nature of the accident.

2. The exact nature of the injury: Concussion? Skull fracture? Unconsciousness? Urinary or fecal incontinence? Convulsions? Headache? Vertigo?

3. The neurological residuals.

4. The presence and nature of personality changes.

5. The child's pre-traumatic personality.

6. The contribution of the family's attitudes (overindulgence, fostering of hypochondriacal developments, etc.) to the child's behavior difficulties.

Thereapeutically, in the case of birth injuries, one will receive a good deal of help from orthopedic measures, in addition to patient habit training, school education which is adapted to the child's intellectual capacity, and vocational guidance which would give to the patient a certain degree of usefulness within (that is, neither above nor too far below) the limits of his physical and mental abilities. Where the intellectual retardation does not warrant the expectation of even a relatively small degree of self-dependence on however simple a level, commitment to an institution would be the logical step. Considering the details of the capacities, development, and treatment of birth injured children, we refer to the excellent monographic presentation by Doll, Phelps, and Miss Melcher.[2]

In postnatal head injuries, surgical intervention may become necessary, depending on the nature of the trauma. The personality changes call for the best that mental hygiene and psychotherapy can offer. In the milder

[1] Bailey, Pierce. Fracture at the Base of the Skull; Neurological and Medicolegal Considerations. Medical News. 1903, 82, 919.—Osnato, Michael, and Vincent Giliberti. Postconcussion Neurosis—Traumatic Encephalitis. Archives of Neurology and Psychiatry. 1927, 18, 181.—Kasanin, Jacob. Personality Changes in Children Following Cerebral Trauma. Journal of Nervous and Mental Disease. 1929, 69, 385.—Healy, William. The Individual Delinquent. Boston. 1927.

[2] Doll, Edgar A., Winthrop M. Phelps, and Ruth T. Melcher. Mental Deficiency Due to Birth Injuries. New York, 1932.

cases, adjustment may be attempted in the home with the aid of the family and the school authorities. Sometimes the transfer to a less indulgent and less solicitous environment with simplification of the demands and diminution of temptations is beneficial, such as removing the child from the bad influences of his "gang" associations and from the tempting vicinity of Five-and-Ten Cent Stores and movies and placing him in the tranquillity of farm life. In the severe cases of domestic unmanageableness and incorrigibility, commitment to the stern discipline of a correctional institution will have to be considered.

CHAPTER XX
DYSERGASTIC REACTION FORMS

THE ANERGASTIC reaction forms, based on structural damage to the central nervous system, are usually of a protracted, even permanent, character. They are either progressive, leading to a continuous mental deterioration with or without periods of remission. Or the losses once sustained remain stationary without further impairment. Or there may be a certain degree of spontaneous or therapeutic restoration of the disturbed psychobiological functioning which, however, mostly fails to attain the complete reorganization of the pre-psychotic personality. There exists another group of psychopathological reaction sets which are also, in most instances, bound to somatic disorders, are of a more transient type, and depend on temporary metabolic and toxic damage rather than on more or less irreparable tissue alterations of the brain. The cerebral disturbance is usually of an edematous nature. The resulting mental pictures are those of delirium, hallucinosis, stupor, and coma. These conditions have been grouped together by many authors under the heading of "amentia," but this designation has also been applied to other, altogether different states and has occasioned a good deal of unnecessary terminological confusion. Adolf Meyer speaks of them as *dysergastic reactions*. They may sometimes occur in the course of anergastic dysfunctioning (e.g., delirium in epidemic encephalitis, coma in brain tumors and in meningitis) and as symptoms of some of the "functional" psychoses (hysterical delirium, schizophrenic and depressive stupors), but as a rule they accompany infectious, toxic and auto-toxic diseases of various kinds; this is especially true of delirium and coma. In children, febrile convulsions must also be included in this category.

DELIRIUM

It is astonishing that one rarely finds in the literature satisfactory descriptions of delirious reactions of children despite the fact that they are observed so frequently in the various forms of infantile infections. It is also remarkable that Homburger's *Psychopathologie des Kindesalters* mentions no delirium other than the hysterical. This neglect may be due to the experience, expressed by Bleuler, that "children react quite easily with delirium, so that in them the psychical disturbances do not have a great significance." Ziehen, on the other hand, paid much attention to the occurrence and forms of the delirious reactions in children and collected a most valuable bibliography.

In contradistinction to the French, who use the term delirium for all delusional states with or without clouding of consciousness and with or without hallucinations, German and American psychiatry has reserved this appellation for "a reaction characterized by hallucinatory fancies, usually of a fearsome or worrisome nature, or dreamlike, either with disorientation or at least with a misinterpretation of the situation due to haziness or scare" (Meyer).

It is difficult to state at what earliest age delirious reactions occur. Before disorientation or misinterpretation can take place, the child must have grown old enough to be oriented and capable of correct interpretation and to give evidence of this capacity as well as of its impairment. Typical delirious pictures have been observed in infants as young as sixteen months; they were especially outspoken in cases of atropin poisoning. Those babies, in addition to displaying the specific physical signs of the intoxication, were extremely restless, irritable, and were seen to grasp for imaginary objects and to pick things out of the air. Whether delirium exists or, at any rate, can be clearly recognized before that age, remains an open question.

From an *etiological* point of view, the delirious reactions of children may be divided into the following groups:

Infectious deliria accompanying the period of incubation, the febrile state, or the stage of defervescence.

Toxic deliria.

Deliria connected with nutritional disorders.

Deliria occurring in the course of anergastic conditions.

Hysterical deliria.

Before entering into a discussion of the individual groups, it is well to describe briefly those symptoms which are common to all forms. The outstanding feature consists in a *clouding of consciousness*. The patients are obviously confused, in a dreamlike state, unable to think clearly for any length of time and to fix their attention on the thread of a regular conversation, on their playthings, or on other objects or occupations. They often stray from one thing to another and may keep busying themselves with various incoherent activities, pulling at the bedclothes or making various motions the meaning of which may sometimes be identified with fragments of purposive performances, such as handling toys or doing the home work (*occupational deliria*). The children are *not fully oriented* as to time and space; while sick in bed, they may at times believe that they are playing out in the street or visiting relatives or attending classes. The parents, siblings, doctor, and nurse may be mistaken for other persons and woven into the delirious dream contents. *Hallucinations* occur mainly in the visual sphere. They are usually very vivid. They may be of a simple nature, taking the form of flashes, colors, moving clouds, or people, animals, angels, devils, various freaks are seen. The emotional tone is mostly one of *fear*. The patients imagine that something painful or dangerous is being done to them; the dream assumes a highly dramatic shape in which bizarre tortures and persecutions frighten the child. *Illusions* are often present; the curtains or a towel are mistaken for ghosts or burglars. Imagination and reality are not kept apart and form together a weird mass of fleeting, tormenting, scary, loose, irrational scenes. In exceptional cases, the grotesqueness may evoke amusement in the child; but usually the reaction to the imagination is one of crying, screaming, begging for help, and defensive movements. At other times, a certain paralyzing helplessness is felt, in which the youngster is entirely passive and accepts the flood of experiences which overwhelm him as an inevitable fate.

Infectious deliria are especially common in typhoid fever of older children. They are relatively rare in infants. Under eight years, typhoid fever is often associated with a surprisingly clear sensorium. The delirium is often largely nocturnal. Persecutions and hallucinations play a leading rôle. There is apparently no relation between the occurrence and type of the reaction and the degree of fever. The onset does not depend on any particular stage of the illness.

William G., almost twelve years old, was admitted on March 31, 1931, at the beginning of the second week of his illness. On April 8, it was first noticed that he seemed fearful and spoke incoherently about someone trying to run away with him. He later told the ward physician that someone had attempted to kidnap him. The next morning, upon questioning, he stated that during the night people had come and tried to carry him away. He said, "they have gone out there," pointing to the window. He told of similar experiences every morning. He was disoriented until April 17. He kept speaking of "the Uptons" (his neighbors) "who live over there in the woods." The Uptons put him in a chair and gave him electric shots but the Police Department stopped them from doing that. He saw the policeman march past his room. A nurse, so he said, put a rag over his mouth, "so I couldn't holler." People kept entering through the door and leaving through the window. The nurse sprinkled something over the food that made him sick. On April 18, he was fully clear and recalled all of these experiences, declaring that they were "imaginations," but still insisted that one night when he yelled the doctor came with a gun.

James C., fourteen years old, during the period of defervescence, appeared frightened and had the following experiences, mostly at night: An airplane tried to get him. Once, people wanted to stick him in the back and threw daggers at him but he ducked them. "They took hooks and stuck me up there and tried to make a mummy out of me and told me not to make a secret of it and they would let me go." He feared, when people came toward him that they would split him open; he was afraid to eat for fear of poison; he said he had killed someone who was now in a coffin just outside his room. One evening, he stated that a man had gone after him and thrown a knife into his leg and the doctors put a cast on his leg; he said it was still on but when the covers were removed he remarked that he guessed somebody had taken it away; a little later, he believed that he had three casts on. When asked whether he knew one of the physicians present in the room, he replied: "No . . . Yes, I have seen him before. I don't know which one shoots poison, but there is one that cries all the time when he shoots poison." He thought that his father was outside in the hall: "I saw him. He is Tarzan of the Apes. He is Lord Greystone. I am Jack Greystone."

Sometimes the typhoid confusion is associated with transitory aphasia or with cataleptic phenomena. A boy of not quite five years of our own observation presented for approximately twenty-four hours the picture of waxy flexibility (flexibilitas cerea) on February 7, 1932; the illness had begun on January 20.[1]

[1] Kanner, Leo. The Occurrence of Cataleptic Phenomena in Children. Journal of Pediatrics. 1934, 5, 330–340.

(It is known that typhoid fever in the early years of childhood may sometimes result in the arrest of mental development; this result has been ascribed to meningitic and encephalitic influences. Transient post-typhoid psychoses have been described as depressions, hypomanic states, and hallucinoses).

Delirious episodes have been reported in acute inflammatory rheumatism, scarlet fever (especially on the first day), pneumonia, mumps (very rare), malaria (with visual and auditory hallucinations), diphtheria (relatively infrequent), erysipelas, measles (infrequent, sometimes during the incubation period), typhoid fever, septicemia, typhus, and in other acute infectious diseases. Any febrile illness may at times produce a delirious reaction in children.

The duration of an infectious delirium may vary from a few hours to several days, rarely more than a week. The full-fledged syndrome with disorientation, fear, hallucinations, and dramatic dream production is usually preceded by a state of general malaise, drowsiness, and blunting of the sensorium. The children are in an irritable and whining mood which may persist in the more lucid intervals of the delirious stage. The delirium disappears either when the temperature goes down or when the general condition improves. In the case of aggravation of the sickness, the psychic reaction may assume the form of a stupor or of a comatose state. Occasionally some of the dream experiences may remain for some time after the illness as residual delusions.

Toxic deliria are in children much less frequent than those occurring in the course of febrile diseases. Belladonna and stramonium intoxications are typical examples. The patients show the characteristic physical symptoms of atropin poisoning; the pupils are widely dilated and do not react to light and to accommodation, the mouth is dry, the pulse rapid, and the face is red and flushed. The delirious features are illustrated by the following case reports:

Ida B., a colored girl of not quite three years, drank from a bottle nearly ten drachms of tincture of belladonna at 10:30 A.M. At eleven o'clock she was seen lying on the floor. On being picked up, she was limp, cried and groaned. She grasped for hallucinated objects, went through the motions of putting invisible food into her mouth, and struck at non-existing people who seemed to annoy her. She was extremely restless. Her speech was wild, rapid, and indistinct; she appeared to address imaginary persons. She recovered completely following the administration of an enema and gastric lavage.

James P., two and a half years old, awoke at three o'clock in the afternoon from his nap, could not stand up, reached for objects which did not exist, seemed excited, jerked his arms, and threw himself about in a wild manner. His father discovered near his bed a bottle labeled "Eye drops" which was empty. When admitted at 5:30 P.M., the child was raving; he talked constantly but did not articulate any words, kicked, yelled, made all kinds of noises and went through motions as though reaching for objects out of the air. He was instantly given morphine and a gastric lavage, and pilocarpin at seven o'clock in the evening. He was well the next morning.

A negro child had a cold. Her mother sent to the drug store to get some senna leaves to make "tea" for her. She put a handful of the leaves into a quart of water which she brought to a boil for a few minutes and gave about half a glass each to Geraldine, aged four, and Vessie, aged nine. Geraldine, within thirty minutes, seemed wild and excited and could not walk. The parents then noticed that the druggist had given them "stramonium leaves" by mistake. When admitted a few minutes later, the child's pupils were wide and fixed, her face flushed, her mouth dry, and her pulse rate 140. She thrust her arms about and cried out when she was touched. Her stomach was washed out, she was given morphine immediately and pilocarpin later. She was normal at the end of forty-eight hours. Vessie went to bed soon after drinking her "tea" but got up about forty minutes later, descended the stairs and fell when she reached the kitchen. She seemed unconscious and rolled from side to side. Upon admission, she was wildly excited, spoke rapidly and violently and threw her arms about constantly. She was well the next morning.

It is said that feebleminded children, especially Mongols, are particularly susceptible to atropin poisoning. Cocain delirium is most unusual in children. Cases were reported of intoxication with solanin, santonin (fear, visions, inability to walk and to speak), hyoscin (vision of fire, hearing of noises, motor excitement). Alcoholic intoxication in childhood leads to coma rather than delirium. The very rare cases of children's alcoholic delirium resemble the same condition in the adult.

Delirium *on the basis of nutritional disturbances* is also very unusual. In the adult, it is especially starvation which gives rise to peculiar hallucinatory states, so ingeniously depicted in Knut Hamsun's novel, "Hunger." Sometimes cachectic conditions in tuberculosis and malaria produce similar pictures.

That delirious reactions may be seen in the course of cerebral diseases, has become evident in our discussion of the anergastic illnesses, especially of epidemic encephalitis. Head injuries may produce delirium in adults and, much less often, in children. They have been thus grouped by Adolf Meyer:

Direct post-traumatic deliria

1. Delirium accompanying febrile conditions.
2. "Delirium nervosum" of Dupuytren, not differing from deliria after operations.
3. Delirium as a phase in the slow emergence from coma following trauma.
4. Protracted deliria, usually with numerous confabulations.

Hysterical deliria will be taken up later in the discussion of hysteria.

The *treatment* of the infectious and toxic deliria is naturally directed towards the more significant etiological factors. The patients should be watched closely because in their dream-like hallucinatory experiences there is danger that they might leave the bed and walk about and come perilously near an open window or a stairway. If the child is too excited, a cold pack may be of help. Sometimes sedatives and hypnotics must be resorted to.

HALLUCINOSIS

Hallucinosis is a dysergastic hallucinatory condition which differs from delirium in that orientation is well preserved, the sensorium much clearer, and the whole picture less acute. It usually follows the infectious or toxic illness rather than being chronologically coincident. The prototype in the adult is the acute alcoholic hallucinosis with preponderatingly auditory hallucinations, fear reactions, and persecutory delusions. In children, it is exceedingly rare but has been noticed to occur in the wake of infectious illnesses. The following case is the only one which we had an opportunity to observe personally.

Franklin K., ten years old, came of a very unstable family. His father, an alcoholic, who abandoned his commission of U. S. Army captain to become a mail clerk, deserted his wife, returned after two years and suicided three days later with bichloride of mercury. His mother had little school education. Franklin was the second of three living children; the eldest wet his bed every night at the age of eleven years. The patient had always been considered as peculiar, he had been enuretic all his life, afraid of the dark, disobedient, mischievous, and had pavor nocturnus when he used to scream, "Don't let them get me!" In June, 1931, he and another boy ran away from home intending to "hop a freight train" but returned the same day when it began to rain. From August 16 to September 19, 1931, he was at the Clinic with severe tick bite fever. He had a delirium for several days at the height of the illness, with fearful dreams, terrifying visions, disorientation, and encopresis. He was clear and well behaved when discharged. At home, he gained weight and was in good physical condition. About a week after his return, he became restless and overactive, would not go to sleep until after midnight, and was observed to address imaginary companions. He often seemed frightened. He once stated that he saw a man with a bear in the corner. He developed a slight hacking cough which he said he could not help because "there were spigots being turned on" in his throat. (On examination, his throat and chest were found to be normal.) He was sent to school on October 12, but had to be sent home because he appeared scared, slightly agitated, and drank his ink. The condition cleared up almost overnight about October 20. He had remained oriented during the entire period. When seen two weeks later, he seemed completely recovered, except that his pre-typhus behavior pattern persisted. He returned to school and offered no further problems other than that in November he was caught smoking a pipe. The hallucinosis had lasted approximately four weeks.

STUPOR

In stupor, consciousness is disturbed to a much higher degree than in delirious reactions. The rapport with the environment is almost completely abolished, except that the patient can be roused with some difficulty. Most of the conditions responsible for delirium may occasionally result in stupor. Sphincter control may be preserved but is often lost. Ingestion of food is usually not disturbed. The reflexes mostly are normal. There is little or no change in the respiratory and circulatory functions.

Stuporous pictures are known to occur in catatonia, the affective psychoses, and hysteria. They often follow epileptic and epileptiform convulsions. They may appear as steps in the gradual recovery from various forms of coma or, on the other hand, in the gradual progression towards coma. A mild degree of stupor is often seen in typhoid fever.

COMA

Coma is the profoundest degree of inaccessibility in which all consciousness is totally abolished. Meyer characterizes it as "a state of complete unconsciousness and reduction of reactivity to the minimum, to heart action and respiration with more or less abolition even of nervous reflex responses, and with complete amnesia where the patient recovers." It may be "a reduction from any mental state, from the normal, from the delirious, or from the defective. It is always essentially a condition of very radical suspense of cerebral integration." It occurs in a great variety of conditions and is always a very serious symptom. It may be due to exogenic toxins (opium and most of its derivatives, chloral, sulphonal, trional, veronal, paraldehyde, chloroform, cyanides, carbon monoxide, carbon dioxide, atropin, hyoscin, the various alcohols and phenols, and lead), to infectious and autotoxic influences (typhoid fever, malaria, uremia, diabetes, liver atrophy), to intracranial disorders (traumatism—concussion and compression of the brain, tumor, encephalitis, meningitis, abscess, hemorrhage, thrombosis, embolism), and is the outstanding feature of a convulsive attack.

For differential diagnosis of the various forms of coma we must refer to the pertinent textbooks. One will, of course, be guided by the anamnestic data, inspection of the skin (color, bruises, edema, rash), the type of pulse and respiration, the odor of the breath (urinous, acetone, alcohol, laudanum), the width and reaction of the pupils, the appearance of the eye grounds, the behavior of the reflexes, the general muscle tone, the temperature, the presence or absence of convulsions, the percussion and auscultation of the chest, specific neurological signs, the laboratory examinations as indicated (urine, blood count, spinal fluid, Wassermann, Widal, special chemical analyses, spectroscopic investigation, etc.), and the condition of the patient upon awaking from the coma.

Coma, if it does not end fatally, either passes through sopor and somnolence to awakening as in natural sleep, or through stupor or sopor to delirium with ultimate recovery or transition into some chronic disorder.

The treatment and prognosis depend on the nature and severity of the underlying illness.

CHAPTER XXI

SYDENHAM'S CHOREA

COUNTLESS articles and monographs have been devoted within the past seventy years, especially by French and German authors, to the psychic manifestations of Sydenham's chorea (chorea minor, "St. Vitus's dance"). As a matter of fact, the condition has long been regarded as a mental illness akin to hysteria, until its relation to rheumatism and rheumatic heart affections was given due consideration. Attempts at a cerebral localization of the characteristic motility disorders have so far failed to produce uniform results. Transient "increase in the irritability of the thalamus" (Anton), lesion of the cerebello-thalamic pathways (Bonhoeffer), temporary damage to the corpus striatum, and diffuse toxic meningitis and encephalitis have been made responsible. In consequence of the present-day uncertainties, chorea is sometimes grouped with the organic diseases of the central nervous system, sometimes with the functional neuroses, and sometimes with the rheumatic disorders. It has been variously alluded to as a "functional nervous disorder," an "infectious neurosis," or "cerebral rheumatism." A few authors, prominent among them Kleist, have thought of a possible correlation between the psychic symptoms on the one hand and supposed diffuse cortical lesions on the other.

The motor disturbance consists of gradually developing, involuntary, jerky movements which may be bilateral to start with or begin unilaterally and after a few days or weeks spread to the other side. There is general clumsiness and difficulty of muscular coördination. The first complaint is often that the child drops objects, does not get the food properly into his mouth, and that he cannot button and unbutton his clothes as well as before. Sometimes it is noticed at an early date that the patient drags one leg a little. Sooner or later the facial muscles and the tongue may be involved; this leads to all sorts of grimaces and to an impairment of speech which becomes thick and slurred. In severe cases, the child is totally or almost totally unable to feed himself and to make himself understood. The lack of muscular control may cause the child to bump into furniture and to sustain injuries in various ways. One little girl fell down the cellar steps and hit her head severely on the cemented floor. An eleven-year-old boy who in spite of his "nervousness" was sent out to chop wood hit his head with an axe and fractured his skull. At the height of the illness, there is marked general hypotonicity. The movements usually are more outspoken when the child's attention is directed to them.

Girls are from two to three times oftener affected than boys. The ages of predilection are between five and fifteen years. Adults are by no means immune. Rheumatic diseases present a relatively fertile soil, especially in people who have had chorea before. Chorea sometimes coincides with pregnancy. According to Osler, the condition is most unusual among

186

American Indians. Weir Mitchell's statement that negroes are almost exempt can no longer be upheld.

An attack usually lasts from two to three months, but may extend over a much longer period of time. Relapses are not infrequent, particularly within two years after the first seizure.

Fright has been given a prominent place among the events immediately preceding the onset of the choreic movements. Gowers referred to it as "the only immediate cause that can be traced with any frequency." Sachs found it to be an etiological factor in 56 out of 184 cases. One of our own patients, a nine-year-old girl, developed jerking movements a few hours after opening the door to a drunken man who lurched towards the entrance and scared her so that she acted like a "wild child"; she had chronic tonsillitis, dental caries, and later rheumatic heart disease. A four-year-old boy became very much frightened when his two older brothers jumped at him suddenly in the dark; he began to shrug his shoulders while sitting at the table during the next meal. A nine-year-old girl suddenly started to twitch her right shoulder and leg after an argument at the bedside of her paralyzed mother, in which her father insisted on taking her to live with him; she preferred to live with her grandparents. It must, however, be stated that such, and even more drastic, family quarrels had occurred before that without causing the child to twitch.

Lois McE., twelve years old, developed normally and was a cheerful, lively, affectionate child. She had pertussis at one year, measles at four, diphtheria at six years. Her tonsils and adenoids were removed when she was nine years old. Since her diphtheria, she was considered a frail, delicate girl. She had average intelligence and had always done well in school. At twelve years, she was confronted with a rapid succession of difficulties. Her father, a railroad brakeman, was seriously injured by a locomotive in June; he was in a hospital during June and July. Her mother, who came from an unstable, alcoholic family, used her husband's absence for an escapade from home, leaving her four children entirely alone. For about a year, she had been depressed, brooding, and sitting around for hours at a time chewing her finger nails. She gave as the reason for her desertion her husband's meanness and violent temper. Frequent verbal arguments had culminated in May in his beating her with a cane over her head in the children's presence. Lois became worried over the domestic situation and increasingly sensitive and irritable. When, in the middle of June, she was mildly reprimanded by a teacher for a trifling misdemeanor, she sobbed for a long time, whereas before that she had reacted to criticism calmly and good-naturedly. On July first, a rat bit her finger and she was extremely frightened. On July twelfth, she fainted, and when she regained consciousness, she had involuntary movements of her right arm and leg; a few hours later, the left side was also affected. The jerkings soon increased in frequency, violence, and number of areas involved, until she was in constant motion and almost completely unable to talk and to feed herself. In the hospital, she improved gradually with rest in bed, hydrotherapy, and bromides. She was entirely well by the end of October.

Frightful experiences undoubtedly figure as "exciting causes" in a considerable number of cases. One must, however, remember that the patient may have had a good many scares previously, which had no effect on the motility, and that often choreic disorder is preceded by many days or even by a few weeks of increased irritability and excitability. It is not at all unusual to learn that a sociable and well adjusted child loses interest in his play life, begins to quarrel with the playmates, becomes very sensitive, cries on the slightest provocation, and resents correction. The family and the school teacher are puzzled by the child's "nervousness"; when clumsiness and at first slight incoördinate movements appear, they are often taken for additional indications of a "nervous" condition. It is easy to understand that within these "prodromal" days the patient is much more apt to respond strongly to exciting occurrences than at other times. Furthermore, the lives of quite a few children, as for instance that of Lois McE., are sometimes so replete with various environmental upheavals, that anyone looking for excitement as an etiological factor in chorea or other diseases will be copiously rewarded. It is, therefore, not enough to inquire into specific events of a few days before the onset of the jerkings, but it is necessary to have sufficient biographical and situational data which would permit a proper evaluation of those events. Even then it will be found that in some instances there is indeed a close temporal relation between fright and the beginning of choreic unrest.

Arndt, in 1868, made the statement that there is "no chorea without accompanying mental symptoms." Ziehen went so far as to speak of a *choreic psychopathic constitution.* So much is true and has been accepted by all investigators that the general reactivity of the average choreic child differs more or less perceptibly from that of the average non-choreic child and from his own behavior before and after the illness. The outstanding features are a varying degree of emotional instability, restlessness, and difficulty of attention. The patients are fretful, cross, irritable, sensitive, fault-finding. They often change quickly and without evident reason from tearfulness to hilariousness. It is difficult to keep them in bed. They are hard to please and not easy to manage. Temper tantrums are not unusual. A few of the children even revert to enuresis, and on rare occasions encopresis has been known to occur even in older patients. Attention has been said to be diminished by some authors, while others maintain that there exists an increased vigilance (hyperprosexia) which causes the youngster to change rapidly from one subject or occupation to another. Before attributing any of these behavior deviations to the chorea proper, it is essential to know something about the patient's pre-choreic personality. It would not be correct to make the chorea responsible for irritability, temper outbursts, or fear reactions which had been present for many years previously.

Slight *delirious episodes* are observed occasionally. The patients are fearful, consciousness may be somewhat clouded, and there may be some auditory or visual hallucinations.

One boy had chorea, lasting two months, at eleven years, following a severe fright from a thunderstorm; a year later he had another attack which succeeded a scare from falling on freight car tracks and fear of being run over by a train. On the evening of that day, while thrilled by a moving picture in which he saw an ape attacking a man, he felt that "his right side gave way." He developed right hemichorea which became generalized after a few days. For about forty-eight hours, he had a slight elevation of temperature (100°); during that period he was hilarious, excited, wept a good deal, complained that people were following him to the toilet, and said that he saw green snakes on the floor. This boy had always been mismanaged at home, never had any habit training; he and two brothers were disciplinary cases in school; he had been afraid of the dark, of dogs, and of thunderstorms all his life and had frequently masturbated.

Full-blown *psychoses* are very rare in children's choreas. Viedenz observed them five times among 3.073 cases and only one of them had developed before the age of puberty. Kirby saw one case in 1.200 patients. Diefendorf found not more than three cases in a material of over 5.000 choreas. According to Bernstein, the maximal ratio of combinations of chorea and psychosis amounts to approximately three per cent. Severe delirium seems to be the predominating form. It was first described by Marcé in 1860 as *délire maniaque (maniacal delirium)*. Manic-like excitements are seen occasionally on a non-delirious basis. Stuporous states occur sometimes in chorea complicated with arthritis or endocarditis.

It is interesting in this connection that Knauer reported mental disturbances in 0.1 per cent of cases of acute rheumatic fever: 1. Cases with delirious fear reactions at the beginning, followed by a stuporous-depressive phase. 2. Cases in which excitement, normal behavior, and stupor alternated. 3. Cases which showed a condition of depressive stupor throughout without marked motor excitement. 4. Delirious excitement in the entire course of the psychosis.

Edward N. was second of four children, all of whom had the worst possible habit training. At the age of ten years, he developed rheumatic pains in his legs and arms, particularly in his knees, and, after four weeks, choreic movements involving the entire body. He became extremely restless and irritable, was disturbed by the slightest noise, threw himself on the floor, ran wildly up and down the stairs, did not sleep at night, tore his clothes, urinated and defecated in his clothes, and threw knives and chairs at anyone who came near him. He calmed down in the hospital within a few days with hydrotherapy and luminal. He recovered within a few weeks. He had rheumatic heart disease. He still is a habitual truant, has temper outbursts, and walks in his sleep.

The diagnosis of chorea is usually not difficult. The differentiation between tics, chorea, athetotic movements, and general hyperactivity of children will be discussed in the chapter on tics. Children who have once had chorea may later respond to emotional strain with similar movements. It is then very important to make sure whether one deals with a recurrence of chorea or with a more or less conscious attempt on the part of the patient to escape scholastic responsibilities or other difficulties by means of the movements. Many physicians are too ready to label any sort of motility disorder as "St. Vitus's dance." Just as it is dangerous to overlook a chorea and to expose the child to the strain of school work, so is it harmful to dismiss a youngster with tics with the "diagnosis" of St. Vitus's dance, keeping him in bed and treating him to sedatives. A correct differential diagnosis is therefore of far more than academic importance. The entire manner of treatment is altogether different.

This is not the place to go into the details of the treatment of chorea, which will be found discussed in every textbook of pediatrics. Strict rest in bed and keeping the child isolated from any possible source of excitement has a beneficial effect on the movements, prevents emotional disturbances as much as possible, and is a prophylactic measure against cardiac complications. Hydrotherapy has good results. Various sedatives have been recommended; one should, however, be careful with the dosage. In an illness, which in itself has a tendency to produce delirious reactions, they are even more apt to arise on the basis of overdoses of drugs. One case was brought to the Henry Phipps Psychiatric Clinic with a severe delirium due to bromide intoxication rather than chorea. Injection of typhoid vaccine in increasing doses has proved to be helpful in many instances. Management of the child during the period of convalescence is as important as the treatment during the illness proper. The usual activities, play, and school attendance, should be entered into gradually and under supervision. Wherever necessary, domestic and scholastic maladjustments should be straightened out while the child is isolated in bed at home or in a hospital.[1]

[1] A brief selected bibliography concerning the psychopathology of chorea follows:

Marcé. De l'état mental dans les chorées. Mémoirs de l'Académie Impériale de Médecine de Paris. 1860, 24, 1.

Arndt. Chorea und Psychose. Archiv für Psychiatrie. 1868, 1, 509.

Bernstein, A. N. Die psychischen Äusserungen der Chorea minor. Allgemeine Zeitschrift für Psychiatrie. 1897, 53, 538.

Zinn, Karl. Beziehungen der Chorea zu Geistesstörung. Archiv für Psychiatrie. 1896, 28, 411.

Viedenz, F. Über Geistesstörung bei Chorea. Archiv für Psychiatrie. 1910, 46, 171.

Kleist, Karl. Über die psychischen Störungen bei der Chorea minor nebst Bemerkungen zur Symptomatologie der Chorea. Allgemeine Zeitschrift für Psychiatrie. 1907, 64, 769.

Burr, Charles W. The Mental State in Chorea and Choreiform Affections. Journal of Nervous and Mental Diseases. 1908, 35, 353.

Diefendorf, Allen R. Mental Symptoms of Acute Chorea. Journal of Nervous and Mental Diseases. 1912, 39, 161.

Davies, Elizabeth, and T. W. Richards. The Psychological Manifestations of Postchoreic Conditions as Shown in Five Case Studies. Psychological Clinic. 1931, 20, 129.

Knauer, A. Die im Gefolge des akuten Gelenkrheumatismus auftretenden psychischen Störungen. Zeitschrift für die gesamte Neurologie und Psychiatrie. 1914, 21, 491.

CHAPTER XXII
THE ENDOCRINOPATHIES

PROMINENT among the many forward strides of recent medical progress has been the discovery of the functions and dysfunctions of the glands of internal secretion and the study of their rôle in the economy of the human and animal body. Endocrinological research has opened up new pathways and vistas of inestimable significance. Already a mass of facts has been accumulated which not only has contributed vastly to our knowledge of biochemistry and of the autonomic mechanisms but also manifoldly increased our therapeutic resourcefulness. It has been learned that certain endocrine glands have a share in the somatic participation of emotional reactions and that certain diseases of these organs may be directly or indirectly associated with psychopathological features. Just as other newly acquired fragments of knowledge have been seized upon by enthusiasts to serve as cornerstones for huge hypothetical skyscrapers, so the innersecretory glands were elevated one-sidedly and not too critically to the rank of "regulators of personality." To the psychoanalysts, the inferiority fighters, the focal infectionists, and those who immediately refer all behavior deviations to special brain centers was added another group which would reduce a considerable portion of psychiatric activity to the administration of glandular extracts and hormones. It is needless to assert that any sensible physician should and does endeavor to treat specifically endocrine disorders whenever in a given case there is evidence of their existence. Beyond that, a pluralistic inclusion and evaluation of all the factors involved will keep his vision unrestrained by theoretical blinders.

In this chapter we are concerned with the well-known and fairly circumscribed dysfunctions of the innersecretory glands so far as they have a bearing on the intellectual development and emotional reactivity of the children affected.

THE THYROID GLAND

Hyperthyroidism. Little attention has been paid in the literature to a form of hyperthyroidism to which Sir Robert Graves referred as early as in 1835, when he wrote (*Clinical Lectures Delivered During the Session of 1834-35 and 1836-38. Philadelphia. 1839, page 134*): "The well known connection which exists between the uterine functions of the female and the development of the thyroid, observed at puberty, renders this affection worthy of attention, particularly when we find it so closely related by sympathy to those palpitations of the heart which are of so frequent occurrence in hysterical and nervous females." Diffuse enlargement of the thyroid with tachycardia, with or without digital tremors, with shining eyes, but without exophthalmos and without the ocular signs characteristic of Graves' disease, is not at all uncommon in girls at the age of between eleven and fourteen years. Boys are much less frequently affected. The condition is usually transient. It is accompanied by excitability and irritability. The patients are easily fatigued and often very sensitive and there is a tendency to hypochondriacal complaints. Sometimes the children are reported to have presented behavior difficulties for many years previously. Rest, avoidance of exciting books and moving pictures, and relief from domestic and scholastic strain are the chief therapeutic measures.

Exophthalmic goiter is very rare in children before puberty. In some cases, fright or other strong emotional experiences have been mentioned as "precipitating causes." In addition to the personality disorders one encounters in the hyperthyroidism of pubescence, one may occasionally observe delirious reaction pictures, moodiness with rapid transitions from sadness to hilariousness, and in single instances even protracted states of depression or manic-like elations.

Hypothyroidism. Congenital deficiency of thyroid secretion, in the form of sporadic or endemic *cretinism*, is associated with varying degrees of a general stunting of physical and mental development. Endemic cretinism is most common in the regions of the Alps and the Himalayas; in this country, the environs of the Great Lakes, the States of Washington, Oregon, California, and Nevada are said to show a relatively high incidence. Some investigators would strongly object to one's treating the endemic and the sporadic forms together; they are the "Dualists" who consider the two as being essentially different, in contrast to the "Unitarians" who regard them as identical. Sporadic cretinism has sometimes been termed "congenital myxedema," while the endemic form has been designated by Falta as "cretinic degeneration."

The typical anomalies usually become recognizable at about the fourth month of life, sometimes as early as at one or two months. Dentition is delayed and is acquired late or not at all. Longitudinal growth is incomplete. The extremities are short and pudgy; the hands are broad, thick, and short, and the fingers square at the ends. The movements are awkward and incoordinate, and the gait is often clumsy at the beginning. The head is large, mostly dolichocephalic; the anterior fontanelle may remain open for many years. The neck is short and thick. The skin is dry, scaly, redundant, and "baggy," the hair scanty and coarse, the tongue thick, the lower lip often everted, and the forehead wrinkled. There may be pseudolipomata in the supraclavicular region and in the posterior triangle of the neck. The abdomen is bulky and prominent; umbilical hernia is frequent. The facial expression is dull, immobile, and apathetic. The voice is coarse and harsh. The patients have a low basal metabolic rate.

Some authors speak of "cretins" only if the patients are totally idiotic, have no reproductive powers, are unable to express themselves and incapable of any habit training. Other patients who reach a slightly higher level, have a limited vocabulary, attain puberty, even though later than usual, and learn to feed and dress themselves, are referred to as "semicretins." Those who develop fair linguistic capacities, who can be taught to adapt themselves to the simple demands of the environment, and even are amenable to some little scholastic and vocational education, are called "cretinoids." The patients are mostly calm and placid and seem at peace with the world. Judgment is impaired in proportion to the degree of the intellectual defect. There is a decided lack of spontaneity which, together with timidity, accounts for the fact that cretins as a group, in spite of their feeblemindedness, figure to a surprisingly small extent in the annals of delinquency. They are, however, known for their stubbornness and selfishness, though it is remarkable how rarely one sees temper tantrums in children with hypothyroidism.

Thyroid medication, carefully administered and supervised, has done wonders for some of these children, as regards both physical growth and intellectual improvement, especially in cases of sporadic cretinism. The earlier the treatment is begun, the better are the opportunities usually. If it is started later than in the sixth or seventh year, the prognosis is less favorable. Though optimism is therefore strongly indicated if the disease is attacked in infancy, one should nevertheless refrain from too pointed prognostications because, in addition to the drug and to the time of its prescription, there is an unknown individual quantity in the equation, which is, after all, responsible for the great differences in the degree of retardation of untreated cases. Sometimes one observes most astonishing progress. A girl who had only two teeth at eighteen months, walked at two years, formed words at about three and a half and sentences at four and a half years, at which time thyroid was first given, had at nine a mental age of eight and a half years and did very well in school. But as a rule, even in the average successful case, there remains a retardation of from one to two to three years as the child approaches the termination of grammar school. It is also important to know that an interruption of the medication may sometimes bitterly revenge itself and result in developmental standstill or even in a dropping out of abilities already possessed. Some children who are either too seriously retarded at the onset or whose families cannot be relied upon to provide and dispense the thyroid extract are best taken care of in appropriate institutions. Since most patients, even after marked improvement has set in, are poor critics of their limitations, judicious vocational guidance is essential to prevent them from embarking on academic or other preparations in which failure would be inevitable. Thus one boy of sixteen years, who with a mental age of not quite eleven years had with strenuous effort succeeded in reaching the eighth grade, had the ambition of becoming a pharmacist; it was learned that his very sympathetic and lenient teachers did not even see a possibility of giving him passing marks in the eighth grade. The boy was dissuaded and, as a compromise, his parents found for him a position as a clerk in a drug store where he satisfactorily dispenses soft drinks and sandwiches.

Endemic cretinism is often associated with deafness due to a myxomatous swelling of the mucous membranes of the middle ear; the hearing defect results in mutism. While thyroid medication generally has a good effect on the general myxedema, it does not improve the deafness.

THE PARATHYROID GLANDS

Manifest and latent *tetany* (*spasmophilia*) ordinarily have no psychiatric implications. The differential diagnosis between the convulsions of tetany and those of epilepsy will be taken up in a later chapter. The distinction between congenital stridor, laryngospasm of tetany, and breathholding spells will be discussed in connection with the latter.

THE PITUITARY GLAND

Hyperpituitarism. In *acromegaly* one finds complaints of fatigue, lack of concentration and of initiative, sluggishness, sleepiness, convulsions, slowness of speech, and sometimes mental retardation. That, on the other hand, the intellectual faculties may be well preserved, is best shown by the case of an acromegalic man who has for many years held a position as associate in mathematics in a leading university.

Hypopituitarism. In *Fröhlich's syndrome* (dystrophia adiposo-genitalis) one may encounter signs of general emotional and intellectual immaturity, and sometimes the condition is associated with convulsions. Some cases show no personality difficulties whatever. So-called "adiposo-genital idiocy" or "idiotie polysarcique" or "idiotie avec obésité" of Bourneville is very rare.

THE PINEAL GLAND

The relations between pineal dysfunctions and psychopathology are not well known. Pineal tumors, which are extremely rare, have been said to result in boys in sexual precocity, massive development of the secondary sex characteristics (pubic and axillary hair, deep masculine voice, etc.) as early as at three or four years of age, and in rapid intellectual development.

THE SUPRARENAL GLANDS

Hyperadrenalemia has been reported to be associated with a number of sexual anomalies: 1. *Suprarenal pseudohermaphroditism*, characterized by feminine hermaphroditism with virile secondary sex characteristics. 2. *Suprarenal virilism*, developing in girls from ten to fourteen years of age and marked by obesity, restlessness, irritability, flightiness, and homosexual trends. The girls may develop mustaches. In later years, marked muscular weakness complicates the picture. 3. The *"infant Hercules"* (Jelliffe, Smith Ely, and William A. White. *Diseases of the Nervous System. Philadelphia and New York. 1919, page 257*): the children "at the ages of from four to eleven years develop genital hair, beards, general hypertrichosis and markedly older skeletons. Sometimes the intelligence is precocious, again they are imbeciles." The monograph by Alfred Gallais (*Le syndrome génito-surrénal; étude anatomo-clinique. Paris. 1912*) furnishes good descriptions of all these forms.

THE THYMUS

H. Vogt, in 1911, described as *idiotia thymica* a condition of mental defect with dwarfism, weakness, almost complete loss of motility, and fragility of the bones, similar to the findings in dogs in which the thymus had been removed at the age of a few days. The relation between the illness reported by Vogt and the supposed absence of thymus function has not been demonstrated.[1]

[1] Vogt, H. Idiotia thymica (Schwachsinn durch Thymusausschaltung). Zeitschrift für jugendlichen Schwachsinn. 1911, 4, 548.

THE SEX GLANDS

Disorders of the innersecretory functioning of the reproductive organs (*dysgenitalism*), due to developmental anomalies, traumatic influences, inflammatory processes, or neoplasms, may greatly affect the general somatic configuration in the sense of gigantism, obesity, and disproportion of the body. The shape of the sex organs themselves may be abnormal, and especially the secondary sex characteristics may be variously altered. Precocious puberty and nubility may appear as early as in the second year of life. (A girl described by Albrecht von Haller menstruated at two years and was pregnant at eight; she lived to be seventy-five years old.) There are no specific psychopathological patterns associated with any of the changes. The example of the Skoptsy, a religious sect in Russia practising castration, often quoted to illustrate the effects on the mental condition of the deprivation of the procreative glands, is not well chosen, because there the operation is a result rather than the cause of a superstitious, fanatical, and morbid attitude.

Abnormality of sexual functioning is in itself an event of the first magnitude, affecting the total personality of the individual, especially since it is almost always accompanied by more or less conspicuous peculiarities of the general appearance and calls for an adjustment to life very much different from that of the normal person. It must also be kept in mind that dysgenitalism is usually combined with dysfunctions of some of the other endocrine glands. It is therefore easily understood that eunuchs, eunuchoids, hermaphrodites, etc., may develop various more or less outspoken personality difficulties. Eunuchs are said to be generally dependent, timid, lacking initiative, and to have a rich fantasy life. The historical example of Narses, the Byzantine statesman and war-lord, shows that castrates may indeed attain high achievements.

Various studies have been undertaken to throw some light on the possible relations between the functions of the sex glands and schizophrenia. Kraepelin assumed that there might be an autointoxication on the basis of disordered secretion of the procreative organs; in support of his theory, he cited the frequency with which the onset of the mental disturbance seemed to be connected with pubescence, pregnancy, and menstrual disorders. Mott described pathological changes in the ovaries and testicles of schizophrenic patients, also in their pituitary and suprarenal glands. Nolan D. C. Lewis reported atrophy of the glands of reproduction, in addition to other endocrine abnormalities. Gibbs found in many of the male patients a feminine hair distribution and in many female patients a masculine one. Kretschmer felt that there are similarities in the hair distribution and personality make-up of schizophrenics and eunuchoids. Some of these observations could not be confirmed by a number of other investigators. Certainly they are not always present, nor are they specific for schizophrenia, nor has one a right, if they are present, to jump immediately to the conclusion that they alone are etiologically responsible. It is quite understandable that so profound and sweeping a disturbance of the total personality might in one case or another be associated with various forms of incidental metabolic, endocrine, and autonomic nervous system disorders.

Henderson and Gillespie sum up the relation between mental health and the procreative functions with these words: "There are numerous evidences of an intimate connection between the gonads, as a part of the whole psychophysical organization, and mental disorder, but the evidences of a direct causal relationship between disorders of the generative glands and mental disturbance are so far very indefinite. We know that mental disease commonly breaks out soon after puberty is reached, at pregnancy and at the menopause; that the thought content of a psychosis is often predominantly sexually colored; and that disturbance of the sexual function and sexual paraesthesiae are common symptoms. But most of these are more easily explained on psychological grounds. . . . Something more than disease of the gonads is apparently necessary to produce a mental illness."

PERSONALITY DIFFICULTIES EXPRESSING THEMSELVES IN THE FORM OF INVOLUNTARY PART-DYSFUNCTIONS

CHAPTER XXIII

GENERAL CONSIDERATIONS

A DISTINCTIVE group of personality disorders, constituting a considerable and clinically conspicuous portion of the psychopathology of infancy and childhood, is made up of localized functional disturbances seemingly limited to a specific organ or organ system. They are sufficiently characterized by a number of common fundamental qualities.

The essential uniting feature consists in the highly significant fact that, in spite of vast laboratory research, organic lesions cannot be objectively demonstrated. We fully realize and, as a matter of fact, wish to draw attention to the negative version of our statement of the principal common denominator. This version is practically inevitable at a time when contemporaneous medical thinking finds it so difficult to rid itself of the notion that the term "functional" is an embarrassing excuse for ignorance and that at some future time ultrachemical and ultramicroscopical discoveries will reveal mysteries hitherto unsolved. This may indeed be so. Yet meanwhile it certainly does not do either to abandon oneself to unproductive shoulder-shrugging from a feeling of hopelessness or to reach out into the nebulous realm of unproven and unprovable hypotheses which are sometimes given out as convictions and assertions. Even the too frequent use of words, such as "perhaps," "probably," "possibly," "in some way," and the like, intended to mitigate and to avoid the semblance of theoretical dogmatism, is doubtless devoid of the foremost criterion of truly scientific endeavor, namely, that of objectivity.

It is fortunate that the recent advances in psychiatric knowledge have provided factual material which, built up on a sound and concrete basis, is well suited to dispel both despair and speculation with regard to some of the so-called functional disorders. One is no longer compelled to accept the finding of physico-chemical inadequacy or of anatomo-pathological tissue alterations as the one and only legitimate explanation for anything that goes on within the human organism. A systematic approach with psychobiological methods of investigation has given ample, and, because of strict adherence to facts, incontestable evidence of the eminent rôle which psychogenic factors may play in the development and maintenance of somatic dysfunctions. Pavlov's work with animals and Krasnogorsky's experiments on children have established beyond a trace of doubt the dependence on emotional factors of physiological functioning. It was reserved to Adolf Meyer to clear the horizon, obscured until then by dualistic and pseudo-monistic trends, by introducing into medicine the concept of the mentally integrated individual in whom life expresses itself in the forms of involuntary, automatic part functioning on a vegetative level (the "parts," to be sure, being closely interrelated) and of more or less conscious, symbolizing, overt or implicit performances of the organism as a whole on a psycho-biological level. The integrated whole has a pathology of its own, a psycho-pathology.

The integration concept makes it understandable that on many occasions one or another part may participate in dysfunctions of the total personality. Thus we come to deal with one type of complaints which are clearly and unmistakably personality-determined (e.g., stealing, fear reactions, temper tantrums, masturbation, sensitiveness) and another group of complaints which are centered around certain organs and which experience and the examination of individual cases prove to be anchored not in the organs themselves but rooted in psychopathological difficulties of the organism as an integrated unit (e.g., certain types of enuresis, a facial tic, blushing, an hysterical paralysis).

Thus we are in a position to go one significant step further and to add to the negative feature of absence of organic lesions a more constructive and workable and therapeutically inestimable positive property inherent in the second group of complaints. They are somatic part manifestations of a more or less obvious psychobiological or psychopathological reaction involving the total personality of the patient. Hence, they are best understood and treated not *per se*, not locally, not detached from a consideration of the patient, but by means of studying the child in his entirety, with attention to his physical, emotional, intellectual, constitutional, and environmental peculiarities.

Many physicians find it difficult to realize these facts because they cannot conceive of an unquestionably involuntary function of the urinary bladder or of a selective group of muscles as being of psychogenic origin. They do not usually look for an organic interpretation of thumbsucking or nose-picking since these performances appear to be subject to volition; they can see the child in action; they can perceive how a threat or distraction causes the youngster to remove the finger from his mouth. But if it comes to an apparently uncontrollable act, such as wetting the bed during sleep, the connection with psychogenic features is not so easily recognized. It is hoped that the following chapters will, on the basis of factual case material, convincingly demonstrate the psychogenic origin of the reactions of which they treat.

A good deal of thought has been given to the questions why it is that personality difficulties have an outlet in physical part-dysfunctions and why it is that specific organs are selected by different individuals. Freud has expressed the opinion that psychogenic symptoms of a somatic nature represent an unconscious *flight into disease* from which the patient derives an emotional gain (*Krankheitsgewinn*). Richards has coined the term *body protest* to indicate that the physical disorder serves as an outlet for worries, disappointments, frustrations, and other affective difficulties. The symbolical significance of the symptom is sometimes easily traced, at other times its meaning and the original purpose are less evident. The example of tics developing from primarily purposive, defensive or expressive, movements reminds one of Darwin's ingenious theory with regard to the evolution of emotional expressions and gestures from movements which were once useful to the animal series when in the presence of conditions which excited a particular emotion. It would lead too far to refer even to a selection of the recent studies which have succeeded in demonstrating experimentally and clinically the somatic participation in emotional reactions

We do, however, think it necessary to enumerate some of the outstanding theories anent the choice of the participating organ, since they are frequently quoted in the literature and since they developed concepts and terminologies, the acquaintance with which is indispensable for their critical evaluation:

Partial infantilism. The term "infantilism" was introduced by Lasègue in 1864. Since then the concept has undergone considerable changes. Especially the French school has worked with it intensively. For some time it was looked upon as a disease *sui generis*. General lack or slowness of development in growth, intelligence, and behavior has been described as *universal infantilism* or, after its first observer, as the *type of Lorain*. Dwarfism and, since Peritz, eunuchoidism and later, especially under the influence of Hirschfeld and Kronfeld, "psychosexual" retardation have been described as some of the prototypes. There was a good deal of controversy as to whether or not all forms of infantilism are caused by endocrine dysfunctions. The problem was complicated by the distinction between somatic and psychic infantilism. To the concept of universal infantilism was added that of *partial infantilism* (Anton), denoting that certain organs or organ systems did not keep pace with the general evolution of the individual. Congenital malformations of the heart, coeliac disease, faulty or retarded speech development, and cirrhotic kidney are often cited as specific examples. Some authors were tempted to consider partial infantilism as responsible for certain "functional" disorders, such as encopresis or enuresis. According to them, the infantilistic organ, on account of its subevolution, is more than any other apt to succumb under the strain of psychogenic disorders.

Organ inferiority. According to the Adlerian theory of organ inferiority, not all organs and organ systems are equally endowed in every individual; almost all people are said to have a "weak spot" somewhere, which is more susceptible to endogenic and especially to exogenic damage than the rest of the body. In one person it may be the digestive apparatus which represents a congenital and often inherited *locus minoris resistentiae*, in another it is the circulatory, respiratory, or motor system, the genitourinary organs, the central nervous tissues, the external integument, or the special sense organs, etc. Sometimes an inferiority of two or more systems may be present in the same person. If a child reacts with enuresis to some situational difficulties, this is explained by the existence of an organ inferiority of the urinary apparatus. If he vomits, the alimentary tract is inferior. If he responds to personality difficulties with a tic, the muscular apparatus or a certain part of it has had a lower vitality from the very beginning. This inferiority may be passively accepted by the patient. He may compensate for it by aiming at a greater general capacity through cultivation of the organs which are not inferior or by increasing the vitality of the inferior organ itself through persistent training. Or he may even over-compensate for the defect and reach an unusually high proficiency in the use of the originally inferior organ (Demosthenes who overcame his speech defect and became a famous orator furnishes a classical example). The attempts at compensation or over-compensation are often accompanied by or, if not quite successful, result in additional conflicts which again are mirrored in the functions of the weak organ. Thus, according to Adler, the individual, besides his verbal language, has an *organ vocabulary* of his own, which is an expression of his struggles and furnishes a key to the understanding of the choice of his neurotic symptoms (*Symptomenwahl*).

Neurologizing trends. While the assumption of partial infantilism or the congenital inferiority of specific organs tries to explain functional disorders by finding fault with the misbehaving part itself, there are many investigators who would project the source of the disturbance on existing or postulated areas of the central nervous system. The method of preference is analogy with findings in organic cerebral diseases. Since alexia and agraphia are known to occur in certain brain lesions, children's reading and writing disabilities are promptly referred to identical lesions even though not the slightest objective proof can be offered for their actual existence. Since tic-like movements have been observed in encephalitis and (hypothetically) localized in the basal ganglia, all tics are promptly projected on the striate body. In the case of enuresis, occult spina bifida or myelodysplasia are held responsible, whether they are really there or not.

Conditioned reflexes. Pavlov, in the course of his well-known studies, came to the conclusion that "all nervous activity of the dog appears to us as reflex—that is, a reaction of the animal to the external world through the nervous system." He distinguishes two types of reflexes: a. The unconditioned reflex—"a reaction in which an external phenomenon is united with a certain response of the organism by a constant and unalterable connection. For example, every time a mechanical body impinges on the eye, there follows without fail a defensive movement." b. The conditioned reflex—"where the union of the external phenomenon with the corresponding activity of the organism is of a temporary nature, is formed in the presence of certain conditions, continues in the presence of those and other conditions, and under certain other circumstances can be later destroyed." The production of saliva upon the ingestion of food is an unconditioned reflex; it is a law of nature. But salivary secretion upon the mere sight or smell of food is a conditioned reflex because the association has been acquired in the course of life's experiences. The sight of food acts as a conditioned stimulus. If the offer of food is preceded a sufficient number of times by another stimulus, such as the sounding of a bell or the flashing of a light, then the sound or flash may come to evoke the secretion of saliva, just as the sight or smell of food did. Pavlov calls them indifferent stimuli so long as the conditioning has not taken place; after that, they become positive conditioned stimuli. If a metronome of one hundred beats has thus been made a positive conditioned stimulus, then a metronome of fifty beats will, because of the close resemblance, also result in a flow of saliva; but if the latter is often repeated without the ensuing offer of food, the flow becomes less and less until it finally stops. Thus a negative conditioned stimulus has been established. Positive conditioning, according to Pavlov, is due to cortical stimulation, negative conditioning to cortical inhibition.

"By his method of conditioned reflexes Pavlov thinks he has discovered the nature of sleep and of neurasthenia. Both of these he has produced artificially in his dogs, by giving them too difficult problems of differentiation. For example, suppose a tone of a distinctly lower pitch is made a negative conditioned stimulus (that is, it is not accompanied by food), then let a third tone be taken so close in pitch to the first that the dog cannot distinguish between them; there results a lack of balance of the processes of stimulation and of inhibition, and the animal develops symptoms of neurasthenia, refusing to eat, whining, etc. Pavlov has cured such dogs by rest and bromides" (Gantt). In this manner, Pavlov comes to view all activity in the light of positive and negative conditioned reflexes. What to us appears as psychogenic organ dysfunctions, is invariably reduced to physiological processes in a variously stimulated and inhibited brain. The organ selection depends on the specific mode of conditioning which in the given individual has given rise to headache, vomiting, tics, or enuresis, as a response to certain situations.

Substitution, conversion. If a child gags long enough until he vomits in demonstration of his alleged inability to eat cabbage or spinach, the meaning of the ejection of food is quite clear and can be easily understood by the patient as well as by the observers. The motive and the aim are transparent without further analysis of the act. With his vomiting, the youngster indicates this: "I do not want to eat spinach. I do not like it. If you eat things that you do not like, they should come out. This will show mother how sick the spinach makes me. She will not give it to me again. Besides, she will be worried about me. She will tell everybody something about my eating. She will give me a nickel or candy if I keep it up long enough." He does, of course, not verbalize these things as we have just done it for him. But if he is old and intelligent enough and were willing to reason clearly and sincerely, he would formulate the situation in those or similar terms. An entirely different reaction is the vomiting of the retarded but very conscientious girl on the eve of a decisive school test. She is in a state of tension and fearful anticipation. Failure will mean repetition of the grade, scoldings or beatings from the parents, teasing on the part of her playmates. The girl goes on hammering the lesson into her head but, with the mounting difficulties and realization of inability, she develops nausea, stomachache, and finally vomits. The vomiting is a substitutive reaction: "It is not that I am not capable of doing the work, I am too sick to do it"; furthermore: "It is not the fear of the test that has made me sick, it must have been something that I have eaten." Again it is we who verbalize the situation, and not the child, who merely knows that she is sick at her stomach and vomits. Here, at least, we still have a definite chronological connection between the substitution and the emotional strain which has been substituted. This relation is not always so obvious and so near the actual difficulty in time or in logical association. The substitutive reaction may become so remote from the underlying problem that only a searching analysis can uncover the relationship between the two. The incident or incidents giving rise to the emotional difficulty for which a somatic symptom has been substituted may be well remembered and consciously allied with the symptom, or may be remembered but not at all recognized as having anything to do with the symptom, or not be remembered in the least. In the last case, the memory lives on in a disguised and unidentified form in the psychopathological "symptom." Thus we have three types of substitution.:

Substitution with clear association of the symptom with a well-remembered emotionally loaded situation.

Substitution with no conscious association of the symptom with a well-remembered emotionally loaded situation.

Substitution with no conscious association of the symptom with a suppressed, "forgotten," emotionally loaded situation (amnesic or dysmnesic substitution).

The third form, which is especially frequent in hysteria, has been designated by Freud as "conversion," or "a process by which sums of emotion become transformed into physical manifestations" (Brill). Freud, however, assumes that the forgotten or "repressed" situation is always of a sexual nature. Although it is quite true that "sexual traumata" may indeed be forgotten and the emotional conflict arising from them substituted by all sorts of physical symptoms, the psychoanalytic generalization is not justified. Everyone working with children knows how many and varied situations, such as fright occasioned by a dog bite, a drunken father's wife-beating, the witnessing of an automobile accident, failure in school, etc., may lead to any of the three forms of substitution. If one does not insist dogmatically on the sexual implications of the term, the word "conversion" can be accepted as an excellently chosen designation.

CHAPTER XXIV

THE CENTRAL NERVOUS SYSTEM

· HEADACHE

HEADACHE is a common complaint of children as well as of adults. It is either an indicator of somatic illness, a part manifestation of fatigue, a reaction to worry or disappointment, or of a hypochondriacal nature. There is hardly a physical illness that may not be occasionally accompanied by headache. In some diseases, headache may be one of the outstanding and most disturbing symptoms. It is, in conjunction with vomiting and optic neuritis, a constant feature in intracranial tumors. It is present in tuberculous and epidemic cerebro-spinal meningitis. It is not infrequent in acute anterior poliomyelitis. It occurs in cardiac, renal, gastric, and hepatic disorders. It is often associated with refractive errors and may become quite distressing if the visual defect is not corrected. It is met with in the prodromal stage and in the course of acute febrile conditions. It is a well-known complaint of children with tonsillar and adenoid hypertrophy and with sinus infections. Every experienced parent knows that headache often goes with a common cold and more especially with coryza. It may be caused by sleep in an overheated and poorly ventilated room. Congenitally luetic children sometimes complain of severe nocturnal occipital headaches.

Fatigue plays a considerable part in the production of children's headaches.

One eleven-year-old boy was reported as "suffering dreadfully with headaches" every time after hard play or returning from the school's gymnasium. A short period of rest brought relief. The cephalalgia was obviously not simulated nor hypochondriacal, since the child was well adjusted otherwise and there was no gain to be expected from his complaint. After a short relaxation, he went to do his home work willingly.

With some children, it is not acute exertion that leads to headache complaints but a constant strain due to *lack of adequate recreation*.

A boy of twelve years, slightly obese, normally intelligent, came to the clinic with the request, "I want you to take my headache away." He had had frontal headaches for approximately six months. The boy was very conscientious and ambitious and somewhat submissive. In addition to his school work, he went to a religious school for two hours each day, also during vacation periods. He took music lessions and practiced thirty minutes daily. Being good-natured, he was engaged in helping his younger sister with her arithmetic problems and in running errands for his parents and two older brothers. On Saturdays, he was sent to help out in his uncle's store. There was no time left for play. The type of work itself which he did was not particularly exerting. But the steady and uninterrupted activity created a state of permanent fatigue with headache, which promptly disappeared when sufficient time and opportunity for recreational outlets were provided.

Headache is more frequent in undernourished than in well fed children. It is often produced by *hunger* in youngsters who are in the habit of going to school without breakfast. The pain usually starts in the late hours of the forenoon and makes the child incapable of following the lessons. We have seen a considerable number of pupils whose headaches, occurring every day but Saturday and Sunday at the same time, were due to no other cause than the habitual omission of breakfast before going to school.

Another form of headache originating in school is based on the *strain of retarded pupils* who are expected to do work which is far beyond their capacity. It is usually the conscientious child who responds with headache to the increased effort involved in his attempt to keep up with the class requirements, and to the inevitable frustration. Cimbal designates this form as *school headache* (*Schulkopfschmerz*) and defines it as "those pains in the region of the head, nape of the neck, and face, which are produced under the exertions of school and home work and fade away in the hours of relaxation." It is often wrongly interpreted as an alibi by parents and teachers. Placement of the child in a grade better adapted to his capacities or in an ungraded class with removal of the strain tends to do away with the headache more effectively than the prescription of drugs or the unjust accusation that the patient's complaint is merely an excuse for "laziness."

Leroy B. was twelve years old. According to his mother, "he has had headaches all the time for the past four or five years. I have given him aspirin tablets and made him lie down. The teacher sends him home from school with them. He complains of them three or four times a week. My doctor told me maybe it is the tonsils and adenoids." Tonsillectomy and adenoidectomy, however, had no better results than the aspirin. The boy had a mental age of nine years and had been pushed up to the fifth grade. He had been working until late at night in order to compete successfully with his classmates. He reacted to the strain also by means of blinking and jerking his hands (for which he was beaten severely). Adequate school adjustment did away with all of his difficulties.

Children with *hypochondriacal* tendencies most frequently complain of stomachaches and of headaches. Very often the two go together. The pattern is usually furnished by other members of the household.

A thirteen-year-old girl, in the fifth grade at a mental age of nine years, had headaches and also pain in her chest and stomach. Her father complained of weakness in his legs. Her mother had headaches, sometimes with vomiting, and pains in her chest and abdomen. Two sisters, aged seventeen and ten, and a brother, fifteen years old, had "bad" headaches. This child could hardly be said to be under a strain in school. She was phlegmatic and indifferent and made not the slightest attempt to do her work. She had simply "given up," and by doing so had perhaps shown greater wisdom than those who wanted her to perform the impossible task of conforming to fifth grade requirements. Her headache was of a characteristically hypochondriacal nature. Her description of it ("It feels like somebody is beating it and sometimes like I am going around") was a literal repetition of her mother's recital of her own headache complaints.

The *headache of convenience*, to use an expression coined by Robey,[1] who

[1] Robey, William H. Headache. Philadelphia and London. 1931, p. 129.

calls it a manifestation of dishonesty, is met with in children as well as in adults from whom they usually learn it. So many mothers, in the child's presence, are in the habit of excusing with a headache their absence at a party or obtaining quiet by asking those about them to please consider their headache. The youngster is apt to make a mental note of that and use the same plea when he does not like to go on an errand or to go to school on the day of a dreaded test. The complaint comes always at a time when it is most convenient to the child, on Sunday morning before Sunday school, on Monday morning when he wishes to stay in bed a little longer and defer the new week's contact with the school, or just before the music teacher is to arrive. One boy of twelve was said by his mother to have "Nine o'clock headaches, nine o'clock toothaches, and nine o'clock pains." The obvious treatment of this sort of headache is kind disregard, at the same time trying to find out why the child does not like to return to school after the weekend or to have his piano lesson.

Headache is occasionally one of the features of a reaction associated with the mild hyperthyroidism of some pubescent girls in whom one finds slight enlargement of the thyroid gland, rapid pulse, sometimes fine digital tremors, and general unrest. In two girls, headache began on the occasion of the first menstruation when the children, entirely unprepared by their elders, became frightened. The headache then returned with each flow until the girls were sufficiently informed and reassured; the headache then left them.

MIGRAINE

Migraine is a specific form of headache characterized by acute onset, periodicity, violent pain, extreme malaise, association with more or less pronounced gastric disturbances, and sudden and complete recovery. In intervals of varying duration, usually in the morning hours at the time of, or soon after, awakening, the child complains of severe headache, mostly unilateral (hence the name, derived from *hemi*—half and *crania*, from *cranium*—skull). The pain occasionally begins in school and becomes so excruciating that the patient is sent home. Some authors insist on the one-sidedness of the pain, while others rightly feel that bilateral headaches may well be termed migrainous if some of the other criteria are present. But to include any form of recurrent headache unaccompanied by other pathognomonic signs, would be stretching the concept too much.

Several types have been distinguished: simple, ophthalmic, ophthalmoplegic, and symptomatic migraine.

The description given in the first paragraph applies to the *simple type*.

Richard D., ten years old, has had since the age of two years attacks of headaches with malaise, followed by nausea and anorexia, accompanied by profuse sweating, and culminating after twenty-four hours to four days in vomiting after which there was instantaneous recovery. The attacks began during convalescence from poisoning with "deadly nightshade." The child was undernourished and had a functional systolic murmur at the apex. He was cheerful, normally intelligent, and did well in school. He had enuresis almost every night.

Edward A., nine years old, had severe headaches over the left eye for the past three years, associated with nausea and terminated by vomiting which afforded immediate relief. They occurred about once every two weeks and lasted approximately twelve hours. "When he rises in the morning he knows that he is going to have a headache." Edward was undernourished, had a flattened chest, poor posture, and orthostatic albuminuria. He was a boy of superior intelligence (I.Q. 118) but emotionally unstable, excitable, easily upset. He was said to have an unhappy disposition and to "worry and cry over everything." He had enuresis until seven years old. His mother nagged him a good deal and contrasted him with his younger brother. His father had sinus trouble, was hard of hearing, and complained of ringing in his ears. His mother described herself as "nervous, fidgety, and bothered by noises." The paternal grandmother had for many years been an inmate of a state institution for mental diseases. A paternal aunt also was psychotic. Another had transitory mental disturbance following the "flu."

The *ophthalmic type* of migraine seems to be at least as frequent in children as the simple form. Any sort of visual disturbance may precede or initiate or accompany the attack. These are a few of the characteristic complaints: "The headaches are ushered in by flashes of zigzag light in front of his eyes. Sometimes he thinks he sees animals." "She sees colored spots with her headaches." "Sometimes he sees stars before and during the attacks." "He sees spots, stars, and bright sparks." "He often sees yellow specks before his eyes two or three days before the attacks." "When I have the headaches, I can see red dots dance up and down in front of my eyes." "Frequently he sees dark spots prior to the headaches." "He complains of black spots in front of his left eye before the attacks." "While she has the headaches, she can see only half of what she tries to read."

Ophthalmoplegic migraine is comparatively rare in children. It is characterized by paralysis or weakness of the eye muscles at the beginning, in the course, or at the end of the attack. Few cases have been reported as occurring at an early age (e.g., by Schulhoff in a "psychically abnormal" eight-year old boy, whose migraine started following a cerebral trauma two years previously, and whose father and maternal uncle suffered from migraine; by Prochazka in a girl of ten years; by Van Romunde and Engelhard in a four-year-old child who had a ptosis of the right upper lid six days after birth, lasting for two weeks, and later migraine attacks with oculomotor paralysis; by Heilbronner in a patient who at five years began to have attacks of simple migraine and at seven years started to have ophthalmoplegic symptoms).[1] In view of the relative scarcity of case reports in the literature, it is interesting to note that, according to Flatau, not less than 58.5 per cent of all ophthalmoplegic migraines begin during childhood.

Symptomatic migraine is that form of migraine-like headaches which occurs in patients with definite organic cerebral lesions. According to Ziehen, tuberous sclerosis (Bourneville's disease) often begins with migrainous headaches.

The distinction of four groups does in no way exhaust the range of the

[1] Schulhoff, K. Ophthalmoplegic Migraine. Časopis českych lekaruv. 1914, 53, 998. Prochazka, V. On Ophthalmoplegic Migraine and Recurrent Ophthalmoplegia. Ibidem. 1913, 52, 1550. Van Romunde, L. H., and C. F. Engelhard. On Ophthalmoplegic Migraine. Nederl. Tijdschr. v. Geneesk. 1915, 59, 1029. Heilbronner, K. Demonstration of Patients. Psych. en Neurol. Bladen. 1914, 18, 194.

possible varieties. Flatau adds a *facioplegic*, *epileptic*, and *psychic form*. Dizziness is often associated with the attacks, sometimes as a sort of "aural vertigo." Sensory disturbances are not infrequent. One child felt numbness in his tongue. Another had a sensation "as if someone kept tugging at his hair." The feeling of a lump in the throat, similar to the globus hystericus, was reported in two of our cases. In one child, the headaches were often combined with earache. In another, the attacks were preceded by "watering of the eyes." It is of interest that sometimes, in addition to the typical periodical attacks, there is a more or less constant dull headache present. Sachs and Hausman (*Nervous and Mental Disorders from Birth through Adolescence. New York. 1926, pp. 643-644*) report the occurrence of temporary aphasia in a ten-year-old girl who had inherited migraine from her mother. "The girl when spoken to was able to mumble a few words indistinctly, but could not find the word she wished to say. She was in intense pain and extremely irritable, but, after a good night's rest, the headache disappeared and with it the aphasia. This aphasia is associated with right-sided hemiplegia in right-handed persons."

Until not so long ago, migraine was considered unusually rare in childhood. Flatau, Comby, Fabre, Curschmann, and Hamburger paid especial attention to its occurrence in the early years of life.[1] Flatau was able to trace the onset of the condition in 307 adults; he found that in 21 per cent of the cases the headaches began before the fifteenth year. S.E. Lachman had the kindness to place at my disposal his as yet unpublished review of the migraine material of the Harriet Lane Home; in twenty-four undoubted cases the age of onset was given and compared with Comby's and Fabre's figures as follows:

Age of Onset	Comby		Fabre		Lachman	
	Boys	Girls	Boys	Girls	Boys	Girls
Under 1	1		2			
1		2		1		
2		2		1	1	1
3			1	1	2	
4	2			1	1	
5	1		2		1	1
6	3					3
7	1			2	2	1
8	1			1	3	
9		1				2
10		1	1			2
11				1	1	1
12						
13						2
Total	9	6	6	8	11	13

[1] Flatau, E. Die Migräne. Lewandowsky's Handbuch der Neurologie. Volume 5. 1914, p. 342. Comby, J. La migraine chez les enfants. Archives de Medicine des Enfants, 1921, 24, 29 Fabre, E. La Migraine chez les enfants. Thèse de Paris. Curschmann, H. Über Kindermigräne. Münchener medizinische Wochenschrift. 1922, 69, 1747. Hamburger, F. M. Münchener medizinische Wochenschrift. 1923, 70, 150.

Constipation was present in not less than ten of the twenty-four cases. In one child, the bowels moved regularly except during and two or three days following the attacks. Another frequent finding was error of refraction (in fully fourteen children); correction of vision, however, invariably failed to check or attenuate the migrainous attacks. Three of the patients had functional systolic murmur and one had occasional extrasystoles. One child had a history of ptomaine poisoning and another of acute phosphorus intoxication from eating matches. Sinusitis and polyp in the right antrum (the migrainous headaches were sometimes right-sided and sometimes left-sided) were found in one case each. One girl was syphilitic. One child had a convulsion at two years, one had "spasms" at the age of one year and fainting spells during the summer at three years, and one had chorea at five years. In view of the fact that most French authors are inclined to assume a close relation between migraine and the so-called arthritic diathesis, it may be of interest to relate that in four of our cases there was a history of rheumatic disorders: one child had erythema nodosum at six; one had a rheumatic mitral insufficiency; one had at four years an attack of rheumatic pain in the lower extremities associated with fever for about a week; the fourth had inflammatory rheumatism since nine years and frequent attacks of pain in the joints with temperature elevations since then. (Both parents had occasional attacks of arthritis in the joints of the arms and legs and a sister had died of valvular heart disease following arthritis.)

In ten of the twenty-four cases, the onset was referred by the parents to definite acute illnesses or other events: 1. Since pneumonia. 2. and 3. Immediately following acute otitis media. 4. After an attack of dysentery at two years. 5. After grippe and "lumbago" with swollen left knee and hip. 6. After poisoning with nightshade. 7. Following an automobile accident. 8. Since he started to go to school. 9. Following a scare. 10. Fright from witnessing an accident (The patient, a luetic girl, had breathholding spells in infancy. At eleven years, she was frightened, whereupon she was sick with a high fever for several days. She was "out of her head" and imagined that she saw skeletons walking around the room and owls flying over her head. Shortly after this undoubtedly delirious episode, she began having typical migrainous attacks with scotomata and color vision, dizziness, nausea, and vomiting.)

Migraine is often quoted as an eminently *hereditary* condition. It is a fact that sick headaches are frequently found in the ascendency. Eleven of the twenty-four cases studied by Lachman had migrainous relatives. Father and son were affected in two instances, father and daughter once, mother and son in three cases, mother and daughter in three, a boy and his paternal aunt once, and a boy, his older brother, and his paternal grandfather once. The father of one of our male patients had epileptic attacks.

Migraine seems to be somewhat more common in girls than in boys.

Numerous theories have been advanced with regard to the *etiology*. Vasomotor changes in the central nervous system in the sense of either angiospastic or angioparalytic conditions due to sympathetic hypertonia or hypotonia have been assumed. Other theories have to do with ocular and nasal pathology; pituitary disturbance (Timme: small sella turcica with erosions; J. H. Fisher: periodic temporary swelling coincident with functional overactivity); error in purin metabolism; intestinal toxemia or bacteriemia; food allergy; sensitization disorder similar to hay-fever; liver dysfunction (Diamond); toxic putrefactive substances in the general circulation with failure of the liver to synthesize and detoxicate them; angioneurotic edema of the brain (Rowe). Others believe that migraine is closely related to epilepsy (e.g., Gowers) or to cyclical vomiting. With regard to the latter, Cameron says: "A close association between cyclic vomiting in children and that form of periodic headache known as migraine has often been observed. It is sometimes found that one or both parents of a child with cyclic vomiting suffer habitually from migraine. In a few instances the one condition has been observed to be gradually replaced by the other, the child with cyclic vomiting becoming in adult life a sufferer from migraine. There is indeed much which is common to the two conditions. The periodic nature of the seizure, often following a time when the general health and vigour appear to have been at their best, the extreme prostration, and the comparatively sudden recovery are found in both. In the cyclic vomiting of children, it is true, little complaint is made of headache, the visual aura is absent, and the vomiting is the most prominent symptom."

Whatever the true etiology of migraine may be, the presence of an endogenic factor can hardly be questioned. At the same time, we learn again and again that emotional difficulties may very well precipitate or influence the course of the individual attacks and, as a matter of fact, may have played a significant part in the setting of the very first seizure. Excessive irritability is almost invariably present during the attacks, even in children who are otherwise cheerful and good-natured.

One ten-year-old boy of superior intelligence was brought with the complaint of "spells" of disobedience and extreme crossness. The mother, who had a long record of sick headaches, noticed that these "spells" coincided with worry over failure in school and, having read a good many popular books and articles on child psychology, decided that the child's complaints of nausea and vomiting could be explained by his ill-humor and should be disregarded, at the same time punishing him for his irritability. In the course of the examination it was found that the boy had periodic episodes of not too severe headaches beginning soon after awakening or later in the forenoon followed by continuous nausea and seeing of red spots. The headache was mostly unilateral over his right eye. The boy knew that he was cross during those periods but he "just cannot help it, just cannot stand anything" (especially not the psychological pseudo-wisdom of his nagging mother). The attack lasted from twelve to thirty-six hours. When it was over, he usually lay down to sleep and, when he got up, he felt "perfectly well."

The *treatment* has to take care of the patient not only during the attacks but also in the interim periods. For the acute episodes, many remedies have been recommended, such as gastric lavage, high colonic irrigation, application of heat or cold, and various drugs, especially aspirin, pyramidon, phenacetin, acetanilid, luminal, and bromides. Jelliffe advised nitroglycerin to be given at the beginning of the seizure which, he feels, is characterized by vasoconstriction, while the latter part is said by him to be accompanied by vasodilatation. Some recommend calcium preparations.

Osler praised the effects of cannabis indica. Complete rest and the avoidance of excitement has been stressed by practically all investigators.

In the intervals, a well balanced diet has been urged. Those whose etiological theories are based on the assumption of specific nutritional damage make, of course, use of them in the therapeutic régime, prescribing, for instance, limitation of carbohydrates, increased protein diet, etc. Regulation of bowel movements is of significance in the many cases of constipation. Wherever there are refractive errors, they need correction which, however, rarely influences the course of the headaches. The same is true of any other physical disorder found during the examination of migrainous patients.

The psychogenic difficulties tending to precipitate, aggravate, or increase the frequency of the attacks should be elicited and remedied. In one of our cases, the undoubtedly migrainous headaches which during the school period occurred as often as two to three times each month did not take place in the course of the entire summer holidays. The child was under a strain having to do scholastic work which was beyond her capacity and having a nagging, unsympathetic teacher. Placement in an ungraded class considerably reduced the number of seizures but did not abolish them altogether. Robey, in his book on *Headache*, states: "Especially in searching for the cause of migraine should the nervous organism, faulty environment, and social habits be studied."

CHAPTER XXV

THE DIGESTIVE SYSTEM

IT HAS BEEN known for a long time that the alimentary tract participates frequently in reactions of a psychogenic origin. Pavlov's famous work and theories on the conditioned reflex had their starting point in the experimental demonstration of the close connection between anticipation of food, "sham feeding," the sight and smell of favorite food, and affective states on the one hand and the flow of salivary and gastric secretion on the other hand. Cannon begins his well-known book on the somatic changes under the influence of pain, hunger, fear, and rage with a chapter on the effect of emotions on digestion; on the basis of animal experimentation, he deals with the emotions favorable and unfavorable to the normal secretion of the digestive juices and to the contractions of the stomach and intestines.[1]

Though most of the work has been done with dogs and cats, some investigators have had an opportunity to study similar situations in children. Bogen reported the case of a three-and-a-half-year-old child with stenosis of the esophagus (due to the swallowing of lye) and gastric fistula, who showed several interesting features. If given milk or meat by mouth, the food, incapable of passing through the closed esophagus, remained in the diverticulum; nevertheless, there was a flow of gastric juice. The same occurred if the ingestion of food was in his presence discussed with his sister. Thereupon, Bogen gave meat to the child forty times, at the same time sounding a certain tune on a toy trumpet. In seven out of ten ensuing experiments, there was a flow of gastric juice containing free hydrochloric acid upon the sounding of the trumpet without an offer of food. The child, however, thwarted in his hope of receiving the food, later failed to react with gastric secretion to actual feeding. In a little boy observed by Hornborg and in a girl studied by Richet (as early as 1878), the chewing or tasting of agreeable substances resulted in a rich flow of gastric juice, which did not take place upon the chewing of insipid objects, such as gutta-percha.[2]

---

[1] Pavlov, Ivan P. The Work of the Digestive Glands. London. 1902. Lectures on Conditioned Reflexes. Translated by W. Horsley Gantt. New York. 1928.

Cannon, Walter B. Bodily Changes in Pain, Hunger, Fear and Rage. New York and London. 1915. The Influence of Emotional States on the Functions of the Alimentary Canal. American Journal of the Medical Sciences. 1909, 137, 480.

[2] Bogen, H. Experimentelle Untersuchung über psychische und assoziative Magensaftsekretion beim Menschen. Pflügers Archiv für die gesamte Physiologie. 1907, 117, 150–160.

Richet, Charles. Des propriétés chimiques et physiologiques du suc gastrique chez l'homme et les animaux. Journal de l'Anatomie et de la Physiologie. 1878, 14, 170–326.

Hornborg, A. F. Beiträge zur Kenntnis der Absonderungsbedingungen des Magensaftes beim Menschen. Skandinavisches Archiv für Physiologie. 1904, 15, 209–258.

A large amount of clinical material has been accumulated, which proves beyond a trace of doubt that personality disorders of an emotional nature may express themselves wholly or partly in functional disturbances of the gastro-intestinal system, affecting either its secretions or its motility or both. A remarkable change has taken place in recent years in the general attitude with regard to the so-called gastric and intestinal neuroses, in that they are no longer studied and treated as isolated local phenomena; the dysfunctions are more properly referred to the underlying emotional states and to the situational background in which they developed. A gastric neurosis is no longer considered a neurosis "of the stomach" but a more or less localized reaction to difficulties rooted in the individual as a whole. However, most of the publications limit themselves to the study of adults. In the following, we shall try to review the psychogenic digestive disturbances of children. The common feeding problems arising from faulty training are discussed in another section of this book.

PSYCHOGENIC DISORDERS OF SALIVATION

Salivary secretion is relatively small in early infancy. It takes some time before the normal baby learns to dispose, by means of deglutition, of the saliva which accumulates in the oral cavity. When there is a large quantity, as is the case in dentition, the saliva is permitted to run out of the mouth. This is done so regularly that some authors speak of "physiological dribbling." Idiotic children may not acquire for many years the mechanism of habitually swallowing the surplus secretion of the salivary glands, which therefore keeps flowing in a slow stream over the chin and down the neck and chest and on the clothes. It is difficult to say whether in cretins and other idiots there is an increase in the amount of production or whether, with average productivity, the difficulty lies mainly in the faulty mode of disposal.

In postencephalitic children there seems to be a definite excess of secretion. One sometimes sees patients who stand there unable to check the steady efflux of a thin fluid from their mouths, which drenches the clothes or forms on the floor a puddle of considerable size.

The "watering of the mouth" in anticipation of pleasant food is so well known as to have become phraseological. A few investigators studied the effect of "mental" activity (solving arithmetic problems) on salivary secretion. While Brunacci and De Sanctis observed a smaller quantity during mental work than during rest, Lashley obtained the opposite result. Krasnogorsky succeeded in establishing conditioned salivary responses in children. Winsor found that "expectation and disturbing experiences such as a shock or the ingestion of distasteful food caused a marked reduction in the quantity of secretion from the parotid gland." Pavlov has demonstrated that even the chemical composition of saliva depends to a certain extent on the nature of the ingested food.[1]

[1] Brunacci, B., e De Sanctis. Sulla funzione secretoria della parotide dell'uomo. Archivio di Fisiologia. 1914, 14, 441.

Lashley, K. S. The Human Salivary Reflex and Its Use in Psychology. Psychological Review. 1916, 23, 446.

Krasnogorsky, N. I. Über die Wirkung mechanischer und chemischer Reizungen

GLOBUS HYSTERICUS

The globus hystericus is the well-known complaint of hysterical adults and some children that something like a ball or a stone (in one of Ziehen's cases even described by the child as a frog) moves from the stomach upward until it reaches the throat. Some authors believe that the sensation is caused by a mild spasm of the esophagus, and there are isolated reports that the spasm could be demonstrated roentgenoscopically.

AËROPHAGIA

Normally, a certain amount of air is always to be found in the gastric cavity and can be seen in the fundus with the aid of X-ray examinations. The suckling swallows some atmospheric air together with the milk and, if held up after the meal, emits it with an audible eructation. Older children sometimes draw air into the stomach when sighing, sobbing, coughing, or hiccoughing. The mechanism of abnormal *air-swallowing* or *aërophagia* (a term coined by Bouveret in 1893), is not exactly known. According to some, the deglutition of air can be explained mechanically by aspiration from the stomach through an easily yielding cardia. Others think of a clonic spasm of the muscles of the pharynx, by means of which air is pressed into the esophagus and immediately expelled through contraction of the esophageal musculature or carried into the stomach. Mathieu (*Archiv für Verdauungs-krankheiten. 1904, 10, 29*) describes the process as follows: Nervous individuals, after having eaten, have a feeling of tension in the epigastric region, which they usually ascribe to the presence of an increased quantity of gas. In their effort to rid themselves of the gas, they make movements (sighing, moaning) which cause them unintentionally to introduce air into the stomach. After a certain quantity of air has been accumulated in the gastric cavity, it is emitted with a good deal of belching. The patients feel relieved temporarily and on the next occasion repeat the procedure until it becomes a habit with them. According to John Thomson, older children sometimes swallow large quantities of air-containing saliva in order to lessen the discomfort arising from undue acidity of the gastric contents.

In some children, the habit begins during a time of acute abdominal uneasiness in the fashion depicted by Mathieu and is then kept up as a habit. Thomson gives a clear picture of the procedure: "The child, if sitting, bends slightly forward; or, if lying raises himself. He then shuts his mouth firmly, lowers his chin, assumes an air of absorption, and settles himself to swallow. As the air goes down, a slight clucking sound may be heard when it passes into the air-containing thoracic portion of the esophagus. Then the mouth is usually opened and the wind comes up . . . When the patient is left undisturbed, the air-gulping goes on until he is tired, or until his supply of saliva is exhausted. While the air is being swallowed, the up-and-down movements of the larynx are easily seen; and on inspection and percussion of the abdomen, the stomach is found to be rapidly distending . . . In some

verschiedener Teile der Mundhöhle auf die Tätigkeit der Speicheldrüsen bei Kindern. Jahrbuch für Kinderheilkunde. 1926, 114, 268.

Winsor, A. L. Factors Which Indirectly Affect Parotid Secretion. Journal of Experimental Psychology. 1930, 13, 423.

cases the air is quickly returned before it has passed beyond the esophagus. In others it goes right down into the stomach. When this occurs, most of it is usually brought up again shortly, provided there is nothing to prevent the child sitting up, but, if he has to remain lying on his back or right side, the necessary eructations do not take place and the air gradually passes through the pylorus. Later, such of it as is not absorbed in the bowel is expelled from the anus."[1]

Aërophagia, though a comparatively harmless habit in most instances, may sometimes lead to more serious difficulties. The gastric distension, if too rapid or too voluminous, may occasion severe abdominal pain and, through upward pressure on the diaphragm, cardiac and respiratory distress. Wyllie has even ascribed cases of sudden death to what he termed "gastric flatulence"; at least, that is what he felt was the cause of death in children whose past-morten examinations showed no other positive findings than extreme gastric distension and some collapse of the base of the left lung.[2]

The *diagnosis* of aërophagia is not made often in children because to the patients themselves the habit affords some pleasure and does not give them cause to complain. The parents usually do not consider the eructations significant enough to engage medical help. They are dismissed as "belching," which is taken the more lightly if, as is often the case, the belching is also present in one of the parents or grandparents.

The *treatment* must pay attention to the child's personality and especially to the existence of other habit and behavior disorders. The child should be kept sufficiently occupied with interesting toys and outdoor play with other children and his attention should be instantly distracted whenever he is found indulging in the pleasures of aërophagia and the ensuing eructations.

REGURGITATION AND RUMINATION

Some authors use the two terms almost interchangeably, whereas others are anxious to make careful distinctions, often without much success. Food is not infrequently regurgitated by infants and older children if they have eaten beyond the point of satiation. Particles or larger lumps are brought up into the mouth and spat up. If this is not done too frequently, it rarely forms the content of a complaint.

Rumination, or *merycism*, is a well defined clinical syndrome. It was first described in adults by Fabricius ab Aquapendente (*Opera omnia anatomica et physiologica. Lipsiae. 1687, p.135*).

His two case reports are delightfully naïve; his ruminating nobleman is said to have had two horns on his forehead, and his Paduan monk had a father who had "a little horn on his forehead." Since then, the literature on rumination with case descriptions, etiological theories, and therapeutic suggestions has assumed vast proportions. It was noticed that especially intellectual people, and more particularly physicians, were subject to the

[1] Thomson, John. The Clinical Study and Treatment of Sick Children. Edinburgh. 1925, pp. 120f.

[2] Wyllie. On Gastric Flatulence. Edinburgh Hospital Reports. 1895, 3, 21.

practice. Brown-Séquard and the famous psychiatrist, Naecke, were ruminators. The occurrence in children has not been published until the latter
half of the nineteenth century.

The act consists of bringing up the food without nausea, retching, or
disgust; the food is then either ejected from the mouth or, if liquid, permitted to run out, or it is reswallowed after chewing has, or has not, taken
place. When observed during the procedure, the child may be seen strain-
ing and arching his back. The mouth is kept wide open, the head held back,
and tongue movements of a sucking nature may be observed. From the
total appearance it becomes quite clear that the patient's attention is absorbed by the performance and that he shows signs of gratification.

Many theories about the *etiology* of rumination have been advanced. We
mention briefly those which are more frequently quoted in modern publications:

Atavistic anology to the rumination of herbivorous mammals. "Evidence of human evolution" (Sinkler). Sign of degeneration. Heredity (occurrence in two or more members of one family is indeed not infrequent;
Brockbank reported six ruminators, father and five children, in the same
family). Dilatation of the lower end of the esophagus (*antrum cardiacum;
gouttière ésophagienne*). Idiopathic esophagus dilatation. Gastric dilatation. Relaxation of the cardia. Cardiospasm (Husler). Pylorospasm. Motor
dynamic affection of the stomach (Lincoln). Overaction of the sphincter
muscles in the upper portions of the alimentary canal (Grulee). Irritation
of the nervus dilatator cardiae on the basis of central, peripheral, or reflex
vagotonia (Zweig). Pathological conditioned reflex (Lust, Curschmann).
Reflex act presided over by a center in the medulla oblongata, the afferent
pathway being represented by the vagus, the efferent by the phrenic nerves
and the motor nerves of the abdominal muscles, the stomach, and the
esophagus (Riesman). "Early symptom of a certain lability of the reflex
mechanism of the pharynx, esophagus, and stomach, under conditions that
point to the influence of a psychoneurotic element" (Strauch). "Effort on
the part of nature to stimulate reflexly the gastric secretions" (Halliday,
himself a ruminator). Movements of the tongue. Hyperacidity of gastric
juice. Achlorhydria. Achylia gastrica. Insufficient mastication. Rapid eating. Overeating. Aërophagia (Ylppö). Fingersucking. Neuropathic constitution. Neurasthenia (Naecke). Gastric neurosis (Lemoine and Linossier;
Freyhan). Motility neurosis (Brüning). Mnemic phenomenon (Aschenheim). Lack of occupation, boredom, ennui, analogous to the "cage sickness" of animals (Göppert). Imitation; a feebleminded child observed by
Peyer is said to have learned the practice through emulation of ruminating
cows.

Rumination is at first acquired incidentally and later taken up as a
pleasurable habit practiced voluntarily. The complete abandon to the performance and the profound gratification derived from it can be observed
quite often. Whatever the primary occasion may have been, the habit
nature of the act in perpetually ruminating children can hardly be questioned. Though undisturbed indulgence may often not impair the patient's
health if the food, or most of it, is reswallowed or if very little has been regurgitated, the usual complaint with which ruminating infants are brought

to the physician's attention is that of failure to gain or loss of weight, which is remedied promptly after cessation of the habit. In some babies, however, there may be so much waste of food through ejection that the condition of health is seriously affected through malnutrition, dehydration, acute gastro-intestinal disturbances, and lessened resistance to inter-current illnesses. Of fifty-two children taken to the Harriet Lane Home, not less than eleven died of the direct results of rumination. It may be added that the children are often not brought because of the habit but because of some other sickness and that the rumination is discovered during the examination or in the course of the patient's residence in the hospital. The flowing out of milk from the mouth is frequently interpreted by the parents as "vomiting."

In older children and in adults, the observation has been made that those addicted to the habit sometimes display a remarkable selectivity in that they only bring up their favorite foods whereas disliked substances are not ruminated. Schippers noticed the occurrence of rumination in infants even during sleep.

Of the fifty-two cases seen at the Harriet Lane Home, there was an equal number of boys and girls. Thirty-two were white and twenty were colored children. One had a duodenal ulcer and ulcerative stomatitis. Acute otitis media was the primary reason for consultation in ten patients. One suffered from acute epidemic encephalitis. Acute primary pneumonia was present in one and pyelonephritis in another. Three had hereditary syphilis. Every one of the children was first seen with rumination in the course of the first year of life, between the ages of two and a half and twelve or thirteen months, and some of them were followed for several years.

The degree of intellectual endowment ranges from idiocy to superior intelligence; this, of course, could in most instances be established only after the patients have reached a sufficiently high age to allow accurate testing. The family background showed instability and feeblemindedness in a considerable number of the cases.

In our attempt to examine the children several years after the infantile rumination had been treated, we were struck by the fact that the present whereabouts of the families could be located in a surprisingly small group only. In the course of time, the parents and their children evaporated without leaving any trace which would lead to finding them at their new residence; inquiries among relatives, former neighbors, and postal authorities were frequently unsuccessful. This in itself throws some light on the type of the patients' ascendency. One child was a foundling. Two others were illegitimate, of unknown fathers. In one case, a colored mother left her infant with an acquaintance and did not come back for him; she left the city for regions unknown. One mother was recommended for the State Training School for the Feebleminded. On the other hand, a few of the children came from stable, well-adjusted homes in which there were no personality difficulties in the occupants.

Of those that could be located and reëxamined, one girl, now fourteen years old, is physically healthy, normally intelligent, does well at home and in school, and never offered any behavior problems. She comes of stable parents and has several normal and bright siblings. A colored girl was brought back to the clinic at the age of six years with gonorrheal vaginitis.

Paul C., seven years and seven months old, ruminated until the age of seven months (note in the record at that time: "He was a typical ruminator, being of the wide-awake, alert type, who took delight in vomiting)." He was in good health when reëxamined. He had a mental age of seven years. He had, since infancy, had sick headaches two to three times each year. He got easily excited. He ate and slept well, played well with other children and was quite popular among them. His father a moderate drinker, suffered from attacks of sciatica; a daughter from a former marriage was totally blind. His mother complained of "quivering all over"; she had typical migraine attacks; before marrying the boy's father, she had an illegitimate child who had infantile paralysis and died of typhoid fever. Paul's oldest full sister eloped and married; both she and her husband "took life easy." A brother of six years was "mischievous" and "a bully." There were only six survivals of the mother's sixteen pregnancies. She stated in the interview: "Me and my husband both got a temper. I have the worst."

Dorothy B., now fourteen years old, ruminated until the age of ten months. She was physically ill with chronic nephritis. She was mentally retarded (mental age slightly below eleven years; I.Q. 77). She had had anxiety attacks for the past three years. She cried a good deal, had a jealous disposition, was restless, sullen, and quick-tempered, ("If she gets mad at you, she is liable to kill you"). She presented a feeding problem. At five years, she began to wet the bed every night and stopped rather suddenly after eighteen months. She hated school. Her mother was working, and Dorothy stayed with an aunt whom she did not obey ("You can't make me do anything. You are not my mother"). Her parents had been separated for ten years. Her father, a railroad detective, was said to have a "very bad temper." Her mother, since having chorea at fourteen, had been restless and irritable; she had severe headaches during which she became blind for about twenty minutes and her whole side, either the right or the left, "even half of the tongue and half of the gums," felt numb, "like worms crawling up." Dorothy was an only child.

Roberta D., a colored girl of eight and a half years, ruminated until the age of ten months. She had a marked lordosis, hypertrophied tonsils, and a slightly enlarged thyroid. Her intellectual level was one of over nine years (I.Q. 107). She was an only child of stable and intelligent parents. She did very well in school. She did, however, present a mild feeding problem and wet her bed several times during the week.

Amos S., a colored boy of thirteen, was first seen at the Harriet Lane Home at twelve months with rumination, scabies, and a sty. A few months later, he had acute otitis media and acute primary pneumonia. He was feebleminded (as were his mother and several siblings). He sucked his thumb. His mother felt that "he would do better in school if he did not spend all his time sucking his thumb." He wet his bed until very recently; enuresis, however, was traditional in his family.

A survey of the many curative methods suggested at one time or another yields the following variety of remedies:

Surgical treatment. It sounds almost unbelievable that as late as in the nineties of the past century trephining of the skull was not only advised but actually carried out in a number of instances. Hammond (*Merycism*,

Journal of Nervous and Mental Disease. 1894, 21, 680) followed the report of a case with the words: "Whether the cure of the merycism in this case was directly due to the operations on the cranium or the result of the mental improvement is a question which it would be difficult to answer."

Drug treatment. Hydrochloric acid, atropin, and luminal have been often employed in the treatment of rumination. The gastric juice of pigs has been administered by a few German physicians.

Mechanical devices. So-called ruminating caps are applied to the skull and strings tied tightly around the chin so that the infant could not move his jaw between the feedings. Plugging of the nostrils with wax or cotton wool has been recommended. Ylppö advised to fixate the child for a time so that he should lie on his abdomen. Siegert invented an inflatable balloon consisting of fish-bladder which he inserts into the esophagus with the help of a stomach-tube after each meal in order to block the passage from the cardia. Most of these measures are now of historical interest only.

Dietary measures. Mayerhofer, in 1912, was the first to employ and obtain good results with thick feedings. This method has since then gained the popularity which it indeed deserves. It has proved effective in the great majority of cases.

Psychotherapy. Under this heading, various procedures have been advised. Some plead for a change of climate. Others (so Comby) recommend "waking suggestion" without betraying the secret of how to use it in infants of less than one year.

The most sensible and also the most effective treatment consists in the administration of thick feedings (farina) and in distracting the child's attention whenever he is observed to indulge in the habit. In view of the poor home background of so many of the patients, it is essential that proper ventilation, feeding, and general care are established and, if necessary, supervised. In the case of serious malnutrition, hospital treatment may become imperative.

PSYCHOGENIC VOMITING

Vomiting in general is much more frequent in children than it is in grown-ups. Its origin may be infectious-inflammatory, toxic, cerebrogenic, reflex-determined, or psychogenic. It may arise from local gastric illness, or from a large number of extra-stomachic diseases (of the intestines, the appendix, the liver, the peritoneum; of the heart; of the kidneys; of the respiratory organs associated with paroxysmal cough; of the brain and the meninges; of the ears), or from pathological conditions attacking primarily the entire organism. It marks the termination of migrainous attacks. It may be a reaction to injudicious feeding.

Psychogenic vomiting is rife among youngsters of all age groups. It is important to emphasize that, no matter how obviously the child's personality may seem involved, the omission of a thorough physical examination constitutes a grave error. Though this is true with regard to any sort of complaint, it is especially so in cases of repeated vomiting, since there is hardly an affection of the human body that may not, at least in children, cause the ejection of food *per os*. On the other hand, coincidence with somatic illness does not always spell causal relationship. Vomiting often presents a beautiful example of the integrative psychobiological functioning of the human being, illustrating the emotional unbalance of the autonomic nervous system which, with or without the production of pylorospasm, may manifest itself clinically in the expulsion of food.

Stiller, in his book on gastric neuroses (*Die nervösen Magenerkrankungen. Stuttgart. 1884*), gives the following criteria of "nervous vomiting";

1. The ease with which the patient throws up. (Note: The vomiting arising from feeding difficulties on the basis of poor habit training is, however, often associated with considerable gagging and retching. Ease of vomiting must be clearly distinguished from projectile vomiting of cerebral origin.)

2. Its independence of the quality and quantity of the ingested food. (Note: Here again the same restriction obtains. Children who are "particular" about their food are more apt to vomit if forced to eat the things which they dislike than those of their preference.)

3. The fact that certain, very often bizarre, substances are retained.

4. The sometimes selective ejection of certain substances which are even eliminated from a mixed meal.

5. The indifference with which the patients tolerate the habitual vomiting.

6. The astounding tolerance of the body, based on general reduction of metabolism, for the inanition resulting from habitual vomiting.

7. The extraordinary dependence on the least external and internal situations affecting the mood.

8. The frequent occurrence of the vomiting spells not preceded by the ingestion of food, at a time when the stomach appears to be empty.

9. The presence of other nervous symptoms simultaneously or alternating with the vomiting spells.

To this Boas (*Diagnostik und Therapie der Magenkrankheiten. Leipzig. 1920*) adds as a further point:

10. The absence of essential secretory or motor disturbances of the stomach. (Note: This is not necessarily the case. Increased or diminished acidity and spasms of the pylorus may be sometimes observed in cases of unquestionable psychogenic vomiting.)

There are several types of vomiting in children which interest the psychiatrist. Sometimes one of these reactions may emerge from another. In many instances, the selection of this form of outlet for personality difficulties is based on early gastro-intestinal upsets with vomiting which supplied the pattern. In other cases, imitation of similar parental responses to emotional upheavals furnish the model. Not infrequently, a combination of both factors is obtained from the history.

The outstanding situations in which psychogenic vomiting occurs are listed below:

Gagging, retching, and vomiting may be a culmination of feeding problems which can be referred to poor training. They are taken up in the discussion of faulty feeding habits.

Vomiting may be a part manifestation of hypochondriacal trends. It is considered in connection with hypochondriasis.

A type of vomiting found in children is that which constitutes a reaction to being expected to do mental work which is beyond their capacity. It has been sometimes designated as *school vomiting* (*Schulerbrechen:* Boas). The youngster who is intellectually incapable of conforming to the grade requirements may develop a hatred of school and become so disgusted that he feels nauseated and throws up, sometimes even at the mere thought of school.

"He gets excited and vomits. Towards Sunday night and Monday morning he begins to feel sick and in the morning when there is school he shakes like having chills; they send him home from school because he vomits. He would be able to go two or three days only. Since we are not sending him to school he is all right. Since school began this fall, he has worse spells than ever. In all attacks he complains of pain in the stomach, vomits, and has diarrhea." This eleven-year-old boy, who also blinked, bit his nails, was afraid of the dark, and became upset when called to recite in the class room, had summer complaint with vomiting at 22 months and several gastro-intestinal upsets between two and four years of age. His mother had "nervous indigestion" all her life; it worked "in spells" related to excitement and worry; she vomited occasionally. The boy had a mental age of nine years and was expected to accomplish promotion to the fifth grade. He was placed in an ungraded class, whereupon the vomiting ceased.

It is true that this boy did not vomit during school holidays and when kept at home on regular school days. But it is erroneous to conclude from that, as is often done, that the therapy consists simply in having the patient stay at home. This form of management stops the vomiting, to be sure; but it does not attack the fundamental problem. Through placement in a class in which he can do the required work the hatred of school is remedied. It may also become necessary to treat or to arrange for the treatment of a parent or sibling who reacts similarly to other difficulties.

Vomiting may also occur as a response to acute excitement.

"Loud noises or excitement causes her to be cross; she shows it up in digestion, too; when she is excited, she has vomiting spells."

"He had attacks of pain in his stomach for about three years. At first they were six to twelve months apart, this year he had three or four. They usually begin in the afternoon. He would look pale and lie down. He would then start to vomit and lie curled up. He may keep up for a day or two, getting gradually over. He cries a great deal during the attack." The spells were always preceded by strong excitement. Several attacks followed the visits to moving pictures with "scary" contents.

In some spoiled children, usually of high intelligence, the vomiting is clearly a pleasurable procedure which is enjoyed by the patient because it provides him with a tool to dominate and terrorize the family.

A little adopted girl of five years, of superior intelligence, in excellent physical condition, enjoyed alarming her overindulgent foster mother with frequent vomiting, often self-induced by the introduction of her finger into her throat, and by the repeating of words and sentences which was interpreted as stammering. As soon as both of these performances were disregarded and failed to produce the desired results, they were given up.

Car-sickness. Nausea and vomiting in trains, streetcars, and automobiles are not infrequent in children. They are often related to seasickness (the term "nausea" itself originally meant sea-sickness) and to vertigo. It is difficult to say and must be determined in each case, whether the frequent occurrence in a parent of the same reaction is to be interpreted as an indication of heredity or furnishes the child with a pattern which he imitates. We are reminded of the little boy who saw his sea-sick mother vomit on the boat and, stating that he would not do such a thing, instantly vomited; since then, he threw up at home a good many times, causing his parents to fear that he had a cancer. In some children, we had an opportunity to obtain the history of situational factors etiologically connected with the car-sickness.

John I., eleven years old, lost his father in an automobile accident one year ago. Since then, he always vomited in automobiles and street cars. He also vomited once when he heard his aunt tell of an accident in which a truck driver was killed and the car burned in a ditch.

Care is indicated in the evaluation of so-called *cyclic vomiting*. It is quite true that children with this type of periodic vomiting show often behavior difficulties because of or in addition to the illness. One girl who had attacks of cyclical vomiting in her childhood also suffered from enuresis, developed mild depressive states during puberty and, at sixteen, had a full-fledged manic excitement. The condition itself, however, which is in some features related to migraine, seems to be based mainly on physiogenic factors and is best considered and treated on its own merits.

LOCALIZED "NEUROPATHIC" DISORDERS OF THE DIGESTIVE TRACT

There exists in children a group of localized dysfunctions of the alimentary canal which rarely come to the psychiatrist's attention and which many pediatricians have linked up more or less closely and consistently with a "neuropathic" disposition and ascendency of the patients. This is especially true of the spastic conditions of the various sections of the gastro-intestinal system and of the disorder known as mucous colitis. Thus, for example, Finkelstein and L.F. Meyer, in Feer's textbook, deal with congenital hypertrophic pyloric stenosis under the heading of *Die nervösen Magendarmerkrankungen*. The preponderance in boys of this disease and of cardiospasms (Hertz's achalasia of the cardia; idiopathic dilatation of the esophagus) has been explained on the basis that the male sex is generally more vagotonic than the female. We have, on the one hand, the knowledge that the four-or five-week-old baby with a hypertrophy of the pylorus, whether it be primary or compensatory, is accessible to no other than a local attack and that, to judge from John Thomson's follow-up studies, the surviving patients develop normally and, as a matter of fact, "doubtless owing to the special care that they had had, were above the average in vigor and development."

It is quite certain that spasms of the colon and perhaps also of the cardia in school children, adolescents, and adults have sometimes a psychogenic origin and are benefited by adequate psychotherapy. Visceral participation in normal emotional life has been demonstrated experimentally. It is therefore quite understandable that in both acute affective upheavals and more protracted "dysphoric" states there should be, through the medium of the autonomic nervous system, an increase or a diminution of the physiological co-functions of the splanchnic integrants. Cannon speaks of a "psychic tone" or "psychic contraction" of the gastro-intestinal muscles. Its modifications under the influence of emotional disturbances can be looked upon as near-physiological alterations.

We have had the experience that of the cases of spastic colon and of mu-co-membranaceous colitis only a certain number had to be referred for psychiatric consultation. In the others, careful inquiry into the children's personality reactions and environmental conditions disclosed no need for other than ordinary medical care. Where behavior difficulties are found to exist, it seems rather futile, even from a purely academical point of view, to theorize on whether the psychiatric problem is the cause or the result of the gastro-intestinal dysfunction or whether they are merely coincidental. A rational approach will deal with the child and all his difficulties in a manner which would tend to remedy his faulty reaction tendencies and the underlying situational and personal maladjustments and at the same time relieve the local disorder through hygienic, dietary, and pharmocological means. With this sort of régime, we are certain to reach all that calls for correction in the individual case, without having to succumb to theoretical generalizations. A routine psychiatric examination of children with colo-spasms and mucous colitis would undoubtedly be of great value and throw some light on the problem. Since only those with complaints of behavior disorders have been referred to us, we are unable to draw definite conclusions applicable to all cases.

CONSTIPATION AND DIARRHEA

Next to the proper feeding of infants and older children, their bowel movements are an item of great concern in the minds of their mothers. Attention to the establishment of regular defecation is undoubtedly an important factor in child training. It is, however, essential that the educator should know which mode of nutrition is conducive to the desirable regulation and what the child's normal excretory rhythm is. Some individuals empty their bowels once in twenty-four hours, others twice within the same period, others again once in two days or twice in three days. Oversolicitous parents often become alarmed if the number of stools does not come up to their expectations and are too ready to blame the bowels instead of the type of food or the youngster's natural inclinations. They immediately become obsessed with the fear of chronic constipation, and then laxatives and enemas are made a matter of daily routine. After several years of such a management everyone concerned, including the patient himself, is convinced that drugs and "syringes" are the only means of "keeping the bowels open." Many cases of chronic constipation are in reality cases of habitual constipation. Newspaper advertisements with their dire prophesies continue to worry the already overanxious mothers; constipation is therefore a frequent complaint in the pediatrician's office and in children's dispensaries. It goes without saying that in every instance a thorough physical examination must precede the recommendation of any remedial plan.

Habitual constipation may have its origin in a temporary somatic condition which so alarms the parents and concentrates the child's attention on his bowel movements, that the protracted medications and too frequent attempts to defecate and urges to "press" create in his mind the conviction that he is chronically constipated. Or it may begin with the youngster's refusal to go to the toilet as a part manifestation of general negativism and obstinacy which also manifests itself in the stubborn refusal to eat and to go to bed. Or the foundation may be laid by a number of situational factors which do not permit the child to empty his bowels at a time when there is a need for it. This happens if he does not get his breakfast early enough and must rush to school without having time to defecate; in the class room, he does not ask for leave, either because of his own prudishness or on account of the teacher's unreasonable attitude or owing to the fear that he might miss some of the instruction given in his absence. In homes where the toilet is in the yard, the child may be unwilling to go out in cold weather or fearing the dark in the evening. There are families where the complaint of constipation is traditional in several generations; its existence is expected in the children on the assumption that it is "hereditary" and, in order to prevent it, suppositories and *per os* medications are administered at an early age. We have seen ten and twelve-year-old youngsters who had been given purgatives routinely since infancy without it ever occurring to their mothers to discontinue the drugs; often castor oil, senna leaves, "family physician," Ex-lax, Nujol, etc., were given with or without medical advice; in some cases the prescription was momentarily justified but the parents took it upon themselves to keep the medation up indefinitely.

Prophylaxis and treatment of habitual constipation are based upon the same principles: a well-balanced diet, regularity of feeding, sufficient exercise in the open, going to the toilet at the same hour every day at a time which is free from distractions and haste. It is best to leave the business of emptying to the youngster, avoiding admonitions while he is on the stool and anxious inquiries the minute he rises. Dangling toys before the child and making dramatic scenes of each session only gives him a welcome opportunity for occupying the center of attention, with which he may be loath to part for a long time; the sessions become prolonged, the mother solicitous, to the tragicomedy of the toilet procedure is added that of getting the tot to take the laxative, and the "constipation" becomes habitual.

It is known that constipation is quite frequent in epileptic and in migrainous children.

Diarrhea on an emotional or habitual basis is rather uncommon in children. Anxious anticipation may be accompanied by increased peristalsis and frequent evacuations. The so-called "examination diarrhea" is a well-known phenomenon. It may well be that the diarrhea in young babies in hospital wards following a change of nurses, reported by Finkelstein, was due to no other factors than the arrival of a new and unwelcome nurse; it is, of course, also possible that in that case dietary causes were at play.

The psychoanalysts, having their own specific way of "interpreting" things, claim that constipation is an expression of "anal eroticism," that the patients are unconsciously averse to "giving away" anything, and that they are disposed to avarice, hoarding, and pedantry. Identification of defecation with giving birth to a baby and of feces with gold plays a rôle in the psychoanalysts' mode of thinking.

ENCOPRESIS

The term *encopresis* denotes, since Weissenberg,[1] the act of involuntary defecation which is not directly due to organic illness. The term fecal incontinence, or incontinentia alvi, is reserved for the occurrence of soiling in connection with local abnormalities of the rectum and anus, in children with acute or chronic cerebral or spinal diseases or injuries, and during acute infections in which the patient's otherwise normal bowel control is temporarily suspended because of weakness, delirious reaction, or general irresponsiveness, ranging from mild lethargy to deep coma. The diagnosis of encopresis, therefore, can be made only after demonstrable organic lesions that may be logically made responsible have been excluded. Soiling with bowel contents sometimes occurs during an epileptic or epileptiform convulsion.

Normally, any child at two years may be reasonably expected to have established adequate habits of intestinal elimination. Persistence of soiling beyond the end of the second year of life may be due to serious mental retardation, or to lack of proper training, or both. In these patients encopresis is always associated with enuresis.

Morton F., three years and five months old, had a developmental level of a little more than twelve months, as determined by the Gesell test. He was a badly spoiled only child of feebleminded parents. His mother had frequent temper tantrums. The child, his parents, a paternal grandfather, grandmother and great-grandmother lived together in a small, filthy, ill-ventilated apartment, in which the women's main occupation consisted in ministering to the boy. He wet and soiled himself both in day time and at night, did not say more than three words (and those very indistinctly), cried almost constantly, sucked his fingers, ate dirt and feces, and was destructive. During the first interview, the mother jumped up from her chair dozens of times to see after the child, who was playing quietly in the adjoining room, or in response to any slightest noise or move that he made. Training of toilet or other habits had never been attempted.

Howard J., a colored boy of four years and eight months, presented the rather unusual combination of diurnal enuresis and nocturnal encopresis ("every other night"). He had just begun to use monosyllables. He was the retarded illegitimate child of an unknown father and a feebleminded mother. He had been spoiled and received no habit training in the home, which consisted of three rooms and housed ten people. Howard still used a nipple ("for comfort") and had temper tantrums.

Shirley B., a girl of four years and nine months, physically healthy, came from a fairly stable family. She had a developmental age of less than two years. She wet her bed every night, often had enuresis in daytime, and often soiled both her bed and her clothes. She had temper tantrums in which she bit her hands.

Frankie L., a girl of three years and eight months, epileptic, with large infected tonsils and chronic otitis media, still wore diapers because she wet and soiled herself "all the time." She had a developmental level of approxi-

---

[1] Weissenberg, S. Über Enkopresis. Zeitschrift für Kinderheilkunde. 1926, 40, 674-677.

mately eighteen months. She had temper tantrums in which she bit and screamed and kicked.

Serious developmental retardation is a common feature in the cases which we have quoted so far. It is present in the greater majority of instances of encopresis. We have seen many idiotic and imbecile children who, with good training, had established good fecal and urinary habits at an early age, and again others in whom the training had had but little effect. Usually, at about five years of age, even the imbecile (and, sometimes, the idiotic) child has ceased to soil himself.

This was not the case with Irene L., who wet and soiled her bed and her clothes at the age of almost eleven years. She often wandered away from her home. She had a mental age of five years. She was not in any way concerned about any of her difficulties. Her father, an alcoholic, deserted the family, her mother was illiterate and feebleminded. The child had leucoderma, dental caries, and right external strabismus. She was committed to the State Training School for the Feebleminded, where within a few days she was rid of her encopresis and, some time later, also of her enuresis.

The mentally retarded encopretic child is not as trying by far as are the more intelligent patients addicted to the habit of soiling themselves. Thom says of them: "One can only say that these cases call for a careful psychiatric examination by the best qualified person available. And it will often test all his skill and ingenuity to understand the mental processes at work that result in such conduct."[1] These instances are rare, it is true, but not so infrequent as to deserve the total neglect which they receive in most pediatric textbooks. Of our material, all but two of the children belonging in this category have had competent habit training in infancy. The underlying motives were found to be different in each individual case. The encopresis is much oftener diurnal than in the imbecile patients. Treatment has sometimes instantaneous success, but in other cases it takes a long time before the practice can be eradicated. Occasionally, the soiling with bowel contents is a voluntary spite reaction against the parents; such cases have been reported by Thom and by Pototzky.[2] According to Stier,[3] most encopretic children present features of cruelty and brutality. Thom's patient, a seven-year-old girl, reacted to a jealousy situation not only with encopresis but also by smearing with her feces the walls of her room, clean linen, and even her food and dishes. Pototzky's case was that of an eleven-year-old boy whose trousers were found filled with feces about one hour after each scolding by his parents; he delighted in their embarrassment and disgust which was caused by their handling of his soiled clothing.

Charles H., a nine-year-old boy with chronic dacryocystitis and congenital malformation of both hands and both feet used to soil his clothes

[1] Thom, Douglas A. Everyday Problems of the Everyday Child. New York, 1928, p. 102.

[2] Pototzky, C. Psychogenese und Psychotherapie von Organsymptomen beim Kinde. In Oswald Schwarz's Psychogenese und Psychotherapie körperlicher Symptome. Berlin. 1925.

[3] Stier, E. Das Einschmutzen der Kinder, seine Beziehungen zum Einnässen. Zeitschrift für Kinderforschung. 1925, 30, 125–144.

until he was six years old. He was the son of an alcoholic, vindictive father
and a hypochondriacal mother. Charles received practically no habit training in infancy. Someone had told the parents that, on account of his de-
formity, he would not live long. They did not feel like teaching him "if he
had such a short life ahead of him." He therefore started out in life with no
bowel or bladder control established. He was considered constipated if his
clothes were not soiled as often as his mother expected; he was therefore
given laxatives and enemas every day. Thus, defecation was made a
major issue in the child's activities and, through his fight against the purgatives and syringes, in his family relations. It was one of his tobacco-chewing
father's favorite occupations to spit about everywhere, and he was especially delighted if the practice aroused his wife's anger. The boy modified
this pattern to suit his own status and soiled himself more or less voluntarily to spite his mother or to extricate himself from the need of carrying
out some order unsatisfactory to him. Poor home environment, faulty training, concentration of attention to the child's bowel movements, and sometimes spite reaction formed the basis of his encopresis.

Melvin T., eight and a half years old, had good toilet habits as long as
he was with his parents. When he began to go to school, his grandmother,
whose husband had just suicided, took him to her home "because she took
a liking to him and wanted him to stay with her." Since then he had been
soiling his clothes: "Instead of going to the toilet he does it in his pants.
At times when you scold him for it he does not do it for a while and then he
goes on out and does it again. The only thing I can lay it to is laziness. I
try by talking to him to bring him out of it. I've beat him a couple of
times with my hand. We talk to him and try to shame him. Since he has
been over here to the hospital, he does not do it so much. You would think
it would come out soft, but it doesn't, it is just like anyone else's. He does
not soil himself when he is in school. It is generally in the evening when he
comes home from school. It is about the same time every day. When he
gets out to play he just does not come in." The last sentence contains a
partial clue to the situation. His grandmother had made every effort to
usurp for herself and to absorb the child's whole being. She made him sleep
with her, bathed him, would not let him go out to play, was jealous of his
little playmates, and derived a peculiar enjoyment from cleaning his soiled
clothes. The boy had to sneak out of the house after school and delayed his
return as much as possible. He hated his grandmother and her sometimes
really disgusting proofs of her affection. He was returned to his parents'
home and given opportunity for recreational outlets, and his encopresis
ceased promptly. He was physically healthy and had an intelligence quotient of 99.

Wilbur G., seven and a half years old, in good health and normally intelligent, suffered from the continued hostilities, coupled with peculiar
"educational" practices, of an untruthful, indifferent, self-righteous mother,
who was eager to make herself appear in the best possible light and her boy
in the worst possible light. Some of her complaints, offered as accusations,
were found to be outright inventions. She presented him as a "feeding problem" and later on, apparently forgetting what she had said, stated
that he ate everything nicely. She complained of his being enuretic but "I
always get him up at night at about eleven o'clock since he was a baby. He
would wet the bed if I didn't." It had, however, never occurred to her to
give him an opportunity to demonstrate whether or not he was really enuretic. The child masturbated. Because of constipation in early infancy, his

mother "had to" syringe him every morning; she had often expressed surprise that so bad a boy did not soil his clothes. He finally did accommodate her, beginning about a month before she took him to the dispensary: "I wanted to have him examined to see if it was only laziness or weakness. The examination showed it wasn't." What it really was, was a protest against the daily enemas, the nightly waking, and the fact that the syringing with its effect often caused this intelligent and conscientious child to be late in school. It seemed of little use to try to influence the mother's attitude, except that she did give up the syringing and waking. There was also little coöperation to be expected from the father who was much too preoccupied with his "fight" for government compensation. Our efforts were therefore limited to direct work with the child, whose soiling ceased immediately. He never wet his bed after the habit of waking him was given up.

It is probably only incidental that all of our patients with encopresis, who belong to the second group (that is, not seriously retarded), were boys. We have seen several more such children besides those reported above. All of them showed signs of emotional instability and immaturity, and it is especially interesting to note the frequent occurrence of temper tantrums in connection with the complaint of encopresis. Constipation, in the sense of habitual lack of the bowel contents, is also a not uncommon feature. One child was not permitted to change from the use of the chamber pot to that of the toilet until the age of four years and, when he insisted, he was told that he would "go down to the ground"; he developed a morbid fear of the toilet, and when the pot was discarded, he preferred to soil his clothes to running the risk of going down to the ground. After this fear was dispelled, normal habits of elimination were easily established.

CHAPTER XXVI

THE CIRCULATORY SYSTEM

IT IS REMARKABLE to notice the contrast between the relative frequency of psychogenic circulatory affections in the adult and their scarcity in children. A fair portion of the internist's practice is made up of so-called *cardiac neuroses;* emotionally determined heart sensations are especially numerous during the years of climacteric involution. Most youngsters have not yet learned to share with their elders the age-old interpretation of the heart as being the principal organ of life and the seat of their feelings. It is therefore hardly surprising to observe that, if such complaints as pain around the heart or palpitations do occur in the early years, they are mostly traceable to direct parental or medical influence. Hypochondriacal attitudes in some older member of the family, centered about the heart, may lend themselves to imitation and the formation of similar trends in one or another of the children. The custom of some oversolicitous mothers of feeling and counting their own pulse or that of their offspring at the slightest suspicion of illness may direct a child's preoccupations toward self-observation and the employment of the same method.

A further, by no means negligible etiological factor consists in the peculiar and obviously harmful, yet wide-spread habit of discussing children's physical conditions with their parents in the patients' presence. It is one of the most astounding phenomena in the general practice of medicine that diagnoses, prognoses, and impressions are often given out right in front of a child, apparently with the assumption that he will not be more affected by what he hears than a piece of office furniture. Remarks, such as, "She has a systolic murmur but it is probably not due to a leakage of the heart," or, "His heart seems to be a little affected," or unfounded prescriptions of digitalis or rest cures have started quite a few children on the road to chronic invalidism. Even where an organic cardiac ailment really exists, there is hardly a justification for blurting out everything, and especially pessimistic predictions, within the child's hearing. But what of the girl who for a long time, declared by a physician to have a "leaking heart" which she did not have, was treated daily to digitalis, kept out of school, kept in bed for weeks at a time, forbidden to go out and play, and deprived of all the activities and associations of a normal youngster? It is true that about two weeks after the revision of the "diagnosis" and after a radical clearing of the morbid atmosphere the child was as vigorous, happy, and playful as any healthy child could be. But the two years of invalidism imposed upon her by injudicious management, the family's anxiety, her own constant fear of death (the physician had said she "might drop dead some day"), all the unnecessary anguish and wasted time cannot be made undone. It is, of course, needless to say that real cardiac illness must be handled with the utmost care which, however, does not include dire prophecies nor the need of making the patient a witness of the discussions of his illness.

Some children have for many months or even for years a tendency to respond to any kind of excitement with a greater or lesser degree of tachycardia with or without palpitations; functional murmurs and even a slight degree of cardiac dilatation may be present. The pulse rate, under the emotional influence of the examination, may be as high as 140 to 160 beats per minute. Physical effort and change of posture have no marked effect on the pulse frequency. The tachycardia is never present during sleep. Often, but not always, the condition is a part manifestation of pre-pubescent or pubescent hyperthyroidism. It usually disappears gradually during the second decade of life. The treatment consists of the establishment of a well-balanced distribution of work, rest, and sleep over the twenty-four hours of the day, adjustment of the child at home and in school, and the creation of a calm environment. Digitalis and other medications, giving to the parents or to the patient the impression as if there were a pathological heart condition, are strongly counterindicated. One should be most careful about advising removal from the school or prolonged rest in bed and about curbing the youngster's usual occupations and recreations.

Palpitations and pain in the cardiac region are frequent concomitants of anxiety attacks.

The vasomotor participation in emotional responses often expresses itself externally in the form of noticeable *blushing* or *pallor*. Facial reddening may accompany joyful excitement or shame or embarrassment or may be an indication of physical effort, as in the case of stuttering children whose attempts to speak are sometimes associated with considerable blushing. In some youngsters, especially during adolescence, this reaction may be so frequent that the boys or girls are apt to become self-conscious and constantly preoccupied with the fear of its recurrence in public; this condition has been referred to as erythrophobia. Occasionally the emotional vasodilatation may extend over the neck and chest.

Pallor, with or without "goose flesh," is often a complication of fear and fright. It is, above all, an outstanding symptom of syncopal attacks ("fainting spells").

Heim has studied the blood pressure of "neuropathic" children and found that it was variously affected by excitement. He quotes the example of two boys (their ages are not given) whose average blood pressure was between 80 and 95 mm.; when they had severe toothache, they reacted (to the pain or to the fear of the dentist or to both?) with a pressure of 140 to 160, lasting for a few days before and shortly after the extraction of their teeth. Federn ascribed the blood pressure changes in "neurasthenic" individuals to a "partial atonia of the large intestines."[1]

[1] Heim, Paul. Das Verhalten des Blutdruckes bei neuropathischen Kindern. Deutsche medizinische Wochenschrift. 1900, 26, 320.—Federn, S. Blutdruck und Darmatonie. Wien. 1894.

CHAPTER XXVII

THE RESPIRATORY SYSTEM

THE RESPIRATORY apparatus lends itself much less than most of the other organ systems of the body to the expression of psychogenic part-dysfunctions in children. The breathing mechanisms are involved in the visceral participation of certain emotional reactions, especially those of fear and surprise. Even popular phraseology knows of the attitude of "breathless" interest. The sighs of sorrow, yearning, and relief are common occurrences.

We know that some children who have derived the advantages of special attention as a result of an upper respiratory infection may continue to *cough* in order to keep enjoying the concomitant parental solicitude. This is especially the case in certain families in which a member has been ill with tuberculosis and any cough is immediately viewed with alarm as a possible indicator of the dreaded disease. It is, however, interesting that psychogenic cough is much less frequent than psychogenic vomiting. In one of our cases, a baby had once been kissed by a neighbor who a few months later was admitted to a sanatorium for tuberculous patients; the mother began to worry that her child might have been infected and for years interpreted every little cough or clearing of the throat as a danger signal; the child, at five years, acquired the habit of coughing which stamped him as an invalid and gave him a *carte blanche* for all sorts of misbehavior.

Another form of peculiar respiratory disorder was brought to our attention by a mother who was alarmed by her seven-year-old son's "smothering spells." It was learned that she was in the habit of hugging the boy so vigorously that he was incapable of breathing during the procedure; the "smothering" was caused by the mechanical compression of the thorax and not by "nervousness," as the mother had thought.

Hiccoughing is sometimes met with as a special variety of tic in children and in adults. The respiratory disorders following in the wake of epidemic encephalitis have been described in connection with that disease. The manifold relations between asthma and personality difficulties of children have been discussed in the chapter on the somatic factor. The breathholding spells of infants will be taken up together with the other attack disorders.

CHAPTER XXVIII

THE URINARY SYSTEM

ENURESIS

ENURESIS is the involuntary and, at least at the inception of the act, unconscious passage of urine by persons more than three years of age. It has been established that approximately ten per cent of all one-year-old children have acquired the dry habit; at eighteen months, about thirty per cent have good bladder control; at two years, from sixty-five to eighty per cent have ceased to wet themselves; at three years, the average child is expected to keep his clothes and bed entirely clean. Some authors are accustomed to refer to the mode of micturition during the first two or three years of life as *physiological enuresis*.

For the sake of clearness, it is advisable to follow the example of those who in cases of demonstrable organic involvement use the term "incontinence of the bladder" or "urinary incontinence." The designation of "enuresis" should be reserved for diurnal or nocturnal wetting in which a more or less direct causal relation to known anatomical, inflammatory, or neuropathological disorders cannot be obtained by the most painstaking physical examination.

The frequency of enuresis is well known to every pediatrician, general practitioner, child psychiatrist, and to those engaged in the institutional care of children. Of all the patients referred to us for psychiatric consultation, not less than twenty-six per cent came with enuresis as a major difficulty. The age distribution, expressed in percentages, was as follows:

Years	Per cent.
3	6
4	9
5	6
6	12
7	6
8	12
9	16
10	12
11	11
12	5
13	1
14	4

Sixty-two per cent of the patients were boys, and thirty-eight per cent were girls. This figure corresponds quite well to the observations made by most authors who offer statistical data. According to Thom, enuresis is found in both sexes with about the same frequency. Thursfield, however, reports preponderance in girls. It is true that some parents are less reluctant to disclose the fact of a son's bedwetting than that of a daughter's.

All degrees of intelligence were represented, quite in harmony with the general distribution of the I.Q. among the children seen in our department.

Idiocy and imbecility: 8 per cent
Morons: 15 per cent
Borderline intelligence: 40 per cent
Average intelligence: 30 per cent
Superior intelligence: 7 per cent

In most instances (78 per cent), the enuresis has been lifelong, that is, it has continued beyond the period of physiological wetting and was still present at the time of the first consultation. In nine per cent, the children had acquired proper toilet habits but later relapsed. Thirteen per cent had ceased to wet before they were taken to the clinic because of some other personality difficulties. The ages at either onset or cessation are given below:

Onset at 3 years	2 per cent
Onset at 4 years	1 per cent
Onset at 5 years	3 per cent
Onset at 6 years	1 per cent
Onset at 9 years	1 per cent
Total	9 per cent

Cessation at 4 years	1 per cent
Cessation at 5 years	2 per cent
Cessation at 6 years	2 per cent
Cessation at 7 years	4 per cent
Cessation at 8 years	1 per cent
Cessation at 9 years	1 per cent
Cessation at 10 years	2 per cent
Total	13 per cent

As regards the incidence of wetting in the individual children, the following information was obtained:

Daily	50 per cent	Once a month	2 per cent
Almost daily	5 per cent	"Occasionally"	11 per cent
Frequently	7 per cent	"Off and on"	2 per cent
3–4 times weekly	3 per cent	"In spells"	2 per cent
Twice weekly	4 per cent	"Infrequently"	1 per cent
Once a week	4 per cent		

Nocturnal enuresis is the commonest form. It usually occurs only once during the night, but in a small number of instances the child may wet as many as three or four times in one night. The diurnal type is relatively rare. Wetting of the clothes in daytime is not infrequently associated with nightly passage of urine. These are the figures obtained from our material:

Nocturnal enuresis only: 63 per cent
Nocturnal and diurnal enuresis: 30 per cent
Diurnal enuresis only: 7 per cent

It is interesting that so many parents who take the bedwetting for granted look upon the diurnal form as something much more serious. As regards the circumstances under which enuresis occurs during the waking hours, we quote the following statements contained in the complaints:

"Whenever he has a cold."
"Only when he laughs."
"When she laughs heartily."
"When frightened or upset."
"When out playing."
"When he plays too hard."
"When he plays outdoors and does not want to come in."
"From waiting too long."
"If she can't run to the toilet right away when she feels the urge."
"Only when he is frightened."
"He still forgets himself sometimes when he is playing."
"I think sometimes he is just lazy, that he plays and forgets about it. You have to remind him all the time. I tried to whip him, to shame him, to promise him things, but it is just the same."

Diurnal wetting is most apt to occur while the child is playing excitedly and fully absorbed by the game. In patients who are of school age, it is more common to hear of wet clothes in the after-school hours and during recess than in the class room, although enuresis during study periods is not so very infrequent and taxes the educational and therapeutic skill of many a teacher and school physician. Second in frequency is the diurnal wetting which happens under the direct and immediate influence of a strong emotional experience, especially laughter and fright.

In most of those cases in which there is a combination of nocturnal and diurnal enuresis, the bedwetting is much more frequent than the wetting in daytime. But occasionally the opposite holds true. It also often happens that a child may cease to wet his bed but continue to wet his clothes, or vice versa.

These facts are expressed in the following statements:

"He often wets himself at night but more often in daytime."
"At night always, during the day only when he laughs."
"Mostly at night, in daytime only when she is frightened."
"At night always, in daytime often."
"At night always, during the day until two years ago."
"At night in spells of two to three weeks' duration, in daytime only when away from home."
"She still wets herself every day (at 12 years); she used to wet the bed until three years ago."
"At night all his life, in daytime several times each day, for the past year only."

There exists a considerable variety of conditions which have been described as the actual, or predisposing, or exciting causes of involuntary micturition. External irritations due to phimosis, adherent prepuce, balanitis, vulvitis, eczema and pruritus in the region of the genitalia, and oxyuris vermicularis, anatomical anomalies and subacute or chronic inflammatory processes of the internal urinary organs, such as cystitis, pyelitis, and nephritis, and bacteriuria have been found responsible in many instances and believed by some to be responsible in practically all cases. Spina bifida occulta and myelodysplasia (Fuchs) have been accused. Nutritional factors (diets rich in salt and fluids), the concentration and chemical composition (high acidity) of the urine, and hypertrophy of the tonsils and adenoids have been blamed. The depth of sleep has been proclaimed as an outstanding etiological feature. Others have identified enuresis with epileptic equivalents. Some have declared it to be an early monosymptomatic manifestation of hysteria, the expression of a certain type of organ inferiority, an unconscious substitute for masturbation, the result of thyroid dysfunction, or a "stigma of degeneration."

There is not the slightest doubt that most of the conditions just enumerated may, in individual cases, give rise to and maintain urinary incontinence and that their oversight or neglect will strongly interfere with correct adjustment. To treat as a habit the wetting of a child, which is intimately associated with a chronic or recurrent pyuria, is as grave a medical error as would be to treat psychogenically determined enuresis on the basis of a postulated but not demonstrated local or "reflex" irritation of some sort or another. It must, on the other hand, be emphasized that coincidence does not always spell causal relationship and that the wetting may sometimes persist as a habit after the clearing up of the physical factors which have caused it or contributed to its origin.

It is believed in some quarters that occult *spina bifida* plays an eminent rôle in the etiology of enuresis. After reviewing a representative number of cases of both enuresis and spina bifida, we may state safely that, while enuresis is often present in children with spina bifida, the finding of spina bifida is quite rare in enuretic patients (1.5 per cent). We have seen two children of one family, of whom the younger sister, six and a half years old, had no spina bifida and was enuretic (she had tics, feeding difficulties with vomiting, nightmares, and headaches; her vulva was adherent in the midline), while her brother, eight and a half years old, had spina bifida and no enuresis (he offered a feeding problem, vomited, bit his finger nails, and had a history of night terrors).

The possible relations between an existing spina bifida and the functions of the bladder and bowels may be seen in the following cases:

a. Spina bifida without any disturbance of the excretory functions:
  1. Girl, eight years. Recurrent vomiting.
  2. Boy, colored, two years, ten months. Congenital malformation of the hip. Early hereditary lues. Rickets. Inguinal hernia.
  3. Girl, six years. Pyuria. Dental caries. Chronic tonsillitis.
  4. Girl, six years. Crying spells, nightmares, feeding problem with vomiting.
  5. Girl, six years. All sacral segments were open. Little's disease. Serious mental retardation.
  6. Boy, seven and a half years. Dental caries.
  7. Boy, twelve years. Obesity. Pain in back.
  8. Boy, seven years, eight months. Spastic paraplegia. Defective speech.

b. Spina bifida with retention of urine.
  1. Boy, three years. Paralysis of the bladder with attacks of urinary retention.

c. Spina bifida with enuresis.
1. Boy, four years. Temper tantrums. Poor habit training. Nocturnal type.
2. Boy, four years, seven months. Dental caries. Restlessness. Blinking. Nocturnal.
3. Girl, three years, seven months. Nocturnal.
4. Boy, nine years. Diurnal only: "always wet, always dripping." It began as soon as he was dressed. It never occurred during school hours (9–12; 1–3), always at home or while out playing. It disappeared under psychiatric treatment.
5. Boy, five years, three months. Right testis undescended. Right buttock larger than left. Diurnal only, began immediately upon waking. Constipation treated by mother with daily enemas and laxatives.
6. Boy, twelve years. Nocturnal; disappeared entirely after home adjustment.
7. Girl, seven and a half years. Oxyuris vermicularis. Temper tantrums, feeding problem, faulty training. Nocturnal and diurnal. Overindulgent, unintelligent mother.
8. Boy, nine years. Mentally retarded. Redundant prepuce. Diurnal. He had stopped wetting at two years; since six years, he urinated in his underwear during after-school periods of excitement.

d. Spina bifida with urinary and fecal incontinence.
1. Girl, nine and half years. Mentally retarded.
2. Boy, ten years. Nocturnal and diurnal, more often at night.
3. Boy, six years.
4. Boy, eleven years, nine months. Wetting until seven years, soiling still persisted, "even though the bathroom was at hand." Temper tantrums. Had been excluded from school because of his soiling. Pneumonia with delirium of several days' duration at ten years.
5. Girl, six years. Congenital malformation of the heart. Microcephalic. Mental retardation (I.Q. 70). Temper tantrums, lying, cruelty to smaller children. Committed to State Training School for the Feebleminded.

e. Spina bifida with fecal incontinence.
1. Boy, ten years. Lifelong encopresis. Enuresis had never been a problem.

Groups c and d could be further subdivided into such cases in which the incontinence of bowels and bladder were obviously the result of the cord anomaly, and others in which a causal relationship did not exist. The best criterion lies in the circumstances surrounding the wetting and soiling (the spina bifida cannot reasonably be made responsible for enuresis which consistently misses the school period and occurs during play only) and in their prompt cessation after the adjustment of personal and environmental difficulties (as in cases c 4 and c 6).

The *myelodysplasia* theory, propounded by Fuchs, bases the occurrence of enuresis on the existence of a more or less rudimentary non-union of the sacrum and other anomalies in the lower section of the spinal column, often associated with asymmetries of the rima ani, fistular contractions in the sacro-coccygeal region, flat feet (explained by lessening of the muscle tone), sluggish knee jerks and ankle jerks, lipomata or hypertrichosis over the sacrum, sensibility disorders in the lower extremities, especially the big toes, and syndactylia. The occurrence of this clinical syndrome, if it exists at all, is exceedingly rare, and it would certainly not do to refer to it with a sweeping generalization all or most instances of so common a complaint as enuresis. We have utterly failed to find in any of our numerous cases an indication for the diagnosis of myelodysplasia, although we were willing to make liberal allowances.[1]

Phimosis is sometimes associated with nocturnal and diurnal wetting. In a small number of instances it cannot be denied etiological significance. We know, on the other hand, the case of a six-year-old boy with phimosis, who had acquired good urinary habits in early infancy and whose enuresis began immediately after a well performed circumcision at the age of three years. We may also mention the two brothers, of whom one, fourteen years old, had pronounced phimosis without ever having been enuretic, while the other wet the bed but had no phimosis. Three per cent of our own cases of wetting were found to have phimosis; irritation, edema, hyperemia of the foreskin were present in another three per cent; balanitis, preputial adhesions, gonorrhea, excoriation and gaping of the vaginal orifice, atresia vulvae, and fissura ani in one per cent each.

The *specific gravity and acidity of the urine* was normal in practically all cases (that is, of course, after exclusion of patients suffering from demonstrable inflammations or infections of the genito-urinary organs; as cases of "incontinence," we did not deal with them in our analyses of "enuresis").

Adenoid vegetations were held responsible for enuresis on the assumption that they interfere with proper respiration and, therefore, lead to an overabundance of CO_2 in the blood; this, in turn, is said to result in abnormal depth of the sleep, making the child unmindful of the urge to void. Others have thought of the possibility of a reflex irritation of the vesicular centers from the nasopharynx. No proof has ever been offered for these assumptions. It is true that adenoid vegetations were present in not less than twenty-three per cent of our cases. But they are, after all, very common in non-enuretic children also.

The *depth of sleep* has been found to be considerable in many patients who wet the bed. To speak of "abnormal" depth is hardly justified. Sound sleepers and light sleepers are reported also among non-enuretic children and adults. Besides, there is a sufficiently large number of bedwetters whose sleep is described as restless; talking, tossing about, and moaning, and gritting the teeth during sleep is a not infrequent observation in these children. Of other sleep disturbances, the following have been complained of by the mothers of some of our enuretic children.

> Nightmares: 5 per cent
> Night terrors: 3 per cent
> Sleep walking: 4 per cent
> Crying during sleep: 2 per cent
> Sleeplessness: 1 per cent

It is a great exaggeration to designate all instances of involuntary urination as *epileptic equivalents*. It is a well-known fact that incontinence

---

[1] Fuchs, A. Über Beziehungen der Enuresis nocturna zu Rudimentärformen der Spina bifida occulta (Myelodysplasie). Wiener medizinische Wochenschrift. 1909.

may occur in the course of a grand mal episode and also in a state of fugue. Enuresis, because of its very frequency, is, of course, apt to exist in epileptic children. Seven per cent of our bed or clothes wetters were epileptics. In the others, there was nothing in the history or in the clinical picture that would warrant even a suspicion of epilepsy. It is, therefore, unnecessary to look upon the wetting as one of several "epileptoid symptoms," as did Binswanger. On the other hand, one should always make sure that the patient has not had convulsions or anything in the nature of petit mal attacks; in the presence of lingual scars and of the complaint of the child's falling out of bed or unusual weakness upon awakening during or after the nights when the bed has been soaked, the possibility of an epileptic condition must be carefully considered.

One will also hesitate to agree with those who regard the wetting as a monosymptomatic sign of an *hysterical reaction*. In the first place, enuresis is very rarely a "monosymptomatic" affair. It is almost always combined with other expressions of personality maladjustment. Secondly, it is conceded by all investigators that hysteria is practically absent in infancy. Yet most instances of wetting are carried over without interruption from the time of physiological incontinence. Furthermore, there are many stable, well adjusted, and certainly not hysterical adults who present a history of bedwetting, extending sometimes to and even beyond the years of puberty.

Considering the claim that *thyroid deficiency* is at the bottom of the condition, there is hardly anything to be said beyond the statement that any such dysfunction has yet to be objectively demonstrated.

One could not well expect the psychoanalytic school to pass up a reaction which seems to be so close to its pet preoccupations. It was quick to evolve a theory of its own, or rather, one of the several theories it evolved has been more widely accepted by its adherents than the others. For almost every author has something original to contribute, not so much in the realm of factual observation as in the field of "interpretation." Thus we are told that enuresis represents a wishfulfilling regression to the early stages of infancy; that it serves women and girls as an expression of the castration complex, since urine symbolizes semen, and the wetting therefore is an unconscious outlet for the unconscious wish to be a man; that in boys it is a form of identification with the father, in that it symbolizes ejaculation and thus unconsciously fulfils the unconscious desire for potency. The most popular psychoanalytic theory claims that enuresis is a substitute for masturbation. Klaesi has given it the name of *anticatastasis*, or guilt substitute: the "unconscious" replaces the real delinquency (namely, masturbation), which must not be betrayed, by another, less offensive misdemeanor.[1] Even a urethral erotic character has been described, the principal features of which are supposed to be ambition and bashfulness.[2] We cannot refrain from handing on to our readers the psychoanalytic "interpretation" of the story of the Deluge as an enuretic fantasy.

[1] Klaesi, J. Über die psychogenen Ursachen der essentiellen Enuresis nocturna infantum. Zeitschrift für die gesamte Neurologie und Psychiatrie. 1917, 35, 371.

[2] Sadger, J. Über Urethralerotik. Internationale Zeitschrift für Psychoanalyse. 1910, 2, 409.

According to the Adlerian school, enuresis is determined by an inherent inferiority of the urinary organs plus the realization of a goal which is best served by this particular form of reaction. The child may wish to assure in this manner the extension to the night hours of parental affection and occupation with him; or he may want to distract the attention of the adults from a disliked rival; or he may need a convenient excuse for being relieved of disagreeable responsibilities. The wetting is looked upon as an expression of the patient's feeling of insecurity with regard to his position in life and a defensive compensatory continuation of, or return to, an infantile mode of behavior, to assure better protection.

There exist several interesting studies of the personalities of enuretic children. Among them, the work of Pototzky has been quoted most extensively. He distinguishes several types, the knowledge of which he feels is important from the point of view of therapeutic planning:

1. The spiteful-uninhibited children, who wet themselves in order to tease the parents and educators.

2. The shy-inhibited children, who wet themselves upon the slightest unpleasant occasion and often because of fear.

3. The restless, absentminded children, who are so easily distracted that they forget their urinary needs because of lack of concentration.

4. The indifferent children, who are not at all concerned about the habit and do not care whether or not they are relieved of it.[1]

Pototzky finds these types mostly in "psychopathic" children, whom he contrasts with a "neuropathic" and an intellectually deficient group. Our own attitude with regard to such a separation of neuropathic and psychopathic has been set forth in the chapter on "Diagnostic Synthesis."

Bissell divides enuretic children into two sections: those who are hyperactive, excitable, hypersensitive and mostly precocious, and those who are hypoactive, inclined to be lazy, drowsy, and mostly retarded in intelligence.[2]

Behm has three groups:

1. Degenerated, 2. Phlegmatic, 3. Excitable.[3]

Even though such differentiations are interesting and those quoted above are based on good observation, the analysis of our material has so strongly impressed us with the great manifoldness of the personal and environmental features, that we prefer to deal with individuals rather than with groups. It is inevitable that any rules laid down for groups will have to be modified according to the specific factors involved in each case.

Holt and Howland, in their textbook on the *Diseases of Infancy and Childhood*, state that in 68 per cent of the cases of enuresis no physical etiology can be found. It is these patients with whom we are now concerning ourselves. We shall try to examine our case material with the aim of determining the concrete and objectively demonstrated facts which were found to be operating in our enuretic patients.

Beginning with a consideration of the children's personalities, we perceive that in a small number an *ingrained incapacity for training* of urinary

[1] Pototzky, Carl. Die diagnostische und therapeutische Differenzierung der Enuresisfälle. Zeitschrift für Kinderheilkunde. 1924, 37, 12–23.

[2] Bissell, J. B. Daytime Enuresis in Children. Medical Record. 1892, 42, 697.

[3] Behm, Karl. Das Bettnässleiden, seine Behandlung und Bekämpfung. Leipzig. 1924.

habits was a predominant feature. We have reference especially to patients
with an extremely limited intellectual endowment. It must, however, be
conceded that there are idiotic and imbecile children in whom enuresis or
encopresis has never been a problem. Feeblemindedness is not synonymous
with lack of training capacity with regard to toilet habits. But very often
the late development of walking and talking and comprehension seriously
interferes with the acquisition of proper bladder control. In other children,
illness with long stay in bed and periods of weakness or drowsiness or apathy has helped to establish an enuretic condition.

In the majority of our patients, one may observe a *general immaturity*
which expresses itself in a variety of combinations of personality difficulties. It is these children that are usually termed "neurotic" or "neuropathic" or "psychopathic" or "constitutionally inferior," depending on the preferred terminology of those who are accustomed to work with such designations. The enuresis is one of several manifestations of a general habit
disorder. Poor endowment, poor upbringing, and poor example may all
contribute their share to the undesirable conduct. The following personality traits were present in our enuretic children, alone or in combinations:

Timid, shy, bashful, seclusive, unusually quiet .... 8 per cent
Hypersensitive, self-conscious, touchy .... 9 per cent
Overconscientious, serious-minded .... 3 per cent
Restless, hyperactive, fidgety, easily excited .... 24 per cent
Whining, complaining, moody, grouchy, irritable .... 39 per cent
Aggressive, fighting, mischievous, cruel .... 8 per cent
Disobedient, impudent, spiteful, stubborn .... 14 per cent
Listless, indifferent, apathetic .... 4 per cent

Some of the behavior problems which are found in association with enuresis are enumerated below, in order of the frequency of their occurrence:

Behavior problem	Per cent
Feeding difficulties	32
Temper tantrums	26
Nailbiting	24
Fear reactions	12
Encopresis	10
Masturbation	9
Blinking	7
Hypochondriasis	7
Thumbsucking	6
Stuttering	6
Stealing	6
Truancy	4

This list of associated difficulties demonstrates better than anything else
the futility of treating "enuresis" rather than the child in toto with all his
problems and peculiarities and traits. In doing so, a knowledge of the environmental factors influencing his conduct is indispensable. Of these, three
main features are of especial significance. They are:

Lack of adequate training.
General carelessness concerning regularity of habits.
Lack of proper opportunity for the establishment of the dry habit.

Lack of adequate training may result from parental overindulgence. The enuresis is apt to be excused on the ground that the child is too small or too delicate to be educated. Behind this rationalization there is usually the mother's desire to keep her offspring wholly dependent on her for as long a time as possible. Under these circumstances, we cannot very well expect a child to emancipate himself from the infantile mode of micturition, when he has been kept persistently from growing up in every other respect, when he has never been taught to dress himself, when his shoes have always been laced and his hair has always been combed by someone else, when he has not been given a chance to go to bed or to cross the street alone, and when all of this is sanctioned and even fostered by an overprotective mother or grandmother. The mother of a twelve-year-old enuretic girl stated frankly, when questioned about the details of habit training: "I never made her do anything because she is so weak"; she has another daughter, six years old, whom she did not "break" from wetting the bed "because she is so nervous."

Indifference and carelessness on the part of the parents is often another reason for improper training. The care of elimination is left from the beginning entirely to the child, with the attitude that some day in the future he will "outgrow" the habit. Many children really do that sooner or later, but untold damage may be done in the meantime, and the faulty education may later show itself in more serious behavior difficulties in adult life.

Quite common is what one might speak of as *traditional enuresis*. There are families in which bedwetting is accepted as a matter-of-fact experience which several members "have to" undergo. The notion that it is inherited and therefore not accessible to external influence often enters strongly into the situation. One mother reported: "I did not do anything about it because it is inherited from her father; he was twenty-two when he stopped (during war time service in the army)."

The incidence of enuresis in members of the same family is much more frequent than is usually assumed. It was reported in not less than fifty-two per cent of our patients. The distribution was as follows:

Enuretic relatives	Per Cent
One sibling	20
Two siblings	9
Three siblings	1
Four siblings	3
Father	1
Mother	3
Father and one sibling	3
Father and two siblings	1
Father, one sibling, two uncles	2
Mother and one sibling	2
Mother, one sibling, and aunt	1
Mother, uncle, and cousin	1
Two siblings and an uncle	1
Uncle and cousin	1
Aunt	2
Two cousins	1
Total	52

This, of course, does not spell "heredity," nor does it signify an "organ inferiority" which in some mysterious way has been transmitted from generation to generation, nor a *stigma hereditatis* in the sense of Pfister,[1] who tries to prove his assumption by the relative frequency of psychoses and psychoneuroses in the ascendency of enuretic patients. But it does provide a reaction pattern, establishes a sort of family tradition (witness the question of a mother, who has herself been enuretic as was her sister: "Aren't those things to be expected to a certain extent?"), and instils into the parents the wrong idea of the futility of any educational or corrective efforts. In some households, the enuretic siblings, sometimes with utter disregard of age and sex, are simply made to sleep in the same bed, in order to save on the laundry bill and also with the attitude that the culprits ought to stand the wetness and the odor of the other's urine as well as of their own.

Another belief which keeps parents from training their children to acquire healthy toilet habits consists in a wide-spread piece of medical folklore, which refers bedwetting once and for all to a "weak bladder" or a "weak kidney." One often hears statements, such as these: "I think his kidneys are bad." "O my goodness, she wets the bed terribly, every night. I think maybe her kidneys must be bad or something." "We thought that she had kidney trouble but they examined her and took her urine and said that she didn't have no kidney trouble. Doctor, I don't understand it." "He asked me why he does it, and I told him that he has a weak bladder." Being possessed of a weak kidney or bladder, the child, of course, "cannot help it" (and he is told as much), nor is any help expected from educational measures; one simply waits until the organ will become stronger in the course of years or until some clever doctor will happen to prescribe the "fitting medicine."

There are physicians who, in their struggle to speak to the parents in their own language, or because of indifference about matters not strictly "organic," or from a desire not to "waste time" with "neurotic" complaints, help to develop or to maintain faulty notions in the family.

"She wets herself every night. She does not like it but she says she cannot help it. When she was smaller, I took her to a doctor and he said that she cannot be cured." (After treatment had been instituted, this fourteen-year-old girl wet only five times during the first three weeks.) The same attitude had been transferred to her six-year-old sister, who also was enuretic but ceased to wet automatically, without personal examination or treatment, when the attitude of the family and the elder sister had changed.

"I had broke her from wetting when she was a baby but after she had that sick spell (fever and listlessness for about a week at the age of three years), she started again. I took her to the doctor and he said she had a complete nervous breakdown and I should not cross her. It just could not be helped." On the strength of this advice, she was spoiled in every respect, treated like a baby (like an untrained baby) all her life, and not sent to school.

In many instances, it is not so much the enuresis pattern itself which

[1] Pfister, H. Enuresis nocturna and ähnliche Störungen in neuropathologischer Bewertung. Monatsschrift für Neurologie. 1904, 15, 113.

the child sees at home as general carelessness with regard to habit formation and habit regularity. A considerable number of enuretic children comes from untidy, ill-kept homes and from parents who "let themselves go" in many ways. Alcoholism was reported in fully one-fourth of the fathers of our wetting patients, and in two per cent of the mothers. Signs of serious emotional instability or social maladjustment of one or both of the parents were present in not less than eighty per cent. Twenty-one per cent of the children had illiterate or feebleminded parents (moron or below). Major psychoses in parents, grandparents, uncles, or aunts were reported in twenty-two per cent of our enuretic patients.

Four per cent of the children had a history of suicide in a near relative. Epilepsy was reported in the families of seven per cent, criminal records in the parents or siblings of ten per cent, and sex delinquencies in four per cent of the parents. Twenty-seven per cent of the children were raised in broken homes, six per cent were illegitimate.

Under these circumstances, one certainly does not have to think of some mysterious form of heredity via the bladder or the kidney. With such type of ascendency, we are apt to deal with human material which does not adjust as easily as children of healthy and stable parentage. It is easily seen that in such homes habit training with regular meal times and retiring hours and attention to cleanliness can hardly be expected to be carried out consistently and intelligently by people who have not learned to train or control themselves. To many of them, the wetting will appear a relatively small problem or no problem at all in comparison with the major difficulties in the life of the family. As a matter of fact, in a number of instances the enuresis was not offered as a complaint at all and was brought out only incidentally in the course of the examination. It sometimes took a sore throat or an otitis media to bring the child to the clinic where the occurrence of the wetting was discovered. We have seen parents who, after reporting enuresis upon specific inquiry, later "withdrew" their statements when, much to their surprise, they were expected to do something about it. They simply considered the matter too unimportant and did not wish to be bothered. This attitude is at the bottom of many informations to the effect that the child had wet himself every day or every night "until two weeks ago" or "until a month ago," or that it happens "very seldom"; it is then mostly the child himself who, when interviewed alone, supplies the real facts. One finds a parallel in the assertions of many alcoholics that they quit drinking just a short time before the interview or that they drink "very seldom."

Another difficulty met with occasionally, especially in children who live in a rural environment, consists in the *lack of an opportunity for adequate training* of urinary habits. The toilet is not within easy reach. It is in the cellar or in the back yard. In the cold winter nights, the child does not care and is not really expected to go out. Many children sleep in unheated rooms. It has been commonly accepted that cold weather has a diuretic influence. Hence, there is an increased urge to urinate with no convenient opportunity for voiding; the bed is then made to serve the purpose. Once the habit is established, the "weak bladder" theory or other factors may contribute to its persistence also in the summer.

The *effect on the patient* of the enuretic habit may be of great significance for his entire life situation and for his character formation. The conscientious child may develop a feeling of utter hopelessness; he may lie awake for hours fearing to go to sleep and to wet himself; shame and lack of self-confidence and, in the day wetter, also the fear of an "accident" may drive him into seclusiveness. The notion of having a weak bladder or kidney will give any child the wrong conviction that he is sick. Punishments and scoldings may make him sense that he does something morally bad and establish a feeling of guilt. Preoccupation with his problem may interfere with the quality of his school achievements. The entire constellation is apt to bring about unhappiness and irritability. It is, indeed, often difficult to determine whether the enuresis seems to be a personality problem in an inherently seclusive or irritable youngster or, which is more probable and more frequent, these personality traits are results of the enuresis and of its management.

This should not make one unaware of the fact that in some cases certain traits are definitely connected with the child's wetting. This is especially true of the incidence of enuresis as *a spite or jealousy reaction*. In one child the onset was obviously associated with the arrival of a new (the second) baby; the boy, who had been an only child until then, showed his resentment also in many other ways.

Before we enter into a discussion of the treatment, we may be permitted to say a few words about some undesirable forms of home management and their results. "Shaming" the child is a common practice. This is done either verbally, or by letting a big boy or girl wear diapers, or by having the patient stand during breakfast, or by having him stand in a corner facing the wall, or by "telling on him." We know of a case where an interne ordered girls' clothes to be put on a seven-year-old boy and to call him "Lizzie." In a convalescent home a child was taken during the visiting period into the lobby and displayed before a large group of strangers as the bad youngster who disgraces the place by wetting his bed. Often the more indirect method of complaining about the odor or the high laundry bill is chosen. An alcoholic father indulged in the dubious pleasure of pressing his daughter's face into the soaked bedding, although he himself had been enuretic until the age of twelve years. One sometimes hears mothers relate proudly how they have sewn colored strips on some conspicuous part of the child's clothing, or how they let their offspring wash the wetted linen. None of these modes of humiliation has ever done away with the enuresis, but they all help to make the child much unhappier than he has often already been. This is equally true of the many forms of "punishment," which are based on the wrong notion that "meanness" or "laziness" is the source of the difficulty. Sometimes bribing is attempted with equal results as regards the expected cessation of the habit.

Any *therapeutic planning* must be preceded by the realization that it is impossible and unnecessary to reduce all instances of enuresis to a uniform etiological formula. We have tried to demonstrate that in the individual cases different factors may be at work, combining themselves in practically every imaginable manner. We must further be prepared to treat not the enuresis but the enuretic child with all of his difficulties; everything else is not even patchwork. Symptomatic therapy which does not care what the complaint is a "symptom" of is rarely successful and leads to unwarranted pessimism. This is true of the indiscriminate prescription of atropin, belladonna, thyroid extract, urotropin, camphor, strychnin, rhus aromaticum, chloral, bromides, quinine, papaverin, amidopyrin, antipyrin, phenacetin, lycopodium, ergotin, tetrodotoxin, and the many other drugs recommended by a greater or smaller number of authors. It is also true of the invariable resorting to surgical procedures, to circumcision, tonsillectomy, catheterization, bladder irrigations, paraffin injections into the bladder, epidural injections with cocain or physiological salt solution, lumbar puncture, and retrorectal injections. It is true of the use of massage, diathermy, and electricity, of the distension of the bladder by hydrostatic pressure, cold or warm baths, and elevation of the foot end of the bed. All these measures are based on assumptions or on actual findings in a very small number of cases only. They forget that *a living person happens to be attached to the urinating bladder.*

In dealing with the child, we first attempt to treat all physical difficulties which are really present (not those which are postulated by this or that hypothesis). Where the tonsils are in need of removal, the necessary arrangements are made. Where dental caries exists, care of the teeth is recommended. The proper treatment of cystitis, phimosis, refractive error, otitis media, scabies, worms, or anything else that calls for medicinal or orthopedic or surgical adjustment is advised, and we try to see to it that the advice is carried out. We do that regardless of whether or not the condition has anything to do with the enuresis, directly or indirectly. This part of the treatment would be the same in every child, enuretic or not enuretic.

In equal manner, we try to help the patient in his emotional and situational adjustment. We try to relieve him of his feeling of shame or guilt which he may have developed. We make him see that the wetting is not a crime or an expression of badness and that we wish to discuss the problem with him in an unprejudiced manner. Above all, after disrobing the issue of unjustified moral connotations, we dispel the attitude of hopelessness which may have taken root in the child; he is given more self-confidence by presenting to him the cessation of the enuresis as something that can be achieved and that is worthy of achievement. Erroneous beliefs with regard to a weak bladder or kidney or "nerves" or "heredity" are corrected; medicines and manipulations are discontinued (with tactful consideration of the reputation of the physician who has prescribed them; anyone criticizing another physician before the patient or his parents is apt to undermine their confidence in the whole profession). As long as he takes drugs, or as long as he feels that it is some organ which is entirely responsible, we cannot expect him to make a personal matter of the problem, beyond taking the pills or tablespoonfuls. We shall also deal with whatever associated difficulties the child presents, general lack of self-dependence, feeding problems, stuttering, or anything else that calls for psychiatric assistance. Wherever indicated, proper school adjustment is recommended.

At the same time, we must deal with the family situation. We shall discourage and try to do away with punishments and scoldings and shaming and bribing. We shall, as we did with the child himself, also have to correct the folkloristic and pseudo-medical notions of the parents. We shall insist on being given an opportunity to see also the other enuretic children of the household, so that the wetting ceases to be a problem not only in the one child who happens to be our patient, but in the home. We shall try, usually with the social worker's aid, to assure better conditions of cleanliness and better habit regularity in the patient's daily surroundings.

Then, and only then, are we ready to employ more specific educational or suggestive measures. It is customary to advise restriction of fluids after a certain hour in the afternoon. This procedure has the advantage that it may decrease the urge to urinate, that it takes care of those instances of an "irritable small contracted" bladder which one finds discussed so much in the literature, and that, after taking away the patent medicine or the shaming, the parents still are left with the feeling that there is something to be watched and prohibited. But one should be openminded enough to make allowances for the hot summer afternoons, when complete restriction may make the child unpleasantly thirsty; swallowing small pieces of ice may then be of help. It is hardly ever necessary to carry the fluid restriction out for longer than two to three weeks.

It is customary to advise that the child be thoroughly awakened in the night and sent to the toilet. This has proved to be a helpful measure (always in addition to the major features of adjustment mentioned above). It helps to establish in the child the habit of getting up and voiding at a certain hour of the night or, as some people like to put it, to "condition" the child. But it is necessary to find out first at about what time the patient usually wets himself and to wake him about a half hour before the expected accident. It has been established that most children wet themselves more or less regularly at definite hours, very often about two to two and a half hours after going to sleep. One must, of course, use common sense; hard working parents who are badly in need of a few hours of sleep will not be reasonably asked to disturb their rest every night for the purpose of waking the child. Sometimes, an alarm clock placed in the patient's room may do the service.

In well-selected cases much benefit may be derived from the use of a star chart, which presupposes a fair degree of intelligence, ambition, and honesty. It is sometimes surprising to see how a child who has wet himself every night during his whole life, of a sudden becomes dry or almost dry and pastes star after star on his chart. It would, however, be incorrect to attribute this result to the star chart. For its application has in every instance been preceded by an attempt at thorough personality and situational adjustment. The chart is mainly of educational value. In a chronically enuretic youngster, even one star in a week or in two weeks is enough to make the child realize that a dry night was possible and that it may recur. Where there is more than one enuretic child in the family, a competitive star chart, strange as it may sound, has often had remarkable success. One boy, who had a history of lifelong nocturnal enuresis, had no wet nights ever since treatment had been instituted several months ago when he was almost seven years old; needless to say that the star chart was only a part of the therapeutic program; he was one of the boys who had been told previously

46 CHILD PSYCHIATRY

that he had a weak kidney and could not help it. Of two sisters, one, fourteen years old, had only five wet nights during the first three weeks of treatment, and the other, six years old, had not more than one "accident" within the same period.

To summarize: The treatment of enuretic children consists in the adjustment of personal and environmental difficulties with correction of faulty notions and practices; in direct work with the patient and the family; whenever advisable, in restriction of fluids to relieve the vesical tension and to decrease the urge to void; in establishment of the dry habit through waking; in education and creation of ambition and enthusiasm through the star chart; in the care of all physical ills; and in any other additional adjustment that the individual case may call for.

It is in order to hold out a goal to the child to make his efforts appear worthwhile and attractive. The enuretic youngster has usually been deprived of such pleasures as visits to friends or relatives, spending the summer vacations in a camp, joining a club, etc. A promise to make up for such deprivations as soon as the dry habit will be established often helps matters considerably. But the promise must really be kept, or a relapse may be the penalty.

Success will depend to a large degree upon coöperation on the part of the child and the parents. But it is an essential part of the treatment to secure coöperation. If the child is found to be indifferent, one should try to find the reason for his indifference and to treat it as one of his problems. If parents fail to carry out instructions, it is up to the physician and the social worker to educate them and to help them.

CHAPTER XXIX

THE MUSCULAR SYSTEM

TICS

TICS OR HABIT spasms (sometimes alluded to as habit chorea, following the example of Weir Mitchell, and less distinctively as nervous habits) are sudden, quick, involuntary, and frequently repeated movements of circumscribed groups of muscles, serving no apparent purpose. The regions of face and neck are most frequently affected but there is hardly a part of the body that may not be involved in some cases. The tics may manifest themselves in a practically unlimited number of varieties. They may assume the form of shaking or nodding the head, frowning, wrinkling the forehead, blinking the eyelids, different modes of grimacing, twisting the mouth, sniffing, clearing the throat, moving the ears, swallowing, coughing, jerking the shoulders or arms or legs, sighing, hiccoughing, ejaculation of words, etc. Although quite often there may be only one form present in an individual, it happens that the same patient displays a combination of tics which either are carried out simultaneously or alternate or follow each other.

We quote a few examples of multiple tics from our case material:

Clearing the throat, twisting the mouth, and wrinkling the forehead.
Turning the neck and opening the mouth in a child who had previously been blinking.
Raising the left shoulder and nictitation.
Jerking the head and winking.
Twitching the shoulders, arms, and legs.
Making a noise in the throat, blinking, twitching the neck muscles and at times the mouth and nose.
Twitching the hands, jerking the head, and blinking.
Jerking the arms, jumping, and grimacing.

In the following, we cite literally some of the parents' complaints:

"The teacher said he is highly nervous. At times he has the habit of twitching his neck and at the same time opening his mouth wide. He is restless and would not sit still. He used to blink his eyes until he was given glasses last September."

"He has a habit of drawing his head to the side. If he misses anything in school and the teacher keeps him in to explain things, he gets confused and twitches and bites his nails."

"He twitches his face considerably. He began to make faces since he started school at six years."

"He had St. Vitus's dance six or seven years ago and now once in awhile he gets a headache and before he gets the headaches when he studies he'll come home and shake his head. Anything excitable, when he plays ball, that's when he gets to shake his head. He has not had this shaking all summer, only now since he is back to school again."

"For the last five or six weeks she has been shaking her right arm and sometimes her head; she says that she cannot help it. It lasts from fifteen to thirty minutes. It began after a scare when she heard someone coming up the steps. She was so frightened she could not talk for two minutes."

"He is batting his eyes a great deal. It began last summer. He played with a boy who used to do that, but he had not been around him for some time and he still does it. He used to bat his eyes very much last summer; he would walk around almost with his eyes closed."

"She blinks her eyes, the right eye the most. She has been doing it for about three weeks. A little girl in the neighborhood has had chorea and has been doing it so much. Now she does it, and I don't know if it's that or if it is a habit. She does it so much and the whole side of her face pulls up."

"He seems to be so nervous. So much of his trouble seems to be in his throat. When he eats, it is terrible. He can hardly eat from the way it goes on. He twitches his nose and mouth at times. He jerks quite a bit in his sleep. His throat noises started about a year ago, about a year after he had his tonsils taken out. It is getting worse all the time. It sounds like the clucking of a hen."

Olson, in his book on *The Measurement of Nervous Habits in Normal Children (Minneapolis. 1929)*, gives the following "inventory of tics based upon literature:"

A. Face and Head.
   Twisting hair. Grimacing. Puckering forehead. Raising eyebrows. Blinking eyelids, winking. Wrinkling nose. Trembling nostrils. Twitching mouth. Displaying teeth. Biting lips and other parts. Extruding tongue. Protracting lower jaw. Fingering ear. Picking nose. Sucking thumb or fingers. Biting nails. Nodding, jerking, shaking head. Twisting neck, looking sideways. Head rolling. Head banging.
B. Arms and Hands.
   Jerking hands. Jerking arms; swinging arms. Plucking fingers; writhing fingers. Clenching fists. Striking head or body. Scratching. Manipulating genitalia.
C. Body and Lower Extremities.
   Shrugging shoulders. Shaking shoulders. Shaking foot, knee, or toe. Peculiarities of gait. Body rocking. Body writhing. Jumping.
D. Respiratory and Alimentary.
   Hiccoughing. Coughing. Hysterical laughing. Grunting. Barking. Sobbing. Sighing. Yawning. Snuffing. Blowing through nostrils. Whistling inspiration. Exaggerated breathing. Belching. Sucking or smacking sounds. Vomiting, regurgitating. Swallowing. Spitting and salivation. Clearing throat.
E. Miscellaneous.
   Repeating words, tunes, etc. (Echolalia). Repeating actions seen (Echokinesis). Uttering obscene words (Coprolalia).

Olson included in this list "any movement that any writer would designate as a tic." If, for the sake of a clear delimitation, one wishes to adhere to the distinguishing criteria of suddenness, rapidity, and involuntariness, then such habits as nailbiting and finger sucking and nose picking must be considered separately, since they are certainly not spasmodic and can be controlled by volition much more readily than, for instance, blinking or grimacing.

Tics are much more frequent in children than in adults. Boncour found among 1759 youngsters between two and thirteen years of age not less than 417, or 23 per cent, tiqueurs. All degrees of intelligence and all modes of behavior were represented. There were as many as fifteen per cent tiqueurs among the children between two and four, five per cent between four and five, and three per cent between five and six years. In older children, the distribution was as follows:

Age	Percentage of tiqueurs	
	Boys	Girls
7	27	27
8	23	19
9	39	25
10	19	27
11	14	28
12	50	29
13	11	7

It is important to know that in the pre-school children studied by Boncour the "tics" in most instances consisted of "rudimentary bad habits, easily influenced." Wilder saw six tiqueurs under six years of age. According to Thomson, tics occur in boys and girls "between six years old and puberty." Meige and Feindel assert that the "nervous movements" of children below four years are not tics; tics usually do not appear before the age of between seven and eight years. In our own group, the youngest tiqueurs observed were six years old; there was a slight peak at eight and nine years and again at eleven and twelve years, after which there was a sharp drop in the frequency curve similar to that in Boncour's table.

The distribution of intelligence in our material is of interest. A large majority of cases is to be found in the normal and dull normal groups. There were only few morons and no imbeciles or idiots. We had six tiqueurs of superior intelligence (two with quotients of over 120) who, with the exception of one, were emotionally immature.

Tics have sometimes been spoken of as "monosymptomatic neuroses." In the study of our cases we did not encounter one single patient who did not offer additional personality difficulties. If we furnish a few examples only, we do so with the assertion that in all of our tiqueurs there was a combination of several behavior disorders. This is, at least so far as our material is concerned, a rule that has had no exceptions.

Examples of additional personality difficulties of children with tics:

"He has always been a finicky eater. He has a little temper; he cries and opens his mouth wide when he does not get his way." A restless, very disobedient seven-year-old; slight strabismus.

Restless sleeper. Cried over the least little thing. Mentally retarded. Unexplained absence of knee and ankle jerks, triceps and biceps reflexes very sluggish. Strongly positive Chvostek. Hypertrophied tonsils and adenoids. Hypochondriacal trends. Psychogenic vomiting. Enuresis. Nightmares. Feeding problem.

Timid, afraid of the dark. Tired easily. Occasional complaints of dizziness in the head. Feeding problem. Nailbiting. He liked much excitement and teased other children. Perspired profusely during the examination. Pupils slightly eccentric. Compound hyperopic astigmatism.

Eczema. Vomiting attacks. Pylorospasms and colospasms. History of two asthmatic attacks. Fear of the dark. Disobedience and impudence. Fought with brothers and sisters.

Emotional instability. Mental retardation. Crying spells and enuresis at fourteen years. History of nailbiting. Eight pounds underweight.

Very mischievous. Restless both in daytime ("goes from one thing to another") and at night. Masturbation. Tired very easily. Temper outbursts. Lying. Careless about his appearance. Used to bite his finger nails.

The personality features most commonly observed in children with tics are, in order of their frequency: restlessness, self-consciousness, sensitiveness, spoiled child reaction, over-ambitiousness and over-conscientiousness. Easy excitability and quick fatigability are often reported. There is a distinctive group of shy, seclusive, and readily embarrassed tiqueurs. Wilder points out that he has observed tics both in introverted and extraverted individuals.

Friedreich was the first author to dwell seriously on the *etiology* of tics. He declared them to be *coördinated memory spasms* (*koordinierte Erinnerungskrämpfe*), owing their origin to the involuntary repetition, with consciousness fully preserved, of a primarily purposive reflexogenic or voluntary coördinated action. He found the years of childhood to be particularly predisposed and great intensity of excitement associated with the initial pattern especially prone to produce its spasmodic repetitions. One of his patients, a boy of nine years, was in the woods when his cap was caught in the branches of a tree and tossed upward beyond his reach; he was worried over the loss of his cap and for a time kept turning around and looking up in the futile attempt to locate it. Since then, he had a tic of turning around and grimacing. A ten-year-old girl took a play contest with other children, trying to see who could keep mouth and nose closed longest, so seriously that she became dyspnoeic; she developed an inspiratory tic.[1]

Meige and Feindel, in their classical book on tics, clearly recognized the need of an individual study of each case. They say, "*L'évolution du tic est essentiellement capricieuse. Chaque tic évolue à sa façon et l'on comprendra qu'il en soit ainsi si l'on se rappelle que la réaction motrice réflète l'état mental du tiqueur . . . Il est dont présque impossible de tracer une esquisse d'ensemble de l'évolution des tics.*" The authors built up their studies in pursuance of the work done by Trousseau, Charcot, and Brissaud. Although they make it known that "*nous ne savons rien de l'anatomie pathologique du tic*" and that the reaction does not depend on an acquired cerebral lesion,

[1] Friedreich. Über koordinierte Erinnerungskrämpfe. Virchows Archiv für pathologische Anatomie und Physiologie. 1881, 86, 430.

they cannot refrain from advancing the hypothesis that "we deal with congenital anomalies, with developmental arrests or defects in the cortical association paths or infracortical anastomoses, minute teratological malformations which our anatomical knowledge unfortunately is not yet capable of demonstrating." They do, however, emphasize the genetic-dynamic principles active in the formation of tics, which they define as reflex, defensive, or expressive movements which have become automatic, inopportune, and compulsive, no longer directed toward a definite goal. So long as there is itching, especially if it is chronic, the act of scratching may come to be carried out automatically but is not a tic. After the skin irritation has ceased, the persistence of the scratching movements, which now serve no purpose, has moved them into the category of tics. The understandable defense reaction has become a habit no longer useful in the economy of motility.[1]

The example of scratching is well suited to show the futility of speculating on cerebral localizations. No one would think even remotely of postulating lesions or developmental anomalies of the brain as long as the eczema or pruritus offers a sufficient explanation. It is difficult to see how neuropathological lesions could be created or allegedly preformed deficiencies in the associative pathways jump into activity the minute the cutaneous irritation has been remedied. The same is true, for instance, of blinking originally associated with conjunctivitis and later maintained automatically, or of jerking the shoulders after the guilty tight suspenders have been replaced by more comfortable ones, or of wrinkling the forehead after an unfitting hat has been discarded.

In recent years, tics of an unquestionably organic origin have been studied in postencephalitic patients. Some investigators count to this group also the so-called oculogyric and respiratory crises met with in encephalitis. These tics were referred to lesions in the strio-pallidal system. Since they were often accessible to psychotherapeutic influences, the conclusion was drawn that organic and functional tics are closely related and "make use of the same apparatus" (Schilder and Gerstmann). Wilder and Silbermann state that, "although we do not at the present time have a truly exact proof that the *tic mental* has anything to do with the basal ganglia, this is very probable and we also work with this hypothesis."[2] Others interpret psychogenic tics as based on organic inferiority of the striate apparatus (O.Vogt), or as *psychomotricité centripétale* (Bernadon), regression to an ontogenetically (Freud) or phylogentically (Kretschmer) lower level, congenital or psychogenetically acquired anomalies of the striate body (Moser), etc. All these statements have no other practical value than that of more or less interesting opinions devoid of any concrete proof.

Psychoanalysis, of course, did not stop short of tics. From the crop of theories we gather the following examples: Constitutionally increased muscular eroticism (Sadger); disorders of genital potency with transfer of the libido to another region of the body, creating a narcissistic "compressed" stereotypy similar to catatonia and designated as "cataclonia" (Ferenczi);

[1] Meige, Henry, et E. Feindel. Les tics et leur traitement. Paris. 1902.
[2] Wilder, J., and J. Silbermann. Beiträge zum Ticproblem. Berlin. 1927, p. 25.

conversion symptom on a sadistic-anal erotic basis (Abraham); masturbation equivalent (Helene Deutsch; Melanie Klein; Reich); moral conflict between the ego and superego (Stekel; Vilma Kovacs). Almost every one of these assertions is based on generalizations from the study of one case only.

Braving the danger of appearing much more superficial, we shall indulge neither in neurological nor in other guesswork and limit ourselves to the known and objectively demonstrable facts. We then find that tics occur in children of both sexes, rarely before the sixth year of life, mostly of average or slightly below average intelligence, presenting a number of additional personality disorders, responding to emotional and situational difficulties with involuntary localized movements; these movements arise from habitual repetitions of primarily purposive actions or from imitation of others or from gestures which have always been more or less customary with the child.

The last point is best illustrated by the case of a seven-year-old, mentally retarded girl who, in addition to an affective upheaval caused by the discovery that she was a foster child, developed a horror of school where she could not comply with the requirements. She had always presented a feeding problem which was tremendously exaggerated in the mornings of school days. She had long been in the habit of pushing away with her right arm the food and bribes proffered by her foster mother during breakfast and the clothes with which her foster father tried to dress her, so that she should not be late in her class; upon leaving the house, it was noticed that she continued jerking the right arm (which carried the book bag). She did not jerk it on her way back from school or at any other time of the day. When she was legally adopted by her fond foster parents and placed in an ungraded class, her jerkings disappeared together with her feeding difficulties.

The *diagnosis* of tics is not difficult in the majority of cases if one keeps in mind the criteria enumerated at the beginning of the chapter. There are, however, a few conditions which may sometimes be mistaken for tics, or vice versa:

General motor unrest. Everyone dealing with larger numbers of children has an opportunity to observe that there are differences not only in appearance, body weight, intelligence, emotional attitudes, etc., but also in the motility. The average youngster, after proper motor orientation, must slowly acquire a certain sense of kinetic economy. Before he gets that, he is apt to overdo, to overplay, and to make several excursions where one would be sufficient. The average child learns in the course of the preschool years to limit his motility to purposeful and well-timed activities, though in his play with other children he still likes to revert to the earlier mode of lesser motor control and balance. In his games, he prefers to be "wild," to shout and yell instead of talking quietly, and to run instead of walking. Departures from the gradual adaptation to the adult pattern of finely calculated, timed and precise movements may lead to two opposite extremes. There are youngsters, not always obese ones, who are unusually quiet, "phlegmatic," "lazy," who try to get along with a minimum of actions, who are "hypokinetic." It is much more frequent to see the other extreme of the restless, fidgety, "hyperkinetic" child who "is always on the go," "never can sit still," "always must be doing something." These children are very liberal with the employment of their motility. They may jerk and twist and perform many of the movements which are seen in tics. Many of the cases of tics described in children of pre-school age are probably nothing more than examples of this type of overactivity. They differ from real tics in that they are not so consistently localized, that the restlessness may continue during sleep, and that they do not exist when the child's attention is held.

Chorea. Tics and chorea are very frequently mistaken for each other, both by the profession and by the laity. Children with tics were brought to the clinic with these remarks:

"I think it is his nerves, and I think it is inherited from me. I had St. Vitus's dance when I was his age." (The patient had mild facial tics.)

"The doctor said that he was on the verge of St. Vitus's dance when he started attending him. He used to twitch his mouth, blink his eyes, and jerk. I noticed the last few days he has been jerking again."

"I think it is nerves. He just twists his face and touches his nose and ear. I thought it was St. Vicence (meaning St. Vitus). He has done that for two years."

"He was always twitching his right eye and we thought maybe it was St. Vitus's dance. He has been doing that for the last six months or more. I was sick at the time but the children told me they thought maybe it's a habit and we tried breaking him from it. I used to scold and punish him but my husband told me not to do it; when he was younger, he had St. Vitus's dance himself."

It must be conceded that the distinction from chorea, especially from incipient chorea, is not always easy. Choreic and choreiform movements are ushered in more gradually, last longer, have a greater range of excursion, and are not restricted to a circumscribed group of muscles. Tics are repeated in the same fashion, whereas choreic movements vary irregularly. In chorea, there is often a combination with rheumatic fever or with cardiac involvement.

Athetosis, especially the mild forms of congenital double athethosis. The presence of other neurological findings and the nature of the movements (worm-like, more or less continuous) will help in the differential diagnosis, as will also the history of the onset and course of the condition.

Gilles de la Tourette, in 1885, described in the *Archives de Neurologie* a rare specific type of tics which has been named after him. The *tic de Gilles de la Tourette*, or *"maladie des tics des dégénérés,"* begins in children of seven or eight years, most of whom have psychopathic antecedents, with facial movements and throat noises; the jerks gradually become more generalized and progressive. Later whole words or short sentences are ejaculated spasmodically; they may have obscene contents (coprolalia) or consist of an irresistible repetition of remarks made by others (echolalia). The prognosis is said to be unfavorable.

John E. was seen at the Henry Phipps Psychiatric Clinic in 1929 at the age of seventeen years because of spasmodic inarticulate noises which he made in his throat and because of jerkings of the body. The difficulties began at the age of nine years, two weeks after an operation for the removal of his tonsils and adenoids done without an anaesthetic. He started to make throat noises which were most pronounced during meals. The family physician felt that the reaction was a habit and would go away. As the years went by, however, the noises became worse and other unnatural jerking movements developed. While walking along the street, he made sudden skipping-like steps. At times, he would blink his eyes a great deal. In November, 1927, his sister was given antitoxin injections for scarlet fever and fainted. John, thinking that the doctor had killed her, suddenly began to shout and swear and the jerkings became worse. He calmed down on seeing his sister revive but from then on his symptoms were much more pronounced. He emitted spasmodic expiratory noises, suggestive of gagging or vomiting. Occasional jerkings of the body were centered in the pelvis. There were rare upward pseudo-nystagmoid movements of the eyeballs. The noises were more frequent when he was excited or talking and absent during sleep. He sometimes ejaculated "dirty words that he should not say."

John had enuresis until the age of four years. He had presented a feeding problem and vomited frequently until about ten years old. His parents tried to make him eat by threatening to send him to a reformatory if he refused. He masturbated between eleven and fourteen years. He had always wanted his own way and was angered at restriction and discipline. He had a mental age of fourteen years. He was physically underdeveloped with regard to height, weight, and growth of pubic hair.

Torticollis on the basis of tics is rare in childhood. Most cases of wry neck in early years are of organic origin (either congenital: caput obstipum congenitum, or acquired: intra-partum hematoma of the sternocleidomastoid; rheumatic myositis; caries of the cervical vertebrae; scars from a burn). The distinction between tic-torticollis and spastic torticollis is sometimes difficult but in view of the infrequent occurrence in children of relatively little practical significance. We saw a little girl who developed the habit of holding her head to one side from walking and sitting at the table always on her mother's left side. She was around her mother practically all day and also slept with her, also on her left side. The mother was a tall woman and the child, from looking up to her a good deal of the time, assumed the posture of holding her head turned to the right.

The *treatment* of tics is a difficult task. It is not the tics that must be treated, but the patient who has them. It is a matter of common experience that the more the child's attention is directed toward the movements, either in a therapeutic effort or otherwise, the less they are likely to disappear. This is why parental corrections in the form of admonitions or nagging or warning do not usually result in improvement. This is also why such methods as exercises before the mirror in many cases do not have the desired effect. These measures, as well as massage, electrotherapy, and even suggestions centering on the tics only, disregard the much larger issues of the etiological basis anchored in the child's personality and envionment.

Faulty notions with regard to the tics will have to be straightened out. Terms such as "St. Vitus's dance" where there is no chorea, or "bad nerves," or "nervous wreck" have the effect of a *carte blanche* given to the child. The feeling of being sick and having pathological symptoms is impressed on the patient. It is wise, in speaking to parents, to be rather cautious in the use of the term "habit." It often happens that "habit" is interpreted by lay people as something voluntary, something that the child does on purpose in order to torment the family. This is certainly not true of tics. It has been said that the patient, more or less consciously, derives some degree of pleasure from the movements. It has also been stated that they are a more or less conscious means of obtaining a gain. However this may be, so much is certain that the habit is not a "bad habit" in the sense of wilful mischievousness and deviltry. Yet many tiqueurs are done a grave injustice by their environment which, upon being told that the blinking or jerking is a habit, proceeds on the assumption that it should be "broken" through scoldings and punishment.

The next therapeutic step consists in the improvement of the situational difficulties in which the tics were developed and maintained. This may involve work with the family where parental frictions, fear of an alcoholic father, chronic invalidism, contrasting of children, and problems of a more subtle nature may create the need for advice and guidance. School adjustment may be necessary in some cases. Sometimes boarding home placement may have to be considered.

It is essential that all physical faults should receive adequate medical attention. If the original irritation, leading to the evolution of the tic, is still extant, it should be remedied, whether this be a tight cap, eczema, conjunctivitis, or a poor lighting system in school. Every other somatic defect will be included in the treatment (of any child, tiqueur or no tiqueur). But in doing so, it is advisable to refrain from the practice, not so uncommon, of promising the cure of tics through tonsillectomy or circumcision or the like. Where these operations are indicated, it is significant enough to explain their importance to the parents without creating in their minds wrong ideas of causal relationships. Yet this is the report of a mother of a boy with tics: "Nerves. It is a twitching in the face, mostly in the eyes. He would sit and twitch his shoulders. He has had it for over a year. The family doctor said this is from bad tonsils and that he should be circumcised. So he had his tonsils and adenoids out and he was circumcised with the hope that that would help him. But it did not do him any good. He twitches worse than he did before."

Since most of the children who have tics are of school age, they are accessible to direct contact. We shall try to establish self-confidence with regard to the curability of the movements, remove the notion that organic illness is responsible, and work out a constructive plan for adequate occupation and play and rest for the twenty-four hour period of the day. Since tics are practically always combined with other personality difficulties, it is natural that the therapy will be directed toward a better adjustment of the child as a whole rather than treating the coexisting tics and enuresis or feeding problem as separate things.

The fact that sometimes tics return after several months or years should not make one unduly pessimistic with regard to the prognosis. It is understandable that a person who has once reacted with muscular twitchings to some emotional disorder may again select the same or a similar kind of response when things go wrong at a later time. Personalities and reaction tendencies cannot be made over entirely and the course of events cannot be commanded. But if we have once helped the patient to get over the problems of which the tics were an external manifestation, he is likely to return to us as soon as new danger signals appear.

NODDING SPASMS

A great number of names (*head nodding, head shaking, head rolling, nodding spasm, spasmus nutans, spasmus rotatorius, gyrospasm, nutatio capitis spastica, Nickkrampf, Dunkelzittern, Pendelzittern*) has been employed to designate a relatively infrequent condition to which Herrman,[1] in a most excellent article, prefers to refer more descriptively and fittingly as *head shaking with nystagmus*. Its main characteristics are:

Continuous or intermittent, mostly arhythmic, involuntary *movements of the head*, either horizontal, or vertical, or rotatory. They sometimes present themselves in several forms in the same individual. Of the children seen at the Harriet Lane Home, forty-five per cent had side to side movements only, in twenty-six per cent the head was moved backward and forward, and in thirteen per cent it was rotated. In three per cent there was a combination of nodding plus rotation in quite irregular fashion, and in thirteen per cent lateral and vertical excursions were seen in the same patient. In one case, the head motions were first in negation and, when the child was seen nine days later, in affirmation. In another child, they were always up and down when she was standing or sitting, and from side to side when she was lying down on her back; the head was kept still when she lay on her side. Contrary to the statement of some authors that the motions may be observed also during sleep, every one of our patients showed the picture only while awake; one child was reported to roll his head "when slightly roused from sleep." In the day time, the shaking was either constant, or it occurred only when looking fixedly at an object, or only "when sitting in her mother's arm," or only when walking, standing, or sitting, but never when in horizontal position, or, on the other hand, in one instance "only when he lies down." One child "does it all the time but she never does it when she is crying." In one case, the arms were observed to move, at times together with the head.

Though sometimes the movements of the head may be the only symptom, they are in most cases associated with *nystagmus*, which is usually binocular, but at times also uni-ocular. In our material, bilateral nystagmus was noted in sixty per cent, one-sided in sixteen per cent (equally divided between the right and left eye), and no nystagmus was present in twenty-four per cent. Where there is binocular nystagmus, the two eyes do not necessarily move together all the time, nor always at the same rate. The nystagmus may be horizontal, vertical, diagonal, or rotatory, and may, or may not, follow the direction of the head movements. The lateral form is seen most frequently. The oscillations of the eye bulb may be quick or slow, constant or intermittent, and often appear only upon fixation of objects. In one case, the lateral nystagmus was much more marked on the right

[1] Herrman, Charles. Head Shaking With Nystagmus in Infants. Pediatrics by Various Authors. Edited by Isaac A. Abt. Vol. VII, pp. 384–397. Philadelphia and London. 1925.

side than on the left; in another, horizontal and vertical excursions were seen to follow each other in rapid succession. The head shaking and the nystagmus may begin and end at different times. In one case, oscillations of the left eye were noticed first and the nodding did not follow until three weeks later, and the nodding disappeared before the nystagmus. In another instance, the situation was exactly reversed. Nystagmus may be seen at times when there is no nutation or shaking, and may even be elicited only if the head is held firmly between the examiner's two hands. On the other hand, it was found that bandaging of the oscillating eyes causes a prompt cessation of the excursions of the head. Sometimes nystagmus occurs only if the patient looks to one side.

In a comparatively small number of instances, the children have a *peculiar way of holding the head* to one side ("cocking") and looking out of the opposite corners of their eyes.

The condition is usually seen in small infants only. The age at onset could be definitely established in twenty-five of our cases. The figures are given below:

Age at Onset (in months)	Number
Fourth	2
Fifth	3
Sixth	1
Seventh	3
Eighth	2
Ninth	2
Tenth	2
Eleventh	5
Twelfth	1
Thirteenth	1
Fourteenth	2
Twentieth	1
Total	25

It is a highly interesting fact that head shaking in a great majority of babies begins during the winter months. In the same twenty-five cases, the time of onset showed the following distribution:

Month of the Year	Number of Cases
January	6
February	2
March	5
April	1
May	1
June	0
July	0
August	1
September	1
October	1
November	2
December	5
Total	25

There is a higher incidence of nodding spasms in girls (in our material, sixty-five per cent) than in boys. One of the most astonishing features in our group, which comes from a mixed white and negro population, was the disproportionately high occurrence in negro infants (not less than seventy-eight per cent of the total number; the community consists of 82.5 per cent white and 17.5 per cent colored persons). Most of the white patients came from the insanitary homes of poor immigrants, chiefly Polish and Hebrew.

The condition was combined with rickets in sixty-three per cent of the children. Serious developmental retardation was observed in ten per cent. In four cases, there was unilateral strabismus, strangely enough always on the left side; its relation to the type of nystagmus was as follows:

Left internal strabismus with no nystagmus.
Slight left internal strabismus with bilateral horizontal nystagmus, in two cases.
Left external strabismus with left horizontal nystagmus.

Congenital developmental anomalies were noted in two patients only. One had a congenital club foot, and the other had an undescended right testicle.

Additional complaints were:

Continuous crying with breathholding spells.
Constant erection of the penis.
Peevishness at night and a good deal of vomiting.
Sucking movements with the lips and tongue and occasional regurgitation of food.
Restlessness and jumping in sleep, "as if frightened," in two cases.
Generalized convulsions for one day at the age of four months.

In two patients, there was a definite relation of the onset to skin affections (furuncles) at the back of the neck. The mothers reported that the babies were seen to shake their heads occasionally as a reaction to the pain or itching sensation and then to have kept it up after the boils or pimples had disappeared. The nystagmus followed soon after the beginning of the shaking.

We have seen familial occurrence in three cases. The brother of a ten-month-old girl with horizontal and vertical head movements and no nystagmus had both nodding and nystagmus from the age of eight months to two years. The feebleminded aunt of a little negro girl, who took care of the child, still nods her head and "her eyes jump." In the third case we perhaps do not deal with genuine nodding spasms. Of a family of three boys, the oldest, William, ten years old, and the youngest, Frank, aged four, began to shake their heads and to move their eyeballs in infancy and kept it up since then. Their father and Frank had convulsions between the ages of two and three years. William had a refractive error, an I.Q. of 79, was constipated, a restless sleeper, very stubborn, and afraid of the dark; "his head will show the most if he is annoyed." Frank was also retarded intellectually, was constipated, presented a feeding problem, had temper tantrums, and was badly spoiled.

The condition is confined to the first two or three years of life. It usually lasts a few weeks or months, rarely longer than two years. It is an involuntary reaction and does not seem to be associated with affect disturbances as are, for instance, the breathholding spells, which occur at the same age. One child could stop the head shaking voluntarily whenever she was told to keep quiet. Attracting the child's attention often causes a cessation of the head movements, but not necessarily also of the nystagmus.

Thomson interpreted spasmus nutans as being a "functional coördination neurosis," because it develops at a time when the child learns to control and coördinate his ocular movements by means of visual impressions.[1]

Raudnitz, in 1897, evolved the theory, which has found many followers, that being kept in a dark room is responsible for the development of the condition and that infants with strabismus or general weakness and easy fatigability of the ocular muscles are most likely to be affected; the type of movements is said to depend on the location of the lighter parts of the room, to which the children direct their eyes with a certain degree of strain: "We deal with a reflex spasm produced by the attempts at fixation." Raudnitz felt that similar mechanisms prevail in the causation of miners' nystagmus. Raudnitz and Ohm observed that young dogs (and cats) which were kept in the dark almost invariably developed nystagmus after a period of a few weeks.[2]

Other authors have attributed etiological significance to rickets, dentition, impairment of vision, and temporary disturbances in the vestibular apparatus or the nucleus of Deiters.

No particular *treatment* is necessary beyond the need of reassuring the parents that the condition is transient and does not interfere with the infant's health and development. Where it is learned that the child is kept too much in a dark room, better lighting arrangements and a few hours daily in the open air should be recommended.

There exists a *congenital form of head shaking with nystagmus* which is progressive and persists throughout life; in these cases the eye movements are always bilateral and conjugate. In the instance of one highly intelligent seventeen-year old boy this picture was associated with stuttering; his father and five (of eight) siblings have, or had, the same speech difficulty.

Spasmus nutans is always benign. It must, therefore, be clearly differentiated from two other conditions in which there exists a strong tendency to intellectual deterioration:

The *secousses* (Herpin) or *Blitzkrämpfe* (Asal and Moro) are epileptoid in character. All of a sudden, with the rapidity of lightning, the head is jerked forward and the arms are spread apart and immediately brought together again. The attacks usually occur numerous times during the day and

[1] Thomson, J. Clinical Study and Treatment of Sick Children. Edinburgh. 1925, p. 611.

[2] Raudnitz, R. W. Zur Lehre vom Spasmus nutans. Jahrbuch für Kinderheilkunde. 1897, 45, 145.

Ohm, Johannes. Das Augenzittern als Gehirnstrahlung. Berlin und Wien. 1925, p. 125ff.

Paterson, Donald, and R. W. B. Ellis. Spasmus Nutans (Head-Nodding) as Associated With Defective Lighting in the Home. Lancet. 1931, 2, 736.

sometimes are observed also at night. They may occasionally take the form of twitchings of the entire body. They develop at about the same age as does the nodding spasm. The suddenness and great rapidity, the absence of nystagmus, and the mental deterioration of the children are sufficient pointers for differential diagnosis.[1]

The *salaam spasms* or *salutation spasms* (Moro's *Grusskrämpfe*) or *epilepsia nutans* consist of periodic and rhythmical movements of the head and upper part of the body of about two seconds' duration with intervals of approximately ten seconds, which resemble the Oriental form of greeting. Consciousness may, or may not, be abolished. In the individual attack, the head movements may be repeated as many as thirty to fifty times. Gnashing of the teeth is sometimes observed during the performances. The condition is mostly associated with pathologic neurological findings, such as positive Babinski reflex, spastic hemiparesis, hypertonicity, and contractures. The attacks begin at a very early age, and most of the patients become seriously demented. Nystagmus has not been noted in the salutation spasms.

[1] Asal, B., und E. Moro. Über bösartige Nickkrämpfe im frühen Kindesalter. Jahrbuch für Kinderheilkunde. 1914, 107, 1.

CHAPTER XXX

THE SPECIAL SENSES

THE DISTURBANCES of sense perception, as far as they are not referable to local disorders or to circumscribed lesions in the central nervous system, are in many instances associated with definite psychopathological reaction forms, such as hysteria or schizophrenia. They occur often in anergastic illnesses without being necessarily correlated anatomically to the type and seat of the cerebral tissue alterations. They are observed in dysergastic conditions (deliria) and in the aura of migraine and of epilepsy. They may to a certain extent be normal or near-normal phenomena in pre-school children (imaginary toys and companions), in the state between sleeping and waking and in extreme fear. They may, finally, appear as more or less isolated disorders. Though it is hardly possible or practicable to make a rigid distinction between the various forms of psychosensory abnormalities, one may, for the purposes of organization and of ready orientation, recognize the following groups:

Changes in the quantity of perception: loss, diminution, or exaggeration.

Misinterpretations of actual sense perceptions.

Perceptions of non-existent objects (hallucinations).

QUANTITATIVE CHANGES OF PERCEPTION

It is most frequently the sensibility for touch and pain which may, conjointly or separately, be modified in its intensity. In hysterical individuals one occasionally finds tactile anaesthesia or hypoaesthesia or hyperaesthesia, or changes in the sensation of pain in the sense of analgesia or hypoalgesia or hyperalgesia. These alterations are not determined by the distribution of cutaneous innervation but by the lay notions of body segmentation; a "finger," a "hand," a "foot," an "arm," or a "leg" is insensitive or hypersensitive, regardless of the anatomical features of the nerve supply. Special circumscribed zones (the breasts, the inguinal regions, the small of the back) may be unusually susceptible and extremely painful upon the slightest touch (so-called *topalgias*). Sometimes there is in hysteria a transient loss of vision or a concentric narrowing of the fields of vision, or deafness, or a temporary abolition of olfactation (anosmia) or of taste (ageusia). The insensitiveness of the mucous membranes may show itself in the absence of the pharyngeal reflex and in the failure to elicit a sneezing response upon the irritation of the inner coating of the nasal cavity (though, curiously enough, the accompanying lachrymation and dilatation of the conjunctival blood vessels are always present).

Painful stimulation is never registered in comatose states. Sometimes it evokes no defense reaction in catatonic stupor. There may be a considerable lowering of the threshold for pain sensation, borne out by the results of the electrical skin resistance test, in a small percentage of feebleminded children. Thiemich went so far as to consider general analgesia for pin-pricks in the early years of life as a diagnostic criterion of imbecility, some-times associated with imperfect development of the gustatory functions.[1]

We had an opportunity to observe this phenomenon in a mentally retarded three-and-a-half-year-old boy (with a mental age of slightly above two years), who had a history of bleeding from the navel at six weeks, rickets, chronic constipation, bilateral otitis media, and prolapse of the rectum. His father was feebleminded, alcoholic, brutal, a wife-beater who before his marriage had been arrested for beating his mother. The child's mother spent four years at the State Training School for the Feebleminded, to which she referred as the happiest four years of her life. He had an older brother of four years who had breathholding spells and later had temper tantrums. A two-year-old sister ate coal, dirt, polish, and chewed the paint off the furniture; once she drank some turpentine. The suggestion of bathing came as an unheard of revelation to the parents. The patient himself had a history of three convulsions (one at two months, two at nineteen months), breathholding spells, masturbation since the age of one year, enuresis and encopresis, night terrors, fear of dogs, and persistent crying; his articulation was defective. When blood was taken for a Wasser-mann test, it was noticed that the insertion of the needle was accepted peacefully without the slightest defense movement. Strong pin pricks and vigorous pinching had the same effect; they did not seem to be felt. The psychogalvanic record showed no reaction to painful stimuli; in spite of the fact that he was crying when the record was taken, there was no indi-cation of any sympathetic activity.

In children with marked general irritability, in cases of extreme fatigue, and in the course of migrainous attacks, there is occasionally an inability to stand strong light (photophobia) or loud noices (hyperacusis or oxyacoia). Hyperacusis is also an inconsistent symptom of cerebrospinal meningitis, cerebral diplegia, and amaurotic family idiocy.

MISINTERPRETATION OF ACTUAL PERCEPTIONS

Mild actual sensations or perceived objects may be misinterpreted in the form of paraesthesias or illusions or unreality feelings.

Paraesthesias are perverted sensations. They may appear as complaints of numbness, creeping (feeling of "pins and needles," or formication), itching, pricking, burning, or tingling. They occur especially in hysterical and hypochondriacal children.

Illusions are distorted or mistaken perceptions of real objects. Certain optic illusions have long been known to be normal psychological phenom-ena. Small children, in their play, do not clearly distinguish between reality and the products of their fancy. There is often a vacillating mixture of acceptance of actuality, make-believe, illusional and, in a sense, even hallu-cinatory experiences, depending on the child's imaginativeness, age, and the degree of absorption by the game. Stern says rightly: "It is not always easy to determine where the child's awareness of self-deception begins and where it ends."[2] A child is not lying or merely pretending in the same man-

[1] Thiemich, Martin. Über die Diagnose der Imbecillität im frühen Kindesalter. Deutsche medizinische Wochenschrift. 1900, 26, 34–36.
[2] Stern, W. Psychologie der frühen Kindheit. Leipzig. 1914, p. 189.

ner in which an adult pretends, if, when playing mailman, he distributes scraps of paper or tree leaves for letters. The child, for the moment at least, "is" the mailman, and the scraps or leaves "are" letters. Similarly, buttons "are" coins for which blocks, representing bars of soap, are really "purchased" from another youngster who "is" the grocery clerk. One may, or may not, look upon these playful substitutions as illusions. They do share with illusions the property of being taken for real by the child, at least momentarily; at any rate, the child, while playing, does not take the effort to discriminate between the button as a button and the button as a coin though, if taken to task or not absorbed by the game, he will be well capable of making the proper distinctions.

Fears are an especially frequent source of illusional experiences. After listening before bedtime to "scary" stories told by some older playmates or backstairs by a servant or over the radio, the impressionable and imaginative youngster, alone in the dark bedroom, preoccupied with the yarn, living over the events in his fancy with himself as a participant, may easily transform his room into a scene of spooky activity, vividly mistake the curtain fluttering in a mild breeze for a ghost or for a disguised burglar and interpret any sort of noise as the snorting of a wild animal.

Charles R., ten years old, had a "nervous" mother who had many fears to which she always reacted strongly in the child's presence. She was afraid that something might happen to her husband or to her two sons when they were away from home. Charles adopted all of her fears and added others of his own. He not infrequently ran home "all scared" to see if anything had happened to his parents whom he imagined had been hurt in an accident. He was afraid of mice, as was his mother. He had night terrors (a bootlegger hitting his father over his head, men robbing his father of money). He had a marked apprehensiveness when crossing bridges by auto ("The bridge might break; I scratch my head and pull my face"). His older brother once frightened him by jumping at him in the dark cellar, dressed in a wide robe. When, a short time afterwards, he was sent to the cellar to fetch something, he thought that he saw a "shady figure" and heard it say, "Come here, Charles!" On another occasion, while walking in the street, he saw a man who looked like a burglar to him. He began to run, having all the time the feeling that the man followed him. He looked back once or twice and really thought that he saw the man running behind him, although this was not the case.

Feelings of unreality are exceedingly rare in children. Things seem unreal to the patient, different from what he knows them to be. He is fully aware of the incongruity of his experience which sometimes causes considerable distress.

Robert Z., a slightly retarded boy of almost fourteen years, lost his mother at an early age. His father engaged a housekeeper who, in order to make herself irreplaceable in the home and to be married by the widower, selected Robert for a tool to help her carry out her plans. She tied him to herself in every manner imaginable, slept with him, did not leave him out of her sight, and introduced herself everywhere (also in our dispensary) as the child's "mother." She even told us the details of how she had nursed him. In this setting, aggravated by the woman's keeping him away from all other human contacts, he developed the feeling, which tormented him, that all objects did not seem to him as they should; he saw trees and thought that they should not be there; he definitely felt that his "mother's" hands were shaking when he positively knew that they did not shake; sometimes things seemed to him to be larger than they were. After the woman had left the household, the child's unreality feelings disappeared gradually.

HALLUCINATIONS

Hallucinations are sensory impressions without external stimulation. There exists no outward source for the imagined voices, visions, odors, tastes, or tactile sensations. The dream contents are made up largely of such experiences, which may be said to be normal or near-normal phenomena whenever the individual's consciousness is reduced to a lower level. We find them in the so-called hypnagogic state, that is, in the drowsy, dream-like condition which exists just before falling asleep and sometimes also in the process of waking up. They can be artificially induced through suggestion in hypnotized persons. They play a prominent rôle and are of a frightening nature in night terrors.

In young infants, the same factors that are responsible for illusions may produce reactions to which Stern alludes as *hallucinatory games;* they differ from real hallucinations in that they are actively created by the child instead of being felt as something foreign and passive. The child believes in their actuality only as long as he indulges in them instead of being permanently convinced of their independent existence. He has the feeling that he can do something to the imagined objects instead of considering himself a helpless object. He can be easily "sobered" and made aware of the non-existence of the creations of his own play fantasy. There are many imaginative infants who fetch all sorts of things from the empty space, happily roll an imagined ball, and even carefully avoid the non-drawn chalk marks in an improvised game of hopscotch. Many youngsters have imaginary companions with whom they converse for long periods, exchanging opinions and playing games with them. They will often seriously accept the gift of a "penny" when in reality with an appropriate motion nothing at all is put in their palms; they will close their hands around the "penny," guard it against loss, or hide it, or return it upon request. They may sometimes remark unexpectedly, "Here comes a dog," or, "Here comes an elephant," when no dog or elephant is to be seen; they will be rightly insulted and fail to comprehend the adults' attitude, when they are accused of lying in such an event. There is nothing pathological or undesirable in the situation, though it is wise to explain calmly to the child the difference between a real dog or elephant and the "make-believe" animal.

In recent years, auditory hallucinations have been observed in several non-psychotic children (all boys). Levin published four cases (seven, ten, twelve, and fourteen years old, respectively). The "voices" heard invariably gave expression to a conflict within the children. One boy stated: "My mind tells me to do different things sometimes, and I don't know which to do. . . . Sometimes I hear a voice on this side and it says, 'Don't do it,' and the other side says, 'Do it,' and I can't tell which is the right mind to obey." Another patient stated: "Sometimes when I don't want to go to Hebrew School, the bad voice says, 'Don't go to Hebrew, don't go to

Hebrew.' The good voice says, 'Do go to Hebrew, do go to Hebrew'."
Invariably the "good voice" was perceived in the right ear, the "bad voice"
in the left. The third boy reported: "In school, if I put down my pencil,
my heart tells me to pick it up; I pick it up and then my heart tells me to
put it down; and then I put it down, and it tells me to pick it up again,
and it goes on like that till my heart doesn't tell me any more." The fourth
boy related: "Sometimes, when I sit thinking, something gets in my head
. . . Sometimes I do the wrong thing by listening to what's in my head. . . .
Words saying, 'Do it,' or 'Don't do it'. . . . It sounds quiet, like if you're
whispering in somebody's ear. It gets in my ears and passes through. . .
It comes from Heaven—I don't know where it comes from. . . . I don't
know exactly. It comes from my brain."[1]

One of our own patients, George L., nine years and nine months old when
first seen, the son of illiterate and superstitious but well-meaning Spanish
immigrants, was brought to us by his mother with the complaint that he
had "acted funny" and seemed to be "sick in the head" for the past two
years, since his younger brother had been drowned accidentally. His first
"peculiar" action was noticed when, after a fight with a boy for which he
expected a severe beating from his parents, he refused to come into the
house but sat on the front door step, closed his eyes, and said, "I can't
see, I can't do nothing." He was taken into the house and began to cry
amid great excitement of the family and neighbors around him. He kept
crying for about one hour, refusing to say anything or to open his eyes. A
few weeks later, he went through the same procedure; people around poured
ice and water over him. There followed frequent "spells," partly of a similar nature, partly in the form of angry outbursts, in one of which he ran
up to the roof, while in another he threw a knife at his mother. All of these
episodes were preceded by fights with his playmates or by fear of punishment for some misdeed or by his parents' refusal to comply with his wishes.
His school teacher described the boy as "a stick of dynamite in the room,
who had to be handled with gloves," ready to fight on the slightest provocation; she would not dare to give him a paper marked "failure" because
it would immediately produce a tempest. Sometimes he used to announce
that he will have a temper tantrum by saying that he was "getting hot,"
as an indication that he preferred not to take part in a difficult school test
and that he would vigorously resent the teacher's least criticism of his attitude.

George was a healthy, normally intelligent, and very attractive boy. "If
not cross before he starts a lesson, he will do it real well." He felt that another boy was responsible for his brother's drowning by pushing him off the
wharf and stated several times that he would kill that boy some day. All
his fights usually ended successfully and he managed to make his parents,
the neighbors, the schoolmates, and the teachers afraid of him.

During the examination, it was learned incidentally that he heard
"voices," "ever since he can think." One type of voice, rough and loud,
came in through his left ear, telling him to "curse" or to "be bad"; another type, sweet and kind, entered through the right ear and told him
"not to curse" or to "be good." He felt that these experiences were real,
"or else I would not be hearing them." He named the devil as the origin

[1] Levin, Max. Auditory Hallucinations in "Non-Psychotic" Children. American
Journal of Psychiatry. 1932, 11, 1119–1152.

of the bad voice, and God as the source of the good voice. He had a "hard time deciding which voice to obey." He never heard them during his "spells." Occasionally, after looking at Christ's picture at home for a long time and going to bed soon afterwards, he saw the Lord "in a green dress," "like real," "with a beard," "different from those pictures," and "on places of the wall where those pictures do not hang." He was not so certain of the actuality of these visions, which seemed to disappear suddenly, as he was of the reality of the "voices."

George, during his first contacts with the physicians in the clinic, tried to employ the same methods of intimidation which he had used to his own satisfaction at home and in school. When the questions asked of him were not to his liking, he rose, threatened to strike the examining physician and, when he decided that the other party was much stronger, he simply ran away and sneaked, without pay, into a movie. He did, however, return on another day meekly for further examination. Considerable work was done with George, first for a week at the Henry Phipps Psychiatric Clinic, later ambulatory, and during the summer vacation in a boys' camp. His habit of dominating his environment through the instillation of fear was slowly converted into the ambition of gaining approval and respect through good behavior and satisfactory scholastic achievements. Being bright, imaginative, suggestible, and vain, he was easily accessible to kind and patient guidance. He reported gradually about his progress. His "spells" and the hallucinations have left him entirely. He is still somewhat irascible at times but never to the point of displaying temper tantrums. He does well at home and in school, and during the past few months he has received "Excellent" marks in "conduct" and in "effort."

Sherman and Beverly reported the examination of nineteen hallucinating children below fourteen years of age with ten younger than ten years, referred by school authorities, physicians, charitable agencies, and relatives because of violent outbursts of temper, "nervousness," difficulties in the home and school, and truancy from home. They could trace the hallucinations through several stages of development. A boy who saw God on one side and the devil on the other first argued with himself about being good, then recognized vague images, one saying, "Be good," the other, "Be bad"; he finally perfected the images so that they became God and the devil. The authors state: "Nearly all of the subjects were able to recognize, at first, the pathological or at least unexplainable nature of the hallucinations. In all cases, however, the children were certain of the reality of the experiences as true perceptions, but were usually indifferent to them." They also point out that, in contrast to the hallucinations of adults, those experienced by children are comparatively simple and much less removed from the environmental situations in which they developed.[1]

Hallucinations play a prominent part in delirious reactions of an infectious or toxic origin. Visual hallucinations are as a rule more frequent than auditory ones. They are usually fleeting, changeable, moving, and have a frightening effect upon the child, who may react to them with an expression of fear, defensive movements, screams, and pleas for help. They are more dramatic than those in other conditions, but the "plot,"

[1] Sherman, Mandel, and Bert I. Beverly. Hallucinations in Children. The Journal of Abnormal Psychology and Social Psychology. 1924, 19, 165–170.

mostly weird and inconsistent, is woven very loosely and has little, if any, coherence. Sometimes, the imaginary experiences are accepted with a good deal of fatalism. Occasionally, the child is even amused at their grotesqueness. Flashes of light, fire, people in peculiar robes and with bizarre, often menacing motions, ghosts, angels, the devil, and animals may be seen. The voices may be threatening or sarcastic and seem to be addressed to the patient or the fancied people may be heard discussing the child's fate. In rare instances, the children believe that they smell various odors which are not present in the environment (manure, feces, something burned, and the like). Unpleasant tastes may be hallucinated, sometimes leading to the complaint that the food has been poisoned and to the refusal to take nourishment. The patient may experience peculiar skin sensations and interpret them as bugs or worms crawling over the body or certain parts of it. A six-year-old colored girl whose skin had been grafted after an extensive second degree burn (contracted while attempting to light a cigarette from an oil stove), in her delirium interpreted her itching sensations as worms, which she thought she actually saw crawling out of a sandbag (her blanket) and spreading over her (only on those places which had been scalded or grafted); she saw men on horses coming toward her and the devil rising "from down below." Kinaesthetic hallucinations are sometimes experienced: the child feels that he is flying about or carried away or dropped from considerable height. Infants as young as one year of age may be observed as they grope for imaginary objects in the air or put hallucinated food into their mouths. Overdoses of certain drugs are known to produce more or less specific types of hallucinations (fire, abnormally small, "Lilliputian" etc.).

Hallucinations occur sometimes in epileptic, hysterical, and migrainous twilight states. They are often noticed in post-infectious psychoses. The aura of epilepsy and of migraine may consist of seeing flashes or flames or zigzag lights or color spots or of hearing noises (ringing, shouting, buzzing).

Schizophrenic children often hallucinate. Voices and visions are reported most frequently, in some instances the patients tell of peculiar olfactory or gustatory sensations. The child's attitude with regard to them is usually one of indifference; occasionally, they fit in with the delusional contents or are elaborated by the youngster in a delusional manner; for instance, the smelling of gas or ether may give him the notion that someone is trying to poison him. At times, the patient may become dangerous when he is bent upon carrying out orders which he has "received" by the voices.

Anergastic reaction forms may sometimes give rise to hallucinations. Their nature may depend on the specific localization of the cerebral lesion (olfactory in lesions of the uncinate gyrus, visual in tumors of the occipital lobe). In other cases, there seems to be no demonstrable connection between the type of sensory deception and the anatomical site of the tissue destruction (e.g., in encephalitis and in juvenile paresis).[1]

[1] The only extensive monograph on hallucinations in children was written by Bouchut (Des hallucinations chez les enfants. Thèse de Paris. 1886).

THIRD SECTION

PERSONALITY DIFFICULTIES EXPRESSING THEMSELVES CLEARLY AS WHOLE-DYSFUNCTIONS OF THE INDIVIDUAL

CHAPTER XXXI

INTELLECTUAL INADEQUACY

WE HAVE, in the chapter on the intelligence factor, dealt with the evolution of human intelligence, its measurement, the different stages of its attainment, and its manifold relations to personality development and behavior. We have learned to appreciate the high diagnostic value of mental testing and at the same time to view a person's intellectual capacity together with several other and equally important factors, such as the utilization of one's equipment, the demands with which an individual with a given endowment is confronted, the problem of somatic fitness, the form of emotional reactivity, the facts of habit training, environmental influences, and constitutional background. We must emphasize the fact that the terms *mental deficiency* and *mental retardation* cover as wide a range between the near-normal and the extremely abnormal as does, for example, the word "illness." The designation of *amentia*, employed especially in England to denote feeblemindedness, should best be abandoned because it has been used by different authors, in different countries, and at different times for altogether heterogeneous psychiatric conditions. Sometimes the name *oligophrenia* is used for the whole group, which Adolf Meyer has set apart from the other psychopathological patterns as *oligergastic reaction sets*. The gradated distinction between idiots, imbeciles, morons, borderline cases, and dull normal individuals has been mentioned on a previous occasion.

Mental deficiency furnishes a good example of the futility of wanting always to correlate deviations from the average abilities and performances to definite brain lesions or of trying to separate the "organic" from the "functional." We know that many cases of idiocy and imbecility are undoubtedly cerebrogenic and that others are due to thyroid disorders. The lower the degree of intellectual development, the more frequent is the coincidence with demonstrable anomalies of the central nervous system. On the other hand, there are enough feebleminded persons in whom no structural alterations have been found at autopsy. The milder the degree of the retardation, the less often evidence exists of physical disturbances which could be made directly responsible. Most of the prevailing classifications are based largely on neurological principles, are concerned mainly with the more conspicuous degrees of defect, and combine all instances in which structural damage cannot be found under the heading of "simple" or "genetous" (Ireland) feeblemindedness. We cite only two of these groupings.

Ireland's table considers idiocy only. He has twelve varieties:

1. Genetous idiocy.
2. Microcephalic idiocy.
3. Hydrocephalic idiocy.
4. Eclamptic idiocy.
5. Epileptic idiocy.
6. Paralytic idiocy.
7. Traumatic idiocy.
8. Inflammatory idiocy.
9. Sclerotic idiocy.
10. Syphilitic idiocy.
11. Cretinism.
12. Idiocy by deprivation.[1]

Tredgold defines "amentia" as "a state of restricted potentiality for, or arrest of, cerebral development, in consequence of which the person affected is incapable at maturity of so adapting himself to his environment or to the requirements of the community as to maintain existence independently of external support." Such a delimitation excludes from his grouping all those individuals of limited intelligence who, with proper training, can fully or partly adjust themselves to occupational and communal responsibilities of not too complex a character. Tredgold distinguishes between "primary amentia," based on "a numerical deficiency, irregular arrangement and imperfect development of the cortical neurones," and "secondary amentia," due to "an arrested development of cortical neurones," general or localized. His classification is as follows:

A. Primary amentia.
    1. Simple.
    2. Microcephalic.
    3. Mongolian.
B. Secondary amentia.
  I. Due to gross cerebral lesions.
    4. Syphilitic.
    5. Amaurotic.
    6. Hydrocephalic.
    7. Porencephalic.
    8. Sclerotic.
    9. Paralytic.
    10. Other toxic, inflammatory, and vascular.
  II. Due to defective cerebral nutrition.
    11. Epileptic.
    12. Cretinism.
    13. Nutritional.
    14. Isolation or sense deprivation.[2]

We prefer to speak of *intellectual inadequacy* for several reasons. We feel that one is not quite justified in limiting the term "mental" too narrowly to the cognitive functions only. The emotional and conative functions are

[1] Ireland, William A. Mental Affections of Children. London and Philadelphia. 1898.
[2] Tredgold, A. F. Mental Deficiency (Amentia). New York. 1916.

certainly not less mental. "Deficiency" fails to convey the idea of relativity; "inadequacy" permits of the highly important question: *Inadequate for what?* A person with an intelligence quotient of 85 may be, and surely is, unfit to occupy the chair of professor of economics but well suited to dispense articles in a Five and Ten Cent Store. One with an I.Q. of 75 may not even be capable of doing that but he may well be trained to usefulness as a cog in the wheel of the industrial Taylor System. And one with an I.Q. of 60 may learn to milk cows and wash dishes satisfactorily. "Intellectual inadequacy" therefore allows a more melioristic attitude than "mental deficiency."

Because of this relativity, the therapeutic planning must be fully adapted to the specific needs and abilities of the individual in question. Syphilis, epileptic phenomena, rickets, cretinism, nutritional disturbances, orthopedic requirements of children with birth injuries must be given the benefit of the special modes of treatment devised and found to be helpful in these conditions. Other, more incidental, physical disorders of a chronic, subacute, or acute nature also call for prompt and adequate repair.

One sufficiently impressed by the fact that no two human beings, intelligent or otherwise, are completely alike will easily understand that there is no such thing as treating "intellectual inadequacy" and that therapeutic generalizations cannot be offered. We do not treat conditions in the abstract. We treat people presenting such conditions. Even two patients having exactly the same intelligence quotients or the same structural damage may be found to be so different in many other respects, that methods which are constructive and curative in the one may be of no avail and even downright nonsensical in the other. It is therefore necessary in the first place to formulate the goal common to all psychiatric endeavor concerned with the handling of intellectually inadequate children and then to outline the various ways and means through which this goal can be attained. The naïve question asked by laymen, "Can feeblemindedness be cured?", is slowly becoming obsolete and is replaced by the query, "What can you do for a feebleminded child?" We do not claim that an intelligence quotient is always fixed and stationary; the effect of thyroid medication on children with hypothyroidism, the fact that certain youngsters develop fairly well for five or six years and then slow down in their intellectual evolution, and the observation that some few children show at a later age a smaller discrepancy between chronological and mental age than before, are apt to make one cautious. On the other hand, we must be reconciled to the experience that an individual with limited endowment is and usually remains an individual with limited endowment and that to undertake to make of him a person with different endowment would be equal to wanting to change a female into a male or a Melanesian into an American Indian. This sounds most trivial but must nevertheless be stated emphatically because many parents and even physicians have the erroneous notion that retarded pupils could be speeded up in their intelligence by pounding greater wisdom into their heads through extra tutoring and the like.

What is the common goal in dealing with intellectually inadequate children? We strive to help them in a manner which would secure the optimal use of whatever assets we find them to possess. We want to protect them against any social damage which might be inflicted upon them or which they might inflict upon others because they often lack criticism and the capacity for logical reasoning and for anticipation of consequences. We wish that they receive appropriate habit training through example and guidance. We try to relieve them of the unfair demand to compete in school, at home, and later in life with people with a better intellectual equipment in pursuits for which they are not suited. We aim to segregate those incapable of attaining any reasonable degree of occupational usefulness and to withdraw them from human currency in circulation. And we do our best to mobilize the community's forces to assist in the education and socialization of all the others.

For the purpose of segregation, the commonwealths and private enterprise provide *training schools* in which the children are studied, protected, fed and clothed, and trained by expert teachers. Some individuals will have to remain there for the rest of their lives; the world at large is not a safe place for all idiots, most imbeciles, and many morons. Even a considerable number of those may be taught to fulfil certain functions within the institution; they may help to carry out simple routine duties in the farms, gardens, and dairies, they may aid in the house cleaning and in the kitchen, they may learn to mend clothes and serve at the table. Others, more fortunate, may acquire sufficient skill, comprehension, and conventional behavior to be discharged and placed in circulation under parental guidance. Institutional placement is therefore never an expression of hopelessness and should never be so presented to the parents. It is a practical, constructive, therapeutic measure, holding out a promise rather than pronouncing a doom. The child is guarded against injuries which might be otherwise incurred through inability to avoid dangers and through lack of understanding of traffic regulations, against lead poisoning resulting from the unsupervised habit of chewing paints, against being made the tool of sexual abuse and the victim of gangdom's temptations. The child receives instructions in a manner adapted to his ability, always with the view of returning him to society if and when he is ready to return. Every physician who deals with children should make it his duty to become acquainted, through personal visits, with the work of such institutions, just as he is naturally expected to be familiar with the properties and effects of the drugs which be prescribes.

Intellectually inadequate children who do not need institutionalization call for a different form of adjustment, consisting chiefly of *proper education and vocational guidance*. Aside from domestic habit training which every child, intelligent or unintelligent, must receive either by the parents or, if they are dead or intellectually or emotionally or morally unfit, in a well-selected boarding home, the problem of schooling is highly important. The larger cities nowadays have special schools or special, ungraded classes in which pupils, who because of their limited capacity cannot be expected to do the required grade work, are taught individually and freed from the need of competing with the average group of coëvals. Thus they are spared the feeling of shame and failure resulting from having to repeat the same grade a number of times and from being left behind with children much younger and smaller. It is necessary to explain to the parents and to the child, if he is old enough to understand, the reason for recommending an ungraded class or a special school and to hold it up as a helpful measure. One should point out what such arrangement will do for the child rather than use only the negative statement that the youngster is not sufficiently equipped for the regular grade work. Specific manual and mechanical interests and abilities may be found in many of these pupils, which can be utilized fruitfully in their preparation for life. The smaller towns and the rural communities have no such facilities; but even there the parents and teachers can at least be made to know of the child's problems and to deal with them with understanding, leniency, and emphasis on his assets rather than his limitations. At any rate, it is the physician's own duty to learn to recognize the existing intellectual inadequacy either by acquiring the required methods of examination or by consulting those who have the necessary knowledge.

Child education is a preparation for adult life in which occupational adjustment is a matter of the utmost importance. Intellectual inadequacy therefore calls for special vocational guidance. We can give it only if we have studied the individual sufficiently to know what we can expect him to learn and to achieve. It is both unwise and cruel to push a boy or a girl beyond his or her capacity if one has the means to foresee the inevitable clash. Even the most ambitious parents can be made to realize that it is better to change the direction of their hopes than to make their offspring the victims of unreasonable expectations. No special techniques or unusual skill is required for the proper administration of vocational guidance. Knowledge of the child and of the available opportunities and common sense serve the purpose adequately. It is, however, useful to know that fairly accurate aptitude tests for various occupations have been worked out and can be applied to youngsters if particular interests or opportunities make this advisable.

"Feeblemindedness" as such cannot be prevented. Early treatment of prospective parents who are luetic may in some instances reduce the probability of their begetting defective offspring. Whether or not first-cousin marriages result more often than others in the birth of intellectually inadequate children, is a question which has not been settled definitely; we know that deaf-mutism and retinitis pigmentosa are comparatively frequent in products of parental consanguinity. In general, one may say that the healthier, the more intelligent, and the more stable both parents and their families are, the better are the chances for bringing normal children into the world.

Sterilization has been recommended and in some places actually carried out in recent years with the aim of preventing the unchecked propagation of feebleminded humanity. Quite a few legislatures have considered or are now seriously contemplating its introduction into their juridical areas. Most of these efforts are based on the observation that mentally defective parents often beget mentally defective offspring. The high cost of keeping up and building more custodial institutions for an increasing feebleminded population, the assumption that a low intelligence quotient is in itself a potent factor in the etiology of crime, and the dire prediction that in the course of time a growing proportion of morons, imbeciles, and idiots will crowd out the intelligent section of mankind have suggested the idea of

eliminating such economic and social perils by cutting down through operative measures the fertility of feebleminded individuals. Such a program
would indeed be ideal if only we knew enough about the facts of inheritance.
It is true that several families have been studied which for many generations have contributed to dependency, maladjustment, and to prison and
asylum commitments. The Kallikak family is an eloquent example. Of it
Goddard says:

"The Kallikak family presents a natural example in heredity. A young
man of good family becomes through two different women the ancestor of
two lines of descendants,—the one characterized by thoroughly good, respectable, normal citizenship, with almost no exceptions; the other being
equally characterized by mental defect in every generation. This defect was
transmitted through the father in the first generation. In later generations,
more defect was brought in from other families through marriage. In the
last generation it was transmitted through the mother, so that we have all
combinations of transmission which again proves the truly hereditary character of the defect.

"We find on the good side of the family prominent people in all walks
of life and nearly all of the 496 descendants owners of land or proprietors.
On the bad side we find paupers, criminals, prostitutes, drunkards, and examples of all forms of social pest with which modern society is burdened.

"From this we conclude that feeblemindedness is largely responsible for
these social sores.

"Feeblemindedness is hereditary and transmitted as surely as any other
character. We cannot successfully cope with these conditions until we recognize feeblemindedness and its hereditary nature, recognize it early, and
take care of it.

"In considering the question of care, segregation through colonization
seems in the present state of our knowledge to be the ideal and perfectly
satisfactory method. Sterilization may be accepted as a makeshift, as a
help to solve this problem because the conditions have become so intolerable. But this must at present be regarded only as a makeshift and temporary, for before it can be extensively practiced, a great deal must be
learned about the effects of the operation and about the laws of human inheritance."[1]

There are other highly important factors besides our insufficient information about heredity which must be kept in mind with regard to the sterilization question. Not all intellectually inadequate persons are liabilities to
their communities. There exists a considerable percentage of stable and
well-trained people with low intelligence quotients who adequately fill
their places in society, are dependable laborers and farm hands, housemaids
and waitresses, and make good parents. No one would want to restrict
those people from breeding. It is the ill-educated and unstable feebleminded
that are responsible for some of the "social sores." But before immediately
reaching for surgical tools to sterilize them, let us not overlook the fact
that mental deficiency is not in itself and not solely the "cause" of delinquency, prostitution, alcoholism, etc. It is true that unintelligent persons
are apt to be more suggestible and less critical than intelligent ones. It is
further true that because of the type of occupations accessible to them and

[1] Goddard, Henry Herbert. The Kallikak Family. A Study in the Heredity of
Feeblemindedness. New York. 1923, pp. 116–117.

the small financial returns they often live in poor neighborhoods where there is a good deal of temptation. Court records show that the resistance to such temptations depends not only on the I.Q., but also to an equally large extent on early training and character formation. It is up to the commonwealth and its various agencies to provide proper facilities which would reach the feebleminded child and his parents at the earliest possible date and supervise his training, if possible, at home and, if necessary, in an institution or in a boarding home. Many young girls could have been snatched away from the clutches of prostitution, had their condition, intellectual and environmental, been recognized in time and had they been protected by means of proper placement and education. Prostitution is not synonymous with feeblemindedness. As a matter of fact, many of the girls on the road to sexual promiscuity who are brought before our juvenile courts fall into the groups of the borderline and dull normal children, with intelligence quotients which even the most rigid sterilization law would exclude from its scope. Furthermore, prostitution cannot be simply dismissed as a "social sore" originating in any number of feebleminded or not feebleminded individuals; it is the supply of a demand with which several sociological factors have something to do.

As to the cost of the care and training of mentally defective persons, figures are often quoted to demonstrate the high burden placed on the taxpayers, with the implication that sterilization will relieve future generations of a mounting financial outlay. But we should not be blind to the fact that the expenditure invested in the constructive institutional and extramural work with the feebleminded is a negligible trifle compared to the "social sores and pests" emanating from dishonest diplomats and war agitators and fraudulent financiers, none of whom can be suspected of a low intelligence quotient. Thousands of placid cretins, Mongols, and other idiots, well taken care of in wisely administered institutions, tens of thousands of higher grade "defectives" instructed properly in special schools or classes and prepared for simple though useful occupations do not cost the people the thousandth part of the tribute paid to the ragings of a handful of "intelligent" demagogues exacting countless lives and fortunes from misguided nations.

Sterilization does, however, have a place among our prophylactic resources. If a parent, regardless of the I.Q., has by his or her performances given evidence of utmost instability and inability to raise children without inflicting severe damage upon their physical and habit development, then, after a careful psychiatric examination, the communal authorities should have a right to take away from their custody their offspring already produced and to prevent them, through sterilization, from doing further harm. These factors, rather than the I.Q. alone, should be made the guiding criterion.

It is one thing to want to prevent the birth of feebleminded children. It is another thing to prevent maladjustments and personality disorders of intellectually inadequate youngsters who are brought to our attention. It is through the work with them, their families, and the communal agencies that the physician can contribute a lion's share not only to the development of his patients but also to the general welfare of the community in which he practices.

CHAPTER XXXII

EMOTIONAL DISORDERS

JEALOUSY REACTIONS

"JEALOUSY," says Douglas A. Thom in his "*Everyday Problems of the Everyday Child*" (*New York and London. 1928, p. 168*)," stands out preeminently as the cause of much unrecognized conflict in early life, and from a social point of view is very important. Not only does it stimulate anger, hatred, and inferiority in the child, but in later life it may so influence conduct that the individual is continually at odds with his environment. By jealousy we mean that unpleasant feeling induced by any interference or attempt to thwart us in our efforts to gain a loved object, either a person, power, possession, or position. By the very nature of the emotion, it carries with it a lowering of self-valuation, followed by humiliation, concealment, and shame. Jealousy between the ages of one and five is a normal reaction common to most children; yet often through accident or deliberate fostering, this emotion may become so exaggerated and dominant in the personality, as to make it inevitable that serious difficulty in social adaptability should follow."

The two main sources of jealous behavior in children are *the arrival of a new baby* and *the practice of contrasting siblings with one another*. The birth of a brother or sister is especially apt to set up a feeling of resentment in a youngster who for several years has remained an only child and then finds that he or she has to yield a part of the parental affections and attentions to someone else. Much will depend on the attitude of the elders. Many only children not only welcome the new arrival but sometimes beg the parents naïvely for a long time to get for them as a Christmas or birthday gift a baby brother or a baby sister. "Jealousy" is not there *a priori*, it is not inherent in the child, it is a reaction of certain individuals to situations which, at least in their opinion, threaten to take something away from them and to give it to others. It is not exactly envy, that is, wanting to possess something which another person has. Envy is a more circumscribed emotion; the envious person knows that he is envious, he knows precisely what it is that arouses his feeling, and he realizes that what he covets belongs rightly to the envied person. The jealous child does not know that he is jealous, he is not always capable of recognizing or formulating verbally the basis of his reactions, and he feels definitely that he is deprived of something that he has had previously and that he should possess. He would, if properly directed, be willing to share power, attention, and affection, but he is not ready to "play second fiddle." A wise parent will prevent the development of jealousy by preparing the child for the coming of the new member of the household, make him participate in the plans and arrangements, and when the baby comes, have the older sibling take a part, however small, in the care of the infant, being careful at the same time to make that part a privilege and a pleasure and not a disliked obligation and a burden. Both children, as time goes on, should then be treated, trained, disciplined, and encouraged without a spirit of contrasting or favoritism or creating in either sibling a sense of being compared advantageously or disadvantageously. The same is true of the practice, fortunately not so common, of demonstrative affection between parents with comparative neglect of the child. One does not have to speak in terms of the Oedipus complex to realize that jealousy can be incited by leaving the youngster out in the cold while he is made to witness the warmth of parental love.

Sybil Foster has made a study of the personality make-up and social setting of fifty jealous children. Two out of three in her group were girls. The largest number fell into the three-to-four-year age group. Selfishness and pugnacity were prominent character traits, whereas cruelty was shown very rarely. There was an unusually high proportion of disturbances of sleep, food capriciousness, and enuresis; destructiveness and hyperactivity were also not infrequent, whereas truancy, lying, and stealing occurred seldom. In many of the cases, there was evidence of lack of constructive training and a history of domestic friction because of marital discord or divided discipline. One-fifth of the children were objects of teasing from one source or another.[1]

TEMPER TANTRUMS

The temper tantrum is one of the most frequent habit disorders of children. Sixteen per cent of all patients referred to us for psychiatric advice presented, among other complaints, that of dramatic outbursts of anger, displeasure, or resentment. Of these, sixty-three per cent were boys, and thirty-seven per cent were girls. The age distribution, with consideration of both the chronological and the mental ages, was as follows:

Chronological age Years	Per cent	Mental age Years	Per cent
1	0	1	1
2	4	2	9
3	7	3	15
4	11	4	10
5	8	5	10
6	13	6	10
7	8	7	11
8	9	8	11
9	16	9	15
10	7	10	4
11	7	11	2
12	6	12	1
13	1	13	0
14	2	14	1

The various degrees of intellectual endowment were represented thus:

Superior intelligence	7 per cent
Average intelligence	33 per cent
Borderline intelligence	36 per cent
Morons and imbeciles	23 per cent
Idiots	3 per cent

[1] Foster, Sybil. A Study of the Personality Make-Up and Social Setting of Fifty Jealous Children. Mental Hygiene. 1927, 11, 53–77.

With regard to the position in the family of children with temper tantrums, these figures were obtained:

Oldest children:
   in families of two   15 per cent
   in families of three or more   10 per cent
Youngest children:
   in families of two   17 per cent
   in families of three or more   14 per cent
Middle position: 28 per cent
Only children: 16 per cent

Displeasure may, of course, be expressed by a child in milder forms than that of the full-fledged tantrum. If a mother becomes alarmed over the fact that her offspring frowns or turns away in token of dissatisfaction, yet abides obediently by the order received, she must be made to understand that extreme submissiveness, phlegmatic indifference with regard to the events which concern the child, or feigned acquiescence with a silent grudge are problems far more serious than the open but controlled manifestation of discontent. The emotion of anger, if justified and properly socialized, serves a useful and constructive purpose in life in the forms of righteous indignation, resentment, and criticism. It is the uncontrolled and sweeping outburst that becomes a psychiatric concern and calls for treatment of the child and of the setting in which his behavior has developed.

The commonest shape that the tantrum assumes consists in screaming and kicking. The youngster works himself rapidly or more gradually into a rage in which he may yell out, stamp his feet, throw his arms about, thrust himself and roll on the floor, strike everyone or throw every object within reach, curse, bite, bang his head against the wall or a piece of furniture, fight other children or even the parents, and generally "tear up the house."

We quote a selection of a few more or less characteristic complaints:

"She throws things, bites, and uses terrible language."

"She stamps her feet and kicks. She is terrible when she gets that way. She always fumes and fights with her brothers and sisters."

"She kicks and screams and beats her head against the wall. The other day, she smashed the glass of our china closet with a spoon."

"He gets real wild; he wants to climb and gets into all kinds of devilment."

"She just stands there and hollers. Sometimes she beats her eighteen-month-old sister."

"He bangs his head against the wall and throws the toys across the floor."

"If you want to wash and dress her, she strikes you right hard."

"He'll growl and roll on the floor."

"He just cries to break your heart and kicks."

"She just rears up and takes her fists and hits them. If she doesn't want to do something, she will grab hold of her clothes and say she is going to tear them off."

"He gets those rages and wants to tear his little sister to pieces. He has to be held by force until the rage passes. When he is held forcibly and pinned down for a few minutes, this rage passes off and he goes back to his play

again. At times in his rages he tries to hurt himself and will bang his head through a window pane. Once he tried to bang his head on a cabinet door."
"She screams and pulls her hair and beats her head against the wall."

The individual paroxysm may be precipitated by a variety of situations:
The most frequent immediate cause of a tantrum is the failure on the part of a parent, sibling, or playmate to comply instantly and uncompromisingly with the child's wishes. The outburst is at the same time a drastic expression of the child's disapproval and a means of gaining his end. The child "must have his own way" and dictates the exact manner in which his commands are to be fulfilled.

The same youngster who works himself into a rage whenever his will is crossed and who, with the aid of his tantrums, has secured parental obedience, may not at all be willing to carry out other people's orders. He may react with outbursts whenever he is asked to go to bed, wash his face, eat a dish which he has decided not to eat, or fetch an object from another room or from the store.

Note these complaints:

"He has a temper whenever he is ordered to do something." "He would slam the doors." "He is excited, kicks, screams, and shakes himself; he yells, 'I'll hit you, mother. I don't want to do that'." "He fights and screams if compelled to go to bed before midnight."

Tantrums are sometimes used to prevent anticipated punishment or to interrupt punishment which is in progress.

In some selfish and jealous children, the outbursts occur as responses to any demand that they may share their food, sweets, or toys with another person. One girl of four years was in the habit of throwing herself on the floor and kicking violently whenever her twin brother received the slightest attention from either of the parents. The moment the mother took another child up on her lap or as soon as a playmate barely touched a toy, the protestations were prompt, noisy, and kept up until the cause of the displeasure was removed.

There are children, as there are adults, who are bad losers. Whenever, in a fight provoked by themselves, they are beaten, they fly into a rage, bite, kick about blindly, jump up and down, and scream until they get red in the face; overprotective parents will come to their rescue and revenge them on the victor. Losing in a race or in a peaceful game may have the same effect. "He gets terribly mad," one mother reported, "if he plays a game of marbles and loses." Another boy told in a matter-of-fact manner how he beat his sister cruelly because "she had taken a marble away" from him; he added, upon specific inquiry, that she had won it from him in a game which, his sister asserted, he had forced her to play with him.

Every physician and dentist is acquainted with, and often exasperated by, the temper tantrums of some of his little patients just about to be examined or to take their medicines or to receive some specific kind of treatment, medical or dental.

In a number of children, the tantrum reaction has become so habitual that it may be called forth without any apparent provocation. It occurs wherever and whenever the youngster "feels like it." A characteristic example is contained in this story: "Once I showed him in a show window the picture of George Washington, and I said to him, 'This is George Washington,' and he threw himself on the pavement and kicked and yelled, 'No, it is not George Washington.' And the next time we went by, he said, 'Mother, this is George Washington'."

How do temper tantrums originate and how are they maintained? There is a variety of factors which must be considered and the ignorance of which will seriously interfere with any attempt at therapeutic adjustment.

Many types of physical discomfort, especially those of a chronic or subacute nature, are apt to make the child unduly irritable. Any adult who has worn narrow shoes or whose outing pleasures have been disturbed by a swarm of gnats knows how even such comparatively harmless annoyances may affect a person's mood. We have seen a number of patients whose outbursts of anger coincided chronologically with irritating sickness. In two of our children, tantrums, never experienced before, were concomitant manifestations of scabies and disappeared altogether with the cure of the itching skin sensations. Insufficient sleep and malnutrition are also apt to make an individual especially irascible.

By far the most frequent form of establishing and maintaining the anger habit in a child is the alarm shown at any expression of this emotion particularly in a sick, fatigued, resistive, pampered, jealous, or unhappy youngster, and the tendency to "give in." The child learns to use the tantrum as a means of obtaining his wants and dominating the family.

A few reports from mothers are illuminating in this respect:

"I think I'll go crazy trying to keep him quiet. We try and bribe him with money but he simply will not listen." "We generally give him everything he hollers for." "She has terrible tantrums when she wants to go to the movies. We always send her to get rid of her." "Usually we have to agree to his wants." "On account of her being so little and thin she gets her way." "Since she was sick (with chorea), I try to let her have what she wants with the other children."

The practice of giving in may be due to oversolicitude (fear that the child might suffer physically if permitted to continue crying or shouting; alarm over the red face or over the anticipated ensuing exhaustion), to convenience ("I just can't stand his crying, so I let him have his way. I don't like much crying and contention"), to consideration of neighbors ("It would be different if we did not have other people live in the house"), to the advice from physicians who prescribe "rest" for the "nervous" child and warn the parents not to cross him in any way, or to family dissensions with regard to the management of the child who learns that, if he cannot obtain the desired nickel or piece of candy from his parents, a fond grandmother will be sure to produce it if he shouts long enough for it.

The reaction pattern is often copied from a parent or another member of the household. It is mostly not so that the motions and exclamations are imitated with photographic exactness. It is rather the impulsiveness, the sudden, frequent, and sweeping loss of emotional self-control, and the dramatic vehemence that are taken over by the child, who fashions the response according to the more infantile outlets of screaming, rolling on the floor, and kicking. At the same time, he may also learn from the adults of his environment to add to this equipment the methods used by them, such as striking people, throwing objects, and cursing. In not less than sixty-four per cent of our patients with temper tantrums were we able to correlate these reactions with the presence of drastic manifestations of emotional instability in the home. In 12.7 per cent of these cases it was the father's alcoholism or psychopathic reaction trends or "violent temper," in 31 per cent the mother's temperamental mode of asserting herself or of expressing anger, in 48 per cent both parents contributed liberally to the supply of a pattern to their offspring, and in 8.3 per cent it was some other member of the household.

A study of the personalities of children with temper tantrums shows that the outbursts of anger are almost never the only expressions of emotional immaturity and instability in the patient. All kinds of combinations with fear reactions, feeding problems, disobedience, nightmares and night terrors, enuresis, stuttering, nailbiting, thumbsucking, and tics are the rule rather than the exception. In the early life histories of these children one sometimes finds the occurrence of breathholding spells (which, if not properly managed, are almost always replaced by temper tantrums sooner or later), headbanging, and frequent vomiting. Faulty habit training is an outstanding feature in a great majority of the cases. With very few exceptions, we find tantrums in children of overindulgent, oversolicitous, and overprotective parents. These youngsters show many evidences of a spoiled child reaction, inability to get along with playmates and strangers and general lack of self-dependence. "Excitability" and "irritability" are common characteristics. Selfishness with failure to consider the needs and rights of others and jealousy are traits frequently encountered.

We have made the most interesting observation that, at least in our relatively large case material, the coincidence of temper tantrums and hypochondriacal trends is exceedingly rare. As a matter of fact, we have not seen it in more than one patient only. This was true even of children who came from families in which both patterns were supplied by the parents or other members of the household. It is possible that either the tantrum or the somatic complaint provide a sufficient outlet, though the validity of this deduction is weakened by the fact that both tantrums and hypochondriasis may be seen associated with any other type of personality disorder.

According to Ziehen, outbursts of anger occur in imbeciles, epileptics, in myxedematous (rarely) and Mongoloid children (in mild form), in schizophrenia, mania, hysteria, and "neurasthenia." We must not forget that Ziehen paid little attention to children's behavior difficulties unless they could be accounted for as "symptoms" of some nosological "disease" or "constitution." It is true, however, that a comparatively large number of our patients with temper tantrums (fully nine per cent) were epileptics.

The following brief sketches of children with anger outbursts, selected at random, are presented with the view of giving an idea of the personality makeup, behavior trends, and physical condition found in some of these patients:

Boy, 8; 2. Sensitive, easily fatigued, cried easily, showed favoritism in dealing with playmates. Good formal behavior when away from mother. Spoiled badly (Mother: "I think maybe that's the whole trouble. Too much attention paid to him, I guess"). I.Q. 114. Slight diffuse enlargement of thyroid; cervical adenitis; undernutrition.

Girl, 6; 4. Feeding problem. Afraid of the dark. Feared that she will die of tuberculosis as her sister did. Restless. Not permitted to play with other children, did it "in a sneaky way." "Hopelessly" spoiled. I.Q. 97. Mediastinal tuberculosis; markedly positive tuberculin reaction.

Boy, 7; 3. Did not form sentences until five years. Bowel and urinary control at 4 years. In hospital at one year because of head banging. His singing and whistling were interpreted as abnormal activities. Afraid of children in the neighborhood. Overprotected and overindulged. I.Q. 80. Burdened with French and music lessons and memorizing poems. Good health. Lefthanded. Slept with mother.

Girl, 12; 1. Irritable. Dropped things when excited. Fainting spells. Headaches "most any time." I.Q. 75. Dental caries; hyperactive reflexes; refractive error; tachycardia. Just began to menstruate, scared because not prepared.

Girl, 2; 8. Poor habit training. History of frequent vomiting. Would not go to bed without the bottle. Nightmares. Fear of buzzing flies. Did not play with other children; landlady kept her dogs in the yard to prevent her from playing there. Kept tied on a big rope because mother feared she might run out and be hit by an automobile. She fell once on her nose, and parents feared she will become epileptic because an epileptic aunt fell on her nose when a child. Father thought that the mother's menstruation affected the child's behavior; "he just sees how she looks and says to me (mother), 'It's about your time again'." Developmentally normal. Good health.

Boy, 8; 4. Extremely restless ("Even as a baby he was never quiet; he was always on a rumpus"). Easily frightened. Poor progress in school. Hostile mother. Many minor accidents, due to lack of caution. Family record of epilepsy, "nervousness," tremors, nailbiting, and enuresis. I.Q. 92. Good health. Left internal strabismus.

Boy, 3; 6. Spoiled child reaction; restless, eager to attract attention. Masturbation. Grimacing. Very jealous of his father. Breast fed for 18 months. Dental caries; phimosis; scabies; impetigo; chronic tonsillitis; constipation. Average intelligence.

Boy, 4; 5. Overprotected. Did not talk until four years. Enuresis until recently. Contrasted with younger brother. Very resistive and negativistic ("He always says, No"). Feeding problem with vomiting. Destructive. Poor habit training. About one year retarded. Signs of old rickets; constipation.

Boy, 12; 0. Spoiled child reaction. Breast fed for 17 months. Twitching of head and neck. Poor progress in school. History of two fainting spells in church, following a long fast. Five pounds underweight; dental caries; chronic tonsillitis; calcified mediastinal tuberculosis; positive tuberculin reaction. I.Q. 79.

Boy, 10; 2. Restless ("He never sits still, always has to be moving"). Fear of the dark. Nodding spasm (as had his four-year-old brother). Hypochondriacal pain in legs. I.Q. 79. Spoiled child. Horizontal nystagmus; refractive error.

Girl, 7; 2. Feeding problem; usually very quiet; read "all the time"; occasional enuresis. ("She is slow in becoming angry, but when she does, she gets very heated up, and then she does not care with what she'll hit the children who annoy her.") Insufficient recreational outlets. Mild obsessive tendencies. I.Q. 91. Chronic sinusitis; follicular conjunctivitis; bronchitis; underweight; faulty posture; fallen arches.

The *treatment* of children with temper tantrums will, of course, always depend on the facts obtained during the examination of the individual case. It will aim at the following adjustments:

Creation of an optimal environment. Wherever necessary and at all possible, the therapeutic program should include an attempt at a reduction to conventional forms of the parents' emotional outlets. It is futile to expect of a child calmness and self-control if the adults of his immediate surroundings go on tearing their hair and slamming doors and indulging in fistfights or similar practices. If an alcoholic tyrant rages through the house, it is rather natural for a frightened youngster to scream. If an unhappy, disappointed mother bursts out crying or an impatient parent keeps "yelling" at her offspring, there is little one can do to check the occurrence of analogous reactions in the impressionable child. It may at times be advisable to arrange for psychiatric examination and treatment of an emotionally unstable parent or older sibling. Sometimes the task may be intrusted to a tactful and experienced social worker. At any rate, the fact must be strongly impressed on the parent that improvement in the child's behavior depends largely on the cessation of emotional outbursts in his presence.

Overindulgence, oversolicitude, overprotection, discussion of the child's difficulties before him, contrasting him with a brother or sister, nagging, unreasonably severe methods of discipline must be discouraged and judicious handling advised.

Where a sinister home situation cannot possibly be expected to be modified, removal of the patient from the family and placement in a suitable boarding home must be considered.

Work with the child. Physical disorders of any kind, acute or subacute or chronic, must be corrected, regardless of whether or not they seem to have any direct bearing on the occurrence of the tantrums. Wherever required, proper school and recreational adjustments must be arranged. Existing jealousy should be treated according to the principles outlined in our discussion of this trait.

Above all, the patient, if old and intelligent enough, must be given an opportunity to discuss with the physician his specific problems, meeting sympathy and understanding, but at the same time also made to see, with dispassionate criticism, the unsound and harmful nature of his reactions and attitudes. Some children are genuinely ashamed of their rages, others are rather proud of them and of the power it gives them. One boy declared boastfully, "Do I have a temper? Whew!" Another spoke of the outbursts as an inherited doom for which nothing could or should be done. To another they meant (as he had been told) signs of "nervousness," which served him as a sufficient excuse and explanation. One must know these attitudes and use them constructively in interviewing the patient.

Beware of the dangerous "rest cures" and removals from the school, which even some physicians do not refrain from prescribing! Beware also of the indiscriminate use of sedatives! They really do sin against the principle of *Nil nocere*. They give the child and his parents the wrong impression that he suffers from some "disease" (usually called "nervousness") and that the "rest" or the medicine are the sole therapeutic agents. They are hardly ever successful, because the entire situation remains unaltered, and, as a matter of fact, are apt to aggravate the picture because of the implied notion of sickness and of added privileges and overindulgence.

Management of the tantrum itself. The thou-shalt-nots are at least as significant as the thou-shalts. Most essential is the avoidance of alarm. Consternation adds to the dramatic effect and places the child in the midst of the stage. The parents should be advised that no child has ever become sick or died of a temper tantrum. It is, at the same time, of great importance for the physician to be careful wherever caution is indicated; strenuous shouting and kicking is certainly harmful to a child with a decompensated heart. Here, at least for the time being, the management of the cardiac condition far outweighs in importance the handling of the emotional disturbance. On the whole, however, no danger is involved in the practice of waiting calmly until the storm is over.

The habit of "giving in" should by all means be discouraged. Compliance, as we have pointed out, is the surest way of maintaining the tantrum tendencies in a child. A youngster of any age and any degree of intelligence will soon learn to give up his rages, if he has been sufficiently impressed with their futility as a means of obtaining his wishes or gaining attention.

To react to temper tantrums with similar emotional outbursts is equally harmful. For this reason, parental "yelling" at the child, cruel beating, or helpless agitation should be prohibited.

One should also explain to the parents that "reasoning" or "pleading" with a child during a tantrum is an unwise move. No one in the midst of a major emotional upheaval is accessible to logical argumentations or to sermonizing.

The best mode of procedure is to leave the child alone until he has again become calm. If a parent cannot "stand" the performance, he or she is at liberty to leave the room. The more completely the temper tantrum is ignored, the smaller is the probability of its habitual recurrence. The child who has a tendency to destructiveness during such outbursts will best be removed to a place in the house where breakables are not within easy reach. After the rage is over, it is best to give the child the feeling that the act has made so little impression that it has been entirely forgotten. Display of indifference is a punishment much severer and much more effective than any other disciplinary method.

FEAR REACTIONS

Personal experience, training, and example are the outstanding factors which are involved in the establishment of fear reactions, among which several types or patterns may be distinguished:

1. There is, in the first place, a normal, justified, and biologically indispensable form of fear.

The emotion of fear, if sufficiently controlled and rationalized, is a useful and vitally important reaction of the human organism; it makes for caution in the face of existing or reasonably anticipated danger. All prophylactic measures in medicine are, in a way, founded on the principle of judiciously apprehensive avoidance of conditions which are well known to be perilous to the individual or to the whole community. The total absence of fear may, in certain specific situations, be indeed the expression of admirable heroism, but it may also be a serious problem if it is identical with absolute ignorance or indifference concerning the needs and occasions for self-preservation. We have seen feebleminded and postencephalitic children who incurred grave injuries or inflicted irreparable damage on others because of their inability to appreciate the inevitable consequences of their actions. We have known parents who proudly related that their offspring was "not afraid of anything" and almost in the same breath reported how he goes out in the street and "defies the automobiles" or throws lighted matches into haystacks. One need not go so far as did a certain psychoanalyst who claims that most accidental deaths are the results of an "unconscious death wish" which deprives its victims of their usual watchfulness. But it is true that the absence, based on the non-realization of danger, of a normal fear reaction has cost the lives and limbs of many a child. One retarded boy playfully jumped down from a third story window and sustained a fracture of the skull; a little less than one year later, while "pretending that he was a billy goat," he ran his head with all his might against a stone and again broke his cranium.

2. The commonest type of fear reaction is one which, resting largely on precept and on the imitation of adult patterns, seems justified from the child's own viewpoint, but which lacks an objective basis. The patient sees dangers where there are no dangers. The fear hinges on faulty notions and is comparable to the superstitious apprehensions of older people whose dread of, let us say, walking under a ladder is subjectively well founded by the conviction that doing so would mean certain or, at least, probable death. Even though the belief itself is wrong, its existence makes the reaction understandable.

Fear of the dark is a typical example. It may have its origin in the fact that an older brother or sister or someone else in the family is afraid of the dark and that his or her behavior has imparted to the child the idea that there is something to be afraid of. The youngster may have been put, or threatened to be put, into a dark room or closet for punishment; since isolation and darkness were used as punitive measures, it is easy for the child to associate them with something harmful, something to be afraid of. "Spooky" stories, tales of the dense black woods of the fairy tales in which there are gruesome witches and bad giants, and the practice of children to "scare each other" in the dark may have contributed to the fear. There are unenlightened elders who frighten a naughty child into obedience by going to the door and calling for the bogey man or some such figure; the dark hall or room from which the dangerous bogey man is expected to emerge in order to abduct the youngster is naturally identified in his mind as the dwelling of these unpleasant and injurious fellows. Once such an attitude has been established, any object moved at night by a gentle breeze may heighten this impression and increase the apprehension. The finishing touches are then sometimes applied by the parents themselves, who calm the child by taking him into their bed or leave the light on in his room until he falls asleep. This is rarely interpreted by the child as the "soothing" which it is intended to be, but mostly as an additional proof that there must be some objective ground for the fear, since the knowing adults have taken protective steps. It even happens that the fear receives what amounts to open sanction, if a mother assures the apprehensive child that, of course, her darling could come into her bed and that, of course, she won't let the bogey man come near.

Often children who, because of their fear of the dark, would not go to bed alone or into another room alone sooner or later begin to voice their desire for company also during the day. It is, therefore, not unusual to find the combination in the same patient of fear of the dark and fear of being alone.

In the following, we quote a few complaints for the purpose of illustration:

"She is afraid of the dark. You got to have a light burning all the time. She won't go upstairs alone. I have to go with her. If she gets up and finds the light out, she goes in spasms, she gets scared and cries." An eight-year-old girl, very sensitive, hypochondriacal, crying easily, chronically constipated; her mother was extremely fearful, would not go out after sunset, was afraid she might have a cancer.

"He is afraid of the dark. His sister or his mother has to go in first and put the light on." This nine-year-old boy, normally intelligent, coming of a superstitious family, related that he had seen some people "laid out" which made him fear that he might find something like that when he went alone into his room. The child had been badly spoiled since birth when his parents insisted that he was dead. He was a nailbiter, had temper tantrums, and presented a feeding problem. His father, who believed in ghosts and spirits, used to fear that someone would be sick in the family, "and then I'd come home and, doggone, someone would be sick." The boy's older brother was "born with a caul" and was reputed to have the gift of second sight.

"He does not like to be by himself, especially at night. He goes to sleep with a light in the room." Four-year-old boy with temper tantrums, occasional enuresis, sick headaches, constipation, feeding difficulties; masturbated; talked "baby talk." I.Q. 106. "Passing a truck made him sick."

"She was always afraid of the dark, and so am I," said the mother of a twelve-year-old girl who was enuretic, "delicate," easily tired, "always under a doctor's care," and walked in her sleep.

"She is still (at eight years) afraid of the dark. When she goes into a dark room, we have to switch the light on. She will not sleep alone in her room. For this reason, her sister sleeps in the same room."

"She is so afraid of the dark, and she wouldn't stay alone for a minute. She always has to run after me. All three of 'em have to run after me."

"He is afraid to go to sleep alone, his father has to hold his hands till he goes to sleep." Boy, aged three years and eight months, who had temper tantrums, whined and cried almost incessantly, and presented a feeding problem.

"She is afraid of the dark. She would not go upstairs if I don't go with her and press the button and turn on the light." The mother of this twelve-and-a-half-year-old girl, who was enuretic, restless, bit her fingernails, and had temper tantrums, stated that she needed an operation for her hernia but was scared to death to go; she added, "I guess that is who she takes after."

"She sleeps with a light in her room all the time. I have catered to that and she has gotten used to it."

"She wouldn't stay in a room in the dark." Her mother used to be "scared like the child" and "did not overcome it" until two years ago when her husband dared her to go into a dark room and out into the dark street. Both she and her daughter indulged in "hollering spells," nailbiting, and all sorts of hypochondriacal complaints.

The fear of thunderstorms has been found to be built up on the imitation of the behavior of adults in practically all of our cases:

"He is afraid of thunderstorms, but I think it is natural. I am afraid of thunderstorms myself."

"He is scared of storms. He takes that from me."

"He is terribly afraid of storms, and so am I. I think everybody is afraid of storms. If I see lightning, my hand shakes." When the patient, a boy of twelve years, was interviewed, he used almost exactly the same words, including the reference to manual tremors on the occasion of lightning.

Practically anything may be feared, depending on the experience and example existing in the individual case. Follow a few instances:

Animals

"He used to be deathly afraid of dogs, after having one of his own, he got over that." Stuttering, nailbiting, sleepwalking, grinding of the teeth, and poor appetite were other difficulties of this seven-year-old boy.

"She can't stand the cat. She is so afraid of it. I have to do everything to frighten it off." This child, aged nine years, feared also the dark (a light was kept burning in the bedroom) and loud noises. She cried easily, complained of a lump in her throat, had cardiac and gastric pains of a hypochondriacal nature, vomited at times, and had nightmares. Poorest possible home training.

"She is terribly afraid of grasshoppers." An eight-year-old girl from the country, who was also fearful of the dark. Her mother "could not look at bugs," "simply screamed" if she found a worm in her apple, and was afraid that she might have a cancer.

"As a little thing, ever since she began to walk, she used to be afraid of bugs."

"She is afraid of flies. She jumps up and runs when she hears one buzzing. She has nightmares and then she tells us that she had dreamed of buzzing flies."

Vehicles

"Somebody has to take her across the street; she is afraid of the street cars since she was in an auto accident in 1927." (No serious injuries; just "a couple of scratches.") She was also afraid of the dark, of being alone, of dogs, horses, and strangers. Her mother was herself "deathly" afraid of automobiles and had always warned the child of them.

"He is afraid of the airplanes. He puts his hands over his ears. He is very much relieved when they are gone." The patient, who had also many other fears (storms, pain, disease), stated that the airplanes never bothered him when he was in the movies or out in the street; but he got "all upset" when he was in the house and heard one; "it might crash into the house." He had seen in the newspapers the photograph of such a crash and kept thinking what would happen if an airplane dropped on his own home. He cried easily (at thirteen years), had night terrors, talked in his sleep, and had wet himself until the age of eight years. His mother had many fears, especially of thunderstorms during which she was "simply crazy" and "did not know what to do with herself."

Noises

"She is terribly scared of noises." Nine-year-old girl in a pitiful state of neglect, enuretic, complaining of "pains all over," afraid also of the dark; raised in an atmosphere of domestic friction and brutal beatings on the part of an alcoholic father.

"He is afraid of a loud voice" (and of the dark). Nine-year-old boy, nailbiter, thumbsucker, enuretic, feeding problem, who had temper tantrums and cried easily. His paternal aunt, who lived in the same house, had a large assortment of phobias.

Miscellaneous

An eight-year-old masturbating girl had been told by her parents that, if she continued the habit, she would ruin her life, that all kinds of terrible things were going to happen to her. As a result, she developed night terrors and fears that "she will have to have an operation," that "she will have to have her face lifted," and that "she will have children who will be unable to read."

A boy of eight years, who slept with his mother, had night terrors, and fears of the dark, had been "afraid of Hallowe'en masks since three years when his father gave him a good beating on Hallowe'en night because he was so scared when his brother and a group of children came in with masks."

"She has always been afraid of robbers and kidnappers. She reads papers and gets more scared since the Lindbergh baby affair." She also would not ride in automobiles because she had read so much about hold-ups and "being taken for a ride" by gangsters. A nine-year-old girl, spoiled by oversolicitous parents, who whined and cried a great deal. Her mother had three "nervous breakdowns." The child bit her nails, had nightmares and temper tantrums, and was a poor eater.

"He is afraid of strangers and bigger boys than he is." His mother would not permit him to play with any boys "because they are too rough."

"He is afraid to go to the movies because they always give him bad dreams." He would not go to sleep by himself after coming back from the theater.

"He is always scared of spooks." His sister, aged nineteen, was in the habit of "scaring" this six-year-old boy with stories about spooks and ghosts."

There is no limit to the number of illustrations that could be quoted in this connection. Practically all of them have certain features in common, which are of great etiological and therapeutic significance.

Personal experience and the mode of its elaboration. A child overhears the conversation of adults; she understands that there are rats in the wall and that there is a possibility of their gnawing their way into the rooms. She becomes curious about rats and is told that it has happened that rats have bitten sleeping children in the arm right where the bloodvessels are and that they have bled to death. During the night, she hears a noise which seems to come from within the wall. She runs out of the room and crawls into her mother's bed. The practice is continued. The family moves into another house which is free from murine animals. But the fear of sleeping alone persists. The dread of rats is transferred to other animals, from horses and dogs to bugs and worms. The fear habit has become permanent. A child who has always ridden in father's car witnesses an automobile collision. Someone remarks that there are so many reckless drivers nowadays, that no matter how careful you are, you never know what the other fellow is going to do. Soon afterwards the father relates that someone has slightly scratched his fender. From then on the child is afraid to go for car rides. If he is finally persuaded to do so, he trembles and is agitated and watches suspiciously every passing machine. This repeats itself; street cars are added to the repertory, and the fear becomes a habit. A child hears a "spooky" story or sees a "scary" moving picture immediately before retiring. After the light has been turned off, he hears a sound or mistakes a garment for a ghost or a burglar. He calls for the parents to turn the light on again. The next night he would not go to sleep unless the light is kept on. He would not go up to his room alone at night and, after a while, even in daytime. The fear of the dark and of being alone is established as a permanent reaction.

Information, precept, warning, and threats. Some parents, in their necessary and laudable attempts to train the child for caution and avoidance of danger, are wont to clothe their instruction in the form of prophecies. They say, "Do not go near the window! You will fall out and get killed"; or, "Do not talk to strangers! they may be kidnappers"; or, "God punishes children who do not mind their parents." Some people go even further; they turn perfectly harmless persons and things into objects of fear when they inform their children that the policeman or ragman will get them and do all kinds of injuries to them if they do, or do not do, this or that. The hobgoblins and witches and ghosts and the devil serve as additional ammunition. Thus the youngster's environment becomes populated by all sorts of sources of imaginary perils, the belief in which makes him apprehensive. The treatment must do away with all of these notions and cause the patient to distinguish between the appreciation of real hazards and exaggerated or superstitious fears. One boy, before being registered in school, was told by an aunt that he better behave himself, or else he will be put away in an Old Ladies' Home; he became deathly afraid of school and the teacher. His conduct was good in the sense that he sat quietly (too quietly, hardly daring to move), but he was preoccupied with the idea that anything that might be interpreted as bad behavior would land him in the Old Ladies' Home. After he had been convinced that such a danger did not exist and that good deportment was a thing worth achieving for its own sake, he went willingly and gladly to school and did well in his studies; his fear was gone. Sometimes boys are told more or less jokingly that parts of them will be cut off. The threat of removing the genitals is used jestingly by members of the family and as a scare by neighborhood or classroom bullies and may establish a fear of castration (we mean a conscious fear and not the hypothetical "castration complex" of the Freudian school). One boy became panicky and began to stutter when a bigger boy extorted toys and money from him with the assertion that some day he will cut his ears off.

Example. The fear pattern is often found ready-made in some other members of the family and may be taken over by the child together with the wrong motivations given for it. This is almost always the case with fear of thunderstorms. Often, however, it is not exactly a specific dread that is imitated, but the child is made generally fearful and easily frightened by parental quarrels or the tantrums of an alcoholic father, and the soil is prepared for the attachment of the apprehension to some particular objects or situations. The treatment must, therefore, deal with the entire setting.

The patient's personality. Fear is rarely, if ever, an isolated complaint. The children who present no other personality difficulties than fear of the dark or of something else do perhaps not come to the psychiatrist's attention. It is usually some other problem that is given as the primary reason for the consultation, and the fear problem is brought out additionally or incidentally, or may not be produced spontaneously at all, but come out only in reply to the examiner's special inquiries. There may be fearful children who are fully well adjusted otherwise and whom we, therefore, did not have an opportunity to see in our consultation work. Those whom we did study offered invariably a number of other existing or past behavior disorders. These were the most frequent problems complained of in association with fears, expressed in percentages (sometimes several in the same patient):

> Temper tantrums....................34 per cent
> Feeding problems...................45 per cent
> Enuresis...........................29 per cent
> Nailbiting.........................33 per cent
> Masturbation....................... 8 per cent
> Crying and whining.................18 per cent
> Stuttering......................... 6 per cent
> Sleep disturbances.................65 per cent
> Restless sleep.....................14 per cent

Night terrors.....................13 per cent
Sleepwalking.....................11 per cent
Nightmares....................... 8 per cent
Talking in sleep..................10 per cent
Crying in sleep................... 1 per cent
Grinding of teeth................. 4 per cent
Sleeplessness.................... 4 per cent

The frequency of temper tantrums and of crying and whining bears witness to the presence in the patient of other difficulties of emotional control; the combination with feeding problems and enuresis gives evidence of lack of adequate habit training plus general immaturity; the many instances of sleep disturbances and of nailbiting are signals of a state of tenseness which may be partly due to the child's fears.

Both sexes are represented almost equally. So are the ages and degrees of intelligence. In the older child, the presence of fears may interfere with his school and social adaptations.

The treatment of this type of fear reactions will work for a general adjustment of the patient. It will aim at good physical health. It will try to straighten out faulty notions with regard to the justification and sources of the child's fears. It will concern itself with the establishment of better methods of information and training in the home. It will take care of any other specific factors which have been found to be involved in the case. The child will naturally be treated in a way that will help him to overcome any other difficulty which has been brought out in the complaint or during the examination.

3. In a third group, the fear reaction is not only objectively unwarranted, but the patient himself is fully aware of its unreasonableness; yet, in spite of the full recognition of its being illogical and unfounded, he is unable to overcome it. The fear appears to him as something strange, alien, something forced upon him from within. One usually speaks of this type of fears as of phobias. We shall treat of them in another place under the heading of Obsessive-Ruminative Tension States.

4. An understandable and, for the moment, normal fright reaction may sometimes be continued in a rather sweeping fashion for several days or even weeks. The child, under the influence of the original strong emotion, is agitated, sleeps restlessly, is startled by the least occurrence, has no appetite, may even temporarily lose his excretory control, and is utterly unable to take care of himself. We may designate the condition as a panic reaction. Ziehen has coined for it the name of *ecnoia*, or *protracted lability of affect*. Orientation and memory are fully preserved (in contrast to twilight states and delirious conditions).

Elizabeth W., eight years and three months old, in good physical health, normally intelligent (I.Q. 101), had always been a fearful child. She was afraid to go upstairs in the dark and tried to persuade her mother to go with her. This her mother refused to do, so her little sister was drawn into the service. When she first began to talk, she lisped quite badly; the adults in the family used to tease her by mimicking her; she had never talked as willingly and freely as the other children and was considered rather timid. Her father was a stable electrician. Her mother complained of nervousness and headaches; she cried a great deal "when the children upset her." She got excited if the radio played too much, especially on Sundays, when her husband liked to listen in. She was afraid of hospitals and would not even go there to see a sick friend. Elizabeth was the second of three children. Dorothy, aged thirteen, was a "nervous" child and cried easily, particularly "when spoken to crossly"; she frequently walked in her sleep. Caroline, five years old, offered no problem. The maternal grandparents had been separated for many years. Five years ago, the father lost all his savings; since then, there had always been financial stress in the home.

Elizabeth developed normally. She had chicken-pox and pneumonia at three years and measles at five years. When not quite two years old, she was ill with pyelitis and did not walk for eighteen weeks, having to stay in bed. Her progress in school was satisfactory until June, 1931.

At that time, Elizabeth was playing with some other children in their backyard. One of them must have done something to the house, for the woman who occupied it came running out and, far from questioning her own offspring, immediately began to scold Elizabeth and threatened to have her arrested and sent to jail. The child, who did not even know that anything had happened to rouse the woman's anger, was overcome with fright. That woman's daughter, just a little older than Elizabeth, assisted her mother in scolding and added that she would put the child's parents in jail. It was around this girl that Elizabeth centered her fears. She would not go near the house where the F. girl lived. She would not go to school because the F. girl was a "monitor" on the playground where they had their lunch, and she was afraid that the girl might report something about her that was untrue and she would be blamed for it. After a short time, she became so frightened that she would not leave the house at all. At home, she kept crying violently for hours. She slept poorly; she woke up fifteen to twenty times during the night, especially between three and six o'clock, and called for her mother to sleep with her. Her appetite was very poor. "She is always irritable now and does not seem to be herself. She talks louder and hollers louder than she did before that thing happened." She could not be examined; she kept sobbing all the time. The mother was in another room while the child was interviewed and was almost as agitated as the patient herself and walked back and forth, quite upset.

The condition lasted from June until October (when she was first examined). The situation was talked over with the school and the child taken back to the classroom. At first the teacher stayed in the room with her for lunch, then she was replaced by a classmate, and finally she was lured back to the playground, where she again learned to play normally with other children. With the school routine established, her other difficulties disappeared gradually. The absurdity of the threat that she or her parents would be jailed had been explained to her as soon as she was willing and able to listen. Dorothy was treated at the same time and was no longer troubled with somnambulism. With the improvement in the children's conditions, their mother's headaches and excitability diminished markedly.

5. Another form of fear reactions in children is even more dramatic than the "ecnoic" condition. It is usually referred to as *anxiety attacks*. It occurs very suddenly and lasts from a few minutes to about half an hour. It may take place during the day or, more often, at night. It is characteristically described by Richards: "Added to the background of a tense, easily stimulated, highly imaginative personality is usually found an environment charged with worry and friction. Then comes an episode of

no great moment such as a tonsillectomy, or a too dramatically presented physiology lesson, and in a night or two the child wakes up screaming with terror. Flushed face, rapid pulse, wide staring eyes, and perspiration leave no doubt in the mind of the observer that this small person is really afraid. He does not speak of a bad dream, or of seeing things in dark corners. His cry is usually that he is about to die. Everybody is scared. A doctor comes rushing in, hears some strange noises over the rapidly beating heart, and spreads the news that Johnnie has a leaking heart valve, must stay in bed quietly for a week or two, and probably can never run and play as hard as he always has done. Naturally this has a disturbing effect on everybody, especially on the child who has now a medical confirmation of his worst fears."[1]

The dynamics of the reaction, the factors that may be involved, and the therapeutic procedure are illustrated by the following case:

Dolores K., ten years and eight months old, was the "baby" in a family of three living girls, the other two being above twenty years old. Two children who had been born before the arrival of Dolores died in early infancy. The father, a laborer, had been out of work for two years; the enforced idleness had made him irritable and despondent. The mother was "easily worked up," "got smothery around her heart," and had "nervous spells." The oldest sister was enuretic until the age of six years. All members of the family had contributed generously to the "baby's" spoiling.

At the age of eight and a half years, on January 15, shortly after her father had been laid off and two weeks before the date of school promotion, Dolores had her first anxiety attack. The parents were frightened (even though they had become accustomed to the mother's "smothery spells") and called a doctor, who said that the child had a "leaky heart" and may not live through the summer. He kept her in bed for three months and prescribed digitalis which she took for two years. She was withdrawn from school and not permitted to go out and play. The result was that the attacks became more frequent, until they finally came every evening before she went to bed. She had heard that people with leaky hearts are apt to die suddenly while asleep at night. During the episodes, which lasted about three or four minutes, she breathed heavily and "kind of felt like she wanted to belch"; she felt "tight around her heart" and "could not get her breath." She looked "like she was scared to death."

Dolores had always been treated as a "delicate" and "nervous" child. She was enuretic until the age of seven years. She had always bitten her finger nails. She would never eat without being coaxed. But she had been a sociable girl who had many friends.

The following events immediately preceded the first attack: Due to the father's loss of his position, the family who had lived in a comfortable house, had moved to a small apartment. Dolores had to give up her own room and was made to sleep with her parents. The next morning, she drank some root beer from the bottom of the bottle and was told that it would make her sick. She was late in school that same morning; she had run very fast but "could not make it." She learned that she had failed in a test which was said to be decisive in the consideration of promotions. In the evening of that eventful day, she had an attack.

[1] Richards, Esther Loring. Behavior Aspects of Child Conduct. New York. 1932. p. 189f.

Upon examination, she was found to be in good physical health. She and her parents were relieved of the mistaken idea that she had a cardiac ailment. Digitalis was discontinued. She was sent back to school. The family was referred to a welfare agency, which found a part time position for the father. Dolores was permitted to go out and play. Since the day of the first interview, the child did not have another attack. The mother had herself examined upon our advice, was found to be healthy, and her "smothery feelings" left her.

6. There are children, showing many features of general adaptive immaturity and poor habit training, who are literally *always afraid of everything*. It is not one object or situation or a limited number of them that is feared; there are no specific attacks or episodes of any kind. The fear reaction is a permanent attitude rather than a habit. We may actually speak of a "fear attitude" in these persons. They not only recoil in the presence of strangers; they would not even let friends of the family come near them. The household pet, known to be harmless, is an object of dread. Darkness, being alone in a room even though the parents might be in the adjoining room and the door open, people, animals, storms, bugs, flies, noises, everything is included in the child's suspicions and apprehensions. These children often hardly raise their voices above a whisper. They dare not ask for anything for fear that it would not be granted. Cimbal appropriately refers to this reaction as *Lebensfeigheit*, cowardice with regard to all matters of life. If it is permitted to go on, the child grows up to be a timid, undecided, cowardly, withdrawing individual, who does not have the "nerve" to work his way up, no matter how splendid his abilities are, who keeps away from social contacts, who avoids making new acquaintances, and who will always remain in subordinated positions. It is obvious that such an attitude calls for intensive work with the patient and with his family.

7. Fear reactions are an essential feature of delirious conditions. They are not infrequent in depressive states. They sometimes occur in schizophrenic patients.

8. The hypochrondriacal fears will be taken up in a special section.

9. Sometimes fears are simulated by children in order to gain their ends or to dominate the family.

One eleven-year-old boy was often left alone at home in the evening by his parents. He did not fear being alone or being in the dark. He knew that his parents went to the movies and did not like to give up this pleasure (their only pleasure). So he told them that, whenever they were away, he was so afraid that he saw things and that there was "something in his stomach which started to feel funny, like worms crawling around." From then on, they took him with them to the movies, and the "fear" disappeared.

CHAPTER XXXIII
THINKING DIFFICULTIES
DAYDREAMING

CHILDREN are normally expected, in school and at home, to be capable of responding promptly to questions, instructions, and commands, of carrying on conversations on topics within the natural limits of their interest and comprehension, and of pursuing certain goals, whether they be in the nature of fetching a pound of butter from the grocery store, finishing a game, or solving a problem in arithmetic. Difficulties may arise from a considerable variety of sources. There is a temporary and more or less profound irresponsiveness, sometimes amounting to complete inaccessibility, in delirious, somnolent, stuporous, and comatose conditions. Inadequate native endowment or later impairment of intellectual capacity may seriously interfere with a smooth train of understanding, reasoning, and reacting. Aside from these extremes, one is often confronted with thinking disorders in physically healthy and intellectually average, slightly retarded, or superior children; they appear in the form of complaints of daydreaming, lack of attention, lack of concentration, and absentmindedness.

Daydreaming (or, as the complaint is occasionally worded, "brooding," or "being in a study") has been made the object of several interesting investigations.[1] Kimmins states: "The distinction between the nightdream and the daydream is simply one of degree. In the daydream there is also a withdrawal of the attention, more or less complete, from external sources, and there is also a greater or less degree of mental automatism." However correct this be, a fundamental difference is contained in the fact that any amount of dreaming during sleep, provided it does not assume the forms of nightmares or night terrors and is not enacted in somnambulism or in excessive somniloquy, is always a normal phenomenon which does not stand in the way of the individual's social orientation and adaptation; knowledge of the contents may be of significance in the evaluation of personalities as an accessory to the far more essential features obtained from the life history and from an analysis of the behavior during the waking period.

A certain amount of daydreaming, to be sure, is also a normal occurrence in the life of a child. Green correlated the main imaginative preoccupations in the early years with the various developmental stages. Until approximately ten years of age, they are characterized by an expression of a "self-attitude"; they are then concerned with the trends of a "group-attitude," to be replaced, at puberty and in adolescence, by "romance" fictions.

[1] Green, G. H. The Day-Dream: A Study of Development. London. 1923. Varendonck, J. The Psychology of Day-Dreams. London. 1921. (Analysis of the author's own daydreams). Kimmins, C. W. Children's Dreams. In Murchison's Handbook of Child Psychology. Worcester. 1931, pp. 533–536.

Yet, in marked contrast to nightdreams, they may so influence the child's activities as to create a serious problem bearing all the earmarks of a psychopathological condition. The more or less complete withdrawal of attention and the mental automatism of which Kimmins speaks as being typical of daydreams may hold grave dangers with regard to personality development. It is with daydreams as it is, for example, with blinking. Some nictitation is physiological; its absence is, as a matter of fact, as Stellwag's sign, pathognomonic for Graves' disease; an excess, on the other hand, is one of the commonest forms of tics. Similarly, a total or almost total absence of fanciful thinking is, especially in children, a definite minus born of dullness and poverty of imagination. Too much of it leads to absorption and so engrosses the child's attention that he needs no other sources of satisfaction, renounces the pleasures which others derive from actual external experiences, casts off his duties and responsibilities as clashing with his excursions into an unreal world in which he may shape his destinies at will, shrinks from facing and meeting the minor and major obstacles encountered in the practice of living, avoids the contact of playmates and even the members of the family, and becomes a solitary, self-satisfied, asocial, impractical, disinterested, unpopular, and more or less helpless being. In his fancied adventures, he does not have to rub elbows with anything that is difficult or unpleasant; he easily disposes of the ogres and witches and villains of his own creation, but also of the hated teacher or of a rival or of the parents whenever they are in disfavor. This is done either by means of unlimited self-aggrandizement carrying out heroic deeds with utter disregard of even the simplest laws of nature (for this, the fairy tales have furnished the pattern), or the child removes himself entirely from his real environment and, as prince or princess or general or spirit, roams about the universe with unbridled delight. At a later period, altruistic, or rather pseudo-altruistic, motives come to play a prominent part. Messianic ideas of liberation, Napoleonic conquests with the view of rewarding the righteous and punishing the wicked are favorite themes; the child, of course, is the Messiah or the conqueror and the punishment is meted out none too clemently. At about the same age or a little later, sex preoccupations come into their own, at first against the background of heroism performed in honor or in behalf of an imaginary or secretly admired real girl (who is magnanimously transformed into a higher being), and after a while with emphasis on the coarse details of cohabitation. There are children in whose daydreams, instead of self-glorification, the setting is so selected that self-pity is the outstanding result.

All the while, the youngster sits in school, unmindful of his surroundings, inattentive to the teacher's words. While creating and destroying worlds in his seeming inactivity, he jumps when his name is called and has not the slightest idea what is wanted of him. The same thing happens at home. He is a poor scholar, an absentminded listener and, being loath to give up his fancies too soon, may not go to sleep until late at night.

Boredom is one of the principal *etiological factors*. It may be due to a drab and uneventful home life devoid of the little thrills which children as well as adults need so badly. It may have its origin in a retarded youngster's lack of grasp of the subjects that are being taught in the class or in a superior child's being instructed in things with which he has long been familiar. It may arise from educational methods which doom a child to passivity, making him spend hours at a time in his room, sending him to bed an hour or two before he can be reasonably expected to go to sleep, praising him to neighbors and visitors for being so quiet while in reality he is forming the habit of daydreaming. No one can stand a vacuum, least of all a child. He has no other choice than to fill the emptiness with some sort of activity.

It is, however, true that there are some youngsters who with their daydreaming combine extreme shyness and sensitiveness and an odd behavior which should make one particularly cautious because it points in the direction of schizophrenic possibilities. These patients require especially careful guidance and call for the best that mental hygiene can offer.

The *treatment* consists of a program of daily routine designed to do away with the habit of daydreaming by pushing the child's interests and abilities, of which one must inform himself in the course of the examination, into channels of organized and supervised activities. Daydreaming, more than any other complaint, calls for direct work with the child, in addition to parental instruction and proper school adjustment. It does not do to force the patient to do things which he either cannot do or for which he has no inclinations. It is largely in competitive and other group plays that he can best be restored to contact with reality. It goes without saying that the monotony of home life must be broken. Weekend visits, trips to the circus and to neighboring towns or to the country, little surprises, walks with the parents during which the child is given ample opportunity to take part in the conversation, puzzles and mechanical problems will have the desired effect much more promptly than mere admonitions and sermons which are only apt to create in the child an antagonistic attitude without noticeably improving the situation. The slogan must be not so much to interrupt the fancies as to reduce the time and opportunity for their indulgence. Thus it is the daydreaming child that is adjusted and not the daydreams *per se* that are treated.

LACK OF ATTENTION; LACK OF CONCENTRATION

Attention is of paramount significance in the process of learning. Its smooth functioning depends on the factors of realization of a goal, vigilance, selectivity, and tenacity.

The *awareness of a purpose* is to some extent a matter of training. The infant who is given a bottle at certain hours only and for a certain time only and who, during the period of drinking, is not distracted by talking or singing to him or by the dangling of toys will much sooner become conscious of the expected goal of emptying the bottle than the one who may keep it indefinitely and gets it irregularly and is permitted to play while holding it and to dawdle over it. The same is true of being placed on the chamber pot, the acts of dressing and undressing, going to bed, and the like.

Vigilance is the ability to notice and respond to stimuli of sufficient intensity.

Selectivity is the capacity for discrimination between those visual and auditory and other sensory impressions which have a bearing on the goal and those which are more incidental and irrelevant for the moment.

Tenacity, or *concentration,* is the ability to maintain the pursuit of the goal until it is achieved. The terms attention and concentration are often used interchangeably, and the complaints of inattentiveness and lack of concentration therefore refer frequently to the same difficulty. For practical purposes, it is just as well to follow this example, since the etiological background and the treatment are quite similar in most instances.

Every teacher knows that allowances must be made for the entire class when an airplane is espied through the school room window or when an afternoon visit to the circus is anticipated. Every mother has observed that, no matter how seriously her offspring may be engaged in an interesting game, her return from a shopping tour with bundles and packages immediately turns the child's attention from his toys to the contents of the bundles and packages. The original goal of listening to the geography lesson or solving the block puzzle has been abandoned. Concentration has been disturbed by something which offers greater interest and preoccupies the youngster enough to change the goal of his attention. This is a normal, understandable, and only occasional lack of concentration to which each individual is subjected.

Inattentiveness and lack of concentration become the objects of a complaint if they are habitual and seriously interfere with the child's learning capacity. In each case, a thorough study of the patient's personality and environment is necessary in order to determine the underlying factors. Of the great variety of causes, which may exist alone or in combinations. the outstanding ones are listed below:

Defective sense perception. It is obvious that outspoken blindness or deafness limits the child's vigilance with regard to visual or auditory stimuli. Milder degrees of disturbances of sight (astigmatism, refractive errors) and of hearing are sometimes overlooked and must be brought out in the course of the investigation. Their correction, if no other difficulties exist, will improve the patient's attention. Most modern schools have special classes for the conservation of sight and hearing, in which expert teachers do justice to the pupils' limitations.

Illness. In sick children, though goal realization and selectivity are fully preserved, pain and general systemic discomfort may play havoc with their vigilance and tenacity. This is equally true of prodromal stages, acute or subacute or chronic disease, and of the period of convalescence. The treatment of the child's relative irresponsiveness and impairment of tenacity consists in the medical management of his physical condition.

Fatigue. Exhaustion due to hard work with little or no recreation often weakens the child's ability to concentrate. One boy put his difficulty into these words, which showed a good deal of insight: "I am too tired to think." The same boy, after adequate relaxation had been provided, regained fully his former ability to concentrate.

Hunger. Some children are in the habit of going to school without breakfast. In the late hours of the forenoon, it becomes increasingly difficult for them to follow the teacher. The goal is realized but cannot be pursued tenaciously. Hunger often produces headache which adds to the concentration disorder.

Lack of comprehension. Mental retardation with insufficient grasp of that which is being taught is often mistaken for inattentiveness. The child does not attend because he does not grasp the goal and the methods of its attainment. Vigilance and selectivity suffer because the "stimuli" have no meaning to the pupil, who for this reason turns his attention to things which are more easily accessible to his understanding. He may take to daydreaming or, having no goal whatever, become restless or, trying to divert his classmates' attention from his "dumbness," impress them with clownish or mischievous performances. Placement in an ungraded class or, where this is not extant, in a grade which is better adapted to his intellectual level will help to restore his attention by giving him a comprehensible goal and modes of its pursuit which are commensurate with his capacity.

Lack of interest. The child with advanced intelligence for whom the class work is too easy may become bored and lose interest in the goal. Some schools are in the habit of putting any newcomer back a grade or half a grade on general principles, and the child may find the repetition of the work too dull. Pupils of fourteen or fifteen years of age sometimes lose their interest in the school and its subjects because they prefer to obtain a job and help to increase the family's income. Others have no difficulty in concentrating on the subjects which are to their liking or which an admired teacher knows how to render attractive, whereas in other subjects they do not attend because they are presented by a hated teacher or in an uninteresting fashion. This selective inattentiveness is by no means infrequent and is often based on emotional factors. One very intelligent boy who did well in all other subjects could not concentrate and had no "interest" in history because two years previously during the history lesson the teacher had reprimanded and beaten him in front of the class for making a weird noise which another pupil had made. He did not betray his classmate but transferred his emotional reactions to the subject in which the incident occurred.

Preoccupations. Sometimes, when examining a child brought to us with the complaint of lack of concentration, we find that we do not really deal with a "lack" but that he does not concentrate on his school work because he tenaciously concentrates on something else. He is preoccupied with matters which seem far more important to him or which give him greater pleasure. He is capable of vigilance and selectivity and tenacity. He realizes the goal but withdraws from it. The commonest contents of these preoccupations are:

1. Home conditions. The youngster may be worried over serious illness of a member of the family, father's economic difficulties, constant parental quarrels, or paternal alcoholism and brutality. There may be a visiting relative or friend at home who takes the child with him daily on his or her sight-seeing excursions. Mother or father may have gone away on a trip and promised to bring a surprise upon their return, giving the child an opportunity to ponder over the nature of the anticipated gift.

2. Daydreaming.
3. Sex fancies.
4. Obsessive thinking.

It is easily seen from this enumeration of the main sources of inattentiveness and lack of concentration or, as the complaint is sometimes worded, "absentmindedness," that the treatment must differ in the individual cases according to the factors involved in the development and course of the difficulty.

CHAPTER XXXIV

THE DISORDERS OF SPEECH

As THE PERIOD of elementary socialization we have designated the first stage of the child's development, lasting normally about eighteen months, at the end of which he has entered actively into the life of the family. With proper educational assistance, the rudiments of self-feeding and excretory control have been acquired. Erect posture and locomotion and an increasing amount of manual skill have just begun to change the baby from a helpless being into a moving and exploring individual. During this epoch, he has gradually learned to indicate some of his needs and wants by means of crying, pointing, and reaching. He has accumulated a small store of words, at first simple vocalizations, then single or duplicated monosyllables, and later bisyllabic words. Imitated sounds have come to assume sybolical meanings. The baby has become more and more capable of expressing pleasure and displeasure through his physiognomy.

During the first few months, crying is the only mode of vocal functioning It is based on an inherent physiological capacity which at the very moment of birth is brought into function in the form of the *birth-cry*. The naïve idea that the birth-cry is an utterance of joy or of anger at the entrance into the world has been justly discarded. The birth-cry is now explained as a reflex act devoid of any emotional or intellectual significance. Dorothea McCarthy, whose recent work on language development in children has laid the foundations for an objective and theoretically unbiased study, says, "Whatever interpretation is placed upon it, however, the birth-cry is of interest in the study of language development, for it is the first utilization of the intricate organs of speech."[1]

The infant's *crying* during the first two to four months of life is now usually looked upon as a spontaneous, "reflexogenic" reaction to some discomfort produced mainly by hunger, cold, and pain. Eventually the crying becomes differentiated, not only in its intensity but also in its quality and its dependence on external situations; it becomes more articulate and expressive; its "meaning," to be sure, is still very general and unspecific and could hardly be translated into terms of adult speech, but the older the baby is, the surer there is a meaning in his crying and an indication of different modes of feeling in the different shades of his cry.

The sounds emitted in crying are mostly protracted vowels but sometimes consonants, mostly gutturals and labials, may be distinguished as

[1] McCarthy, Dorothea A. The Language Development of the Preschool Child. Minneapolis. 1930. Language Development. In Handbook of Child Psychology. Edited by Earl Murchison. Worcester. 1931, pp. 278-315. (Extensive bibliography). Other classical works on children's language are: Stern, C., and W. Stern. Die Kindersprache: eine psychologische und sprachtheoretische Untersuchung. Leipzig. 1907. Piaget, J. Le langage et la pensée chez l'enfant. Neuchâtel et Paris. 1924.

incidental by-products. At approximately three months of age, a second form of vocal activity, that of babbling, is added to the infant's behavior. It begins with the formation of vowels which slowly develop resemblance to the alphabetical sounds to which the observers are accustomed and which they can commit to paper. The discrepancies found in the literature with regard to the phonetic qualities of these first sputtering sounds are due partly to individual differences between the children studied and to a remarkable extent to the fact that any form of conventional transcription is apt to meet with difficulties. The sounds are not "pure" enough for alphabetic representation; they may, however, be sufficiently recognized as vowels and later, at about six months or shortly therafter, as two letter syllables consisting of a consonant and a vowel (ma-ma, da-da, ba-ba). From now on, new sounds are added gradually. By this time, the crying and the physiognomy have become capable of a good deal of "meaningful" differentiation but the babbling is still in a stage of playful activity. Gesell observed a baby's linguistic behavior very closely and found that, at six months, three per cent of the waking time was spent in babbling or crying; in the twenty-four hour period, there were 104 separate moments of vocalization, varying from one letter sounds to thirty-two repeated syllables; altogether, not less than seventy-five sounds and combinations of sounds could be differentiated. The same baby, at nine months, devoted 6.66 per cent of his waking time to linguistic performances.

In the course of the babbling stage, certain sound combinations are used with especial frequency by the parents when they speak to the child. These utterances, already present in the babbling "vocabulary," begin, under the influence of the environment, to stand out among the others and in time to be linked up with certain objects as symbolical representations. It is then that the child begins to *talk*. The first meaningful words occur at about eight to ten months of age. It is, of course, utterly impossible to expect that the first symbolizations are in any way equal or even similar to the meaning which the adult connects with the same sound; the baby must slowly acquire all of the elaborations and implications which go with a certain word. Meanings develop. "Bye-bye" at first is merely a sound; then it is connected with the mother's waving her hand, then with the mother's moving the child's hand up and down, then with the child's active waving of his hand, then with mother's going out, then with the child's going out of the house, then with anybody's parting in general, and finally it becomes a conventional form of greeting upon leaving or being left.

The articulation of the consonants is acquired successively. Certain labials (m, b, p) are pronounced much easier and sooner than other sounds, and especially the sibilants and the letters r and l are formed relatively late and either left out or substituted before that.

At one year, the average child says three or four words. His understanding of words spoken to him comprises a much larger degree of symbolization. Gesell includes "adjustment to words" in the "minimum requirements" of the twelve-month level. He states: "We have seen a good many instances in which a child acquired, through training or accidental association, an adaptive response to a word stimulus as early as nine months." Within the next half year the active vocabulary grows very slowly but there is a considerable increase in the number of the things comprehended. Gestures play an important part in this stage. McCarthy states: "Children understand gestures long before they understand words, and similarly they use gestures first to express their needs and desires. Many children develop this gesture language to such a degree that it serves their purposes sufficiently well for a considerable period and they feel no need of developing a verbal expression. Thus gesture-language habits often hinder the development of vocal-language habits."

Hence, at the end of the period of elementary socialization, the normal child has gone through three more or less distinctive stages of vocal evolution: the stage of crying, the stage of crying plus babbling, and the beginning of verbal symbolization, both active and, to a much larger extent, passive (i.e., comprehension). Crying still is utilized as an indicator of emotional attitudes. Facial expression and gestures have gradually become an integral part of the infant's communicative equipment.

As the period of domestic socialization we have designated the second epoch of the child's development, lasting normally about three years, during which, through home training, he is given an opportunity to expand his elementary achievements and thus gain sufficient self-dependence and readiness for communal contacts. In the course of this stage his linguistic attainment progresses with astounding rapidity. "The child," says Mc-Carthy, "at eighteen months of age knows only a few single words, and yet in a short time—three years— he has acquired several thousand words, which he is able to combine into sentences as long and as complex as the adult uses in his everyday conversation; he has a ready command of all the inflections of the language and can use language for communicating all his thoughts, needs, and desires." Dorothea McCarthy's unexcelled work, carried out under carefully controlled conditions on a representative number of well selected children with due consideration of their general mental development and their social backgrounds, has given us a good deal of valuable information, from which we cull the following facts:

Considering the total number of words used, the proportion of nouns in the vocabulary is very large at the younger ages, decreasing with age up to about thirty months. Corresponding to this decrease in the percentage of nouns, there is an increase in the percentage of verbs, with advance in chronological age. The other large increases are to be found in the proportions of adverbs and of pronouns. Conjunctions appear late, as do the prepositions, and both of these categories increase, though slightly, with advance in age. Differences in sex and social status are not especially marked in this respect.

Considering the length of verbal responses, the percentage of comprehensible responses increases rapidly with age, and the girls excelled the boys at nearly all ages. The mean length of response shows an increase with chronological age, an increase which is more rapid at the younger age levels. Children who associate chiefly with adults show a much greater mean length of response than do those who associate with other children. The mean length of response shows clear differences from one occupational group to the other, each group maintaining its proper relative position very consistently.

Considering the construction of sentences, there is a decrease in the relative proportion of the responses that were functionally complete but structurally incomplete, with a more rapid falling off among the girls. There is an initial increase in the number of simple sentences without a phrase; an increase in the use of simple sentences with phrases with increase in age; an increase in the percentages of compound, complex, and elaborated sentences with increase in age; a superiority of the girls over the boys, of the children of the upper occupational classes over those of the lower occupational classes, and of children of higher intelligence over those of lower intelligence.

Considering the function of the response, the three groups, adapted information, questions, and answers, show marked relative increases with advance in chronological age, while the group of emotionally toned responses (wishes, requests, commands, and the like) shows a relative decrease with advance in chronological age. Naming decreases with chronological age, more rapidly among girls; remarks associated with the situation show an increase. Again, a superiority is displayed by girls, children of the upper occupational classes, and those of higher intelligence.

The meaning of children's language has been studied most extensively by Piaget, to whose work we have had occasion to refer elsewhere. It is necessary to emphasize that the "meaning" of a word or of a phrase is not a fixed and ready-made affair accepted by the child *a priori*, but that it is learned and elaborated through exercise and through trial and error. Ignorance of this fact has often induced parents to accuse their children of "lying" and of "talking nonsense." A twenty-month-old baby has learned to say, "Turn it on," when he wanted the lamp lit; but, "Turn it on" also meant to him a good many other activities, such as, "Open the window," or "Wind the toy automobile"; another phrase, "Take it off," referred to undressing as well as to closing the drawer or signified an invitation to leave him alone. This relation between speech and the evolution of meanings calls for further investigation.

As the period of communal socialization we have designated the third phase of childhood, extending throughout the school age, during which the child reaches out into the social texture of his environment. Reading and writing, the rules of grammar, coherent narration and composition, abstract definitions and the memorizing of names and various facts are added to the youngster's linguistic equipment.

MUTISM

Mutism is the absence of articulate speech. In most instances, language has never been acquired. In this case, the defect is due most frequently to the total or almost total lack of sound perception.

Deaf-mutism has been divided into a congenital and an acquired form; it has, however, been pointed out that the seemingly congenital form may have its origin in early postnatal diseases of the auditory apparatus and that, on the other hand, deafness on a constitutional basis may sometimes impress one as being an acquired condition. The congenital form is fifteen per cent more common in boys than it is in girls. Mygge[1] found that a deaf-

[1] Mygge. Er Dövstumheden arvelig? (Is Deaf-Mutism Hereditary?). Nord. Medicinskt Arkiv. 1878

mute child is born of every seventh to eighth matrimony between two deaf-mute parents, and of every fourteenth to fifteenth union in which one parent only is deaf-mute. Consanguinity of the parents is a significant etiological factor; according to Hammerschlag, parental blood relations existed in fourteen per cent of the families in which there was one deaf-mute child, in twenty-nine per cent of the families in which there were two, and in not less than fifty-seven per cent of the families with more than two deaf-mute children. There is said to be a frequent coincidence with feeblemindedness and with cretinism in the affected person himself or in his family. An important rôle is attributed to hereditary syphilis. Switzerland has the highest proportion of deaf-mutes (more than two hundred per 100,000 inhabitants); in the United States of America, there are about sixty to seventy deaf-mutes for every 100,000 inhabitants.

Deafness acquired at a very early age prevents the development of articulate speech. Epidemic meningitis, tuberculosis, scarlet fever, typhoid, and traumatism are the main causes. Under the influence of lost audition, it may happen that the linguistic equipment already possessed at the time of the illness causing the deafness undergoes a more or less complete obliteration.

Until about two centuries ago, the unfortunate deaf-mutes were doomed to a lifelong seclusion from any type of communication with others. In the fifteenth century, the Italian, Girolamo Cardano, made systematic attempts to teach them how to write. He was succeeded in his efforts by the Spaniard, Pedro de Ponce (1570), the German, Johann Camerius (1642), and the Englishmen, John Bulwers (1648) and John Wallis (1653). In 1692, the Swiss, Johann Conrad Amman, published his famous book (*Surdus loquens, seu methodus, qua, qui surdus natus est, loqui discere possit. Amsterdam*), in which for the first time a method of instruction in lip reading and actual formation of audible speech was set forth. In 1760, the French Abbé Charles Michel de l'Epée founded in Paris the first school for the deaf and dumb, in which they were taught to express themselves through writing and through standardized gestures. His approach has been termed "the French school" in contradistinction to "the German school," inaugurated by the teacher, Samuel Heinicke, who, in 1778, on the basis of Amman's work, literally and successfully proceeded to make the patients talk. Since then, many schools were opened, until to-day adequate educational facilities are made available to the speechless deaf in all civilized countries.

Mutism, without deafness, is encountered in many idiots whose mental development has remained on the level of the crying or babbling stage. The ability to comprehend is, in these patients, usually not much better than their capacity for verbal expression. Commitment to an institution for the feebleminded is the best solution of their problems.

Transitory mutism is sometimes met with as a symptom of hysteria. The patients are well capable of communicating through writing and gestures. In schizophrenic individuals, absence of speech is sometimes a part manifestation of their negativistic tendencies. In these types, the speech disorder itself does not call for specific therapeutic measures. It is the hysterical or schizophrenic child that must be treated.

LATE ACQUISITION OF SPEECH

Abnormally slow development of the linguistic faculties is a relatively frequent complaint, usually coupled with the question whether or not it is an indication of general intellectual debility. The backwardness may manifest itself in undue prolongation of the crying and babbling stages, delay in the learning of words, tardiness in forming sentences, or an extension of the infantile mode of articulation. Many instances of mutism due to deafness or to idiocy are regarded by the parents as cases of delayed evolution of speech until the auditory defect or the mental disorder has been diagnosed. In the vast majority, however, the family becomes justly puzzled if a hearing and evidently not idiotic baby does not begin to use words at an age when the onset of this function is normally anticipated. Often a physician is not immediately consulted, because of the common knowledge that there exists a wide range of several months within which the first production of words or of sentences may be considered as average. Other parents, again, are already alarmed if their baby is not capable of carrying on a conversation at less than eighteen months of age.

Occasionally, one finds a familial tendency to tardy speech development. Of the two examples cited below, the first is that of a child of slightly superior endowment and the second that of a feebleminded child.

A boy of not quite nine years, with a mental age of ten years (I.Q. 112), began to say words at nine months; he did not form sentences until five years of age. His speech was slightly indistinct, despite the fact that he had special training in articulation since he had started to go to school. His father never said a word until he was five years old and did not talk plainly until the age of seven years; he and the paternal grandparents, of German origin, spoke broken English and markedly defective German. A paternal cousin (the father's sister's daughter) attended a speech training class at nine years.

A retarded boy of seven and a half years, with a mental age of five (I.Q. 66), used duplicated monosyllables (ma-ma, da-da, bye-bye) as early as at eight months. At two years, it was noticed that he could not enunciate his words clearly. There was no progress within the next four years and a very slight improvement since he attended a speech training class. When examined, he spoke mostly in monosyllables. These are a few illustrations: he said pa for pen, pa-e for paper, a-e for lady, ta for quarter and for ten, sa for cent, da-e for dollar, ba-e for basket, Ba-e-po for Baltimore, dal for girl, peso for pencil. He had bilateral otitis media at fourteen months, which impaired his hearing for approximately half a year. There was marked flattening of the lateral surfaces of his tongue. He had slight ptosis of his left upper eyelid and enophthalmos of his left eye. He was very timid and fearful and gritted his teeth in his sleep. His father had the same speech difficulty until he was eight years old. His mother did not talk plainly until the age of ten years and stuttered when she was excited. Nearly all maternal relatives, whose school records indicated normal intelligence, were retarded in their ability to talk.

It cannot be emphasized strongly enough that there are considerable individual variations in the onset and rapidity of linguistic development especially in the interval between the formation of the first meaningful words and the production of short sentences. The degree of reliability of the parents' statements must, of course, be carefully considered. In the following table, we give a few examples of dependable data reported of children having intelligence quotients of above one hundred, who at the time of examination spoke clearly and fluently:

I.Q.	Words (months)	Sentences (months)
1. 101	10	18
2. 101	12	18
3. 101	13	21
4. 103	10	18
5. 103	9	17
6. 103	8	14
7. 104	9	14
8. 104	10	18
9. 104	8	16
10. 104	10	18
11. 104	8	15
12. 105	8	17
13. 106	9	17
14. 107	11	19
15. 108	9	18
16. 109	16	22
17. 109	5	13
18. 109	10	15
19. 110	8	16
20. 111	11	21
21. 112	10	23
22. 114	11	22
23. 115	12	16
24. 115	7	18
25. 115	11	20
26. 118	8	17
27. 118	12	30
28. 124	8	15
29. 124	9	13

It is of interest to compare these figures with those obtained from the histories of children with quotients of below eighty-five, again considering only those whose speech, when examined, was normal for all practical purposes (excepting that the vocabulary was more or less commensurate with the Binet-Simon requirements for their mental rather than chronological ages):

I.Q.	Words (months)	Sentences (months)
1. 84	24	28
2. 84	13	18
3. 83	14	24
4. 83	10	19
5. 83	9	18
6. 83	18	36
7. 83	12	27
8. 83	10	18
9. 81	12	18

I.Q.	Words (months)	Sentences (months)
10. 81	11	18
11. 80	14	22
12. 80	11	17
13. 80	12	19
14. 80	24	28
15. 78	13	19
16. 77	10	17
17. 77	24	45
18. 75	24	30
19. 74	24	36
20. 73	11	18
21. 72	12	20
22. 71	24	36
23. 69	13	20
24. 69	15	23
25. 69	12	18
26. 67	11	19
27. 66	12	22
28. 63	11	40
29. 58	30	48

In a third group, we tabulate the linguistic development of normally speaking children with intelligence quotients of between eighty-five and one hundred.

I.Q.	Words (months)	Sentences (months)
1. 85	12	18
2. 86	11	18
3. 86	13	24
4. 87	14	24
5. 87	10	17
6. 88	13	20
7. 88	9	18
8. 88	6	18
9. 89	12	20
10. 90	11	24
11. 90	10	16
12. 90	14	18
13. 90	12	18
14. 90	11	17
15. 91	12	23
16. 92	10	18
17. 92	10	16
18. 93	11	18
19. 94	10	17
20. 94	5	14
21. 94	8	15
22. 94	8	16
23. 94	11	24
24. 95	10	17
25. 95	9	17
26. 95	14	22
27. 95	11	18

I.Q.	Words (months)	Sentences (months)
28. 96	9	16
29. 98	11	18
30. 99	10	18
31. 99	11	16
32. 99	9	18
33. 99	12	27
34. 99	8	15
35. 99	10	18
36. 100	12	17

A comparison of the three tables shows that, as a whole, the second group has developed speech at a later time than the first and third groups. But it also brings out the fact that intelligence is certainly not the only factor on which the speed of acquisition of language depends. Thus we see that number 27 of the first group (I.Q. 118) has begun to form words and sentences at a markedly later period than number 5 of the third group (I.Q. 83), or that number 22 of the first table (I.Q. 114) offers almost the same figures as does number 27 of the second table (I.Q. 66). It also becomes evident that persons with the same degree of intelligence show noticeable differences in regard to speech development. This fact becomes very clear if we take, for example, the three children with an I.Q. of 109 (the figures being 16 and 22, 5 and 13, and 10 and 15 respectively).

The delayed onset of speech in backward children may be divided into two groups:

Proportionate delay, corresponding more or less closely to the general level of the mental development. If a child of average intelligence is expected to form sentences at between eighteen and twenty to twenty-two months, one with an I.Q. of 75 is actually fifteen months old mentally at a chronological age of twenty months; it is not until he has reached the age of approximately twenty-eight months that he has the general mental level of a twenty months old child. If, therefore, he forms sentences at twenty-eight months, the delay may be said to be well in proportion to his intellectual growth. The tardiness is evident through comparison with normal babies but, in a sense, "normal" for this particular infant. Such cases are comparatively frequent.

Disproportionate delay. It often happens that the ability to speak grows in retarded (and less frequently, in normally intelligent) children at a much slower rate than all or most of the other psychobiological functions. In this case, to use the same example as before, the child with an I.Q. of 75 would form sentences at, let us say, three to three and a half years instead of at twenty-eight months. This type of backwardness in talking is often associated with faulty articulation. It must, however, be stated that there are surprisingly many feebleminded children who begin to speak at a disproportionately early age. The second table furnishes excellent examples.

Late acquisition of speech is sometimes due to inadequate training. One occasionally sees spoiled children of overprotective mothers, who do not talk at the proper time because they are not given an opportunity to appreciate the need and communicative value of verbal expression. The expedients of pointing, crying, and inarticulate screaming sufficiently serve the purpose of procuring for them everything they desire and of indicating displeasure and unwillingness. Such infants practically always show a good many other evidences of unwise parental management, such as delayed excretory control and long persistence of the early infantile modes of feeding and clothing. In the treatment of this form of linguistic retardation, one will naturally stress the necessity of permitting the child to grow up and to make use of his developmental potentialities in accordance with his age.

More or less outspoken degrees of defective hearing which does not reach the point of deafness or near-deafness may also result in late development of speech.

FAULTY ARTICULATION

Backwardness in talking may show itself not only in the time of word and sentence formation but also in the manner in which the child's utterances are enunciated.

Defective articulation which, as all other speech disorders, shows a preponderance in boys, is based on three outstanding etiological factors which may be present alone or in combinations:

Local conditions, due to either congenital or acquired abnormalities. Defects of the tongue (macroglossia; microglossia; hemiatrophy; "tongue-tie"), the lips (harelip), and the teeth (dental malocclusion; absence) affect chiefly the enunciation of consonants and have been termed dyslalia lingualis, labialis, and dentalis, respectively. Deformities and diseases of the larynx (inflammation; tuberculosis; tumors), the nose (obstruction of the air passages), the palate (especially cleft palate), and the uvula (abnormal length or thickness; bifurcation; duplication) interfere largely with the quality of voice. The laity is accustomed to ascribe particular significance to "tongue-tie" (adhesion of the tongue to the floor of the mouth by means of a long frenulum) as being responsible for all modes of speech difficulties and expects relief from surgical procedures. "Clipping of the tongue" is frequently ordered by the mothers (and, we hate to add, carried out by many physicians) as a panacea for late acquisition of speech, faulty enunciation, and stuttering. The operation is often performed as a routine "prophylactic" measure on the newborn or during the first few months of life, usually on the request of the same type of parents and by the same type of physicians who are ever ready with tonsillectomies and circumcisions. How rare "tongue-tie" really is, is best demonstrated by the statements of such experienced authors as Fröschels,[1] who saw only two cases in one thousand patients with speech disorders, and Greene and Wells,[2] who say: "For the thousands of cases treated our records show that only two patients suffered from genuine tongue-tie that required operative treatment. Consequently, the frequent clipping of the tongue which is so readily advocated by almost everybody for all cases of stammering speech is decidedly un-

[1] Fröschels, Emil. Lehrbuch der Sprachheilkunde (Logopädie). Leipzig und Wien. 1913, p. 134.
[2] Greene, J. S., and E. J. Wells. The Cause and Cure of Speech Disorders. New York. 1927, p. 19.

necessary, and an inhuman mutilation of the sufferer." Travis[1] quotes Faunce's[2] work on the relation of the size of the tongue to its influence on articulation; according to this investigator the distance from the anterior end of the frenum to the tip of the tongue is shorter for defectives than for normals. Another group of his cases had very large tongues in relation to the lower jaw.

The treatment of faulty articulation due to local abnormalities is, of course, directed towards the causative factors. Many cases will have to be referred to the surgeon or to the dentist. In others, operative treatment is not feasible (e.g., macroglossia or microglossia). Often the operation is followed by spontaneous improvement of the speech disorder after the child has become accustomed to the new conditions. Sometimes, however, expert training in articulation is required as a post-operative measure.

Mental retardation. Infants acquire their consonants gradually. It may take a child who is generally backward a long time to learn to pronounce correctly the more difficult sounds, such as s, sh, ch, r, l, g, k, which even normally are formed later than most of the others. A succession of two or three consonants also offers difficulties (thr, str, spr, scl, etc.).

Faulty training. It is self-evident that the child patterns his speech after those about him. He cannot possibly be expected to acquire the correct enunciation of words if he does not hear them articulated correctly. If a child hears his German father say, "shtreet-car," then "shtreet-car" he will say as long as there is no school or neighborhood influence to change this pronunciation. If a careless and uneducated mother and the older siblings say "membry" for memory, "pixture" for picture, or "chimley" (or "chimbley") for chimney, then there is no way for the child to know that this sort of diction is not the right one.

The main sources of defective articulation due to poor education are threefold:

Ignorance on the part of the parents. This is especially true of uneducated (not always unintelligent) immigrants.

Carelessness on the part of the parents, as examplified above. The omission of the g from the present participle suffix is so typical of certain groups as to be almost "normal" for them. The substitution of f for th ("mouf" for mouth) in many words is traditional among low class negroes.

"Baby talk." At the time when the child begins to form words without having learned to articulate the more difficult consonants, many parents are in the habit, when talking to the baby, of imitating his type of speech. It is an injurious custom preventing the youngster from hearing and acquiring in due time a normal enunciation because of the absence of a normal pattern. A particular form of communication develops, which is accessible only to a few people in the home; when the child is old enough to establish outside contacts, difficulties are apt to arise from his unintelligible manner of talking.

Abandon of the adults' indulgence in "baby talk" and linguistic re-education are the logical therapeutic methods.

[1] Travis, L. E. Speech Pathology. New York and London. 1931, pp. 200f.

[2] Faunce, R. O. The Relation of Proportions of the Tongue to its Control in Articulation. University of Iowa Thesis. 1928.

Speech disorders based on faulty articulation are usually referred to as *stammering*. Different usage of this term has often led to unnecessary terminological confusion. Some authors reserve the word stammering for "organic" and the word stuttering for "functional" speech disorders. Fortunately, there is now a healthy trend towards moving away from too rigid a separation of "organic" and "functional." That stuttering is not always "functional," has been demonstrated by Gerstmann and Schilder, who observed it in postencephalitic patients.[1]

Severe degrees of defective articulation have been designated as Hottentotism or *idioglossia* (a name also given to the peculiar productions of patients with congenital word-deafness) or *lalling* (often restricted to the substitution of l for r). *Lisping* often refers to the difficulty in pronouncing sibilants, *burring* to a guttural pronunciation of the r-sound.

Defective articulation has been classified according to the sounds that are most commonly mispronounced or substituted:

Sigmatism (lisping) denotes inability to articulate sibilants correctly (s, sh, z, ch).

Rhotacism (burring) designates wrong enunciation of r or its replacement by l or w.

Lambdacism is a difficulty in forming the l-sound.

Gammacism indicates difficulty with the gutturals (g, k, x), which are most commonly replaced by dentals (d, t).

Often, especially in baby talk, several of these forms are combined. Each one of them is physiological for a short time while the child is learning to talk.

In many of the larger cities, the schools provide special classes for speech training of children with defective articulation. Valuable pioneer work in devising methods of linguistic excercises has been done by Fröschels and especially by Gutzmann (*Sprachheilkunde. Vorlesungen über die Störungen der Sprache mit besonderer Berücksichtigung der Therapie. Berlin. 1912*).[2]

DISORDERS OF PHONATION

The human voice is capable of an unlimited range of individual variations. Besides, there are outspoken national differences in cadence and inflection (compare, for instance, the Scandinavian, Anglo-Saxon, and Chi-

---

[1] Gerstmann, J., and P. Schilder. Studien über Bewegungsstörungen, über die Typen extrapyramidaler Spannungen und über die extrapyramidale Pseudobulbärparalyse. Zeitschrift für die gesamte Neurologie und Psychiatrie. 1921,70,35–54.

[2] In addition to the books already referred to the following publications will be found particularly helpful from the descriptive or therapeutic point of view (or both): Kussmaul, A. Die Störungen der Sprache. (Fourth edition, prepared by H. Gutzmann). Leipzig. 1910. Villiger, E. Sprachentwicklung und Sprachstörungen beim Kinde. Leipzig. 1911. Bluemel, C. S. Stammering and Cognate Defects of Speech. New York. 1913. Nadoleczny, M. Disorders of Speech and Phonation in Childhood. (Translated from the German by C. P. McCord.) Philadelphia. 1914. Scripture, M. K., and E. A. Jackson. Manual of Exercises for the Correction of Speech Disorders. Philadelphia. 1919. Swift, W. B. Speech Defects in School Children and How to Treat Them. Boston. 1918. Blanton, M. G., and S. Blanton. Speech Training for Children: The Hygiene of Speech. New York. 1919. Twitmeyer and Nathanson. Correction of Defective Speech. Philadelphia. 1932.

nese types of rise and fall of the speech). Male and female voices can be told apart with ease. In the same person, the quality of the voice changes gradually in the course of years. Through its tempo, intensity (loudness), and tonal character, it reflects excitement and calm deliberation, indicates questioning and commanding, and may clearly express the emotions of tenderness, anger, surprise, or disappointment. Even the infant's crying slowly assumes different shades according to whether it is produced by pain, resentment, or fear. Between two and three years of age and sometimes even a little before that, babies are capable of a surprising amount of tonal symbolization. "Give me water!" may sound definitely like an impatient order or like a polite entreaty. The development of children's phonation has so far received but scant attention. More is known about the change of voice in puberty, especially among boys. "There may be hoarseness, or change of voice either to falsetto or to abnormal depth. Here again there is danger of the disturbance proving chronic, and if it continues for a protracted period the parent should see that proper curative measures are instituted." (Greene and Wells). Good respiratory control is one of the main requirements for good phonation.

The disorders of phonation are due to four main factors:

Local conditions. Abnormalities of the tongue and the oral organs which lie before the tongue (teeth, dental arches, lips) result mainly in disturbed articulation, while the diseases or deformities of organs that lie behind the tongue may lead to faulty phonation. Hoarseness may be due to laryngitis, pharyngeal irritations, vocal cord tumors, or to overexertion of the voice through screaming, crying, and shouting. Nasal tone (rhinolalia) may be caused by obstruction of the nose through swollen turbinates, adenoid vegetations, and severe "head colds"; the change of phonation may be combined with faulty enunciation of certain sounds (m becomes like b, and n like d). The quality of voice as well as the articulation (particularly of the gutturals, sibilants, and dentals) is impaired considerably in patients with cleft palate and with diphtheritic paralysis of the soft palate.

Diseases of the central nervous system are often accompanied by more or less typical alterations of the voice (affecting its speed, pitch, resonance, or cadence) and of articulation. A few examples may suffice. Well-known is the slow, scanning, monotonous speech in multiple sclerosis, in which each syllable is pronounced separately. In juvenile paresis, the speech may become slurring and stumbling. In the Parkinsonian syndrome, it is usually slow and monotonous, but sometimes as festinate as the gait. In Friedreich's ataxia, there is a frequent change of pitch; the patient speaks "as though he had a hot potato in his mouth." In progressive bulbar paralysis, the speech is indistinct, labored, and high-pitched.

Certain endocrine disorders affect the quality of phonation. This is especially true of the coarse and rough speech of the cretin and of the falsetto-like voice of the eunuch or eunuchoid.

Habitual and emotional disorders of phonation. Even normally, the quality of the voice is different in the shy, timid, retiring youngster than it is in the aggressive, forward, outgoing child. Occasionally one sees little boys and girls who have developed the habit of talking very quietly, with the head drooping or the face turned away, without caring whether or not they are understood; the answers may be given promptly and correctly but, to be heard, the child has to be urged to repeat them more audibly. Other children become accustomed to raise their voices too much; they shout instead of speaking. This is sometimes due to the presence of a deaf person in the home, but often enough it is done in imitation of the adult members of the household who exercise their educational privileges by "hollering" at the children. In hysteria, there is sometimes a total temporary loss of voice or the patient does not talk above a whisper (hysterical aphonia and hypophonia).

STUTTERING

Stuttering is speech of a halting, hesitating nature, with the repetition of the initial sounds of a word or sentence. Articulation and phonation are as a rule not impaired, though children with defective enunciation occasionally do stutter. In most instances, the individual vowels and consonants are neither mispronounced nor substituted. It is the rhythmic, smooth continuity or flow of speech that is broken up by improper respiratory control and by spasms of the muscles participating in the normal mechanism of speech.

Travis, in his recent book on *Speech Pathology* (*New York. Appleton. 1931*), has given an excellent description of the various disturbances which he observed during stuttering and to which he refers as the "primary symptoms" of this reaction:

1. Diametrical opposition of the action of the thorax and abdomen (abdominal inspiration and thoracic expiration occurring simultaneously, and vice versa).

2. The larynx moves synchronously with the abdomen or thorax or both, instead of showing the independent and faster rise and fall which characterizes normal speech.

3. Marked protraction of inspiration.

4. Clonic and tonic spasms in the musculature of the speech mechanism, of which the whole or one or more parts may be affected at one time.

5. Tremors in certain movements of the breathing mechanism.

6. Tremors and tonal rigidity in the voice; periodic fluctuations in pitch.

7. Periodic fluctuation of breath pressure just before and after tones.

8. Bizarre voice-wave forms.

9. Extremely brief approximation of the vocal bands before and between. tones.

10. Periodic approximations of the vocal bands between tones.

11. Extreme abruptness of initiation of tones.

12. Repetition of sounds, words, or phrases.

13. Speech blocks, due to "tonic inactivity." Inability to produce a sound for an appreciable length of time.

14. Disintegration of the movements of the speech mechanism as a whole.

Several forms of stuttering have been distinguished. One of the earliest classificatory attempts is that made by Klencke (*Die Heilung des Stotterns.*

Leipzig. 1860), whose five types were nervous, respiratory, constitutional, emotional, and habitual stuttering. According to the kind of letters that offer difficulties with their initiation, some authors differentiate between vowel and consonant stuttering. Another grouping pays attention to the manner in which the patient utters the stuttered sound. The word "date" may be produced by the patient in three ways:

1. Repetition of the first consonant: d-d-d-date.
2. Repetition of the first consonant plus vowel: da-da-da-date.
3. Protraction, without repetition of the first consonant: ddddate.

The term *situational stuttering* refers to the manifestation of the speech difficulty in certain situations only; we have seen children who speak perfectly well everywhere but in school or who stutter only in the presence of their parents. One of our patients had special difficulty when called in class to read or recite Latin. It is interesting that not a few of the children who were brought to us with the complaint of stuttering, when spoken to quietly without mentioning their handicap, talked normally during the entire length of one or several interviews. But when, at the end of the conversation, the father or mother were called into the room, the youngster almost instantly reverted to his speech disorder. The very fact that the patient has spoken well during the interview could be utilized in the therapeutic approach to the child and to his parents.

So-called *ritual stuttering* is much less common in children than it is in adults. The designation indicates the peculiar habit of speaking correctly only if the patient assumes a certain position or performs a certain action. The "ritual" which makes normal speech possible may consist of keeping one hand in the pocket or pressing upon some part of the body; whenever these conditions do not exist, the individual stutters.

A speech disorder which has been treated as a separate form by most German investigators and neglected somewhat by the French, English, and American authors, is characterized by rapidity and swallowing of syllables or words, sometimes to such a degree that the utterances become unintelligible. When speaking slowly, the child is capable of good articulation, and he never repeats sounds. The difficulty is particularly apt to happen during excited and hasty narration. In contradistinction to stuttering, it is the end of the sentences that suffers mostly. The German name is *Poltern;* the English equivalent is *cluttering speech*. It is sometimes alluded to as *agitolalia* or *agitophasia*.

The act of stuttering is often accompanied by various *associated movements*. The face is most commonly involved; wrinkling of the forehead, frowning, blinking, pressing the eyelids together tightly, and many other forms of grimacing appear as soon as the child makes an effort to speak. The mouth may be drawn over to one side. The head may be thrown backwards. Swallowing movements may occur. The patient may jerk the extremities, or clench his fists, or stamp his feet. The synergisms bear a strong resemblance to tics, except that they never take place independently. They share with tics the fate that they are sometimes mistaken for chorea. A peculiar form of associated activity has been described as *embololalia*. The patient, in order to overcome or to cover up his trouble, interpolates short sounds or words which often are entirely out of place in the structure of the sentence. One of our children developed the habit of introducing into his speech the words "and" and "no," regardless of whether or not they had any meaning in the context of his statements.

It is a strange fact that most (not all) stutterers experience no difficulties when they sing or whisper. Sometimes foreign languages are spoken fluently. There is also a great deal of improvement or even no sign of the disorder when the patients believe that they are alone or unobserved or when they speak while in a dark room.

Cimbal calls stuttering "one of the most frequent neuroses of childhood." According to Nadoleczny, there are 98,000 stuttering children in Germany. Travis estimates the number of affected youngsters in the United States at approximately a quarter of a million and points out that in this country there are nearly three times as many stuttering children as the blind and the deaf-mutes of all ages combined. They make up about one per cent of the school populations practically everywhere. The condition is decidedly more frequent and persists longer in boys than in girls. The ratio varies with the different authors; it is given as 8:1 by Coën, 2:1 by Fröschels, 3:1 by Cimbal. Travis states that about eighty-five per cent of the patients begin to stutter before eight years of age. Gutzmann finds that there are three age levels during which the disorder is most likely to commence:

1. The period of the quickest development of speech during the third and fourth years of life when the child has much more to say than he is capable of expressing and when impatient adults do not give him sufficient time to think of the appropriate words. Of Nadoleczny's 890 cases, not less than sixty per cent began to stutter at the ages of from two to five years.

2. The beginning of school attendance.

3. The time of puberty.

So many and so varied theories have been advanced with regard to the etiology of stuttering from the days of Hippocrates to our own time, that it is no easy task to classify them.

A comparatively small group of authors has thought in terms of local abnormalities. Aristotle accused a too thick and too hard tongue. The same idea recurred in the year 1841 which was destined to play a significant part in the history of the condition which we are now discussing. "A regular mania," say Greene and Wells, "took possession of the surgeons of Europe, each one of note claiming to be the inventor of a new modification of some previous operation. The methods were generally arranged by nationalities, the Germans following Dieffenbach, the French, Velpeau, the English, Yearsley and Braid. Nearly two hundred cases in France alone submitted to the operation in the course of the year. At the end of the year a cry of warning was raised, and those who had tried the experiment found the courage to acknowledge their grave error." The notion that tongue-tie is responsible for stuttering is still prevalent in the thinking of the laity.

A considerable portion of investigators makes the condition dependent on some sort or another of disorder of the central nervous system. Klencke, himself a stutterer, assumed the existence of a disturbed relation between the activities of the brain and spinal cord. Coën blamed anomalies, "which cannot be demonstrated anatomically," of the medulla and the spinal cord. Ruff (1885) accused a deranged innervation of the muscles of articulation as a result of a quantitative change in the blood supply of the brain, especially the speech center. Kussmaul (1881) introduced the concept, taken over later by Gutzmann with some slight modification, that stuttering is a spastic coördination neurosis based on congenital weakness and irritability of the syllabic coördinating apparatus; psychic features are declared to have secondary significance. As late as in 1903, Maas referred stuttering which begins sooner or later after some acute infectious disease to an inflammatory process in the speech center.[1] Schilder's observations of stuttering in postencephalitic conditions have caused some people to look to the striate body as the source of every type of stuttering, which they call a "striatal neurosis." The theory which has been evolved in recent years in this country by Orton and his collaborators has been thus summarized by Travis in his book on *Speech Pathology:* "My point of view is that in most cases the act of stuttering is a neuromuscular derangement secondary to general reduction in cortical lead control. The latter is conceived to be due to transient and mutually inhibitive activities of the right and left cerebral hemispheres. In the stutterer, instead of nervous energy being mobilized by one center of greatest potential, it is mobilized by two centers of comparable potential. Because both of these centers when operating singly function in reaction patterns of opposite motor orientation and configuration, there is produced in the peripheral speech organ an undesirable competition in the resulting muscular movements. The symptoms of stuttering are then mainly the peripheral signs of the rivalry between the two sides of the brain." This rivalry is either congenital or, in the majority of cases, acquired through the training of an originally lefthanded individual to use his right hand. It is quite true that a considerable number of cases of stuttering and of specific reading disability present a history of changed handedness, but it is equally true that a large number of stutterers does not present such a history and that there are many persons whose sinistrality has been converted to dextrality without ever leading to the slightest degree of speech disorder or reading difficulty.

A comparatively small group of authors has claimed that stuttering is due to general physical disorders other than those of a local or cerebral origin. Hieronymus Mercurialis, in the sixteenth century, blamed excessive humidity of the body and recommended as a cure the avoidance of bathing and of washing the head. Others, at a much later period, held the view that the condition is due to too rapid exhalation.

A great number of existing etiological theories is based on the view that stuttering is a "functional" disturbance which, depending on the individual investigators, is, or is not, founded on some primary cerebral "weakness" or "susceptibility" or "irritability" or "inferiority." Hippocrates spoke of an incoördination between thinking and speaking, combined with changes in the speech organs. Fröschels and Hoepfner interpret the condition as an associative defect, analogous to the aphasias, characterized by an anomaly

---

[1] Maas, O. Einige Bemerkungen über das Stottern. Deutsche Zeitschrift für Nervenheilkunde. 1903, 24, 390.

of the connection between ideation and verbalization, which has been disrupted and is linked together by the patient in a pathological manner.[1]

According to the main emphasis placed on various factors which have been found to play a part in the onset of the difficulty or in its manifestations, stuttering has been designated as an anxiety neurosis, an obsessive neurosis, an expectation neurosis, an intention neurosis, an inferiority neurosis, an imitative neurosis, and a variety of tic. The psychoanalytic school stresses the importance of sexual traumata and of guilt feelings arising from masturbation. The Adlerian school concentrates on the child's feeling of insecurity and desire for power as the leading etiological moment, the choice of the symptom being influenced by a specific inferiority of some of the organs involved in the speech mechanism.

Heredity has been proclaimed as a major etiological factor. According to Nadoleczny, not less than fifty per cent of all patients developed their stuttering on the basis of an inherited predisposition. One is, however, hardly entitled to speak of heredity every time that one learns that a parent or another relative is, or has been, stuttering. We know that at an early period of speech acquisition there is a natural reduplication of syllables. We also know that at that time the average child goes through a stage of groping for words which would adequately express his desires and experiences. If, at that age, there is a stuttering person in the house, it is easy for the child to avail himself of the same pattern through imitation, partly using it as a cover reaction for his inability to find immediately the proper words. The family looks upon the speech disorder as an inherited condition and often the following children are expected to stutter.

A characteristic example is presented by the S. family. Sidney S., aged thirteen years, came to us with the following complaint, offered with a considerable amount of stuttering and many associated movements: "I came over to correct my speech. Sometimes when I stand up in class I can hardly speak out what I want to say. Sometimes when I am at home, the words seem to stick in my throat, just like a stone wall. It bothers most in class or in clubs. In social meetings. Right now, when I am talking to you, it is not so bad. Sometimes when I am excited it is like that. In school, when I have the correct answer I speak too fast and try to hurry it out. If I could speak right, I would be going twice as fast as I do now. I don't volunteer much. If I grow up and still have the speech defect, it will stop me from doing my best work and making a living. If I apply for a job and cannot talk about my qualifications, I won't get the job. It might interfere in social things. I am doing well in languages and would like to be an interpreter. It's a funny thing, I talk pretty well in Latin and French but not in English. I have been stuttering ever since I can remember." The boy's father stuttered badly when he was younger and still does so when he is angry. "Sometimes he gets so mad he cannot speak a word." When the oldest son, Harry, now twenty years old, began to stutter at about three years of age, the parents attributed the condition to an inherited doom. When the next child, Frank, now eighteen, began to speak, he was

[1] Fröschels, Emil. Lehrbuch der Sprachheilkunde für Ärzte, Pädagogen und Studierende. Leipzig und Wien. 1925.—Hoepfner, Theodor. Grundriss der psychogenen Störungen der Sprache. In Schwarz: Psychogenese und Psychotherapie Körperlicher Symptome. Berlin. 1925.

expected to stutter and did so indeed. The notion of heredity became firmly intrenched. No wonder, then, that Sam, now sixteen, promptly developed the same speech disorder. Then came Sidney, our patient. Contrary to all family tradition, Lillian, eleven, never stuttered. But Milton, nine years old, has a cluttering speech, and Shirley, five, went through a short period of mild stuttering. Harry lost his difficulty at eight years, Sam at twelve, and Shirley lost hers at four years. Frank and Sidney stuttered considerably at the time of Sidney's first interview. In addition to the family's attitude that the speech disorder was an inevitable inheritance, the situation was aggravated by the fact that Harry and Sam, who themselves had overcome their speech difficulties, constantly teased their two stuttering brothers and that Frank had a congenital nystagmus, which was interpreted as a definite proof of the organic origin of the whole family's tendency to stutter. Frank, therefore, had to be approached first. The fact that Harry and Sam now spoke well served as a demonstration that the condition could be overcome. The dogmata of heredity and of cerebral defect were examined together and Frank soon decided that he had no proof for them and that they were much in the way of his improvement. He began to look at his stuttering as a remediable difficulty of a psychogenic nature. His optimistic attitude was transmitted to the family. Within less than three months, Frank's speech was practically normal. This change in Frank, aided by similar work with Sidney, gradually improved Sidney's condition within the same time. Sidney then went to a summer camp, where for several weeks he spoke as well as all the other boys in the camp. He now stutters only on very rare occasions, decreasing in frequency, when he is excited. Stuttering has ceased to be a family preoccupation.

Even some of those authors who look for a neurological interpretation of stuttering emphasize that it is impossible to reduce all instances to one single etiological formula and that the patient deserves individual consideration. Travis states repeatedly that "the etiology of speech disorders must be pluralistically conceived." If one has seen a sufficient number of stuttering children, one is impressed by the large variety of situations which have given rise to the disorder and helped to maintain it. The factor of imitation is evident in some cases. One patient stuttered only as long as a stuttering visitor was in the house. In another case not only the sister's stuttering but also a great-aunt's "hawking way of clearing her throat" was adopted by a boy of superior intelligence and considerable emotional immaturity (enuresis, feeding problem, blinking, habits of wetting fingers and touching objects). Fright or other affective upheavals played a significant part in this boy's sister, who began to stutter after some firecrackers exploded near her; in a boy who was threatened that his ear will be cut off; in a boy whose father also stuttered and whose own speech disorder began when he and his parents were told that he had tuberculosis; in a boy who began to stutter when he was frightened by a dog; in a youngster whose speech trouble followed immediately a fall down the stairs (with no other injuries than a black mark on his nose); in a boy whose perfectly normal speech was changed to stuttering on the morning after his first public recitation before a large audience. Interference with the use of the hand of preference was reported in a considerable number of our stutterers. In one girl, there was a peculiar discrepancy between right and left; the left pupil was larger, the left eye ball was less prominent, there was left internal strabismus, and the left hand was smaller than the right; three other members of the family stuttered and the inheritance notion was prevalent in the home. In some of our cases the onset of stuttering coincided with the time when the children began to go to school. Most of the patients had additional personality difficulties.

Any *therapeutic attempt* must be preceded by a thorough knowledge of the patient's personality and environment, his physical condition, his home management, the school situation, and the mode of onset of his stuttering and of any other behavior difficulties which he may have. It is not the speech disorder which must be treated but the child who presents the speech disorder. If the youngster is found to have any sort of physical ailment, this should be corrected, not because of any direct causal relationship to the stuttering, but because it should be remedied in any individual, stuttering or not stuttering, and because we wish to create optimal conditions of health and composure. The child and the family must be relieved of the feeling of consternation and hopelessness which often goes with notions of organic origin and inheritance and which may have been increased by by the inefficiency of tonics and sedatives and surgical procedures (clipping the tongue, tonsillectomy, dental interventions). The domestic atmosphere must be cleared of the habits of deploring and pitying the patient in his presence, interrupting him impatiently, teasing and ridiculing him, scolding or beating him. Such methods heighten his tension and his self-consciousness and reduce his self-confidence which has already suffered a remarkable loss. They increase rather than reduce the difficulty. The child should be listened to calmly and unemotionally by the physician, by the parents and siblings, and by the teachers. He should be given all the time he needs to say what he wishes to say. Fear reactions should be traced to their sources and treated accordingly. Any additional personality disorders should be treated simultaneously. Whereas the child with faulty articulation may be benefited a great deal by special speech training, the stutterer in most instances is better left alone because these exercises, like the "mirror exercises" which have sometimes been recommended in the therapy of tics, often tend to center his attention on the speech disorder even more than before and to aggravate his condition. It does, however, help occasionally to make use of his ability to sing or whisper without hesitation. Where school adjustment is needed, it should be arranged. Where sexual problems play a part, as in the cases of fear of the results of masturbation quoted by Stekel,[1] they must, of course, be handled properly. Hypnotic procedures should be resorted to only in those cases in which despite every effort parental coöperation cannot be established or in which for some weighty reasons unhappy home situations cannot be modified nor the child removed from the home.

CONGENITAL WORD-BLINDNESS
(Visual Aphasia. Dyslexia. Reading Disability. Strephosymbolia)

Kussmaul, in 1877, called attention to a phenomenon which he termed *word-blindness* and in which "a complete text-blindness may exist, although

[1] Stekel, Wilhelm. Nervöse Angstzustände und ihre Behandlung. Wien und Berlin. 1912, p. 300.

the power of sight, the intellect, and the powers of speech are intact." Hinshelwood later defined the concept as "a condition in which with normal vision and therefore seeing the letters and words distinctly, an individual is no longer able to interpret written or printed language." Following Kussmaul's contribution, several cases were reported, in which the inability to read, with or without the coincidence of right homonymous hemianopsia was acquired by adult patients in the course of their lives and based on demonstrable cerebral lesions, mostly involving the angular and supramarginal gyri of the left hemispheres of the brains of righthanded people. In 1896, W. P. Morgan published in the British Medical Journal the case of a normally intelligent and physically healthy fourteen-year-old boy who had enormous difficulty to acquire a knowledge of the letters of the alphabet and, when this was ultimately achieved, could only with the greatest effort spell out monosyllabic words. "Words written or printed seemed to convey no impression to his mind, and it was only after laboriously spelling them that he was able by the sound of the letters to discover their import." There was not the slightest impairment of his capacity for identifying figures and he had good arithmetical abilities and a good memory for oral information. This, according to Hinshelwood, is the earliest communication in medical literature of reading disability which was not acquired but appeared as a congenitally ingrained defect. Since then, numerous instances have been observed. The concept has been broadened. Orton included in his *strephosymbolia* not only cases of typical "word-blindness" but also "the demonstrably much larger group of children who are retarded in reading much below their achievement in other subjects (notably arithmetic) and whose attempts at reading are characterized by frequent reversals in reading, by confusion between reversible words and who show a greater facility in mirror reading than do normal readers."

With regard to the *etiology*, Hinshelwood[1] looked for an analogy between acquired and congenital dyslexia.

"The defect in these children," he wrote, "is a strictly specialized one, viz., a difficulty in acquiring and storing up in the brain the visual memories of words and letters. It may not extend beyond this special group of visual images. The power of retaining and storing up the visual memories of numbers and musical notes may be quite normal, though in some cases the defect may extend to these also. Such symptoms, although puzzling and inexplicable to those without a knowledge of word-blindness due to disease, become clear and explicable in the light of our knowledge regarding the latter. We have seen that the visual memories of words and letters, of numbers and of musical notes, must be stored up in distinct cerebral areas, as we find that each of these groups may be lost whilst the others are preserved, but since they are frequently lost simultaneously they are probably very close together and may even be contiguous. Hence we infer that in the case of these defective children their difficulties in learning to read can most readily be explained on the ground of some defect in the special area of the brain where are stored the visual memories of words and letters. There is now a general agreement that this area is in the angular and supramarginal gyri of the left side of the brain in right-handed people, and the

[1] Hinshelwood, James. Congenital Word-Blindness. London. 1917.

more important part of the center is situated in the angular gyrus. If there be any abnormality within this area due either to disease, to injury at birth, or to faulty development, it is easily conceivable how such a child should experience abnormal difficulty in learning to read. Any condition diminishing the number of cortical cells within this area or interfering with the blood supply would lower the functional activity of the center, and hence would diminish the power of retention of the visual images of words and letters which is absolutely essential for the successful accomplishment of the act of reading. Varying degrees of damage to this cerebral center would account for the varying degrees of defect manifested by the different cases."

Lucy G. Fildes subjected a representable number of non-readers and of normal controls to various psychological tests, some of which were indeed quite ingenious, and came, on the basis of her experiments, to the following conclusions:

"There is nothing in the results of the experiments to indicate the existence of any such region as a 'visual-word' center, the absence of or injury to which will make the visual recognition of words impossible. The defects found are not so strictly localized as such a hypothesis would demand, for the word-blind individuals reveal special difficulties in dealing with material other than words. Further, the implication of this theory that ability to read depends on the power to store up images of words has no psychological support; the recall of images is not in question. The theory that the experiments do support is that 'word-blindness' is but one aspect of a more general, yet still in itself specific, defect in either the visual or auditory regions or in both. All the non-readers examined showed a reduction of the normal power in dealing with forms visually presented—especially when these forms were very like each other, their defect being shown most definitely in their failure to remember such forms. Further, certain of the non-readers showed corresponding defects in the auditory region—they could not readily discriminate or retain similar sounds. Some of the worst cases had defects of both kinds. Taking the group of non-readers as a whole, however, no correlation could be found between auditory and visual ability, i.e., these defects appeared also to be specific, although occasionally found together in one subject."[1]

Orton ascribes the difficulty to a confusion arising from the failure to establish a clear-cut unilateral dominance of one of the cerebral hemispheres and preventing the immediately successive linkage of the visual impression with its meaning. He states:

"From the fact that loss of the capacity to read follows a unilateral lesion only when this occurs in the dominant hemisphere may we assume that irradiation is necessary into one of the two third (associative) level cortices to produce a linkage between visually presented symbols and their meaning. That one or the other hemisphere or one locus in one hemisphere must have an initiatory function for all volitional motor responses seems obvious. Were it not for this placing of the lead or control in one side, the two hemispheres might originate opposed or conflicting responses to a given situation. In man's brain the entire initiatory control of certain major

[1] Fildes, Lucy G. A Psychological Inquiry Into the Nature of the Condition Known as Congenital Word-Blindness. Brain. 1921, 44, 286-307.

functions, such as speech, writing, and reading, seems to be in one hemisphere, as is illustrated by the occurrence of the alpha-privative symptoms —aphasia, agraphia, alexia, etc., following unilateral lesions. Dominance of this degree has not, I believe, been demonstrated in the lower animals, but some form of initiatory control would seem necessary to prevent confusion of responses such as would result if either hemisphere were competent to lead without reference to the activities of the other."[1]

Orton advances the hypothesis that the process of learning to read entails the elision from the focus of attention of the confusing memory images of the nondominant hemisphere which are said to be in reversed form and order, and the selection of those which are correctly oriented and in correct sequence. This training for proper elision and selection may operate in either hemisphere; dominantly lefthanded children have apparently no greater difficulty in learning to read than dominantly righthanded children. The confusion, and especially the trouble with reversal of letters, arises, according to Orton, in those youngsters "who are neither dominantly righthanded nor lefthanded, or in whom clear dominance has not been established before they begin to learn to read." The term "strephosymbolia" which he has coined in preference to the older designation of "word-blindness" is derived from the Greek words, *strepho*, twist, and *symbolon*, symbol, to indicate the turning or reversals of "words," "signs," or "tokens." "Strephosymbolia thus seems nicely suited to our cases in which our analysis points to confusion, because of reversals, in the memory images of symbols resulting in a failure of association between the visually presented stimulus and its concept" (Orton). The dominance theory does not quite explain why some children who frequently read "*on*" for "*no*" or "*was*" for "*saw*," and vice versa, rarely make the mistake of confusing "*79*" with "*97*" or "*IV*" with "*VI*."

Perhaps the largest number of non-readers with varying degrees of dyslexia was analyzed by Marion Monroe. With reference to hand-and-eye preferences, she found that there was in her material a significantly greater incidence of left-eye preference and of left-eye preference with right-hand preference among the reading-defect cases than among the controls; that left-eye preference was associated with fluent mirror-reading and fluent mirror-reading was associated with reading disabilities; that there was a slight tendency for left-eye preference to be associated with reversal errors in reading; and that reading-defect cases reported a larger incidence of changed handedness (mostly from left to right), and of lefthandedness among members of the immediate family than did the controls.[2]

The occurrence of "congenital word-blindness" is very rare if one adheres to Hinshelwood's two criteria of severity and purity. Monroe has worked out a "reading index" which she obtained by comparing the child's composite reading grade with his average chronological, mental, and arithmetic grade. If, for example, a pupil's chronological age gives him a grade placement of 3.5, his mental age gives him a placement of 4.0, and his arith-

[1] Orton, Samuel T. "Word-Blindness" in School Children. Archives of Neurology and Psychiatry. 1925, 14, 581–615.

[2] Monroe, Marion. Children Who Cannot Read. Chicago. 1932.

metic is 3.6, then the average of these accomplishments is 3.7. If his grade scores on four reading tests were 2.1, 2.5, 1.8, and 2.0, with an average of 2.1, then the reading index is only 2.1/3.7 of his expectation, or 0.56. Monroe found that pupils with indices below 0.80 were always so seriously maladjusted in their reading as to need correctional work. She assumes that approximately twelve per cent of the general population have reading disabilities as indicated by an index of below 0.80. This high rate of distribution renders the problem highly significant from the point of view of diagnosis and treatment.

It is not at all difficult to recognize the specific reading disability of school children if one keeps in mind the following points: In a pupil who in all other subjects, including arithmetic and oral instruction in history and geography, progresses in accordance with his general level of intellectual development, there is found to exist a more or less marked inability to acquire the skill of reading. In everything else, he may be equal to or even excel his classmates, but in reading he is behind his coëvals and behind his own general mental capacity. Those children usually have a good memory for things heard. It is therefore interesting that they are often brought to the clinic with the seemingly paradoxical complaint of "forgetfulness." The reason for this becomes obvious if one obtains the details of the case history. When the child begins to go to school, only a few words or a few lines are being taught at one time. The child hears them often repeated in school and may have them read and reread to him at home. When called upon by the teacher, he reads his lines fairly well, not because he has learned to read them, but because he "remembers" them, that is, he has retained an auditory instead of a visual memory of his lesson. But when the required text becomes longer, it becomes increasingly difficult for him to retain the entire contents, and it is then really the inability to remember, the "forgetfulness," that brings out the underlying dyslexia. The astounding discrepancy between helplessness when confronted with words and sentences on the one hand and normal capacity for learning to decipher figures and musical notes on the other hand is pathognomonic for the condition, as are also the reversals of letters, syllables, or whole words (interchange of *b* and *d*, *p* and *q*, *u* and *n*, *on* and *no*, *left* and *felt*, *he said* and *said he*, *once there was* and *there once was*), use of faulty vowels (*left* for *lift*, *dug* for *dig*) and faulty consonants, and absolute failure to make any sense of the word to be read. One of our patients read *could* for *called*, *under* for *uniform*, *steady* for *straight*, without having the subjective feeling of making a mistake, though on account of his errors the whole context of the story seemed somewhat weird to him; it is remarkable that once he recognized the word *wagon* almost instantly, but when it recurred in the next line, he was unable to make out what it meant. (This inconsistency is rather typical. Normal children, of course, may also make mistakes in reading. But they either can or cannot identify a word, whereas the non-reader sometimes stumbles over a word which at other times offers no difficulties.) This boy had an I.Q. of 99. Correction of a mild refractive error had no influence on the situation. His three-year-old sister and a maternal uncle were lefthanded. He got "excellent" marks in arithmetic but failed three times because of his reading disability.

Another boy of nine years, two months, and a mental age of eight years, eight months, was still in the low first grade when first seen. He characteristically read and wrote *doy* for *boy*, and in spite of a nine year arithmetic ability, found it extremely difficult to read from the primer. He had a slight degree of red-green blindness. A paternal aunt was lefthanded. When asked to read, he fabricated words, sometimes substituting as many as four words for one three- or four-letter word, without becoming aware of this spatial incongruity. When shown a text with a picture on the same page, he simply described the picture while pretending to read from the book.

The *ability to spell* is always impaired in the severe cases. In the milder forms, the children may spell words correctly without being able to read them; they first spell them out aloud and then may, or may not, pronounce them correctly. One of our patients made the same type of errors in spelling as he did in reading (*mali* for *mail, chcat* for *catch, tacher* for *teach, afrid* for *afraid, tarvel* for *travel, carn* for *card, mear* for *measure, gril* for *girl, chil* for *chair, was* for *saw*). His paternal aunt never could read fluently. A maternal uncle was feebleminded.

The condition is found much more frequently in boys than in girls (from 84 to 94 per cent in boys, from 6 to 16 per cent in girls).

It is natural that personality difficulties are to be expected in children who, in spite of their effort, are doomed to failure as long as they are not treated adequately. Marion Monroe, in comparing one hundred cases each of behavior problems in non-readers and in satisfactory readers, found that among the "word-blind" children there was a predominance of school problems, temper tantrums, daydreaming, and enuresis, while disobedience, stealing, truancy, sex offenses, and other social maladjustments were more frequent in the others.

Of one of our boys his mother said, "All the other children take books from the library, and he can't, and this makes him mad. That sort of thing preys on his mind and he wonders what it is all about. His nerves are so bad that he has recently begun to stutter; he never did that before. I don't know if the trouble is in what he gets at school. He can see movies all right." The boy was very irritable and had temper tantrums before the correction of his dyslexia.

John R., aged nine and a half years, colorblind, ambidextrous (used his right hand in eating and writing and combed his hair and threw a ball with his left), had occasional enuresis, was restless, sometimes walked in his sleep, and had attacks of "shortness of breath" and of "sick headaches," as did his father.

Irvin McG., ten years old, son of an alcoholic father and a stuttering mother, "gets along nicely in spelling and arithmetic but cannot read. He has failed four times, this is his third half year in the high third grade." He had an I.Q. of 103. His fourteen-year-old brother had reached the seventh grade, did not talk until over three years of age, and is reported to have a definite reading disability.

Dyslexia is usually associated with *dysgraphia*. The patients learn to form characters rather well, at least with about the same speed and skill as the average child of equal intelligence. They usually copy well and some children are capable of translating the printed word symbols into cursive writing. But if it comes to writing to dictation, the same difficulties are encountered as in reading, with the same type of errors. It is interesting that that even in severe cases of dysgraphia to the point of an almost complete agraphia (upon dictation), the children may have a good capacity for drawing of fairly complex patterns not only from copy but also from memory.

Originally, children's reading disabilities were thought to be "incurable." But already Hinshelwood had sounded a more optimistic note with regard to their improvement. At the present time, methods are available which make it possible to remedy the difficulty through individual training. The principles of remedial instruction are described excellently in Monroe's monograph. It is from there that we quote the following remarks:

"We tried to teach the children who had trouble in learning to read to utilize the possible secondary or vicarious steps in word-recognition which are not usually presented in ordinary instruction. For example, the child whose visual discriminations were precise for small patterns, such as letters, but not for large ones, such as words, was taught by a method which began with the small units and built up the larger ones gradually. The child who had trouble in recognizing the spatial orientation of patterns was taught to use a manual one to give the position of the pattern. The child who failed to discriminate precisely the sounds of words was taught the movements of placing the speech organs to obtain the desired sounds and hence to rely on the kinesthetic cues of articulation rather than on audition. The child who had difficulty in recalling an auditory symbol (the word as heard) when presented with a visual symbol (the word as seen) was taught to associate each with the same overt response, and hence to build up the desired associations by a secondary link. The child whose motor control of the eyes was inaccurate for keeping the place of reading was taught to utilize a combination of eye-and-hand movement in developing the desired habit."

The great importance of recognizing and treating adequately the reading disabilities of children is quite obvious. It becomes especially clear if one learns that many of the patients with normal or even superior intelligence have been declared to be feebleminded and in some instances actually commited to institutions maintained for the training of the mentally retarded. The treatment must be carried out by experienced teachers. The would-be individual tutoring by well-meaning but untrained people is apt to add to, instead of relieving, the child's difficulties.

CONGENITAL WORD-DEAFNESS

There exists a very small number of children whose failure to develop the functions of language is based on an innate inability to comprehend the symbolic meaning of spoken words. The condition is usually designated as congenital word-deafness (auditory aphasia). The term is somewhat misleading, inasmuch as deafness in the ordinary sense is not present. It was assumed that the auditory perception as such is entirely unimpaired in all cases, but recent studies by Ewing have shown that six out of his series of ten patients manifesting gross defects of speech in childhood suffered from a marked, binaural, and evenly progressive lack of hearing for ascending orders of frequency in sound above 256 v.d. (double vibrations). The hearing of sounds of lower frequency was relatively intact. (The average values for audible frequency were found to be 20,000 v.d. as the upper limit and 20 v.d. as the lower.) Ewing felt that the defect may be in the cochlea, along the auditory path, or possibly due to late myelination of nerve fibers associated with hearing. He found that the lack of auditory acuity for the higher frequencies had abolished the characteristic differences of the sound of speech and most noises.[1]

"Word-deafness," or rather the resulting speech difficulty, is naturally not discovered before the time when the expected linguistic development fails to appear. Even then the parents usually think of a simple delay, especially since the patients go through the babbling stage quite normally and may in due time or a little later form consonants as any healthy infant does. The discrepancies become more noticeable when the babies, not comprehending the significance of things said to them, do not attach the conventional meanings to their own utterances, which remain conspicuously few in number and variety. At the same time, the children are capable of understanding and expressing themselves through gestures and signs. As the years go on, they may either restrict their verbal activities to a few sounds, simply because their words are not meaningful and therefore not useful to them, or they may evolve a language of their own, entirely different from and unrelated to that spoken in their environment and sounding to the family like an unknown foreign tongue (idioglossia, idiolalia). This mode of speech may for a long time be mistaken for "baby talk" and the child unsuccessfully "corrected." Writing, in the sense of copying letters, words, and sentences, is learned easily. Some of the more intelligent youngsters can be taught, with the application of great patience, to get the significance of a limited number of word combinations, to write the correct answers to simple written questions ("What is your name?"; "How old are you?" "Where do you live?"), and even to pronounce a few written words and indirectly, through the medium of "reading," to connect the right meaning with those utterances.

There exist varying degrees of the difficulty, from complete "aphasia" to the milder forms of lack of comprehension with confusion of vowels and consonants. It is understandable that the patients, not responding to spoken words, are thought to be deaf or sometimes considered feebleminded. They are unhappy creatures, often shy, meek, and fearful. When they grow older and realize to a certain extent their unusual situation, they must feel as though they move in a peculiar world in which all others communicate in a manner which is closed to them. They may learn to obtain their wants through crying or temper tantrums.

In the treatment, the children's ability to connect visual impressions of motions and gestures with their proper meanings can be utilized by the instruction in lip reading and in the use of sign language. In the cases of high-frequency deafness, Ewing has evolved a method of daily "listening practices" with the aim of improving the auditory acuity.

Vera H., an extremely shy girl of twelve years, in good physical health,

[1] Ewing, Alex. W. G. Aphasia in Children. London. 1930.

was brought to the clinic with the complaint that she must be deaf because she did not react to spoken words. She came of sound and stable stock. She was a full term child, born spontaneously. She held up her head at about four months, sat alone at seven months, and walked without support at fourteen months. As an infant, she babbled normally and at two years articulated a few consonants. Then she failed to show any further progress. Her parents attributed this to a fright the accounts of which were very vague: "One evening, while in the same room with her father, she appeared frightened and cried." No advances were noticed in the following years. She learned at the proper ages to wash herself, to dress and undress, to have good table manners, to handle her toys adequately, and to help with the household duties. She remained enuretic throughout her life. She was righthanded.

Otological examination was extraordinarily difficult because of the child's timidity, whining, and lack of coöperation. The ear drums were found to be essentially normal. During the interviews she responded to low spoken and clearly enunciated words but was unaware of high-pitched sounds. She always, even in the waiting room, sat in a huddled position with her chin close to her chest. She never reacted to the calling of her name but when taken by her hand got up and followed meekly to the examining office. She wept noiselessly with profuse lachrymation and many sobs. Her attention to movements and gestures of others in the room was good. She never spoke spontaneously. Several times she responded in a whisper, using single words, usually monosyllables, and then only on urging. She could not vocally count or enumerate the letters of the alphabet or the days of the week or the months. She would not repeat letters, words, or phrases. Spoken commands were not heeded but orders given through pointing or gestures were carried out slowly but correctly. She did not react to mewing, barking, whistling (unless low-pitched), the ticking of a clock, the counting of money, or a knock at the door. But she did pick out the pretty faces in the Binet-Simon test on verbal order. "Hello" was the only word she repeated on request. She understood well the motions of beckoning, threatening, disgust, and the like. She wrote the following answers to written problems of arithmetic: $2+2=9$; $10-4=11$; $5+1=4$; $3-2=8$. She copied drawings from sight and from memory but not upon oral request. She copied written and printed matter quite well but with little or no perceptible understanding. She once made a mistake while copying and immediately used the eraser on the other end of the pencil properly. She was shown a printed word and asked through gestures to write it from memory. For *water* she wrote *uatea*, *hame* for *home*, and *smal* for *smeared*. When pictures were shown, she could not name them but immediately began to draw them. When motioned to write their names, she clearly and correctly wrote *cat*, *girl*, *bird*, and *pig* (for *bear*). For *horse* she wrote *stepa*. When asked to read what she had written, she said in a barely audible whisper, with a tremendous amount of effort, *cat*, *girl*, *bird*, and *pig*, but could not make out what she had meant by *stepa*. There was a mild degree of red-green blindness (*21* for *74* in the Ishihara test for color vision). All motor functions were normal.

The child entered school at eight years. She remained in the first grade. From time to time, she was sent to special classes for deaf children but the teachers refused to keep her there because they felt that she was not deaf. She was regarded as feebleminded. In the absence of adequate facilities for Vera's type of disorder in the community, it is not an easy task to map out a constructive program by which she could be helped but we are working at present for a satisfactory arrangement to give her the benefit of special training.

MOTOR APHASIA

In motor aphasia (or aphemia), the patient can comprehend spoken and written language yet is incapable of expressing himself through the medium of speech. It is a condition which may be found in a variety of disorders of the central nervous system affecting Broca's area and the adjacent parts of the precentral gyrus and the insula. In very severe cases of chorea, loss of the functions of speech may be a part manifestation of the general and extreme muscular weakness.

Transient loss of the ability to utter words, with good preservation of understanding, may occur on a purely psychogenic basis. It is well known that strong emotional upheavals are apt to render a person "speechless" for a few seconds or minutes. This is especially true of fright, anger, and surprise. The phenomenon of "stage-fright" is a specific example. It seems that children are much more disposed to this type of response than are adults. The features of "hysterical aphasia" will be discussed in connection with hysteria. The speechlessness of catatonics is spoken of as mutism rather than aphasia.

This is perhaps the place to mention the peculiar experience to which one might refer as "nightmare aphasia." At the height of a fearful dream, the child may have the tormenting feeling of general motionlessness with the inability to flee from a threatening person or animal and at the same time be tortured by a paralysis of the speech functions making it impossible for him to talk or shout for help. There is, at the end of the dream, a desperate struggle for verbal expression which is successful only at the moment of, or soon after, awakening.

CHAPTER XXXV

HABITUAL MANIPULATIONS OF THE BODY

Two TYPES of similar, yet sufficiently differentiated modes of reactions or habit formations have often been thrown together and confused with one another. Although we can hardly be suspected of wishing to indulge in unnecessary nomenclatures, the phenomenological efforts and insights of recent years have made us aware of the need for a clear descriptive formulation of human performances which, then, can and should be studied from their dynamic angles. It is from this point of view that we do not approve of the indiscriminate identification of the phenomena known as tics or habit spasms and those behavior patterns which are characterized by habitual manipulations of certain parts of the body, such as thumbsucking, nailbiting, nose picking, or tongue sucking.

The following table lists the essential differences between the two reaction forms by listing the essential distinguishing features.

Tics	Habitual Manipulations of the Body
1. They are automatisms, carried out involuntarily.	1. They are carried out on a much higher level of awareness.
2. They are ushered in suddenly, without any preparation whatsoever.	2. They are initiated very much more slowly and sometimes require a relatively complicated and deliberate preparation (e.g., assuming the proper position enabling the child to bite his toenails; curling up the hair before pulling it out; taking the hand out of the pocket or putting away a toy before introducing the finger into the mouth).
3. They last a few seconds only.	3. There is no limit to their possible duration.
4. They are localized twitchings of a circumscribed muscle group.	4. The performances involve the combined and successive activity of at least two parts of the body, the hand most frequently being one of them.
5. Although originally purposive (expressive or defensive), they seem to serve no obvious purpose after they have become automatized.	5. They appear to be purposive, in that the biting or pulling or sucking itself is the desired goal, usually felt and recognized as pleasurable.
6. The repetitions resemble each other to the point of cinematographic identity with regard to their duration, intensity, and course.	6. The repetitions may vary greatly with regard to their duration, intensity, and course. (The choice of the fingernails to be bitten may depend on their length, on which hand happens to be unoccupied, etc.)
7. Once the single tic has been started, it cannot be interrupted.	7. They may be interrupted at any stage of the single performance.

Tics	Habitual Manipulations of the body
8. They are felt subjectively by the patient as something alien, irresistible, and uncontrollable, for which he does not consider himself responsible.	8. They are felt subjectively by the patient as actions for which he is responsible and which are subject to his volitional control.
9. There is rarely a subject-object relation between parts of the body.	9. One part of the body does something to another (the teeth bite the lips and fingernails; the hand pulls the ear or picks the nose.)
10. They are personality disorders bearing the earmarks of unintended part-dysfunctions.	10. They are personality disorders appearing clearly as behavior dysfunctions of the individual as a whole.

It is, of course, true that, as anywhere else where one deals with human reactions, there are transitions between these two forms of behavior. As a whole, however, the differences are too numerous and too essential to be overlooked. It also becomes evident that the habit of masturbation shows every one of the characteristics enumerated in the right hand column. Yet, for practical purposes of organization, we have preferred to discuss it together with the other difficulties of a sexual nature.

The best grouping of habitual manipulations is that offered by Olson[1] who, however, does not distinguish between tics and the other forms and comprises them under the name of *nervous habits*. He therefore includes in his list blinking, grimacing, and twiching of facial muscles, with which we have dealt elsewhere as "tics." He has observed school children during class hours and recorded the occurrence of the various habits within certain time limits. His classification is as follows:

1. Oral (sucking thumb, sucking fingers, biting nails, protruding tongue).
2. Nasal (picking nose, scratching nose, wrinkling nose).
3. Hirsutal (pulling and twisting hair, scratching head).
4. Irritational (scratching body).
5. Manual (picking fingers, writhing hands, clenching fists).
6. Ocular (rubbing eyes, blinking eyelids, winking).
7. Aural (pulling ear, picking ear).
8. Genital (manipulating genitalia, thigh rubbing).
9. Facial (grimacing, twitching muscles).

Another form of grouping would be one which, excluding tics entirely, is based on the parts of the body which are involved in the manipulations, both actively and passively:

1. Hands and mouth: pulling the lips; rubbing the lips.
2. Mouth and hands: sucking the fingers; biting the nails; biting the hand.
3. Hands and nose: picking; scratching.
4. Hands and eyes: rubbing; pulling at eyebrows and eyelashes.
5. Hands and ears: pulling; rubbing; scratching.
6. Hands and hair: pulling; twisting.

[1] Olson, Willard C. The Measurement of Nervous Habits in Normal Children. Minneapolis. 1929.

7. Hand and hand: picking; rubbing; twisting; scratching.
8. Teeth and lips: biting.
9. Tongue and lips: sucking.
10. Mouth and feet: sucking toes; biting toenails.
11. Hands and feet: picking; rubbing; scratching.
12. Hands and trunk: scratching; rubbing.
13. Hands and genitals: pulling; stroking; rubbing.
14. Thigh and thigh: rubbing.

THUMBSUCKING

Thumbsucking is the earliest form of habitual manipulations of the body. As a matter of fact, rare instances of babies born sucking their thumbs have been reported. Levy[1] thinks that the congenital form can be theoretically explained "as reflex sucking of fingers which through accident of foetal position and movements have stroked the lips. The position being favorable for insertion, the fingers would then be sucked before birth. This would be in conformity with the observations of Minkowski, who noted lip movements in response to stroking fingers on the lips of the two to five months old human embryos."

The incidence of congenital sucking, however, is so unusual as to be negligible from a practical clinical point of view. The habit is almost always acquired during the first year of life and may be said to be near-physiological during the earlier months when any available objects, including the fingers and toes, are conveyed to the oral cavity. It is only after the inhibition of "hand-to-mouth reaction" which, according to Gesell, occurs at approximately twelve months of age, that the sucking may, through its persistence, assume the proportions of an undesirable habit. It most frequently involves the thumbs and the term thumbsucking has for this reason become more popular both in common usage and in literature than the designation of fingersucking. Lindner[2] was the first to call attention to the fact that in a relatively large number of cases thumbsucking is associated with simultaneous indulgence in other manipulations with the unoccupied hand. Levy refers to this phenomenon as *accessory movements*. The following examples are taken partly from his cases and partly from our own material.

Movements accessory to thumbsucking:

She either keeps a toy in the other hand or strokes the ear; while sucking her index finger, she rubs the adjacent finger lightly over the upper lip. (Levy.)

She places her left hand on the genitals with some pressure, often sucking the right thumb at the same time. (Levy.)

During the sucking of the fourth and fifth digits of the right hand, there is a pulling movement of the left ear with the left index finger. (Levy.)

A twelve-year-old girl with many signs of immaturity (enuresis, feeding problem, cries easily), while sucking her thumb, pulls her ear or twists her

---

[1] Levy, David M. Fingersucking and Accessory Movements in Early Infancy. An Etiologic Study. American Journal of Psychiatry. 1928, 7, 881–918.

[2] Lindner, S. L. Das Saugen an den Fingern, Lippen u.s.w. bei den Kindern. Jahrbuch für Kinderheilkunde. 1879, 14, 68.

hair with the other hand. She also rubs the fingers around her lips until they are sore.

Some children suck the right or left thumb or any other digit or digits indiscriminately; in others the habit is sufficiently stereotyped to be limited to one certain thumb or finger all the time. According to Levy, "certain case studies suggest the possibility that the specific thumb selected for sucking is of the hand that makes free movements in the first position at the breast feeding, the other hand (the locked hand) making the accessory movements." Some children indulge constantly and almost uninterruptedly. When this is not the case, the time shortly before going to sleep is a preferred occasion; some mothers diagnosticate sleepiness from their offspring's putting the thumb into his mouth. Hunger, embarrassment, shame, fatigue, boredom, any sort of unpleasantness may result in thumbsucking in children who are so inclined. One nine-year-old boy did it "when he is deeply interested," another, three years old, "will not go to sleep unless we let him suck his thumb"; a girl of twelve years "always goes to sleep with her thumb in her mouth; she also does it when she does her homework or when she is engrossed." The practice is most common in early infancy and mostly disappears in pre-school age. Its continuation after the sixth or seventh year is a manifestation of a general emotional immaturity.

Thelma B., nine years old, normally intelligent, who "sucked her thumb although she was able to get along for two days without doing it," offered a feeding problem and had temper tantrums; she had always been badly spoiled. Her brother, seven and a half years of age, who also had the habit, was a daydreamer, masturbated, talked "baby talk," and had a specific reading disability; he had numerous fears and was hyperactive.

Bertha B., who "sucked her thumb all the time" at ten, normally intelligent, had a history of pica, offered a feeding problem, and had temper outbursts.

Laura S., aged seven years and nine months, had enuresis, temper tantrums, fear reactions, bit and picked her nails, and picked her nose, in addition to her thumbsucking.

Harvey M., nine and a half, was a restless sleeper, enuretic, bit his nails, had temper tantrums, hypochondriacal complaints, and crying spells, and presented a feeding problem. He was badly spoiled and came of an unstable family.

"Sucking," says Thom, "is one of the most common habits that children develop. It is brought about by a well organized system of muscular movements, which serves a most useful purpose in the early life of the child, and is a natural instinctive reaction. The only difference between the child's sucking his mother's breast and its own fingers or toes is that the first act is both pleasurable and useful, while the latter, though pleasurable, not only serves no useful purpose but at times may do harm by malforming the jaw. All of these sucking, biting, and picking habits may be looked upon as organic, pleasurable sensations; that is, sensations aroused by stimulating various parts of the body from which the individual gets varying degrees of satisfaction. It depends upon the intensity of this pleasure how tenaciously the child will cling to his undesirable habit. Children vary greatly, as do adults, in respect to the reluctance with which they relinquish their hold on pleasure."

The degree of seriousness with which thumbsucking should be regarded depends largely on the circumstances accompanying the individual case. There are several factors which may serve as reliable guides:

Age. There is no cause for parental alarm if the habit is practiced by a healthy and well developed infant during the first two years of life. Persistent and intensive sucking in which the thumb is held in a position causing it to push the upper jaw forward may sometimes result in dental malocclusion in the form of mild prognathism; this, however, happens much less frequently than is commonly believed. The longer the habit is kept up, the more it assumes the character of a personality disorder. The great significance of correcting infantile sucking lies perhaps less in the immediate results than in the prevention of the child's carrying over into later years exquisitely infantile modes of reaction.

Local damage to fingers and mouth. The sucking may become a problem of local disease calling for immediate medical attention. The thumb may become flattened out from constant pressure between the lips and jaws or wrinkled from moisture. Stomatitis may develop. A seven-year-old girl had multiple ulcers on her tongue and lips from persistent indulgence.

Aesthetic considerations. Any sort of habitual manipulation is apt sooner or later to bring the child into conflict with the aesthetic conventions of the environment. An indifferent or overindulgent parent may put up with the spectacle but the playmates and classmates and teachers may refer to the ugliness of the practice in unmistakable terms and the children may tease the sucking youngster.

Influence on the character formation. The teasing, in turn, may, and often does, cause the youngster to seek the pleasure of fingersucking in solitary places, unobserved by others. Parental nagging may have the same effect. Some children resort to peculiar performances in order to hide the sucking. Thomson reports a small boy who covered his mouth with the other hand to hide what he was doing; he found an added gratification from this "complication and always used it even when alone." One of our patients acquired the habit of burying her mouth and hand inside her blouse or sweater or at night under the blanket even when she was not watched. Thus an element of secrecy and sneakiness enters into the child's personality. There is the knowledge of deriving pleasure from something which does not meet the approval of the elders. The youngster becomes soon enough acquainted not only with the attitudes of his parents and teachers but also with the current and incorrect terminology which brands all manipulations of the body as "bad" habits; he learns to accept his "badness" as a matter of course and to live up to his reputation also in other things. Although there was originally no reason for any moral implication, the very designation of thumbsucking as a bad habit may soon, in the child's own mind, make a moral issue of it, unfortunately not always in the sense of becoming "good" by abandoning the practice. There are parents whose desire for convenience causes them to tolerate or even encourage the sucking, since the child, while engaged in the act, is suffi-

ciently absorbed to leave them alone, to sit quietly in his place, not to require their attention, not to disturb them in their own activities. In this
case, the situation has exactly the opposite effect; the youngster knows
that he is considered "good" as long as he placidly occupies himself with
his thumb but "gets on mother's nerves" if he does anything to disrupt
her train of thought, conversation, or work.

A good deal has been said and written with regard to the *etiology* of
thumbsucking. It did not escape the attention of those who are ever-ready
to apply the term "neuropathy" to any behavior which in any way deviates
from the (non-existent) perfect model of a human being. After the observation of countless normal and problem children and adults, I must confess that I know of not one individual who has not at one time or another
of his life displayed some mode of performance which has been designated
as "neuropathic" by some authority. If this is so, then there is no person
who does not have a history of presenting "neuropathic" traits, and the
entire concept, if too liberally applied, becomes useless, superfluous, and
outright harmful.

The psychoanalytic school sees in thumbsucking an autoerotic phenomenon, an expression of infantile sexuality through stimulation of the oral
erogenic zone. If "autoerotic" simply means derivation of pleasure from
certain sensations of the body, we are compelled to register our full agreement. The hedonic component of thumbsucking and all other manipulations cannot be denied or minimized. Nor would one wish to deny that
there is a certain lack of self-control common to all of them. Homburger's
term, *perverse pleasure sensations* (*perverse Lustgefühle*) is well-chosen. But
this is something entirely different from attributing a sexual significance to
the practice and even identifying it with "larvated masturbation." Masturbation is beyond doubt one of the many forms of pleasurable manipulations of the body which are open to the child. Instead of declaring all
other forms to be disguised masturbation, one may perhaps wonder whether the early handling of the genitals may not after all, like the rest of the
manipulations, afford an unspecific, undifferentiated, non-sexual pleasure,
to become more specifically sexual in later years. If, on the other hand,
someone insists on the sexual nature of all hedonic sensations, then to him
thumbsucking must, of course, seem sexual.

Levy, in recent years, has in an interesting study come to the conclusion
that in a majority of instances insufficient lip movements, or incomplete-
ness of the sucking phase of the feeding act, regardless of the type of feeding (breast, bottle, or mixed), is responsible for the development of fingersucking; the most frequent etiological factors he found to be: 1. Spontaneous withdrawal from a too rapidly flowing breast or bottle. 2. Forced withdrawal from sucking at the termination of a too short period of time. 3.
Changing feeding schedules with increasing intervals between feedings and
diminished duration of the feeding time.

The *treatment* of thumbsucking is the treatment of the thumbsucking
child. It will depend a good deal on the child's age and degree of coöperation and on whether the sucking is an isolated phenomenon or associated
with other behavior problems. The radical methods of mechanical restraint,
for which ever new devices are described and illustrated in the current med-

ical journals, are usually ineffective; the patients return to the practice as soon as the metal or cardboard splint or sleeve is removed. Some children learn to suck the protective mittens which they are made to wear as eagerly as they sucked the fingers. The application of quinine or aloes meets similar difficulties; the children either resume the sucking at a later time or learn to indulge in spite of the bitter taste. In all of these "cures" the children's attention is centered more than ever on the habit and, besides, they sense a certain parental force and hostility which is bound to make them contrary. They are made aware of the fact that the practice gives them an opportunity to attract attention and to worry their elders. The introduction of a power contest may, even in "successful" cases, create difficulties much more serious than the thumbsucking ever has been. Nevertheless, mechanical means or anointment with bitters may occasionally be justified if the youngster himself expresses his desire to overcome the habit and needs a reminder which would immediately stop the hand on its way to the mouth. In this case the glove or quinine is welcomed by the child as a helpful assistance in his attempt at self-correction.

The futility of restraint or anointments is shown in the following examples:

One mother said of her two-and-a-half-year-old boy: "I have put his thumb in a wire cage; but then he put all the other fingers in his mouth." Another parent stated: "She used to suck her thumb only at night, but now she does it all the time. I try hard to break her. Once we put something on her thumb and said it was poison. She stopped a while but started again."

In children too small to coöperate in this manner or in older thumbsuckers not intelligent or willing enough to take the initiative, the treatment must be gradual. Even though the child should be made to know that the habit is not approved and that it is unbecoming, punishments and nagging should be discarded. No alarm should be shown; it is unjustified and educationally harmful. It is much better to keep the youngster busy with toys which interest him and provide ample manual occupation. He is less apt to indulge in the sucking habit when playing with other children. Nursery schools are therefore decidedly helpful. If the child is found with the thumb in his mouth, it is best not to refer directly to the situation but to change it indirectly by offering him some toy or another object which he is likely to accept and to play with. A star chart with the holding out of a prize first for two or three days, then for a week and longer, in which there would be no thumbsucking, is sometimes of advantage in ambitious children.

In older children, in whom thumbsucking is almost never an isolated complaint, an adequate program of personality and environmental adjustment is of paramount importance.

NAILBITING

Biting the fingernails is the most widespread of all forms of habitual manipulations of the body. It is encountered in numerous children and quite a few adults of all ages and all degrees of intelligence and social status. Sometimes whole families are known to indulge. Without wanting even for a moment to minimize its aesthetic undesirability or its value as an indicator of some more or less outspoken personality difficulty, we certainly cannot consider it as "an exquisitely psychopathic symptom," as does Cramer,[1] nor are we sufficiently alarmed by it to ponder with Bérillon[2] over the question, much discussed by French authors, whether or not onychophagia is a sign of "degeneration." Our attitude with regard to the psychoanalytic claim that it represents larvated masturbation has been set forth in our discussion of thumbsucking.

In contrast to such habits as temper tantrums or feeding difficulties or tics, nailbiting should not be approached largely from the clinician's point of view. By this we mean that it much less frequently becomes the cause for a primary, spontaneous complaint with which the child is brought to the physician's attention, It is, to use the term which Douglas A. Thom has made popular by introducing it as the title of one of his books, an "everyday problem of the everyday child," which the parents usually try to tackle themselves. In most instances, only in those patients who are examined for some other reason, does the physician discover incidentally, through inquiry or inspection, that the nails are being bitten, unless the practice has led to festering or other local disorders. Hence a clinical study of the habit does not reach the vast number of nailbiters whose freedom from major or more disturbing behavior disorders keeps them away from medical examination.

Usually thumbsucking is a leisurely habit, indulged in a state of serene satisfaction when the child is otherwise unoccupied or getting ready for the night's rest; nailbiting is mostly an *expression of tenseness*, produced by anticipation of a difficult test in school or of parental punishment or by any kind of excitement. It is often interesting to see how a youngster in the course of an interview sits quietly and refrains from nailbiting until the moment when the conversation turns to his own difficulties or when the questions of the intelligence test begin to overreach his capacity; then his self-control gradually diminishes and the intensity of the performance grows with the unpleasantness of the situation and he begins to chew his nails. This may be also observed when he listens to the radio rendition of a mystery story or excitedly devours a thrilling book. If he is pleasantly occupied and fully at ease, he is less apt to bite his fingernails.

Thom states correctly that "many of the thumbsuckers are calm, placid, unemotional children, while the nailbiters are apt to be hyperactive, quick, fidgety, energetic individuals." In our own case material we found nailbiting to be associated with motor restlessness in twenty-seven per cent of the children, with restless sleep (jerking, tossing, gritting the teeth, talking, crying out, walking) in twenty-three per cent, with tics in nineteen per cent, and with other forms of manipulations of the body in approximately fifty per cent (especially with thumbsucking—eleven per cent, and nose picking—ten per cent). Nailbiting, therefore, must be viewed as one of

[1] Cramer, A. Funktionelle Neurosen im Kindesalter. In Handbuch der Nervenkrankheiten im Kindesalter. (L. Bruns, A. Cramer und Th. Ziehen.) Berlin. 1912. pp. 40.

[2] Bérillon, E. L'onychophagie est-elle un signe de dégénérescence? Revue de l'hypnotisme et psychologie physiologique. 1908, 23, 27.

several forms of motor discharges of inner tension; Homburger justly refers to it as *motorische Spannungsentäusserung* (motor discharge of tension).

How closely indulgence in the habit of nailbiting may depend on the tenseness of the situation, is best shown by the following example: Pauline B., ten years old, has been under an enormous burden of too much home responsibility, house work, too difficult school requirements with insufficient intellectual endowment and not enough time, and fear imposed by an ignorant, superstitious mother. When relieved of some of her responsibilities, she stopped biting her nails, and there was also a decided improvement in her other personality difficulties. Her pride in her appearance was easily stimulated and she wanted to let her nails grow. Some time afterwards, a sick sister who had been in a convalescent home and her younger brother who had been away returned home and the whole burden of caring for them again fell on Pauline's shoulders, and she promptly resumed her nailbiting. This happened especially when she had the task of watching her brother: "When Sonny gets away from me, I am nervous and bite my nails."

Tension is especially apt to express itself in the form of nailbiting if the pattern has been furnished by older members of the family. We often had the experience, when inquiring about the existence of this habit in the patient, that the parent stated, "Yes, he does that, but I have always done that myself." One mother said: "He bites his fingernails constantly. Of course, I do that myself. I don't know whether he takes after me or whether it is caused from his nervousness."

The intensity varies with the degree of tension and with the occasion. One frequently hears reports, such as this: "She bites her fingernails. She bites it all off, she doesn't leave hardly anything on." Or: "One of his fingers was festered last week from biting." One boy practiced the habit only when watching others play ball. Another boy "got confused and bit his nails if he missed his lessons and the teacher kept him in to explain things to him." A little girl indulged mainly when she met strangers. Any excitement causes some youngsters to lose all self-control in this respect. Many children bite the skin of the end phalanges or of other parts of the fingers or hands instead of the nails, producing excoriations and scars. Sometimes a small cut or a mosquito bite is a place of predilection, and keloids are known to have formed on such spots from continuous biting.

Threats, punishments, mechanical restraint, and application of pepper or quinine have the same results as in thumbsucking. Occasionally such drastic measures have done away with the practice. Thus one mother reported: "He quit biting his nails when the finger once bled and I put iodine on them. The pain was sharp and this made him stop biting his nails." In most cases, however, these modes of treatment suffer from the disadvantage that more attention is paid to the nailbiting than to the nailbiter. One parent tried to attack the problem by telling her daughter that "it was poison; but she cannot control herself just the same." The treatment must begin with the removal of the causes of the tension or tensions responsible for the origin and maintenance of the habit. Appeal to the child's pride is often a surprisingly strong therapeutic factor. One mother stated: "She used to bite her fingernails whenever she was nervous, but she has taken a pride in her nails and wants them to look nice, so she no longer bites them." The appeal through sermons has little effect. It is better to have the child manicured a few times and then to purchase a manicuring set which the youngster should own and use regularly. This method is especially helpful if the mother or some of the siblings do the same thing. A star chart is sometimes useful. Experience shows that of several personality disorders the habit of nailbiting is the most difficult to overcome. We have seen children in whom adequate handling has managed to do away with lifelong enuresis or with frequent temper tantrums much sooner than with the coexisting nailbiting. As in thumbsucking, occupations and toys which really intrigue the patient and healthy association with other children will essentially help in the treatment.

In a number of our patients, the biting of the fingernails was associated with the *biting of the toenails*, which was performed at night after retiring. This certainly is a "perverse" enough source of pleasure. It is usually, but not always, connected with rather severe personality problems and calls for a more energetic attack. One of those children also masturbated, had peculiar spells of running wildly about the house, wet the bed every night, had temper tantrum, and was extremely restless. Another, a girl of four years and eight months, normally intelligent, jerked in her sleep, was enuretic, unruly, stubborn, disobedient, and presented a feeding problem. A three-and-a-half-year-old girl, badly spoiled, masturbated, pulled her ears, had vomiting spells in connection with forced feeding, had the habit of stuffing paper into her nose, and cried out in her sleep. On the other hand, we have seen a ten-year-old girl of superior intelligence, in good physical health, well adjusted at home and in school, popular with her playmates, who had the habit of biting her fingernails and toenails. It is especially interesting to mention that almost all of our patients who indulged in this practice were girls; we have seen only very few boys who bit their toenails.

OTHER MANIPULATIONS

Sucking the tongue. This is a relatively rare habit which seems to afford the infants who practice it an enormous amount of pleasure, to judge from their absorption and expression of extreme gratification. It is found less frequently in intelligent babies than in mental defectives, cretins, and Mongols. It is especially common among the latter and, according to John Thomson, it is responsible for the peculiar fissuring of the tongue which is almost pathognomonic for Mongolism. Thomson adds that "the same condition will be found in any child who has practiced this habit energetically for a sufficiently long time." The parents can do practically nothing to remedy the situation as long as the infants are too small for coöperation. The habit is usually harmless, except that some babies are sometimes so engrossed that they would rather go without food than interrupt the sucking of the tongue.

Sucking the lips is of little practical importance.

Biting the lips, cheilophagia, may follow the habit of sucking the lips or develop independently. It is sometimes done so vigorously that small patches of the mucous membrane are gnawed off and small hemorrhages occur; in extreme cases the lips may be deformed by numerous scars and cracks and scabs.

Picking the nose is not infrequent in children. It is sometimes associated with the very ugly habit of conveying the contents of the nose to the mouth and swallowing them. Occasionally, the picking is only a temporary reaction to a local irritation, but in many instances it is done for many years, by some youngsters so violently that nosebleeds are the result.

Pulling the ear often is a continuation of movements accessory to thumb-sucking. It is the least objectionable habit both from a medical and aesthetic point of view and usually consists in a mild and pleasurable playing with the earlobes. Pulling and scratching of the ears and rubbing and scratching behind the ears in babies should always make one think of the possibility of acute otitis media. Scratching of the ears to the point of bleeding has been reported to occur in patients with erythredema.

Pulling the hair is a behavior problem calling for much more careful attention. In a seriously retarded five-year-old girl it led to almost complete alopecia; the child also bit her toenails; her family background was very poor; her father was a wife beater, her mother emotionally unstable, her nine-year-old sister had enuresis, temper tantrums, and bit her fingernails. A deaf and feebleminded girl of seven and a half years had the habit of pulling her hair with one hand and biting the fingers of the other; she curled her hair up with her fingers and then pulled it out. She also picked her nose, pulled at both ears (she had chronic otitis media), and masturbated; all five children of the family were enuretic. Some children are seen with bald patches on their heads resulting from the practice of rubbing their heads always in the same spot. It is interesting that children suffering from erythredema during the illness pull their hair out in large quantities.

All these, and any other, manipulations may occur singly, but more frequently they are found to exist in any number and variety of combinations, of which we quote two examples:

Biting the fingernails, picking the nose, rubbing the hand over the mouth, stretching the eyelids, performed by a physically and intellectually normal ten-year-old boy who was badly spoiled. He had been raised with the notion that he was doomed to inherit St. Vitus's dance from a maternal aunt who had had it for three months at the age of nineteen and "was cured by getting married." Any of his movements was immediately interpreted as a "threat of St. Vitus's dance." The parents were completely dominated by him, since they felt that crossing him would hasten the arrival of the expected disease. His father had the habit of "twisting his mouth and nose," but to this, strangely enough, no significance was ever attached by himself or the family; nor did anyone in the home think anything of the father's occasional stuttering.

Wringing the hands, pulling the hair, turning the ring around the finger, nailbiting, pulling at the clothes, general restlessness in daytime and during sleep, headaches, irritability, and feeding difficulties in a thirteen-year-old girl who was handicapped physically by a congenital dislocation of her right hip, intellectually by a mental level of less than nine years and school requirements far above that level, and environmentally by a nagging, excitable mother who had an exophthalmic goiter. Proper school and home adjustment and orthopedic treatment improved the child in many ways and reduced her manipulations considerably.

CHAPTER XXXVI

FAULTY FEEDING HABITS

FAULTY feeding habits are among the most frequent complaints with which physicians, parents, and anyone else dealing with children is confronted. Twenty per cent of the patients referred to us for psychiatric consultation offered feeding difficulties. All ages and all degrees of intelligence were represented.

It seems convenient to divide the complaints of habit disorders connected with eating into the following groups:

Faulty table manners.

Ravenous appetite.

Perverted appetite.

Lack of appetite.

Gagging and vomiting.

FAULTY TABLE MANNERS

Children fail to acquire adequate table manners either because they cannot be trained, or, if they can, because they have not been trained.

The imbecile and idiotic child cannot be expected to learn how to use a spoon or fork at the same age as an individual of higher intelligence. It would, as a matter of fact, be dangerous to intrust him with tools which may imperil him or others. We have had an opportunity to quote elsewhere the example of the feebleminded boy who stuck a paring knife into his eye, which had to be eventually enucleated, and of the retarded boy who cut up his baby brother's face with a kitchen knife. It is essential to guard a child against the unsupervised handling of forks, knives, glasses, or breakable dishes until he has been found capable of avoiding the dangers that are connected with their use.

In the same type of children, it may also take a long time before the food, once in the oral cavity, will be chewed and swallowed, without being kept in the mouth almost indefinitely or spilled over the clothes or on the floor together with a large amount of saliva.

In another group, it is the oversolicitous or the indifferent parents who have failed to establish proper eating manners in the child. There are mothers who nurse their infants for one and a half to two years or even longer, or feed them from the bottle for as long as the fourth or fifth year of life. The normal task of domestic socialization is thus unnecessarily and unduly delayed. Others keep spoonfeeding their children for an abnormally protracted period, keeping them in this manner dependent on adults in their elementary social functions. In such cases, the delayed weaning of the child from parental assistance usually shows itself also with regard to clothing and elimination.

RAVENOUS APPETITE

Some feebleminded individuals, persons with general paresis, and retarded epileptics are known to have enormous appetites. The increased nutritional needs of rapidly growing children and adolescents do not constitute a psychiatric problem, nor does the casual overeating at a party or during holidays, with or without subsequent gastro-intestinal upsets. Occasionally, the destitute economic situation of the family induces a parent to bring her offspring with the complaint of "eating too much," at any rate, more than the meager budget can stand.

PERVERTED APPETITE

The complaint, not so rarely as is sometimes assumed, centers around the fact that the little patients eat everything they pick up from the floor, dirt, polish, even feces, that they scrape paint off the walls and furniture and put it into their mouths, that they swallow hair and wool and cotton, etc. These actions are usually referred to as *perverted appetite*, or *pica* (from the Latin name of the magpie), or "a craving for unnatural articles of food." They are compared to the unusual appetences of some pregnant women and to the geophagism of certain savage tribes. But the analysis of any number of cases convinces one easily that we deal here with an entirely different reaction. In pregnancy, the desire for unusual food exists during the period of gestation only; it is a demand for some very definite things; there is discomfort if the appetite is not satisfied. In geophagy, we deal with an established tribal custom; it consists of the ingestion of certain kinds of clay found in the banks of rivers.

Both in pregnancy and geophagy, the "perverted appetite" is highly discriminative. In children, this is not the case. Between the ages of four and nine or ten months, the normal infant has a tendency, which may be referred to as physiological, to put his hand to the mouth. Generally, this reaction loses in frequency and intensity at the end of the first year. In the developmentally retarded child, it may persist much longer. During this period and also some time after, children, especially when they are hungry, convey to their oral cavities any objects which they may have in their hands, whether it is a cracker, or a spoon, or a toy. If the object is too heavy or cannot be grasped with the hand, such as the bed or the play yard, the Mohammed-mountain principle is applied; the infant brings his mouth close to the object and licks or, in the case of clothing or bibs or blankets, sucks at it. It is a matter of training to wean a child from these habits. They are sometimes encouraged, fortunately to a limited extent, by the superstitious notion that dentition is facilitated by chewing on hard objects, such as keys, rings, or wood. On the other hand, if the practice of introducing things into the mouth or licking at things indiscriminately is grossly neglected and the children are not sufficiently supervised, the habit may assume the proportions of a routine performance which is, rather falsely, designated as a "craving." If it were a craving, it would not promptly disappear, without any sign of discomfort, as soon as adequate supervision and training are established. Its occurrence is in most instances an indication of faulty habit training. In many cases, it is one of several expressions of serious developmental retardation. If the objects are small enough, they are swallowed; if they are too large for that, they are either chewed, or licked, or sucked. In the house, it is usually the furniture, the doors, the window sills, paper, wall paper, plaster, buttons, strings, hair, soap, shoe polish, enamel ware, clothes, rugs, cotton, wool, etc., that are eaten or gnawed. On the outside, the child may pick up dirt, sand, bugs, worms, leaves, splinters, pebbles, and put them into his mouth. The objects eaten are the objects accessible; accessibility, and not "craving" or "appetite," governs their selection.

Aside from the aesthetic and educational significance of this habit, it has been known to be one of the most common etiological factors in the causation of lead intoxication during the first two or three years of life. Accumulation in the colon of hair and threads and rags has, on rare occasions, resulted in intestinal obstruction. Constipation is a frequent feature, owing, at least in part, to the type of substances ingested. Because of parental neglect, without which the practice would hardly have become a habit, most of these children are fed improperly and irregularly and suffer from nutritional anemia.

The reaction can always be prevented by adequate supervision and training. Judicious management is also the best mode of treatment; it has proved successful in every case in which it could be arranged. When it cannot be obtained in the home, it is necessary to change the patient's environment, in order to establish better habits and to preclude saturnism and serious nutritional disturbances. Mechanical restraint is a poor substitute, rarely effective beyond the period of its employment, and offers to the parents an excuse for the continuation of their carelessness or overindulgence.

In the following, we quote a few examples from the Harriet Lane Home material:

"Pica" in children

Number, Sex, Age	Substances eaten or gnawed	Additional facts
1. M. 3 yrs. 4 mos.	Anything found on the floor or grounds: dirt, sand, rags, splinters.	Developmentally retarded epileptic child.
2. F. 2 yrs. 1 mo.	Dirt and sand; often vomits them.	Fed irregularly and inadequately from birth. Severe attacks of gastric pain. Chronic constipation; once had a convulsion after being given castor oil. Clinical symptoms of lead poisoning.
3. F. 4 yrs. 10 mos.	Dirt. Onset at one year. Talked to and whipped with little effect.	Child has had diphtheria, scarlet fever and influenza. Positive tuberculin. Constipated. Badly spoiled. Very cross and fretful.
4. F. 1 yr. 11 mos. (Negress)	Dirt, coal, ashes, sand, plaster "on all occasions." Onset at 15 months.	Serious developmental retardation. Cyanotic at birth. First tooth at 18 months. Just beginning to stand up. Does not talk. Fontanelles not quite closed. Hemorrhoids. Constipation. Only child. Very restless.

"Pica" in children

Number, Sex, Age	Substances eaten or gnawed	Additional facts
5. M. 2 yrs. 4 mos.	Dirt "with apparent relish." Refused regular food.	Died at 2 years and 5 months after operation for renal sarcoma.
6. M. 2 yrs. 4 mos.	Everything he gets hold of, esp. paints and match heads. Refuses all regular food except milk.	Developmental retardation.
7. M. 2 yrs. (Negro)	Wood, furniture, paint on doors, chairs, and enamel, shoe strings, hair.	Only child. He had diphtheria, pertussis, acute otitis media, tonsillitis, rhinopharyngitis. Developmental retardation. Constipation.
8. M. 1 yr. 11 mos.	Everything "that contains paint"; chews on wood. Has a ravenous appetite also for regular foods ("eats like a little pig").	Only child. Developmental retardation. Had acute gastro-intestinal indigestion, furunculosis, otitis media. Chronic tonsillitis. Frequent nausea and vomiting.
9. M. 2 yrs. 11 mos.	Plaster, wall paper, dresses. Once ate a small rubber mat.	Traumatic intracranial hemorrhage, with spastic paralysis of both legs, right arm, and right side of face. Serious developmental retardation. Only child. Constipation.
10. F. 2 yrs. 3 mos.	Paper, strings, sand.	Only child. Feeding has always been irregular. Constipation. Frequent colds. Weekly attacks of fever with vomiting.
11. F. 2 yrs. 8 mos. (Negress)	Dirt; plaster which she digs out of the walls. Very early onset.	Congenital lues. Serious developmental retardation. Undernourished. History of generalized convulsions, pertussis, varicella, otitis media. Secondary anemia. Extreme poverty of parents.
12. F. 1 yr. 7 mos.	Wood, paint, dirt, coal, stones, toys. Onset at 5 mos. Did not indulge while in convalescent home, but was soon removed by mother.	Only child (a brother died at six months of malnutrition). Undernourished; nutritional anemia. Refused food, vomited when forced or displeased. Had never been fed properly. Spoiled badly; aunt played piano, grandfather rang bell, mother spanked her when she was fed. Untrained in use of chair and toilet. Drank water out of bottle only. Cried and screamed. Father presented feeding problem and ate dirt in infancy. Mother had attacks of "nervous vomiting." Child had bilateral otitis media.
13. F. 2 yrs. 6 mos.	All kinds of filth from the garbage can; sticks. Did splendidly in convalescent home.	Badly neglected by the woman (not her mother) with whom her father lived. Malnutrition. Positive tuberculin. Slept with mother until the very day when she died of consumption. Enuresis. Fecal incontinence. Serious developmental retardation. History of diphtheria and scarlet fever.

"Pica" in children

Number, Sex, Age	Substances eaten or gnawed	Additional facts
14. F. 2 yrs. 7 mos.	"Everything," esp. paint and plaster. Onset at six months.	Only child. Constipation. Daily attacks of abdominal pain. Weekly attacks of fever. Abdomen frequently distended. History of one generalized convulsion.
15. F. 3 yrs. 1 mo.	Dirt, egg shells, paper, splinters. Chews on rubber heels and frying pans.	Breast fed for over two years. Chronic tonsillitis. Father alcoholic. Slept in one bed with both parents and two siblings. Vomited often, but only in presence of mother.
16. M. 4 yrs. 7 mos. (Negro)	Beads, strings, buttons, handkerchiefs, blankets, clothing. Refused to eat regular food for past eight months.	Adopted illegitimate only child. Serious mental retardation. Undernourished. Constant masturbation. Temper tantrums. Enuresis. Destructiveness. Paroxysms of laughter. Sleeplessness. Profuse nose bleeds. Marked scoliosis. Spina bifida. Rudimentary vertebra between twelfth thoracic and first lumbar. Small movable subcutaneous tumor over left parietal prominence. Rachitic rosary. Father unknown. Mother alcoholic.
17. F. 3 yrs. 6 mos.	Dirt. Onset at two years.	Chronic tonsillitis. Nutritional anemia. Bilateral otitis media. Deafness. Scabies. History of perinephritic abscess.
18. F. 2 yrs. 7 mos. (Negress)	"Variety of things," including dirt, card board, sticks, soap.	"Born with caul." Genu valgum. Pin worms. Frequent abdominal pain, treated with peppermint.
19. M. 1 yr. 8 mos.	Dirt; tears off the wall paper and eats plaster. Prefers plaster to candy or other food.	Youngest of nine children. Badly spoiled. Slight developmental retardation. Nutritional anemia. Mild rickets.
20. M. 1 yr. 10 mos.	"Everything he can get hold of," especially paint from toys, bed, and furniture. Ceased "when not given a chance," but remains a feeding problem.	Spoiled only child, fed irregularly and inadequately, chiefly on sweets. Constipation. Sleeplessness. Chronic tonsillitis.
21. F. 2 yrs. 3 mos.	Window sills, doors, beds, furniture, wall plaster, rugs, thread, clothing. Ceased promptly when placed in suitable boarding home.	Greatly emaciated, fretful, irritable. Constipation (receives enema daily). Developmental retardation. Unexplained glycosuria. History of acute gastro-intestinal indigestion, bronchitis, otitis media. Slight rickets. Utterly neglected by aunt who "raised her."
22. F. 2 yrs. 1 mo.	Wall paper, newspapers.	Nutritional anemia, weakness, crying spells. Spoiled only child. Since age of six months, was given sweetened foods only, demands sugar in her water.

"Pica" in children

Number, Sex, Age	Substances eaten or gnawed	Additional facts
23. M. 2 yrs. 2 mos.	Sticks, bugs, "anything." Ceased when mother, who had been working out, remarried and stayed at home.	Only child. Yelling spells. Serious developmental retardation. History of otitis media, pharyngitis, measles, diarrhea, diphtheria with intubation.
24. M. 3 yrs. 5 mos.	Dirt, polish, feces. "Ravenous appetite" for all foods.	Idiot. Only child, badly spoiled by feeble-minded parents. Enuresis, fecal incontinence. Thumbsucking. Crying spells. Undernourished.
25. F. 2 yrs. 11 mos.	Picks up everything from the floor and eats it. Used to eat plaster off the walls.	Spoiled only child. Screaming spells. Hair-pulling. Headbanging. Night terrors. Vomiting spells. Slight developmental retardation. Father psychotic. Extreme poverty.
26. M. 3 yrs. 3 mos.	Has been nibbling paint for a long time, demolished the porch railing, and "eaten up" the window screens.	Encephalopathy from lead poisoning.
27. F. 3 yrs. 5 mos. (Negress)	"Everything within reach," plaster, paint, paper, dirt, coal, ashes.	Badly mismanaged. Constipation. Vomiting spells. Attacks of abdominal pain. Severe developmental retardation. Saturnism. Lead encephalitis.
28. M. 2 yrs.	"All kinds of things," chairs, doors, oil cloth, rugs, clothes.	A brother died of lead poisoning from eating paint off furniture. History of summer complaint and appendectomy. Child died of lead poisoning with encephalopathy. Autopsy: Cloudy swelling of viscera; general thymico-lymphatic hyperplasia, with necrosis in germinal centers; chronic fibrous perisplenitis and pleurisy.
29. F. 2 yrs. 2 mos. (Negress)	Paint off the window sill and toys.	Tetany. Serious developmental retardation. Died of lead encephalitis.
30. M. 3 yrs. 3 mos.	Dirt, polish, furniture, crib, doors, buttons, clothes.	Badly mismanaged, given strong tea and coffee, fed cake, candy, and ice cream. Lead intoxication with encephalopathy.

If, in non-idiotic children, dirt eating persists after the fourth year of life, it must be regarded as a prognostically ominous phenomenon, especially if it is limited to the practice of *coprophagia* (eating of feces). Of several cases, which have come to our attention at the Harriet Lane Home, one is especially instructive:

Herman R., a negro boy, was brought to the clinic by an aunt with the complaints of odd behavior, truancy, masturbation since the age of two years (of which he openly boasted as "milking the cow"), temper tantrums, disobedience, forgetfulness, sexual advances to boys and girls, constant fighting, enuresis, fecal incontinence (every night), cruelty to children and to animals, and eating dirt. He played with his own feces. "He will mix salt with all kinds of dirt and fry it and eat it. If you give him milk, he will fry dirt from dogs and put it in. If you give him bread, he will put some dirt on it first." Herman is the product of an alcoholic and psychotic father, who is now in a State Hospital for the Insane, and a mother who spent the last 19 years of her life in a mental institution. Herman was conceived in a State Hospital, while the father visited his sick wife. The number of his siblings is not known. A sister, now 27 years old, spent four years in a girls' reformatory to which she had been committed by the Juvenile Court; she had periods of depression in which she attempted suicide. A brother, 19, was in jail for stealing. Herman lived with two feebleminded uncles, who whipped him brutally. He was mentally retarded (baseline of four years, mental age below six years); his chronological age was not known, he was probably between nine and ten years old. He had been told that his mother, on her deathbed, had said that she knew the boy was crazy and that she would come to see him every night; he woke up at night, "hollering," then went always to the same corner of the room and hugged the corner and said he could see his mother. This child was definitely in need of institutional training and supervision.

LACK OF APPETITE

The Complaint. The vast majority of children presenting feeding problems is brought to the clinic with the complaint, in an endless variety of forms, of lack of appetite. In medical terminology, it is often designated as "anorexia," and sometimes the adjective "nervosa" is added to indicate the absence of demonstrable physical factors which might be responsible for the child's reaction.

In the following, we present a selection of the mothers' complaints with regard to the eating habits of their children:

"I do not think she eats as she ought to. She won't eat cereals, except if it is cornflakes. She never gets tired of meat. When she does not eat at meal time, she gets something between meals. If she does not get it, she gets in such a nervous tension, that I give it to her to quiet my nerves, just as much as I give it to her to quiet her nerves."

"She does not eat very well. When she does not, I prepare special food for her."

"She had a chronic colitis for years and developed very bad habits of eating. The doctor told us to force her to eat, and when we tried to force her, she has developed the habit of saying 'No!' to everything."

"She does not eat well. She wants it, and when she gets it, she'll just take a few bites and turn it over to the other children to eat."

"He does not want to eat; everything has to be forced. When he sees food, he runs. I get it down him with force. He never feeds himself and always has to be forced. Up until last summer, he used to vomit frequently. Every meal it is the same thing, and he does not like any food. He has to be threatened and often whipped. If his mind can be kept off his food, he will eat; I have to read him stories when he eats no matter how hungry he may be."

"He has always been particular about his food. He eats raw vegetables (potatoes, carrots), but not meat or cooked vegetables. He only eats one kind of ice cream (chocolate) and only certain kinds of candy. He gags very easily and often vomits when I brush his teeth for him; he always does that unless a particular kind of toothpaste (Calodont) is used. He also vomits if he is near anyone who chews gum."

"She has always been a feeding problem. She has a craving for sweet stuff, but would not eat fruit or vegetables. The only fruit she will eat is orange but I have to strain the juice carefully so that no pulp would get in."

"Lack of appetite. He has never eaten properly. I tried to plead with him, to beg him. I tried to punish him, and that did not work. If I try to force him to eat he just gets stubborn. He does like corn cakes, lollypops, and ice cream; he gets those between meals."

"My husband has to force her to eat by holding her head and nose."

"He is a poor eater. There are only a few things that he would eat. He only eats warm bread and butter, but not cold bread and butter, unless it is toast."

"She drinks milk only when I put vanilla in it. She does not like tomatoes when I give them to her, but she gets up in the middle of the night and asks for tomatoes, and then she cannot get enough of them."

"He does not eat large meals. He has a tendency to be particular about his food. We sent him to camp last summer, and there they did not even notice he was there; he behaved so well and ate everything."

As is easily seen in a number of these examples as well as in many cases which come almost daily to the physician's attention, the "lack of appetite" is often not really an anorexia in the sense of a physiological or physiopathological absence of the normal desire or liking for the usual foods. Nor is it so that certain things are refused because there is a "craving" for others. It is, of course, easy to assume that children like candy and other sweets because of a supposed hypoglycemia. Where there is clinical or laboratory evidence of a glycopenic condition, it doubtless needs careful attention. But the "craving" for candy in most cases is quite proportionate to the parents' propensity for coming across with nickels. One also occasionally hears mothers complain that their children have a "craving" for tea or coffee. It is further of interest to note in the reports the frequent recurrence of the term, "I have to . . ." It is almost typical to hear remarks, such as: "I have to force him"; "I have to coax him"; "I have to threaten him"; "I have to fight with him"; "I have to read stories to him to make him eat."

Causation. Refusal of food may arise from a considerable number of different situations, the most frequent of which are:

Physical discomfort.
Part manifestation of general resistiveness.
Part manifestation of a spoiled child reaction.
Reaction to overfeeding.
Imitation of parental reaction patterns.
Excitement.

Unhappiness.

Hypochondriasis.

Daydreaming and obsessive trends.

If a child who has never presented a feeding problem of a sudden loses his appetite, one must primarily think of the reaction as an early sign of some physical illness. It is a common observation that sick people do not eat as well as healthy people. Under these conditions, the anorexia is temporary and general. The sick child does not discriminate between hot bread and cold bread, between mashed potatoes and baked potatoes, between soft boiled eggs and scrambled eggs, or between milk served from a glass and milk served from a bottle. The more or less abrupt onset and the absence of "fussiness" serve as the best criteria for the determination as to whether we deal with poor appetite as an expression of physical discomfort or with a habit disorder.

In a large number of instances, the refusal to eat is one of several expressions of general resistiveness in the child. We have pointed out that almost every child goes through a period of resistance, spitefulness, or "negativism." In addition to the feeding problem, we find that children belonging in this group also refuse to go to bed at night and to dress in the morning and that they are reported to be contrary, uncoöperative, disobedient, and to say, "No!" to everything.

In the greatest percentage of cases, it is the spoiled, overprotected child who is brought with the complaint of being "fussy," "finicky," "choicy," or "particular" about his food. The faulty habits of eating are the result of, and maintained by, parental mismanagement. The child is made to occupy the center of attention in the home. There is hardly any opportunity that lends itself better for this purpose than the customary three meals, during which the entire family is assembled around the dining table. The scene is rendered as dramatic as possible by constant admonitions, instructions, warnings, threats, comparison with others, coaxing, pleading, punishing, bribing, timing, and mechanical force. The child is urged to take a bite for father, another for mother, and so on, all through the family members; a great deal of ingenuity is spent on thinking up any number of persons, real or imaginary, for whom the youngster is to take another spoonful or morsel, including the President of the United States, Santa Claus, and Little Red Riding Hood. Stories are read or told in order to make Johnnie or Elsie eat. The piano is played, bells are rung, father makes faces, mother wrings her hands in despair, while auntie advises to leave the child alone. Only children and youngest children figure most prominently in this sort of arrangement, which one may find in the mansions of the rich and in the shacks of the poor alike. Special foods are prepared according to the child's prescriptions. The youngster, in turn, whines, gags, vomits, screams, fights, criticizes each dish, extorts promises and nickels, and thoroughly enjoys the entire performance.

Refusal to eat everything that is offered is not always due to the child's capriciousness. It is sometimes an understandable and not at all unjustified reaction to overfeeding or "stuffing." Popularization of the ideal weight charts is not infrequently the source of the practice of "throwing into the child" food *ad nauseam* and *ultra nauseam* in order to have him conform exactly to the standards of the weight chart. There are families, especially Jewish, Italian, and Southern United States families, that delight in plump children. If they do not live up to this expectation, they are fed rich cream and other fats. The average child will learn, to his advantage, to rebel first against the abnormal quantity, but later also, to his disadvantage, against any quantity.

Any child, but more especially the resistive, spoiled, or overfed child, may be initiated into faulty feeding habits by other members of the household who, because of real or hypochondriacal alimentary ailments, are particular about their own nutritional régime. The youngster finds a ready pattern which he imitates, until it becomes thoroughly a part of himself. In some cases, the child's feeding problem is in reality only a reproduction of the entire family's feeding problems.

That excitement may lessen the appetite, is an observation made in children as well as in adults. It is especially difficult to get the excited youngster away from some play in which he is entirely absorbed; father's shouting and whistling in vain for Junior to come to the table, with Junior paying not the slightest attention or even hiding, is an occurrence so common, that it is made use of frequently in the newspaper cartoons.

The same is true of general unhappiness or unusual tension. This may be due to a multitude of factors, such as constant nagging, family quarrels, being contrasted with a brother or sister, and school difficulties. The child who is not well adjusted in school and either dislikes or fears it will most frequently show his lack of appetite at breakfast. One often hears the complaint that children refuse their food and gag or vomit in the morning, whereas they offer no feeding difficulties for the rest of the day. Sometimes undue rush because of getting ready too late will have similar effects.

Refusal to eat, with or without the complaint of stomachache, may be met with as an expression of hypochondriacal trends. In these patients, we may expect to find any number and combination of other ailments which are usually copied from patterns seen in the environment.

There is, finally, a group of children, who are reported to eat very slowly, to "dawdle over their food." In some instances, this habit is a part manifestation of general slowness in all of the child's reactions, showing itself in dressing, in speech, and in play life as well. In others, it is a means of prolonging the pleasure which the youngster derives from occupying the center of the stage during meal periods. Occasionally, the child fails to keep on eating because he is preoccupied. He may so thoroughly indulge in daydreaming fancies that he has no interest in any activity which would interrupt his dreams. One must also think in this connection of the obsessive child who, during the meal as well as during play and during class hours, seems "absentminded" because his entire attention is taken up by his ruminative mode of thinking.

Forms. "Lack of appetite" may express itself in any variety of modes of behavior. The most typical and most frequently recurring forms are:

Refusal of practically all food.

Eating under certain conditions only (water from a bottle; telling stories; counting; in a certain place only; from a certain person only).

Eating small amounts at a time ("getting filled up quickly").

Making up between meals for food refused at meal time.

Eating too slowly.

Being "particular" about food; preferring some foods to others.

Onset. Eating at the proper age must be learned just as much as dressing or reading is learned at the opportune time. Many feeding problems begin when the child ceases to be taught properly. This may be accomplished by preserving for too long the arrangements which are necessary and correct at an earlier period but undesirable in later years. Or it may be due to ignorance, convenience, or neglect on the part of the parents. Often the difficulties are developed during the insufficiently understood and therefore not wisely managed period of resistance. Sometimes the first manifestations of "capricious" appetite coincide quite closely with the beginning of discrepancies between grade work requirements and the child's capacity or with the onset of other emotional strain. Special privileges and abolition of routine during an illness is in some instances sufficient to create in the patient the desire to make a habit of something which he has learned to enjoy better than the regular régime, entailing much less attention. One child had never presented any feeding difficulties until the whole family went to visit relatives in the country during the summer months; they disliked the food and criticized its quality and preparation among themselves. The patient took part in the condemnations and, when they returned, transferred this attitude to the home cooking, much to his parents' alarm. In a few instances, the trouble began when death in the near family from gastric carcinoma or gastric ulcer caused an oversolicitous mother to put the child on a "diet," lest "heredity" might harm him. In another instance, a child who had eaten well until the age of four years began to offer difficulties on the occasion of the arrival of a younger sister.

Prevention. Prophylactic measures for the avoidance of undesirable feeding habits presuppose a good knowledge of the child's physical condition, best obtained by means of periodic examinations; especially information about possibly existing idiosyncrasies for certain foods (eggs, strawberries, etc.), hernias, spastic colon, spastic pylorus, visceroptosis, and secretory anomalies; judicious management of any tendency to constipation; regularity of meals, both as to time and place; appetizing and well-balanced food served in clean containers on a clean table; wise guidance of the child during the period of resistance; establishment of adequate domestication at the time when the average child is expected to acquire it; knowledge of the quality and quantity of food which he may be normally required to consume; teaching good eating habits at the proper age; abstaining from the prolongation of breast, bottle, or spoon feeding beyond the period in which these methods are natural; avoidance of oversolicitude and overindulgence; unwillingness to criticize, discuss, or "pick at" foods in the child's presence; introduction of a brief period of rest between exciting play and the meal; ample time, so that the child would not be rushed unnecessarily; desisting from quarrels or other emotional scenes at least while the child is around; agreement between the adult members of the household as to his training; removal of any heavy strain from which he may suffer; treatment of daydreaming or obsessional thinking wherever they exist.

Treatment. When the faulty habits have already been more or less firmly established, a thorough physical examination must exclude the existence of gastro-intestinal disturbances and of any other illness. Wherever found, the discomfort must be alleviated. Idiosyncrasies must be properly treated. The parents must be instructed with regard to the desirable type and amount of nutrition. Where it is necessary, the situation should be modified in the sense of doing away with emotional upsets in the child's presence, with the practice of overfeeding, and with the many manifestations of overindulgence, oversolicitude, and overprotection. The child must be taught to understand that the parents' part consists solely in providing and preparing the food, whereas its consumption is the child's own concern just as much as theirs. This cannot be accomplished through the medium of sermons which, if at all comprehended, usually have only the effect of taking the place of the former "coaxing." It is best simply to put the food before the child at the regular meal time (and always in the same place) and then to withdraw; after thirty minutes the dishes should be removed without the slightest comment. No nourishment of any kind should be given between meals. It must be explained to the parents that there is no danger involved if the child misses one meal or two meals or even several meals, but that there is considerable danger in crippling the patient emotionally for life by permitting the coaxing, etc., to go on indefinitely. The habits of forcing or punishing the child should be entirely discarded. The case should be followed in short intervals. The social worker will be of definite help in visiting the home and helping the parents to carry out the instructions. Sometimes educational star charts may prove to be of benefit in the intelligent older child. Peculiar notions about "heredity" must be corrected. It is also essential to convince the mother that she does not "have to" do this or that trick in order to "make" her offspring eat. In those cases where she cannot be expected to exercise sufficient emotional self-control, it will be best to remove the youngster to a healthier environment until he has learned to establish good feeding habits and until, through continued instruction, the parents or the spoiling grandmother have been able to notice the results of adequate training in a suitable convalescent or foster home; it is then that often the most unreasonable and uncoöperative parents, convinced by the success, come to their senses.

Sometimes the child's own negativistic attitude has been utilized successfully in the treatment of his eating difficulties. Without receiving any food between meals, he is given at the regular meal time minimal quantities of the type of things which he likes best and equally small amounts of other foods. If he begins to ask for more of anything, the battle is often half won. He is then given another minimal portion. When he gets into the habit of asking for more, his favorite dishes are slowly replaced by other things which he has previously refused. Never should he be given an opportunity to notice the intention underlying this kind of régime, or he may immediately use it for his own purposes and revert to his former mode of behavior. The main purpose is to have the youngster derive as much pleasure from refusing to be satisfied with such small amounts as he has derived previously from refusing to accept any food at all.

GAGGING AND VOMITING

Habit disorders connected with feeding are often associated with gagging, or vomiting, or both. We have spoken elsewhere of the types of psychogenic vomiting which have no close relation to faulty nutritional practices. We, therefore, limit our attention in this place to the complaints of gagging, nausea, and vomiting coincident with so-called "nervous anorexia." Ejection of food occurred in a little more than one-third of our patients presented with feeding problems. It is most frequently a reaction to being forced to eat.

"Since the onset of school in September, the child has refused her breakfast. If she is forced into taking it, she immediately vomits and goes off to school. She refuses milk, and eats very little throughout the day." She had always been "coaxed" to eat, especially by her mother and grandmother. She was physically healthy and of high average intelligence. The setting was one of domestic friction between an irresponsible, shiftless father and a "nervous" mother, and of maternal oversolicitude.

"He does not eat. He throws up in school, also at home before going to school." This almost eight-year-old boy was an orphan, whose parents both died of tuberculosis. He had a positive tuberculin reaction and chronic tonsillitis. He was spoiled by his grandparents, who pitied his plight of being an orphan and were very solicitous. They thought that he had no appetite because "his stomach was so weak." He was highly intelligent.

"She has been sick a lot. She will get along with hospital people, and she will get along with the home doctor, but she won't get along with us. We can't make her eat. When we try to make her eat, she gags and vomits." Normally intelligent, eight-year-old, asthmatic daughter of an alcoholic father and a hypochondriacal mother. Spoiled by grandparents. She had crying spells, refused to go to bed, was afraid of the dark and of being alone, bit her fingernails, picked her nose, and had mild obsessive tendencies. Change of the domestic feeding régime did away with the gagging and vomiting.

The treatment of gagging and vomiting connected with faulty eating habits is essentially that of the feeding problem itself. It is of especial importance to explain to the parents and to the child, if he is old and intelligent enough to comprehend, the principles involved. After the physical investigation has made certain that organic disturbances are not responsible for the reaction, the parents' idea of underlying "ulcer" or "cancer" or "weak stomach" must be corrected and their unjustified alarm over the habit alleviated. Treatment of coincident somatic ailments, situational adjustment, and adequate training are imperative.

Emil K., 7 years and 3 months old, was referred for psychiatric consultation because of his vomiting. He was physically underdeveloped and had old rachitic deformities (enlargement of epiphyses; slight bowing of legs). His tonsils and adenoids were removed in early childhood. He had a mental age two years in advance of his chronological age; he had "skipped" two grades in school and brought excellent reports home. The father, an intelligent, kindly man, had always been oversolicitous about him. The mother, who was troubled with hay fever, was very precise in her manner and particular about every little detail. She worried considerably about

Emil, because of her conviction that something was wrong with his stomach; she was sure it was smaller than other children's stomachs and in some way different. The parents were very devoted to each other. Emil was their only child. His feeding difficulties began at the age of one year; he was taken to a hospital but after a few days removed against advice by his father, who did not agree with the ward régime. Since then, his mother always "had" to coax him to eat. He ate very slowly and put very little into his mouth at a time. He was dreamy and preoccupied while eating. If urged to hurry at all, he vomited. However, when there was some real necessity for hurrying, such as drinking milk quickly so that someone else could use the glass, he had no trouble. The mother felt that she must sit and direct the entire procedure, lest he might not have enough. He was given candy between meals when he asked for it. He was slow in dressing and in answering questions. He did not play well with other children: "He won't fight back or stand up for himself. He runs from boys of five or six years who tease him and chase him with a lasso. He plays usually with girls or with smaller boys or alone." He ran to his mother for protection when attacked by smaller children. It took several months to change the home management of the child. It was finally possible to convince the parents that the physical examination, which included a gastric analysis, had shown no abnormalities whatever and that the real difficulty consisted in the failure to establish proper habit training. The mother began to carry out the instructions given her at the clinic. Emil ceased to present a feeding problem, did not gag nor vomit, and gained weight. His mode of contact with other children also improved considerably. The mother, who had acquired confidence in physicians and medicine, decided, to her advantage, to undergo treatment of her hay fever.

CHAPTER XXXVII
SLEEP DISTURBANCES

SLEEP IS ONE of the primary vital necessities. No matter how widely the various theories of its causation, nature, and purpose may differ, they all agree on its basic significance in the economy of life. The regular alternation of wakefulness and sleep, coinciding with the cosmic succession of day and night, is one of the most fundamental and lawful expressions of psychobiological periodicity, being as conspicuous and showing as little variability as the sequence of growth, maturity, and involution, and the rhythm of the sex cycles. Serious disruptions or inversions of the natural arrangement are indicative of dangerous changes occurring within the organism. The knowledge and proper regulation of major and minor sleep disturbances is therefore not less important than that of the anomalies of nutrition and elimination.

The principal types of sleep disorders may best be divided into the following groups:

Insufficient and restless sleep.

Nightmares and night terrors.

Sleepwalking.

Excessive sleepiness and drowsiness.

Narcolepsy and cataplexy.

Inversion of the natural order of sleeping and waking.

INSUFFICIENT AND RESTLESS SLEEP

Insomnia and restless sleep in early infancy are mostly the result of bodily discomfort produced by hunger and thirst, wetness, indigestion, tightness of the diapers, cold, or excessive heat. The baby gives vent to his malaise through the medium of crying, which is maintained until adequate relief is given or until his restlessness has been ultimately conquered by the physiological need of sleep. Both in the infant and in the older child, any sort of physical illness may lead to conditions which by means of continuous irritation interfere with the required composure. The itching sensations of eczema or scabies, breathing difficulties due to adenoid vegetations or head colds, alimentary disorders, and pain arising from otitis media and other acute or subacute diseases may so influence the child that he either has difficulty in falling asleep or that he wakes up during the night or, if he does manage to sleep through, tosses about in his bed and does not in the morning have the feeling of freshness and vigor which is the natural effect of healthy sleep. The comparative dullness, irritability, and poor scholastic achievements of the adenoid mouthbreather are well known to school physicians; at least a portion of this reaction is based on those children's restlessness at night and consequent uneasiness in the classroom. The therapeutic approach to these types of inadequate sleep is self-evident. It rests on the removal of the primary etiological disorder.

354

Restless sleep may be evidenced by a number of reactions which may occur singly or in combinations. They are:

Jumping, tossing, jerking movements of a purposeless character. The child may just keep turning from one side to the other. Or he may suddenly draw up his legs, wave his arms, or make all sorts of motions without waking and without remembering anything about them in the morning.

Crying out and screaming in the sleep. It is often reported by the parents of children who are usually also hyperactive during the day.

Gritting or grinding of the teeth.

Waking easily and going to sleep again several times in the course of the night.

Talking in the sleep. This is much more common than is usually believed to be the case. Although Ziehen considers somniloquy as a symptom of a degenerative or hysterical constitution, it may be safely stated that a considerable percentage of children who are otherwise normal at one time or another talk during their sleep. The parents usually are unable to get the contents, since the speech is mostly indistinct and fragmentary. In other instances, the observers catch statements or exclamations which seem to indicate that the child lives over the experiences, mostly play situations, of the preceding day.

A more unusual form is that referred to as *jactatio capitis nocturna*. It consists of a rhythmical rolling of the head from side to side on the pillow, which occurs mostly in the hypnagogic state (that is, when the child is just about to fall asleep) and at times also after sleep has reached its maximal depth. In some cases, the movements take place only if the child in his sleep has assumed a certain position. Homburger thinks that their etiology and mechanism are similar to those of tics. The French, as a matter of fact, allude to the reaction sometimes as *tic de sommeil (sleep tic)*. It must not be confused with the habit of head banging which is seen occasionally in infants and in imbecile and idiotic children, who beat their heads more or less rhythmically against the walls of their beds while fully awake, either as a somewhat weird source of pleasure or as an expression of anger.

Moser recently described the occurrence of nocturnal head jerks in adults; they take place on lying down just prior to falling asleep. There may be only a few mild jerks, or two or several severe jerks, sometimes associated with an occasional tonic spasm of the abdominal muscles sufficiently vigorous to shake the bed. They are more apt to happen in men of advanced years.[1]

The *hypnalgias* which Oppenheim described in adults are occasionally, though very rarely, seen also in children. They consist of pains occurring during sleep only. Strauch reported a case of oneirogenic (that is, dream-determined) gastralgia with vomiting, which disappeared "on a merely suggestive medication with verbal assurance of cure."[2]

In the majority of our case material, insufficient or restless sleep was not

[1] Moser, W. The Nocturnal Head Jerk. Medical Journal and Record. 1932, 135, 222.

[2] Strauch, August. Sleep in Children and Its Disturbances. American Journal of Diseases of Children. 1919, 17, 118–139.

the chief complaint for which the children were taken to the clinic or referred for psychiatric consultation. Where bodily discomfort was not directly or indirectly responsible, the patients who jerk and jump and talk and cry in their sleep are usually children who are also restless, hyperactive, and easily excited during the day. The nocturnal fidgetiness appears as an attentuated continuation of the child's diurnal reaction tendencies. The treatment, therefore, instead of immediately taking refuge in hypnotics or sedatives, must attack the factors and situations which have driven the patient in the direction of hypermotility. In addition to physical causes, we may find general emotional and habit immaturity as the result of improper training. The youngster may be under a heavy strain by being expected to do better work in school than his capacity permits. Or the home setting exerts a disconcerting influence upon him. Hence, even though the tossing and somniloquy occur in the unconscious state of sleeping, only a study of the patient's total personality and environment will help us to make the proper plans for their relief by means of a satisfactory adjustment.

In dealing with children's sleeplessness, we cannot afford to omit a certain, not at all uncommon complaint of "insomnia" which really does not deserve this designation. Under insomnia, one usually understands the inability to sleep; this is rarely found in children unless they suffer from pain or itching which keeps them awake; occasionally obsessive trends or masturbatory fancies may have the same effect. But in the rank and file of "sleepless" children we are confronted with unwillingness rather than inability. We often find the sleep difficulty to be a part manifestation of general resistiveness and of a spoiled child reaction, based on faulty parental management. The youngster who "has to" be told stories and coaxed in order to take another sip of milk or another spoonful of spinach learns that the act of going to bed is another means of securing his mother's attention and gaining his wants. The problem may begin at an early age. At the very minute that the baby cries at night someone is sure to rush to the crib and to rock it, to pick him up and carry him about until he again is quiet, to take him into the parents' bed, or to turn on the light and dispense reassurances. These services, given voluntarily at first, may later be demanded persistently for many years. There are the children who wake in the middle of the night and call for mother "because they cannot sleep"; the mother goes to her offspring's bedroom and calms him or sits down near him or invites him to spend the rest of the night with her and, presto!, the insomnia is over. The time of retiring is frequently made as dramatic as the meal time with all the discussing, bribing, punishing, cajoling, and pleading attending each morsel. The child will not go to bed unless certain rituals are performed. Father must go upstairs with him and hold his hands until he has gone to sleep. Mother, grandmother, or sister must read to him. The door must be left open to make sure that he does not miss the arrival of any visitors. If any of these desires are not complied with, he either cries or "fusses" or runs about in the room if he does not go to the length of throwing a full-fledged temper tantrum. The parents, "for the sake of peace" or in fear of what the neighbors might say, ultimately give in, and the bedtime performances are kept up indefinitely. Other children are unwilling to retire under any circumstances. The histrionics begin as soon as the very word bed or sleep is mentioned. The discovery is made that part of the homework has been forgotten, or toilet sessions are unnecessarily interpolated or, when really needed, unduly protracted. The youngster pleads for "just ten more minutes" and, when they are granted, for "another ten minutes." Most of this time is taken up with haggling in which the child usually is the winner. When he finally withdraws, it is with the victorious feeling that he is bestowing a special favor upon his family. Thus we have three equally dramatic scenes, some or all of which may be enacted in the individual case, as part features of the spoiled child "insomnia":

Refusal to go to bed, with all sorts of argumentations, excuses, and delays.

Rituals, crying, calling, playing after the child has gone to bed.

Waking at night and calling for mother or father until the child has been "calmed" or taken into the parents' bed.

Drugs are decidedly out of place in the *treatment* of this type of "sleeplessness." Here, as everywhere else in medicine and in mental hygiene, prevention is at least as important as therapy. Many people are in the habit of punishing their children by putting them to bed, thus impressing upon their minds the wrong notion that the bed is something undesirable, a punitive measure, something he has good reasons to resent. This idea is often strengthened by the would-be educational method of locking naughty children in dark rooms or closets and creating or suggesting as a valid alibi the fear of the dark. Regularity of retiring and getting up is as necessary as regularity of feeding. If it is introduced at the very beginning, it becomes an integral portion of the child's habit equipment. At the moment of withdrawal, parental contact should be cut off completely, at least as far as the youngster's awareness of it is concerned. Adults should not brag in his presence about the late hours which they keep, nor should they speak of the wonderful time they had with their visitors after the child had retired. Many people are in the habit of "making themselves interesting" or inviting sympathy by complaining that they did not sleep a wink last night; if they receive the desired commiseration and are excused from this or that duty and given this or that privilege, the child finds a pattern which he thinks worthy of imitation. The youngster who is admonished to talk in whispers and walk on tiptoes because father takes his nap in a remote part of the house, will soon learn to use any noise as a pretext for not falling asleep and demand similar considerations for his own person. One should not, of course, expect a child to find the necessary tranquillity and composure in the midst of great ado and hilarity (many are the children who are taken to noisy parties and, when they are sleepy, left on a couch or davenport and then, in the small hours, picked up and driven home, shaken in the automobile, until they finally find their peace at home). On the other hand, if Junior learns to pay attention to any slightest noise, lying awake and listening to the crickets and frogs and the neighbors' late homecomings and the honking of automobiles in the street, he is more than likely to suffer from insomnia in later life.

After these difficulties have entrenched themselves, the treatment must begin with the fundamentals of habit training. It will include the methods of feeding and dressing and establishment of greater self-dependence as well. Sources of unusual excitement should be removed at least an hour before going to bed. Sending the child to sleep immediately after he comes in from play or in the middle of a lively party will make it difficult for him to exclude instantly all stimulations and preoccupations. Strict regularity should be maintained and insisted upon at any reasonable cost.

Sometimes parents complain that their children do not readily go to sleep when they have made them take protracted naps far beyond the time when they are really needed. The child simply cannot go to sleep early and may spend two or three hours in bed indulging in daydreams or discovering the unhealthy pleasures of masturbation.

NIGHTMARES AND NIGHT TERRORS

Both the *nightmare* (*ephialtes, incubus*) and *night terror* (*pavor nocturnus*) are nocturnal fear or fright reactions occurring during sleep. Both terms are are often used interchangeably, but they really designate two forms of behavior which differ in several respects. Neither of them is in any way harmful to the child, in the same sense that breathholding spells or hypochondriacal pains do not impair his health. But they are more or less drastic indications that something is wrong with the youngster and that it is his personality that is in need of psychiatric investigation and adjustment. The outstanding differences between nightmares and night terrors are enumerated in the following table.

Nightmare	Night Terror
1. Fearful sleep experience after which the child wakes. The fear may persist for a while, giving way to good orientation and clear realization.	1. Fearful experience taking place in the sleep or in a somnolent twilight state, not followed by waking.
2. Slight defense movements or moaning immediately before waking are the only noticeable activities.	2. The features are distorted and express terror. The eyes stare, wide open. The child sits up in bed or even jumps to the floor in great agitation, runs helplessly about, clutches at persons or objects, cries out that someone is after him, implores an imaginary dog or burglar to leave him alone, shouts for help, or screams inarticulately.
3. The child is already awake when the parents notice his distress and, after he has been calmed, is able to give a coherent account of what has happened.	3. The child, sleeping through the episode, is unable to give any account of his distress which he is living out in all details while the parents look on and infer from his shouts and actions only what might go on within the child. The attack cannot be cut short by any amount of calming and reassurance.
4. The child, after waking, knows all the persons and objects of his surroundings.	4. The persons and objects of the environment are often not recognized and may be mistaken for others and woven into the dream content.
5. No hallucinations ever occur.	5. The child hallucinates the frightening dream objects into the room.

Nightmare	Night Terror
6. There is usually no perspiration.	6. The attack is usually accompanied by perspiration.
7. A long period of waking and conscious going over of the dream situation may follow.	7. Peaceful sleep instantly follows the termination of the reaction.
8. The entire episode rarely lasts longer than one or two minutes.	8. The terror may last for some time, up to fifteen or twenty minutes.
9. The contents are remembered more or less clearly. The incident itself is always recalled.	9. There is a complete amnesia for the contents as well as for the very occurrence of the episode.

We quote a few descriptions of night terrors given by the children's mothers:

"He doesn't sleep at all good. He has nightmares (nightmares and night terrors are often confused by lay people), hollers and runs all around. He is asleep while he has that and does not seem to remember anything later." A seven-year-old boy with migraine-like headaches, defective speech, and feeding difficulties, whose father was "shell,shocked" and was definitely psychotic and whose mother had migraine and a history of a "nervous breakdown." The child was intellectually retarded.

"About one half hour after retiring he cries and raves in his sleep for about ten minutes. He cries that the children are after him." Seven-year-old boy, who was a restless sleeper, had been crying at night for several years; his father deserted the family three years ago. Only child, spoiled a great deal and fed irregularly. Dental caries and chronic tonsillitis. I.Q. 88.

"He has had night terrors since the age of two years, cries about two hours after being put to bed. The cry sounds like he is terribly afraid. He does not remember the affair afterwards. When he was younger he used to get them four to five at night, now only when he runs around an awful lot or if he has a temperature. Last winter when he had the flu he had three attacks in one night. When he has the attacks he jumps out of bed. He grabs me around my neck, puts his feet around my body, and keeps crying for me, not realizing that I am right there." Eight-and-a-half-year-old boy, premature at eight months, with a history of many illnesses and several operations (herniotomy, circumcision, mastoidectomy, tonsillectomy). He had spina bifida. Emotionally immature, with hypochondriacal trends, psychogenic vomiting, nailbiting, and restlessness. He had always been a restless sleeper. His mother was easily excited; his younger sister was enuretic; a paternal cousin had a cerebral tumor. I.Q. 109.

"He has had night terrors for about two years. He has them from one every night to once in two or three weeks. He sits up in bed, looks very scared, tries to get out of bed, perspires heavily, and cries or screams. I sleep in the same bed and try to wake him as soon as he moves. When I try to quiet him he seems to want to get away but after a while he would calm down and go back to sleep." The father of this eight-year-old, badly spoiled, normally intelligent boy was schizophrenic and an inmate of a State Hospital; his mother was oversolicitous; his older brother wet the bed at fourteen years. Fear that the two boys might inherit the father's mental illness was uppermost in the minds of all members of the family. The child had hypertrophied tonsils and adenoids.

It is only incidental that the cases quoted all happen to be boys. One finds night terrors with equal frequency in girls. We like to contrast these descriptions of pavor nocturnus with the account of nightmares as given in the following instance:

A thirteen-year-old boy with astigmatism, dental caries, enlarged cervical glands, and a functional systolic murmur, slightly retarded in intelligence, of a fairly stable family, the only child of overambitious parents, had many fears, cried easily, had been fidgety all his life and especially since he began to go to school. He often woke up at night complaining of being afraid and reporting that he had just had a bad dream which frightened him. Something was coming after him, cats grew larger and larger until they seemed like elephants, or a huge ball was rolling towards him increasing in size as it came nearer. He would give a vivid picture of what had happened in the dream and was easily reassured. It would, however, take some time before he went to sleep again. The incident roused his interest and he would keep discussing it with his mother asking questions about the nature and prophetic meaning of dreams.

In conformity with the prevailing trends in medicine, different factors were named at different times as the uniform *causes* of night terrors. They have been ascribed to carbon dioxide intoxication on the basis of breathing disturbances due to adenoid vegetations. All children with pavor nocturnus were declared to be epileptics. Other authors speak of night terrors as hysterical reactions. Still others feel that observation of parental intercourse is a strong factor in their causation. Recently the theory has been advanced that they are brought about by a hypoglycemic state and should be treated by large doses of dextrose. The majority of patients with night terrors certainly display no evidence of an epileptic nature. How many hysterical children are subject to the pavor attacks will, of course, depend upon one's conception of hysteria. If one postulates that night terrors are hysterical "symptoms," then there is no other inference possible than the one that all children who have these symptoms are hysterical. Hypertrophy of the tonsils and adenoids are not less common in children with terrors than in any other group of children. As to the effect of witnessing parental sex relations, there are doubtless cases in which the patients have slept in the parents' bedroom and had opportunity to see intimate marital situations. But there also exist many equally doubtless cases in which the sleeping arrangements have definitely precluded such experiences. It is further difficult to be too positive about the exact causal relationship between those observations and the night terrors.

Wherever, in children with or without pavor nocturnus, one finds a glycopenic condition or adenoid growths or unsatisfactory sleeping arrangements, they should unquestionably be remedied. But attention must also be paid to other difficulties of the child's personality of a physical, constitutional, emotional, intellectual, or environmental nature. It is also interesting to note that often night terrors are linked with other sleep disturbances, such as restlessness, somniloquence and crying out in the sleep.

Night terrors rarely occur beyond the age of puberty. In later years, especially in the period of adolescence, nightmares predominate among the frightful sleep experiences.

Fear reactions, completely analogous to night terrors, occur sometimes, though very infrequently, during the afternoon nap. They are then referred to as day terrors, or pavor diurnus. They are reported to happen particularly if the child falls asleep in an uncomfortable position on the davenport, on the hard floor, or on a wooden bench.

SLEEPWALKING

It is only natural that folklore should dwell with great predilection upon *sleepwalking*, or *somnambulism*, and attach mysterious significance to it; it is usually believed to be caused by the influence of the full moon shining on the sleeping child, especially at the time before the closure of the fontanelles. All sorts of impossible activities are ascribed to the somnambulist; he is supposed to have the ability to walk securely on ropes and narrow planks, to climb high walls, and even to decipher letters through closed and not transparent envelopes.

Sleepwalking is nothing more than an enacted dream. In a way, as we have mentioned, there may be a certain amount of walking, or rather agitated running about, in connection with night terrors. Sometimes the parents' report that the child walks in his sleep must later be revised as really describing an attack of pavor nocturnus. A mother complained that her eight-year-old daughter (who also had occasional anxiety attacks) "walks in her sleep most every night; she began to do that about a year ago"; she went on to state that the girl was extremely frightened, jumped out of her bed, and screamed that someone was after her. There are certain features that sleepwalking shares with night terrors; in both cases consciousness is clouded, the child does not wake from his sleep, and there is an amnesia for the episode, except that the activities during somnabulism are sometimes remembered as the contents of a dream the motor enactment of which, however, is not recalled. The outstanding difference between the two reactions is that in night terrors there is physiognomic and often verbal evidence of terror, whereas in sleepwalking the motions are carried out without any display of affect and have a more purposive appearance. The eyes are mostly held open, the gait is somewhat unsteady and swaying. The child leaves his bed slowly and seems to have a definite goal. The senses are blunted, excepting that of equilibrium and locomotion. The patient usually avoids obstacles, though occasionally he may stumble over a carpet or run against a piece of furniture. The activities may be limited to walking, jumping, or climbing, but often they are much more complicated. The dangers have undoubtedly been exaggerated, though at times the child gets into hazardous situations; he may risk falling or jumping down the stairs or the roof, walk out into the street on a cold night, scantily clad, or even in very rare instances set fire to the house.

Lydia C., ten years and seven months old, had always been restless in her sleep; she was in the habit of rolling her head at night; she had occasional nightmares. She began to walk in her sleep at the age of six years, soon after she had been entered in school. She usually got up quietly, walked to an adjoining room, mostly the kitchen, and then went back to bed. On one occasion, while trying to go into the cellar, she fell down a whole flight of stairs. She was slightly retarded in intelligence (I.Q. 88). She bit her finger nails. She had chronic pyelitis and nycturia, once or twice each night. She came of an unstable family. Her father complained of a "bad heart," though upon examination he was found to be healthy. Her brother was feebleminded and "nervous." One sister was enuretic. Another sister, sexually promiscuous at thirteen, was committed to a correctional institution by the juvenile court. Both paternal grandparents were alcoholic, the grandmother was burnt to death through her own negligence. Her mother was easily excited and had "nervous headaches." The maternal grandfather, alcoholic, was killed by a taxicab. A paternal uncle died in a State Hospital of an organic cerebral condition.

Dorothy B., eight years and eleven months, had a frightening experience at the age of seven years when she once went to the store and, on her way home, a stranger offered to carry her basket; she ran away and he followed her. Several months previously she had willingly submitted to intercourse with an older boy and contracted gonorrhea for which (for the gonorrhea, not for the intercourse) she was severely beaten by her mother. Shortly after the basket experience, she had measles with high fever and mild delirium. Three weeks after recovery, in the night before she was to take the first communion, she walked in her sleep for the first time. According to her mother, "she walked to the window and she might have killed herself. I asked her, 'Dorothy, where do you go?' and she said 'I am going home'." Once she went into the living room. At one time she was discovered standing at the foot of her bed. Twice she just sat up in her bed and then lay down after awhile and went back to sleep. There were six episodes altogether. The last time, "she sat up at night and I thought she was awake and I wanted to give her some argyrol drops in her nose, but she was asleep. She got up and walked in the kitchen and stood before the sink and then got back to bed." Occasionally she talked in her sleep; most of the time she would say "Let me go home! Let me go home!" These were the words that she had kept saying to the strange man who had followed her from the store. The child had a poor appetite. She was very restless. She had hypertrophied tonsils and adenoids. Her intelligence was normal. She sucked her thumb until the age of six years. Her father died of tuberculosis when she was not quite one year old. Her mother remarried. The stepfather, a drinker and "loafer," deserted the family soon after marriage and after laying the foundation for a child who now is in an institution for feebleminded children. One of her brothers was, at thirteen, in a boys' reformatory for burglary. Her mother was illiterate, uncoöperative, and hardly a fit person to raise children. Frequent changes of residence never took the family out of the slums. She was placed in a boarding home where she adjusted well and was soon rid of all of her behavior difficulties.

Myrtle R., aged eight years and six months, had dental caries and chronic tonsillitis. She was intellectually retarded (I.Q. 80, with a baseline of four years only). She was generally restless, fidgety, enuretic, talked and "kicked" in her sleep. About half a year ago, before the time of school promotion, she got up several times during the night and walked about the room. Somnambulism did not recur after her failure of promotion had become a certainty. Her parents were divorced when Myrtle was a few months old; her father, an ex-Navy man, disappeared and had never been heard from since then. Myrtle's older sister, aged nine, was enuretic, very stubborn, and presented a feeding problem.

The *treatment* of somnambulism will be governed essentially by the same considerations as that of nightmares and night terrors. Necessary precautions must be taken to prevent the sleepwalking child from injuries during the episode. Though serious accidents are relatively infrequent, they are known to have occurred (compare the incidence of falling down the stairs in the first case quoted, and walking to the window and almost dropping out in the second instance). Superstitious notions, so often connected with somnambulism, will have to be corrected.

EXCESSIVE SLEEPINESS AND DROWSINESS

The simplest form of increased sleepiness is that to which Ziehen refers as *Schlaftrunkenheit*. It is, according to him, "that peculiar state, preceding the acts of going to sleep or of definite waking, which in normal individuals lasts a short time only and is not accompanied by any actions worth mentioning. In pathologically predisposed persons it may last longer and give rise to complicated performances. Its twilight state character manifests itself in the fact that it is followed by amnesia. Hallucinations and delusions may occur. This pathological *Schlaftrunkenheit* becomes more frequent at puberty."[1] It hardly ever forms the subject of a complaint. It seems to be unusually rare in childhood.

Drowsiness and sleepiness during the day may be found in a large variety of conditions. It often exists in connection with high elevations of temperature. It may be the result of drugs, such as bromides and luminal, or remedies containing a high percentage of alcohol. It is met with in food intoxication and in acid intoxication, sometimes preceded by restlessness and insomnia. It is reported as a symptom of chronic intestinal indigestion, bacillus coli pyelitis, uremia, acute poliomyelitis, acute and subacute liver atrophy, and tuberculous meningitis. It is an outstanding feature in epidemic encephalitis. It follows epileptic and epileptiform convulsions and sometimes petit mal attacks. It may precede, or appear as a mild form of, stuporous and comatose states.

We have seen a considerable number of negro children who were brought to the clinic with the complaint that they spent a great deal of the day sleeping, without losing a minute of their night's sleep. They were physically healthy and intellectually retarded boys and, much less frequently, girls between eight and fifteen years of age. They were not particularly sleepy during the interview. They did not feel compelled to sleep but lay down at home for naps, securing comfortable positions. As far as could be ascertained, the children were very dull and had an extremely limited range of interests. They really did not care, nor did they often know, how to use their time to better advantage. We apparently deal here with a sleep habit, based on lack of interest in school work and home work and association with brighter children and in anything else. In most instances, both parents were out working during the day, or there was one parent only. There

---

[1] Ziehen, Theodor. Die Geisteskrankheiten, etc., im Kindesalter. Berlin. 1926 p. 348.

were little, if any, changes in the monotonous home atmosphere. So the children took to sleeping as a pastime.

NARCOLEPSY AND CATAPLEXY

Gélineau, in 1880, described under the name of *narcolepsy* a condition characterized by diurnal attacks of sleep, lasting from a few minutes to a quarter of an hour or a little more, initiated by a feeling of drowsiness and irresistible fatigue. During the episodes, the patients sleep normally; they are easily wakened, and sometimes there is a feeling of annoyance at being disturbed. They know that they are being overwhelmed by the desire to sleep and may try desperately to fight it, but mostly in vain. When the attack is over, they are usually fresh and wide awake at once. Narcoleptic sleep may, or may not, be accompanied by dreams as normal sleep, and their contents may, or may not, be remembered. The attacks may come at any time of the day, though the hours of the morning and around noon seem to be preferred. They may happen while the patient is resting or walking or in the midst of a conversation or driving an automobile. If he succeeds temporarily in overcoming his somnolence, he has a headache, and the final attack is of longer duration.

The sleep attack is one of two typical features of narcolepsy. The other consists of a peculiar loss of muscle tone upon any stronger emotion, or more selectively upon laughter or, less frequently, anger or fright. The patient experiences a sudden feeling of weakness, his arms sink down, his head falls on the chest, his lower jaw droops, and he collapses. Consciousness is usually not impaired. (On the other hand, the sleep attacks themselves may in some patients also be precipitated by emotions.) The reaction is referred to as *cataplexy*, affective loss of muscle tone (*affektiver Tonusverlust;* Redlich), or *Tonusblockade* (F. Stern), or *emotional asthenia* (Weech). Oppenheim, in 1902, described attacks of loss of consciousness of brief duration, following hearty laughter only, in individuals who are free from the narcoleptic episodes of somnolence; he called the condition *Lachschlag.* Homburger observed it in a fourteen-year-old girl.

Narcolepsy is very rare. About forty cases were reported up to 1926. Of thirty-five instances which Redlich collected from literature and from his own observation, the symptoms began in twenty-two between the ages of ten and twenty years. The only case in which the onset fell before the tenth year is that of an eight-year-old colored girl, published by Weech from the Harriet Lane Home; this communication merits especial attention for the additional reason that narcolepsy seems to be the prerogative of the male sex. It is, in the light of this fact, interesting to note that the above mentioned "sleep habit" of retarded negro children is also vastly predominant in boys.

Narcolepsy is a chronic condition and lasts many years. It makes no inroads on the patient's intelligence. Nocturnal sleep is normal and bears no relations to the frequency or duration of the diurnal episodes. Richter has shown that the electrical palm-to-palm resistance of the skin is unusually high during sleep and mostly not above 100,000 Ohms during the day; in narcolepsy it may remain as high as 400,000 Ohms in the periods of waking.

Very little is known about the *etiology*. "Genuine" narcolepsy has been contrasted with "symptomatic" somnolence. In the symptomatic attacks, which occur chiefly in epidemic encephalitis and further in brain tumors, epilepsy, and hysteria, the cataplectic component is absent.

Adie believes that "narcolepsy is primarily a disorder of an intimately connected endocrine-nervous mechanism, the pituitary 'tween-brain system I shall call it, that is formed by the pituitary body and certain vegetative centers in the base of the 'tween brain."[1]

Recently we had an opportunity to see a case of genuine narcolepsy, which was examined conjointly at the Harriet Lane Home and the Henry Phipps Psychiatric Clinic and in which the early onset was remarkable. Charles T., at the age of eight years and two months, was noticed to become drowsy in the late afternoon. Prior to that time, he had gone to bed at 8 P.M. and slept until 6 A.M., but now he could not keep himself awake at 6 P.M.; he went to bed and woke at 5 A.M. At times he fell asleep at supper, and once he had the same experience in school. His sleepiness came suddenly and it seemed impossible to keep him awake. Thyroid tablets and other glandular extracts had no effect on the condition. When he was excited or on being tickled, he felt a sudden weakness causing him to collapse. It is interesting that the boy's mother was similarly affected to a minor degree. Since the beginning of his somnolence, the parents noticed that he became somewhat irritable, that he started and talked in his nocturnal sleep, and that he gained ten pounds within five months. (His father weighed 125 pounds at the age of ten years.) He had always been slightly constipated and had for some time complained of occasional frontal headaches and of his eyes tiring in school. Examination by Dr. Terry Burger showed a somewhat obese, rather phlegmatic boy, who at first was apprehensive because he feared that an operation would be performed, but easily reassured and coöperative, submitting willingly to venae puncture. There was some glandular enlargement at the angles of the mandible. His hair was a bit dry but not coarse. He had many carious teeth. Thyroid isthmus was palpable. Optic fundi somewhat pale; remains of an old choroiditis on the temporal side of the left disc. Tonsils had been cleanly removed. There was marked tenderness in the intrascapular region over the spinal column. X-ray of the head showed no abnormalities. BMR: − 10. Wassermann reaction negative. His intelligence was normal (I.Q. 101).

[1] This is a list of some of the outstanding publications on narcolepsy:

Gélineau. De la narcolepsie. Gazette des hôpiteaux. 1880, 53, 626–628.

Oppenheim, H. Über Lachschlag. Monatsschrift für Psychiatrie und Neurologie. 1902, 11, 242.

Löwenfeld, L. Über Narkolepsie. Münchener medizinische Wochenschrift. 1902, 49, 1041.

Henneberg, R. Über genuine Narkolepsie. Neurologisches Centralblatt. 1916, 35, 282.

Redlich, E. Über Narkolepsie. Zeitschrift für die gesamte Neurologie und Psychiatrie. 1926, 32, 672.

Weech, A. A. Narcolepsy—A Symptom Complex. American Journal of Diseases of Children. 1926, 32, 672.

Adie, W. J. Idiopathic Narcolepsy: A Disease Sui Generis; With Remarks on the Mechanism of Sleep. Brain. 1926, 49, 258.

Richter, C. P. The Electrical Skin Resistance of the Body During Sleep. Proceedings of the National Academy of Science. 1926, 12, 214.

Ephedrin has been found to be helpful in the treatment of narcolepsy.

INVERSION OF THE NATURAL ORDER OF
SLEEPING AND WAKING

In children with epidemic encephalitis, one may find a reversal of the ordinary sleep curve. The patients stay awake during the night, until three to five o'clock in the morning, in which time they are very restless and behave queerly (whistle, sing, grind their teeth, run around the house, disturb and rearrange the bedding, etc.) They make up for the loss by sleeping soundly during parts of the day. This condition may last for weeks or months and then disappear gradually or more abruptly. In some cases, it may persist indefinitely.

CHAPTER XXXVIII
ANTISOCIAL TRENDS

Two or three decades ago, there might have been a heated debate as to whether medicine had anything to do with children's delinquencies. If they were trifling in their scope, the father's razor strap was deemed sufficient to cope with the problem; if they were more severe, confinement in jails or in reformatories was meted out as appropriate "punishment." The theft of a nickel was within the realm of parental discipline; the illegal abduction of a hundred dollars was a juridical affair. The physician was not in any way concerned, unless a medical diagnosis could be pinned on the child. Coëxisting epileptic, luetic, obviously imbecile, and hysterical conditions brought some of the delinquent youngsters to clinics or private offices where the epilepsy, lues, imbecility, or hysteria, but not the factors underlying the theft, truancy, burglary, or arson were studied and treated. Terms, such as *kleptomania* or *pyromania* usually exhausted the medical interest and wisdom with regard to repeated stealing or incendiarism of children who could not be labeled otherwise. More ambitious attempts to account for such actions of individuals who did not present any symptoms of the enumerated illnesses resulted in the assumption of a nosological entity, a "disease," which was termed *moral imbecility* or *moral insanity*. It was supposed to consist of a selective "ethical defect," a loss of the "power of conscience," with normal development of all other faculties. Already in 1819, Grohmann spoke of "ethical degeneration," and Prichard, in 1830, postulated a "morbid perversion of the feelings, affections, and active powers" as a characteristic feature. So eminent a psychiatrist as Kahlbaum went so far as to speculate on a "faulty development of the moral fiber systems." Lombroso's famous concept of the born criminal (*il delinquente nato*) gave an added impetus to the belief in the existence of moral insanity. The patients were said to be of normal intelligence; with the then rather crude methods of investigation, educational mismanagement was found to be absent, though no one seemed to notice that the report of frequent criminal tendencies, alcoholism, and psychotic reactions in the parents would tend to discredit such a statement. References to somatic "stigmata of degeneration" could not very well be missing in a period when the issue of degeneration was paramount in psychiatry and in criminology. A number of weighty authorities still hold fast to the concept of moral imbecility. Meggendorfer tried to bring the reaction into close relation to schizophrenia and coined the name of *parathymia* which, however, has not been generally accepted. The greater majority of investigators has declined to recognize such a specific condition (Maudsley, Leidesdorf, Krafft-Ebing, Naecke, Binswanger, Berze, and Ziehen, who in some cases still applies the designation of "normal ethical stunting").

The advent of the twentieth century has marked a considerable change in our study of crime; a sober turning away from theorizing on abstract "crime," from measuring the skulls and estimating the brain weights of murderers and prostitutes, and from classifications of groups was inaugurated in these United States of America by the pioneer work of William Healy and by the leaders of the mental hygiene movement. Individuals are now studied instead of imaginary diseases. The antisocial act is not taken as a *fait accompli* to be settled by vengeful retaliation in accordance with the severity of the misdemeanor. It is considered as an indication for an objective and dispassionate study of the personality development of the child who has committed the act. In the place of absolutistic evaluation of right and wrong and of considering the "law" as a rigid measuring rod, a more relativistic attitude is assumed, which attempts to view the act in the light of the child's make-up, his training, the environmental influences which acted upon him, the stratum from which he emerged, the general social structure, the standards prevailing in his home and among his associates, his motives and aims, the particular circumstances in which the misdeed was conceived and carried out, and his after-reactions. The act is dealt with as any other psychiatric complaint. All this is done in preparation for a constructive plan of adjusting the patient and of mapping out with him and for him a future in which the underlying difficulties would be remedied or, at any rate, his own attitude so modified that he would not be likely to react to them in an undesirable manner.

If we so analyze and treat antisocial behavior and antisocial trends, we are under no obligation to accept or create hypothetical diseases. In all our experience with delinquent children in a large psychiatric dispensary, in a much frequented pediatric clinic, and in a juvenile court before which several thousand cases are arraigned annually, we have failed to encounter one single boy or girl who could be classed as suffering from so-called "moral imbecility" or "moral insanity." This is so, not because this "disease" has spared our particular community or because we have missed the diagnosis, but because we have found in every instance a variety of combinations of factors at play, constitutional, intellectual, domestic, educational, gregarious, suggestive, imitative, and other factors which may work differently in different persons and which may, or may not, culminate in a criminal act. Besides, the rôle which opportunity plays in the beginning of many a habit of stealing, lying, or wandering away from home has not been sufficiently emphasized. Money lying around loose in the house with no one noticing the disappearance of small coins has often suggested the first thought of secretly appropriating pennies or nickels. Sending the child to stay with grandmother whenever his presence at home does not seem convenient has not infrequently caused the first experiment of adventurous wandering in the streets, since the parents believed the child to be at his grandmother's, while the grandmother thought he was at home. The initial success then invites further experimentation.

The commonest forms of children's antisocial behavior (sex delinquencies are discussed elsewhere) are:

Disrespect of authority.
Lying.
Stealing (larceny and burglary).
Cruelty.

Destructiveness.

Truancy from school.

Wandering away from home. Vagabondage.

DISRESPECT OF AUTHORITY. DISOBEDIENCE

No training is possible without certain rules laid down and enforced by those who have the experience and the task. The apprentice, the student, the soldier, the medical interne all receive their instructions by means of a system of regulations which they must follow in order to become themselves experts in their respective jobs. Child training is not thinkable without authoritative guidance by the natural instructors, the parents. Obedience on the part of the child is a necessary basis. But obedience is not something which the child either possesses or lacks *a priori*. It is a reaction to other people's orders or suggestions which must be taught and implanted in the youngster. It is logical that when the infant becomes old enough to sense his place in the family texture, the adults in the household, and especially the father and the mother, are recognized as the ones in command. They have always fed the baby, dressed him, put him on the chamber pot, taken him out for walks, and tucked him away in bed. After all these things have been done to him manually, some of them gradually begin to be done to him verbally, in the form of commands. Instead of being fed, he receives the food and is told to ingest it without assistance; he is told to go to the toilet alone. It is this slow change from manual handling to oral direction that marks the transition from the period of elementary socialization to that of domestic socialization. At this time it is relatively easy to establish obedience because the average child enjoys performing the functions which he is just acquiring and because he can learn from very simple experiences that failure to obey works out to his disadvantage.

Disobedience as an habitual response to parental orders may be ushered into the child's mode of behavior in a variety of ways:

Faulty management of the natural and physiological period of resistance or negativism, through which practically every average child passes for a longer or shorter time during the third or fourth year of his life. It is then that he discovers that he has a will of his own. Just as he derives pleasure from exercising any of his new acquisitions, he takes particular delight in practicing the novel function of willing or not willing something. He does, of course, not have a sufficient experiential background to be capable of discriminating between that which is or is not useful for him to will or between that which he is or is not expected to will. Thus his volition soon comes into conflict with that of his elders. For approximately two years, his passive submission has been taken for granted by everyone concerned. Now he has added to his reactive equipment the meaning and application of negation and tries it out to his heart's content, just as he likes to repeat over and over the recent additions to his vocabulary or as he has reveled in his first walking excursions through the rooms. The parents, who have not known the child to act in that manner before, find him "different," "resistant," "disobedient," "negativistic." If they disregard the petty and irrelevant "I won't" and "No, no, no" replies, at the same time insisting with gentle firmness on the more important matters of daily routine and habit regularity, the reaction rarely lasts more than a few months or a year. On the other hand, there are parents who argue with the tot and preach sermons to him or even beat him, thus introducing an element of controversy, of a power contest, in which the youngster, meanwhile growing older, is bent upon being the victor. He is no longer a disciple, duty-bound to accept instruction; his parents, through injudicious management during the period of resistance, have themselves brought in the element of debating and battling which may be perpetuated. They have erroneously assumed that the child, at that age, has reasoning faculties similar to their own. The other extreme is that of delaying any sort of guidance and "giving in" completely, with the false notion that the child is too young or too delicate to be steered into conforming with the parents' precepts or that his "cuteness" precludes firmness.

Inconsistency, based on thoughtlessness or moodiness or both, is another frequent source of disobedience. The child is not given an opportunity to find out what is desired and what is forbidden. To-day he may romp and run about without a word of disapproval; to-morrow, when father comes home tired from work or mother has a headache or grandmother takes a nap, he is scolded for the same activities which were tolerated the day before. To-day he is given an old mail order house catalogue and shown how to busy himself tearing out its pages; to-morrow he is reprimanded for treating the current issue of a magazine in the same manner. It does not occur to the mother or to the maid that the child is not capable of distinguishing between the two and consequently becomes confused about an attitude which to him must appear full of discrepancies.

Parental dissensions anent the training of the child are often a potent factor and probably the commonest origin of disobedience. If mother wishes to put him to bed, father, yielding to his remonstrances, pleads with her to let him stay up a little longer. If both of them refuse to give him a nickel, grandfather or a loving aunt produces the coin. If the one insists that he finish his spinach, the other sides with him and substitutes the desert for the repudiated dish. Divided authority is, of course, no authority. The child does not really disobey because he at the same time obeys the adult who holds the view agreeable to him. At the end, he does very much as he pleases because he has not been taught differently.

Excessive leniency has the same effect. A spoiled, overindulged child is simply not taught to obey. He learns to use crying spells, temper tantrums, and invented stomachaches as sure methods for obtaining his wants if he does not get them otherwise. The little girl who says, "I am going to scream," if mother does not comply, may later be the woman who goes into a faint if the new hat or coat is not forthcoming or threatens to jump out of the window if her husband wishes to give up the vacation trip. The youngster acquires a store of "tricks of the trade" to avoid obedience which, he knows, will not be enforced if he is persistent and tricky enough.

It has been a much discussed fashion in recent years to let the child "assert his individuality" by not interfering with his actions. We hear of youngsters being reared by parents who would not say, "No," to them. This may be all right with some children and harmful to others. It depends to a large extent on the "individuality" which is to assert itself. As a preparation for adult life,—and all training is such a preparation,—the wisdom of such a procedure must be questioned. Every person must meet reasonable (and, often enough unreasonable) restrictions and limitations and learn how to adjust himself to them.

Excessive sternness, trying to obtain submission through the instillation of fear, fails to impress upon the child's mind the justice of the commands, creates meekness and timidity, or spitefulness, or sneaky practices offsetting superficial and seeming compliance, and turns the home into a place of unhappiness and dread. The result is pseudo-obedience which is looked upon as a burden to be thrown off in the absence of the parents or at a future time.

Disobedience is not always a sign of undesirable behavior. The child has a right to resent *unreasonable orders*. He should have a right to dodge the all too frequent osculations of an unshaven uncle or an aunt with halitosis. A normal youngster cannot be expected to "sit still" or "keep quiet" for hours so that father may concentrate on his mystery story or that mother may uninterruptedly discuss the servant question with her visitor. If the mother is too embarrassed to return a cracked egg or a supposedly shortweighted meat order to the grocer's, she should not unload the burden on a sensitive child.

Unreasonable orders are particularly apt to come from what Plant justly calls *unreasonable authority*. So ancient and concise a code of ethics as the decalogue, instead of enjoining obedience, asks the people to honor their parents. Disrespect is not conducive to wilful and intelligent compliance with the precepts of a contemned person. A child who rightly evades the illogical or unfulfillable or outright harmful orders of a drunken father or raging mother or hostile stepmother will sooner or later come to disregard any instruction issuing from those sources. Rigid adhesion to "old country" standards may cause a similar clash in the offspring of immigrant families. So may religious or social narrow-mindedness or fanaticism.

Once the respect of authority has been shattered in the home, the resulting disobedience may be transferred to other authority as well. It may lead to disregard of the teacher's instructions and to impudence in school or even, especially if examples are furnished by the family or the neighborhood, to defiance of legal authority. It is, of course, understood that not all children who are spoiled or too strictly disciplined or otherwise mismanaged are necessarily disobedient. Much will depend on the youngster's own personality make-up which must be studied in each instance, on his health, on his intelligence, the degree of his emotional stability, healthy or unhealthy outside influences, and any number of other factors.

The prevention of disobedience consists in the avoidance of the etiological features enumerated above. The treatment will concern itself with their correction through work with the patient and with his family. Uniformity and consistency of discipline with abstinence from extremes and full parental agreement with regard to policies will be advised. The parents should be urged to give reasonable commands only and to insist on their fulfilment. This should be done in a manner which makes the child realize that it is to his advantage to obey. Bribes and threats should not be employed. But after the child has failed to obey, it is in order to deprive him temporarily of some privileges which he enjoys. On the other hand, good behavior should be acknowledged and rewarded.

Objectionable modes of securing discipline should be discouraged. Corporal punishment has been abolished in the school, in the army, and (it is hoped) in the prisons; the "third degree" method used sometimes by the police deserves public condemnation. But many parents still have the attitude that their children are their property and that they are entitled to beat them as often and as severely as they wish. They work with hands, brushes, and razor straps. The teacher, the psychiatrist, and the pediatrician are often approached with the question whether or not children should be beaten. Whipping is usually a sign of limited educational resourcefulness. It is done either in anger, that is, at a time when the parent who wishes to control the child is not capable of controlling even himself or herself, or from a sense of misunderstood duty, often accompanied by such offsetting remarks as the one, "It hurts me more than it hurts you," and followed by excuses, apologies, regrets, and yielding in the end. A gentle tap as an expression of disapproval may be in order. Even an occasional (a very, very occasional) thrashing may sometimes serve the purpose, even though it is quite certain that better and equally effective measures are always available. But beating as a disciplinary habit may have a number of ill results. It may make the child afraid of his parents. It may put them in the wrong in the youngster's mind and create bitterness, spite, and a spirit of revenge. It may make the child callous and accustomed to the inflicted pain which is accepted as an inevitable aftermath of actions which the child does not think of giving up. It is particularly unreasonable to "punish" infants for things the wrongfulness of which they do not comprehend. One sometimes hears mothers tell that they never chastise their children themselves but wait until father comes home and let him do the whipping; father's homecomings are then dreaded by the youngster for hours or, if his occupation keeps him away longer, for days, and when he does come home, the child may be hiding or pretend sickness or, as was the case in a few of our patients, even run away until they are picked up by the police. The habit of sending the child to bed in daytime as a punitive practice may result in actual or simulated fear of being alone or in vindictive fantasies. One boy related delightedly how he enjoyed being sent up to his room; if he was good, he must stay around the house and ask permission, which was often denied, whenever he wanted to go out. But if he was bad, he was promptly sent to his room from which he let himself down to the back yard; he then ran into another street, returning in time to climb up and be back in his room when he expected to be called to the table. Although this had been going on for many months, he was never found out. He often was intentionally "bad" in order to be relegated to his room. The parents felt that their mode of punishment was very ingenious and effective while in reality it fostered misbehavior and deceit.

LYING

To the average youngster willing falsification of facts is something un-known and unnatural until it is, directly or indirectly, introduced into his reactive equipment from the outside. The first three or four years of life are conspicuously free from lies, though not from apparent misstatements which to the adults may look like intended falsehoods. The two principal criteria of a lie are knowledge of the untruth of the utterance and the goal of gaining advantages or evading unpleasantness. These are absent in the beginning of the period of acquisition of speech. Primarily, the baby asks for milk only if he wishes milk and refuses it if he does not want it. He announces daddy's arrival only if he really sees him com-ing. Nevertheless, he makes numerous incorrect remarks. They are based on a number of reasons inevitably connected with the psychological level commensurate with his age:

The imperfection of his linguistic tools. He may well know his daddy and distinguish him from others. But as long as the word "man" is not a part of his vocabulary, he may announce the approach of any stranger with the remark that "daddy" is coming. "Daddy" is the only available term for men; therefore, every man is "daddy." The child has, from his own point of view, told the truth. Another example: An infant has spilled the milk. The mother looks at him disapprovingly and threaten-ingly. The child says, "No, no, no." With this negation he may not at all deny his action. "No, no, no," may mean, "Mother, do not look at me that way," or, "Mother, do not beat me," or, "I shall not do that any more." To brand the cry of "No, no, no" as a lie may be a grave injustice. Hanselmann aptly pointed out that no one would think of censoring a child's "untrue" drawings; they may evoke amusement but never the reproach that they are dishonest. But his verbal expressions which undergo a similar development are often severely criticized as lies without bother-ing to realize the child's imperfections and to understand the real meaning of his utterances.

Insufficient discrimination between reality and fancy. A child may distress his solicitous parents by declaring that he sees a fox or an elephant or a fairy. This is not an hallucination, nor is it a lie. "Make-believe," which the child really "believes" for the moment, is an essential and, one may say, natural feature of his play activities. It is far more in keeping with fairness to invite the child to explain whether he means a real or a make-believe elephant than to scold him for "lying." No sensible person would think of reprimanding him for not hiding from view if he plays peekaboo. And yet the situation there is very much the same.

Insufficient ability to recognize causal and temporal relation-ships.

Wrong interpretation and immature elaboration of things seen and heard.

It is evident that seeming misstatements arising from these factors in-herent in the child's developmental level are not genuine lies. They do not represent knowing falsehoods, nor do they have the definite purpose of deceiving others in order to gain an end.

Genuine lies are comparatively late in appearing. It is not the truth-fulness that must be learned. The child does not at first know what it means to misrepresent facts intentionally. It is the act of lying that is acquired.

There are various types of lying:

Simple reversal of the truth. The child who has broken a dish insists that he has not broken it. If he has not done his homework or practiced his piano lesson, he states that he has done so.

Exaggerations. The report of teacher's faint praise assumes the proportions of an expansive eulogy. Father's strength or income or influence is magnified in the conversation with playmates.

Fabrications. A child comes home excitedly and depicts a fire or an automobile accident which has not taken place. Or he tells his playmates of vacation trips or adventures which he has not experienced.

Confabulations. A child plays truant or, when sent for an afternoon visit to grandmother's, prefers to wander about the streets. Upon coming home, he is asked what happened in school or at grandmother's. Not knowing the facts, he fills the gap with invented reports.

Wrong accusations. The cat, or the maid, or sister is blamed for spilling the milk which the child has spilled. Here, at least, the fact that milk has been spilled is true. Much more serious signs of a grave personality disorder are the altogether fabricated accusations of sexual assaults or equally severe misdemeanor, as met especially in morbidly cruel and in hysterical youngsters.

A lie may be intelligent, unintelligent, or fantastic. An intelligent lie appears plausible. It is not easily detected. It serves the purpose well, even though the purpose itself is not desirable. An unintelligent lie is easily recognized and misses the point entirely. It is usually a feeble-minded reaction. Fantastic lies are often of a pathological nature. They are well defined by Healy: "Pathological lying is falsification entirely disproportionate to any discernible end in view, engaged in by a person who, at the time of observation, cannot definitely be declared insane, feeble-minded, or epileptic. Such lying rarely, if ever, centers about a single event; it manifests itself most frequently over a considerable period of years, or even a lifetime. Various charges against others, and even self-accusations, are sometimes indulged in, which may prove troublesome matters in courts of law. Extensive, very complicated fabrications may be evolved. This has led to the synonyms: mythomania; pseudologia phantastica."[1] This type of prevarication is usually too complex and requires too much scheming and intriguing to be common in smaller children. It is during the years of puberty and, more frequently, in adolescence that pathological lying assumes its characteristic form.

Lying mostly originates in three types of situations:

Lying in self-defense. A child may have accidentally broken a valued vase. He knows that the parents are upset. He also knows that on previous occasions they have punished him severely for causing lesser

---

[1] Healy, William. The Individual Delinquent. A Text-Book of Diagnosis and Prognosis for All Concerned in Understanding Offenders. Boston. 1915, p. 729.

damage. In fearful anticipation of painful beatings and parental hostility which sometimes hurts even more, he decides to deny his guilt. He learns to lie to save his hide. The severer the parents' punitive measures, the greater is the temptation to lie. In a vengeful environment in which the pettiest misdemeanors are treated with sternness entirely out of proportion to the child's actions, defensive lying may easily become an habitual reaction.

Lying in imitation of adult behavior. Mother notices the approach of an unwelcome visitor or of the instalment collector; she sends her son to the door with the instruction to tell the man that she is not at home. Or the maid answers the telephone; father, when informed who is calling, says, "Tell him I am out of town and won't be back until next week." Or mother is invited to spend a day with a friend; not knowing what to do with Mary when she comes back from school, she takes her with her; the next morning, she sends a note to the teacher that Mary had to stay in bed because of a sore throat. This is how many truthful children receive their first instructions in lying; when they themselves adopt this form of behavior for their own purposes, these same parents are usually very distressed. We have seen many children brought to the clinic with the complaint of lying by mothers who in the ensuing interview do not hesitate to give a deliberately false account of the family situation.

One ten-year-old girl gave the following very instructive report of a family scene. One day they had her father's employer for dinner. This evidently was considered a big event, and Dorothy did her very best to behave herself nicely. Whenever the guest opened his mouth, his hosts exclaimed, "Really?", "You don't say so!", "How interesting!" But when he left, father dropped down in a chair with the expression of a martyr, saying, "Thank God he is gone," and mother added, "Oh, what a bore!" Soon afterwards, they again had company, and the parents praised their employer sky-high. Dorothy remarked, "But isn't he a bore, though?" With the sign of utmost indignation, her parents said, *uni sono,* "Now, Dorothy, you are being naughty. You go right up to your room and stay there!" Dorothy, puzzled, remonstrated, "But, mother, you said so yourself." Whereupon mother, trembling, "How dare you say such a lie? Out you go!" And to the guests, "I do not know what has got into the child. Why, this is outrageous." Bright Dorothy went up to her room, bitter, her faith in her parents shattered. She made up her mind to do likewise. And she did.

Lying in order to receive attention and admiration. Children, in their conversations with each other, like to make themselves interesting, to outdo the others, to be, at least at times, in the limelight. He who has carried water for the circus elephants, just returned from a distant trip, had a death in the family, whose brother has become a minister or a policeman, or whose father has gone up in an airplane, is the hero of the day. The youngster who lives in a drab monotonous environment in which "nothing happens" feels strongly tempted to gain the coveted attention by supplying invented adventures instead of the absent actual events. If their truth is challenged by the audience, he will be driven into furnishing more and more details and, with growing practice, become an expert story teller. Boasting and bragging have often their origin in this desire to be in the center of attention and to make up through the play of imagination for the lack of the little thrills and excitements which give to the playmates such an air of importance.

The principal prophylactic and therapeutic aims lie in the direction of avoiding or correcting the main etiological factors. Fear of cruel punishments is unhealthy in more than one respect. Sensible management will make the child understand that it is to his advantage to tell the truth. He should not be bribed into confession by the promise of indemnity. Any normally intelligent youngster will appreciate fairness and accept reasonable punishment imparted calmly and without hostility. The use of force and trickery is apt to be met with spite and stubbornness. Parents should be careful not to deviate from the truth themselves, at least not in the child's presence. If certain conventional lies seem indicated, it is best to explain them to the youngster. If Dorothy had been told why it was wise not to mention the shortcomings of her father's employer to others, she would have understood and respected her parents instead of despising their treatment of her. Father might take his little boy or girl on his lap and explain that business considerations made it necessary to have the maid tell the caller over the telephone that he is not at home; that he well realized it was a departure from the truth but that sometimes circumstances made this imperative. Such a management would preclude a feeling of bitterness and injustice and, what is more, outright contempt. An occasional trip to the circus or to the shopping district or a birthday party will provide the child with a break in the monotony and with material with which to entertain his playmates, lessening the temptation to fib.

STEALING

In eighty-eight reporting juvenile courts in the United States, not less than 21,000 children and preadolescents (94.76% boys and 5.24% girls) were seen because of stealing in 1930. If one realizes that innumerable petty thieveries at home and in school are never brought to the judge's attention and if one thinks of the many detected and undetected, forbidden appropriations of mothers' pennies and neighbors' apples and classmates' pencils, stealing must indeed be considered a not at all uncommon behavior problem of childhood. Its very frequency, the vast variety of objects taken, the multitude of underlying motives, the occurrence in healthy and unhealthy, intelligent and unintelligent, wealthy and poor, well cared for and neglected youngsters ought to curb one's desire to unite all, or most, or even a selected number of those cases under the term of "kleptomania." A study of individual offenders will further teach us that sometimes the theft of one penny or a relatively worthless eraser may be the expression of a far more serious personality disorder than that of several dollars or an article of high value.

Robert, a physically healthy, only very slightly retarded boy of fourteen years was caught by a policeman riding on a bicycle which had been stolen by another boy. The offense itself looks comparatively trifling, especially if we learn that the bicycle had been "loaned" previously to many other boys by its abductor and that Robert knew how "they had gotten away with it." In the course of the investigation it appeared that he had a very poor home training. His paternal grandfather was a heavy drinker, abusive, and at one time spent eight years in prison for killing a boy. His father, alcoholic, a wife beater who was once arrested for assaulting his wife, had in his youth been committed to a boys' reformatory as "incorrigible minor." He deserted his family several years ago. His mother was forced by her parents to marry the man at fourteen when she was pregnant with Robert; after her husband's desertion (and probably also during their numerous temporary separations preceding the final break), she was sexually promiscuous. Robert's difficulties began when he was nine years old. His father was then living with another woman and his mother worked away from the home and returned late at night. Robert used the occasion to play truant and to roam about the streets. Food was not sufficiently provided at home, so he helped himself to bread and cold meats and fruit and candy in stores and market stalls. He became "hot-headed and unruly" in school, or rather in the many schools which he attended, owing to nine changes of residence (usually evictions) within the past five years. In the court he feared commitment and pleaded tearfully for "another chance," which was given him. Less than two weeks later, he was brought back for stealing small articles from the Five and Ten Cent Store and from an amusement park. This time, he had induced a smaller boy to go with him and gave him the stolen items "to hold." When apprehended, he placed the entire blame on his companion whom he had asked to wait outside telling him that they had been to "buy" a few things and who, therefore, did not even know that they had been stolen. Robert was committed to a reformatory where, for the first time in his life, he learned that there were other standards of behavior than those manifesting themselves in alcoholism, brutality, adultery, and evictions, which he had seen at home. He made a good adjustment in the institution, where he received vocational training, and achieved distinction as a member of its musical band.

Carl, aged thirteen and a half years, was a well-developed, healthy lad of superior intelligence (I.Q. 127) and pleasant manners. He came of a stable family and had always had an excellent school record as regards both conduct and scholastic progress. He had a keen interest in natural science and it was his ambition to become a biologist. He had acquired an astounding knowledge of insects and butterflies. He established a laboratory in the back of his father's office; he denied himself the usual boys' pleasures and invested the nickels which he received sporadically in chemicals, test tubes, boxes for his collections. The head of the nearby branch library, a friend of the family, asked him to display some of his work in the library. His arrangements were so successful and so well spoken of, that a request came from the central library that he loan his material for a special exhibition in one of its show windows. Carl was anxious to make the demonstration complete by adding to it drawings of microscopic slides. For this he needed a microscope. He had heard his father complain of poor business conditions and did not have the courage to ask him for one. He obtained his teacher's permission to remain in the classroom after school hours and to use one of the school's microscopes there. One afternoon, he needed some of the specimens which he had in his laboratory and went to ask the teacher to let him take the instrument with him for the rest of the day. But the teacher had left the building. Carl took the microscope home with the intention to return it the next day. Not having finished his work, he kept it for another day. He now realized that he had "stolen" it. When he found out that its absence was not noticed, the temptation to keep it a little longer and use it at home undisturbed was too great. The display in the central library attracted considerable public attention. A newspaper reporter came to Carl's home and transferred his entire laboratory to the library, where it was added to the exhibition. It was then that the principal who had come to see the work of his popular pupil identified the microscope as school property and, without further inquiry, had him arrested. Carl was made to apologize for the act which he regretted more than anyone else. His father began to give him a regular weekly allowance from which Carl was to buy his own microscope when he had saved up enough money. A local natural scientists' association made him one of its members.

These two examples suffice to demonstrate the variety of situations in which stealing may arise and also the fact that each case requires individual handling. One may roughly distinguish several forms of thefts:

Intelligent stealing, that is, appropriation of articles needed or badly wanted, in a way which would not immediately lead to discovery, and *unintelligent* stealing, that is, appropriation with little or no caution of things which could easily have been obtained in a less objectionable manner.

Casual stealing,—yielding to persuasion or temptation on one occasion only, or very rarely, and *habitual* stealing.

Selective stealing,—taking only objects which may be of use to the child, and *indiscriminate* stealing. Two boys of approximately ten years broke the lock of a freight car from which they removed paint cans, brushes, and piston rings. They hid them under a bush and went about telling their playmates what they had done. They had no intention of either using or selling the articles stolen.

Solitary stealing and *group* stealing. This is an especially significant distinction. In the cases of group stealing it is important to know the rôle which the child has played, whether he had "thought up" the plan, or whether he acted as the real leader, or as one of the followers, or as a "post" to watch for the police or anyone else who might interfere.

Larceny,—theft of things easily accessible; *burglary*,—stealing after breaking into a house; *robbery*,—taking property from another person by force or intimidation.

There is no limit to the number and type of articles which may be and have been, stolen by children. Cataloguing the various objects taken in several thousand thefts would more or less duplicate the contents of a mail order house catalogue. Even furnaces, office desks, and kitchen stoves are among the things taken by some of our patients. There are, however, a few especially desired items which return again and again in the complaints of children's stealing. Money tops the list; it is most frequently taken at home. Snatching pocketbooks is a practice not uncommon among street urchins. Children often help themselves to their classmates' writing utensils. Boys' theft of bicycles is an occurrence recorded almost daily in the juvenile courts of our larger cities. Automobiles are equally popular, particularly among lads between fourteen and eighteen years of age.

Stealing, just as lying, does not exist in infancy. One can speak of stealing only when there is a knowledge of wrongdoing. The infant learns very slowly to comprehend the conventional meaning of property. Everything, including the child himself, seems at first to belong to the adults. For a time he is given things: food, clothes, toys. Then, when he runs around and is big enough to reach for objects on the table or in the cupboard or in the pantry, he practices taking things. Sometimes the adults acquiesce, at other times they prohibit. Thus the baby realizes that some things may be taken and others may not be taken, depending on the rules laid down by the adults. A normal two-year-old knows very well from experience which of the familiar things in the home he may touch, remove from their places, and use in his play and which others he must leave alone. But the idea of property has not entered clearly into his mode of thinking. Parental approval or disapproval and not realization of ownership is the guiding criterion. By the time the concept of possession and a clear distinction between mine and thine is acquired, the well-trained child has, on different grounds, been prepared for a discrimination between things he may have and others that he may not have. It is now that judicious education more plainly allots certain clothes and toys to the child which are his own. It is needless to add that wise employment of his belongings is a further part of child training. The youngster still may have an ill-controlled desire to take a piece of candy from the drawer or a cookie from the pantry or sister's doll from her toy cabinet. This will be particularly the case if mother sends the child to the drawer or to the pantry whenever he asks for candy or cookies and if sister helps herself to his toys without asking his permission. Thus a looseness and confusion is created which makes it difficult for him to orient himself in a rather complicated system. It is this confusion which usually gives rise to the first knowing and intentional stealing. In the period of resistance and obstinacy, if it is improperly managed, taking forbidden objects may become just another means of self-assertion, together with refusal of food and going to bed, the frequent "I won't" replies, and the "cravings" for candy or ice cubes which the child knows mother does not want him to have.

In the older child, stealing may arise from a great number of situations and sources:

Desire of possession is sometimes the main motive in youngsters who are in the habit of getting everything they want or who are denied many things that they need or that they think they need. The spoiled child has not been taught self-denial. He has not been corrected at home when he has taken and broken the older sister's doll or dropped father's wrist watch. His excuses when he had removed a nickel from mother's pocketbook and purchased candy were found so "cute," or the solemn prophecy that God would punish him with a stomachache did not come true. When, in the store with mother, he had helped himself to an orange, mother in her embarrassment bought a whole dozen of them, explaining to the storekeeper that the child simply is wild about oranges. So prepared, the youngster may later not hesitate to appropriate at home, in school, or anywhere else articles which he desires.

The child who because of poverty or carelessness has been denied toys or titbits may find it beyond his will power to resist temptation when an opportunity seems to offer itself. There are such beautiful pen-knives or eversharp pencils or flashlights (a much stolen implement) displayed in the store. The child may go there once, just to look at them and to fancy himself as possessing enough money to buy the coveted luxury. He may return a few times, until sooner or later the desire becomes irresistible. Bicycles are often the culmination of a boy's dream of earthly possession. They are quite easily accessible, in the streets, where boys leave them while they go into a house or a shop, or on porches, or in back yards. The lad who cannot hope ever to be blessed with a bicycle may yield to the temptation of "just borrowing one" for an hour's enjoyment, and then he either fears being caught upon returning it or else he learns to like it so much that he does not wish to part with it.

Loose social standards in the home. In many instances, children's stealing develops, one might almost say, naturally in an environment permeated with asocial or antisocial attitudes. To a minor degree, the child's education in matters of honesty may suffer a blow if mother, for example, to save a half carfare, instructs him to misstate his age to the conductor. But in a considerable number of cases of habitual stealing, utter disregard of accepted moral standards may be found in the children's homes.

Father, alcoholic, desultory worker, mistreated his wife and quarrelled constantly; he died of influenza when the patient was ten months old. He was the mother's second husband. After his death, she married again. She was arrested for brutally abusing her stepchildren, one of whom she burned on the nose with a hot iron as punishment for disobedience. The stepfather was once placed on the adult docket of the juvenile court for failure to support his minor children. One brother ran away from home and was arrested in Oregon for taking a shotgun from a dwelling. A stepbrother was committed to a reformatory for being "incorrigible, a truant, and impudent." The family lived in a crowded, poorly ventilated home. There Joseph, twelve years old, two and a half years retarded, failed to develop a sense of social responsibilities. There was occasional truancy; once he was arrested for throwing stones at windows "for fun." After a series of minor thefts, he organized a "gang" of three boys and, together with the others, broke into thirteen market stalls, feasting on the stolen cold meats and fruit and soft drinks, until they were apprehended.

Andrew G. was the spoiled youngest son of a socially dependent family, raised in a morbid atmosphere of paternal alcoholism and the mother's religious fanaticism. Of his two older brothers, one was arraigned before the juvenile court twice, and the other six times, always for "disorderly conduct." State Hospital commitment had been advised for the mother on a number of occasions. She was paranoid, bothered physicians in the community trying to sell them her "infallible cancer cure," and forced her children to kneel with her in prayer for hours at a time. Andrew had stolen indiscriminately and was finally caught taking pigeons from a coop.

Two intellectually retarded boys, aged fourteen and thirteen, were involved in the same charge. John D. stole a pocketbook containing $143.00, and Calvin W. helped to spend the money. John's parents were temperate and industrious but unintelligent and very poor. They had two boys whom, at an early age, they sent to collect wood and coal from the railroad tracks and the steamboat piers and discarded boxes from stores and back yards. The lads were also sent from house to house selling mother's home made candy. If they managed to make more money by staying away from school, the parents wrote notes to the teachers excusing their children's absence on the ground of sickness. The elder lad, Theodore, was first to broaden the area of these activities by entering into a home and removing an alarm clock. He was arrested a number of times for stealing coal from trucks. John specialized in truancy and gambling in which he did a good deal of cheating. The only reason he could give for the undesirability of stealing was "because you get caught." Calvin's maternal grandparents both died of alcoholism. His father left school at twelve when in the second grade; he was illiterate and decidedly feebleminded. His mother was untidy, unintelligent, untruthful, and deaf. A maternal aunt suicided. Two maternal uncles served a three-year term in the penitentiary for grand larceny. The home was dirty, dark, offensive to olfaction, and located in the slums. When arrested, Calvin gave an assumed name. He had been staying out late at night for years without being corrected. He was dismissed from a boys' organization because he assaulted a girl on their playgrounds.

Feeblemindedness is in itself not a "cause" of stealing. But it is easy to understand that the mentally retarded child, especially if he is not sufficiently trained, is much less able to form adequate social habits than youngsters who have a better grasp. It is especially the "dull normal" who contributes most liberally to the rank of juvenile thieves. The percentage distribution of intelligence quotients of the white boys and girls examined in the psychiatric department of the Baltimore City Juvenile Court between July, 1930, and August, 1932, is as follows:

I.Q.	Per cent
Under 50	1
51–60	2
61–70	9
71–80	35
81–90	27
91–100	18
101–110	6
111–120	1
121–130	1
Total	100

Children not infrequently steal *in order to gain the much coveted recognition and admiration* of their playmates or to avoid isolation from them. A variety of factors may be at play:

Several youngsters plan a picnic to which each is to contribute his share. There is the boy whose parents refuse to give him the money or the food which he is expected to bring. He is ashamed to admit that. He steals what he needs either at home or, if this is not possible, elsewhere. Or a child joins a boys' or a girls' club. The uniforms and ball outfits are expensive. Christmas or the birthday is far off, and even then it is doubtful whether these things will be forthcoming. The child is sent by the parents, a boarder, or a neighbor to pay a grocery bill. Instead of doing that, he procures for the money the desired uniform, hiding it somewhere, and leaving the adults with the impression that the bill has been paid. The theft is committed in order to be able to compete with others.

The unpopular child struggles for acceptance in a group. He bribes his way into companionship by misappropriating money for which he buys toys and sweets, distributing them generously among the others.

The bragging child whose stories are challenged may steal so that he may not lose his reputation of something like a hero and "prove" the "truth" of his previous statements.

The "dare" is a powerful incentive to thefts. An intelligent boy of thirteen stole two rifles from a shooting gallery. He had never before taken anything that was not his. The "gang" with which he associated dared him to "swipe" the rifles: "I did not want to back out and to appear yellow. I had to show off, I had to show them I was not afraid. I am glad they caught me. It showed me I was a fool. It took something like this to break us up."

Group stealing is very frequent. It is often undertaken not so much with the desire of possession as in a spirit of adventure or as a game for which detective stories, moving pictures, and newspaper reports of gangster activities have furnished the pattern. Concepts, such as "being yellow" or "squealing," are taken over and considered with awe. He is a hero who is most aggressive and "gets away with it," either in the sense of evading detection or, if arrested, managing to be dismissed or placed on probation instead of being "put away," that is, committed to a correctional institution. It requires little imagination to realize how disastrous a preparation for adult life such activities and standards are if they are not nipped in the bud through constructive readjustment and reëducation of these children.

In a small number of cases, the first acts of stealing are performed in a mood of *vindictiveness*. The child, embittered on account of severe punishment, "gets even" with the father or teacher by taking objects which he knows are highly valued by them.

Jealousy is another factor in the stealing of some children. This is especially the case where parental gifts are bestowed unevenly or where the youngster is made to feel that one of the playmates has taken away his popularity by the display of more and prettier toys.

Children who stay out late or those who wander away from home are induced to steal by sheer hunger or lack of clothing.

There is an interesting group of girl shoplifters who usually have good records of behavior and who, about the time of puberty, pilfer in department stores. They are rarely alone, mostly two or, less frequently, three together. They are normally intelligent or slightly retarded. In most instances, they readjust very well if properly handled.

Evelyn R., sixteen, and Ann O., fifteen years old, went out together and stole two dresses, two pairs of hose, eight compacts, several lipsticks, two sets of beads, and two bracelets. Evelyn had a mental age of nearly twelve years. In school, she completed the eighth grade with good marks in her studies and conduct in spite of her intellectual limitations. She presented no problems at home. She had always enjoyed a good reputation among her teachers and classmates and in her neighborhood. Her father, a disagreeable alcoholic, divorced by his wife ten years ago, was prompt in contributing to Evelyn's support. The home environment was peaceful and congenial.

A half-sister, from her mother's previous marriage, was stable and well behaved. Ann had an I.Q. of 97. She was of an athletic build. It was her desire to become a pharmacist. Her parents were highly respected people. Her mother was excitable and nagged her a good deal and had sometimes beaten her severely. When brought to court, Evelyn showed deep regret, whereas Ann was defiant at first, but soon changed her attitude and coöperated splendidly. Neither of the girls could give a satisfactory explanation of their actions. Both had good clothes and had allowances permitting them to purchase the little toilet articles which they had stolen. Both had good realization of the anti-social nature of their deeds.

In some of the cases, the stealing coincides more or less closely with the days of or shortly before menstruation. In others, it occurs at any time, independent of the menstrual flow. It would be incorrect to term these girls hysterical, since there is nothing in their life histories to justify such a diagnosis. The incidence of shoplifting in otherwise normal girls is so frequent, however, that it seems in order to single it out as a specific mode of behavior; one cannot very well speak of it as "kleptomania," as some will have it, since there is nothing "irresistible" about it and since it mostly remains a single brief episode in the lives of well adjusted girls who have always been normal and who afterwards go on developing normally. Where we found that there were no other difficulties involved, we invariably recommended dismissal, and not one of those children has ever been brought back to the court. It is, of course, self-understood that considerable work was done with them prior to their being discharged and that they were followed up periodically by the social workers of the court. The pubescent or preadolescent female shoplifter deserves special study which may also throw some light on the peculiar incidence of shoplifting in some older women during the menstrual periods.

A certain analogy to the shoplifting girls is to be found in the boys of approximately the same age, who steal automobiles. Here, an additional factor exists in the laws of some of the states forbidding boys before fifteen or sixteen years to drive motor cars.

Stanley F., a fifteen-year-old boy of superior intelligence (I.Q. 146), coming of a refined and cultured home, was arrested while driving a stolen car. He had an excellent school record, preparing for Princeton College, took active part in athletics, was a member of various clubs and strongly interested in music. He had pleasant manners, got along well with people, and had never presented any behavior problems before. Being below the age limit which would entitle him to a driver's license, his parents, of course, did not let him steer their automobile. He associated with boys over sixteen, most of whom had their own roadsters. He courted the favors of a girl who told him of the many pleasant rides which the others had given her. When she finally consented to give him a date, he appropriated for the great occasion a magnificent car parked in front of a home, with the intention to return it and to park it a few blocks away in order to avoid detection. But his action was observed, the police was notified, and he was followed and arrested.

Roland R., of exactly the same age as Stanley, had an entirely different background and life history. His father never properly supplied the family needs; he was fighting the Government for compensation on the basis of hypochondriacal complaints. His mother was feebleminded and overindulgent. There was a long record of parental separations and reconciliations. Roland was a braggard whose ambition it was to become a gangster and "a real big shot." He was the "philosopher" of the group with which he associated (with an I.Q. of 87), read "deep" books which he did not comprehend, and boasted that he worked on a scheme "how to get to the galaxy." His leadership of his "gang" was challenged by a boy who, after having reached the age of sixteen, got a job as a truck driver and invited his companions to ride with him. Roland promptly took to stealing parked automobiles and treating the boys to joy rides.

Stealing, sometimes, is performed in the course of amnesic fugues and in hysterical conditions.

Sybilla K., a physically healthy and normally intelligent girl of almost sixteen years, had typical hysterical anaesthesias, the characteristic globus complaint, and a history of sudden blindness at twelve years, which disappeared after three months at the onset of menstruation, as her physician had told her it would. Her parents were industrious and intelligent people living in an isolated farm near a large city. The home life was very monotonous; the father was extremely strict with himself as well as with the family; the children had many duties but no privileges. The father "did not believe" in recreation; he felt that going to church on Sunday and reading the Bible ought to offer sufficient relaxation. "Worldly" books were not tolerated in the home. Sybilla was not permitted to visit friends. Her pleas to invite them to her own house were met with stern disapproval. The girl went to business college in the city. She always lived in the hope that something exciting would happen. She finally provided the excitement herself. Instead of going to school, she one day strayed in the streets, then wandered into a department store, went to the clothing department, and when she believed herself unobserved dropped a dress into her bag, went to the lavatory and removed the sales tag, then walked out nonchalantly. Before leaving the building, she was apprehended by a house detective. She at first was very insolent, then screamed, and finally told a fantastic story. While on her way to school, she said, a woman dropped a cameo which she politely picked up and gave back to the woman. The woman told her, "You are the one I have been looking for." She had dropped the cameo with the idea that whoever picked it up would be the person to go with her. She took Sybilla behind a lamp post and there, at the point of a pistol, told her to do as directed. (The designated lamp post was located at a street corner which hundreds of people pass in a steady stream at that time of the day.) The woman then took her to another street where a man was sitting on the foot board of an automobile, and the two exchanged secret motions. She then told Sybilla to go to the department store and steal the dress. There was hardly a doubt that the girl, at least in later interviews, fully believed the contents of her story.

It is quite obvious, in view of the variety of motives and training and backgrounds, that the therapeutic planning depends on the factors involved in the individual cases. The available alternatives, legal and educational, are:

Dismissal. The child whose stealing was promoted by a "dare" and who has always been stable and well behaved, the youngster whose first experience has given him a sufficient insight into the undesirability of ever repeating the act, or the one who just happened to be in a group of stealing companions without participating himself, will best be dismissed after a constructive interview with the patient and the parents, provided that the parents themselves have a healthy social attitude. It does not do, in these cases, to become unduly indignant and, which is even more disastrous, to prophesy a future criminal career for the little offender. Understanding and steering of the patient into good associations and organized recreational activities will help to socialize him sufficiently.

Close observation and follow-up (probation) for a protracted period. Where the stealing has become habitual or where the youngster's social attitudes have suffered through the influence of companions or through laxity in the home, more intensive work becomes necessary. The physician or teacher will keep in close contact with the child and his parents. The modern juvenile courts have especially trained social workers (probation officers) whose duty it is to aid in the supervision and readjustments which should be attractive to the child, who must be made to feel that something worth while is given to him rather than taken away from him. The Boy Scouts, the Y.M.C.A. and Y.W.C.A. groups and other well disciplined clubs for boys and girls offer the best opportunities. Not only the patient but also his family should be guided and induced to coöperate. It is a good plan to supply the child with a regular weekly allowance, however small, which he could call his own and use as he sees fit.

Placement in a boarding home. If an unhealthy and dangerous home situation cannot be modified, removal of the child to a better environment is indicated. After the adjustment has been made, one will keep working constructively with the patient.

Commitment to a reformatory. In those instances where the child's behavior difficulties have grown beyond the control of the family or of a boarding home or in which even the most conscientious probational management does not succeed in socializing the youngster, commitment to a correctional institution remains as *ultima ratio.* The modern and progressive reformatory is not a penal institution but a school which, in addition to wholesome discipline, offers vocational training, musical instruction, athletic and dramatic recreations, etc., and aims at preparing its boys or girls for a smoother adjustment in a socially approved manner in adult life.

Most of the cases of stealing which come to the pediatrician's attention fall under the first two groups. Knowledge of the child's personality and of his environment and educational history is the best and only guide in working out a therapeutic plan.

DESTRUCTIVENESS AND CRUELTY

Just as infants do not really steal before acquiring a sufficient comprehension of ownership rights, so they do not wittingly destroy objects before the understanding of values has dawned upon them. Realizing that it takes some time for a baby to develop, through experience and instruction, the vitally essential caution that makes for self-preservation, it certainly is not in the least surprising that he does not *a priori* possess the capacity for discriminating between things that can and those that cannot be broken or torn. This distinction is decidedly the outcome of gradual learning and the process of trial and error. Very often the damage resulting from a tot's performances is not even due to the direct handling of the object destroyed or it is the incidental and by no means anticipated byproduct of his varied and exploratory play activities. Douglas A. Thom quotes a few illuminating examples: "He pulls at the table cover to help him to get up from the floor; he twists the cat's tail because it results in noise and action; he cuts his stockings to demonstrate his ability to use the scissors; he crushes the flowers to show he is pleased with them; with chalk or pencil he has discovered he can leave his imprint on the wall or woodwork."

As the child grows older and the desirability of maintaining the integrity of objects has been adequately impressed upon his mind, destructiveness naturally assumes a different aspect. Even then the damage may not be precipitated by malicious intent. Of the various factors leading to destruction, we list the commonest ones:

Clumsiness. Some children are less skilful than others and their movements are less graceful and less finely coördinated. They drop things more easily. This applies not only to the choreic and athetotic youngster or the one who loses his grip on things in an epileptic petit mal attack. There are people who retain a certain degree of motor awkwardness, a certain lack of dexterity throughout their lives. There is the familiar example of housewives and servants who are unable to finish a day's work without breaking something.

Impatience and haste. The little girl who must wipe the dishes and is at the same time in a hurry to run out and play may, in her impatience, be less careful than is good for the durability of the glass and chinaware. The arrival of an unexpected visitor may well cause the hasty and excited child to run against a stand adorned with a costly vase.

Mechanical inadequacy will sometimes result in overwinding a wrist watch just received as a birthday present or of a toy locomotive or in breaking off the point of a pen knife.

Curiosity. Children are normally and naturally inquisitive. They want to know what things are made of, what is inside of a doll, what it is that makes the clock tick, etc. The taking apart of these objects, which to the adult appears as destructiveness, in reality represents a quest for information which speaks rather well for the youngster's intellectual desire for better knowledge. It is his first active attempt to learn, to "figure things out," to comprehend mechanical connections. It is, from the point of view of the child, rather a constructive and instructive, than destructive effort, devoid of malevolently injurious designs.

Play. It sometimes occurs that youngsters, especially those who have themselves been beaten severely, in their play with dolls or toy animals inflict on them for their fancied misdeeds such severe "punishments" that in the end they are broken or marred. "Discipline," usually in imitation of methods employed by the elders, and not the accidental harm is the primary purpose.

Anger. Contrary to the preceding situations or motives, there are certain emotional reactions in which a child may be driven to destructiveness with the full intention to destroy. It is not uncommon for people with imflammable dispositions to throw objects in temper tantrums, either aiming at the person who has aroused their ire or transmitting their wrath to the objects themselves as a sort of ventilation of their feelings and a more indirect vindication. Children in their outbursts may tear their clothes, destroy their books, thrust anything that is within easy reach, or kick the table or piano leaving noticeable scars on the furniture.

Spiteful and vengeful destruction in order to "get even" with someone is closely allied to damage done in anger. Here the intention to hurt the hated owner of the injured object is quite obvious. It is not so much the often sneaky and secretive act that calls for a remedy as are the personality traits which it discloses and the factors which have contributed to their evolution.

The same is true of destructiveness arising on the basis of *jealousy*. There are children chivalrous enough to delight in the fact that brother or sister has received a new toy or a new piece of furniture. Others may be trained well enough to hide their jealous feelings. Others again may steal or hide the object. Still others may break or tear it so that it can no longer be enjoyed by anyone.

"Mischievousness." This term is often applied by parents to destructive tendencies of children which may be based on any of the enumerated motives. There is, however, a number of youngsters who, without being angry or vindictive or jealous, derive a peculiar pleasure from deforming objects. Many, but by no means all of these children are mentally retarded. In the juvenile courts one not infrequently has an opportunity to see boys who would not think of harming another child but who have been arrested for throwing stones at windows of private dwellings or public buildings. The desire to show off before the playmates or a challenge may be an incentive. There is always a reason for the "mischievousness," which must be detected in the course of the examination.

Cruelty is the most serious and educationally most difficult cause and form of destructiveness. It makes a great difference whether the harm is done under the immediate influence of a strong emotion or whether the act is performed "in cold blood," with apparent enjoyment of the deed itself as well as of its result. It also makes a difference whether a child is satisfied with the damage which he does to a hated or envied person indirectly through the marring of inanimate objects or whether he goes after an individual or an animal who has done nothing to him. The spiteful, jealous, or angry youngster at least reacts to some definite situation, to be sure, in an undesirable manner calling for correction. The cruel child needs no specific provocation. He derives pleasure from seeing others suffer. He lacks any trace of sympathy. One may differ as to whether sympathy is a congenitally inherent quality or something that is acquired through training. Homburger says: *"Die Anlage der Sympathiegefühle ist eine letzte, nicht weiter zurückführbare Gegebenheit."* At any rate, the family records of the patients whom we have seen because of cruelty almost invariably show that lack of consideration for the feelings and sufferings of others has been present in one or both of the parents and, what is more, that the child himself has been a victim of parental tortures mostly disguised as disciplinary measures. Most of these children offer an unfavorable prognosis with regard to their character formation. To what extent the bullying of younger children, often enough associated with cowardice in the presence of stronger playmates, and the tormenting of animals is an expression of sadistic tendencies, is often difficult to determine and can be decided only by a thorough study of the individual case, unless one wishes to go so far as to consider cruelty always as a sign of sadism, and then it becomes merely a matter of terminology.

Leonhard F., at the age of seven years, was found on the point of trying to burn puppies in an ash can, after having poured gasoline on them. A little later, he set fire to a mattress in his grandmother's back yard. He then attempted to set fire to some hay in a neighbor's barn. He destroyed a tank with five gallons of gasoline which he found in a strange garage. He was suspended from school because he was "very annoying and trying," tortured smaller children, and did "queer things" to get the classmates to laugh. He stole a gun to use when he went to the country hunting raccoons at night; in order to find out if the gun worked, he shot at a window in a dark alley. He supplied himself with candy and fruit through petty thefts in stores. He appropriated balls from golf courses and sold them; sometimes he threw them at children in the street. At fourteen, he broke into a house; he had passed it the day before and noticed a woman putting something into an ice-box; he could not see what it was but thought he heard bottles rattle. In order to enter, he had to climb over a wire fence and to break the lock of a gate. He found two bottles of beer and wine which he drank. He repeated this procedure several times before he was arrested. On one occasion, he even invited a "guest" to go with him, a man who went under the name of "Sleepy Wolf." The boy had always bitten his fingernails, had nightmares and jerked in his sleep, and twitched his face. He was physically healthy and only slightly retarded intellectually. His father was involved in a carnal knowledge case while his wife was pregnant with Leonhard. He deserted the family several times, on one occasion living for four years with a girl to whom he had posed as a single man and leaving her after she had borne three children. He beat his wife cruelly, at one time cut her head and threatened to kill her with a knife. His only contact with the children was established through the medium of his razor strap and, if they were fortunate, it was "only" a manual one. Leonhard's mother married at fifteen. After the first night of married life, she left the bridegroom and stayed away for three years. She contracted lues during one of her husband's absences. The home was nauseatingly filthy; she raised chickens and had incubators in every room. The yard was a depository for excreta and old cans. "The landlord," said the boy, "can never find my mother when he comes to collect rent." She "does not feel like bothering about cooking." It was in such an environment that Leonhard's cruelty and other difficulties originated. He had great admiration for his brutal father and wished to be like him. His mother could not quite comprehend why the boy should be taken away from her and committed to a reformatory "just because he had a little fun; all the boys do that sometimes." In the institution, he was extremely difficult to manage.

The treatment of destructiveness in children depends on the type, frequency, and motives, on the patient's personality, and on the manner of home management. The approach to the correction of anger outbursts has been discussed in a preceding chapter. Where one deals with spite and jealousy reactions, the situations producing them should be remedied in addition to educating the youngster. Instead of punishing a child for his curiosity, he should be encouraged to ask questions and receive information from patient parents; he will then be less tempted to destroy things in order to learn something about them. Much will also depend on the choice of toys. When a child has a plaything, he wants to play with it, not merely look at it and keep thinking of how much money it cost. He appreciates much more an inexpensive toy that he is permitted to use to his heart's desire. It is wise to select toys of a kind that the child would be able to do something with them without being afraid that he might do something to them.

Cruelty must always be looked upon as a serious indicator of personality and environmental difficulties, to be examined and treated with no lesser care and expertness than one would examine and treat pulmonary tuberculosis or rheumatic endocarditis.

TRUANCY FROM SCHOOL

In every civilized country, legislation has made school attendance obligatory for all children between six and at least fourteen years of age. The percentage distribution of illiteracy among the population has come to serve, perhaps a little too one-sidedly, as the measure (instead of as one of several measures) of the cultural level of a nation.

Since the acquisition of elementary knowledge of the "three Rs" has become compulsory and organized education has been provided through public taxation, individual participation has been justly prescribed as a major civic obligation. Dodging this duty is looked upon as an antisocial, or at any event, an asocial act. Parental failure to send a healthy child to school is met with legal punishment. An enrolled pupil's unexcused failure to attend is, as truancy or "unlawful absence," subject to the jurisdiction of the juvenile courts. According to Richards, in one year the school commissioners of a certain city reported twenty thousand instances of unlawful absences.[1] Within a period of six months, one hundred and nineteen children were arraigned before the Baltimore City Juvenile Court on the charge of truancy.[2]

Why do children stay away from school? In analyzing our material, we have found the following etiological factors to be predominant:

Dislike of school in general. It may be based on lack of intelligence to do the work required in the grade to which the child has been pushed up with utter disregard of his limitations. An adult being compelled to listen for several hours each day to, let us say, lectures on higher mathematics for which he is not prepared and which, therefore, he is incapable of grasping, will not exactly be fond of the procedure or of the place in which he feels his time is wasted especially if he is expected to prove to the satisfaction of others that he has acquired knowledge, the

[1] Richards, Esther Loring. Behaviour Aspects of Child Conduct. New York. 1932, p. 54.
[2] Report of the Juvenile Court of the City of Baltimore for the Period of Six Months from October 1, 1929, to April 1, 1930. Baltimore, p. 12.

principles of which he does not comprehend; he will sooner or later develop an understandable and pardonable desire to absent himself and to look for more profitable and pleasurable places and occupations. On the other hand, dislike of school may be due to boredom in a child of superior endowment to whom the subjects taught are too well known and offer no novelty; he may come to feel that occasional absences would not interfere with his scholastic progress. Or a pupil may wish to escape the constant teasing of his classmates by staying away from school.

Fear of punishment or of being ridiculed or berated before the whole class often causes a child, who may have started out from home in time, to change his course and to wander about the streets.

In many households, especially where there are several children to be dispatched to school, the morning activities pertaining to the use of the lavatory, to dressing and combing, and to breakfast are so disorganized, that not infrequently a child may leave his home late and not arrive in the classroom in time. When lateness repeats itself and fear of punishment is added to the experience, the youngster may prefer to remain absent for the rest of the day.

Sometimes children absent themselves from school for the first time owing to the *example* and invitation given them by some classmate. It is, of course, easy to see that persuasion will be the more effective, the greater the number of the factors is that combine themselves to instil into the pupil dislike or fear of school. Where persuasion does not work, children sometimes have a powerful instrument which may induce the best behaved youngster to deviate from the path of duty and righteousness: the "dare." For the ethical code of certain youngsters around the age of puberty, particularly among boys, it is considered unsportsmanlike not to accept a "dare." As a matter of fact, many instances of truancy, especially of first offenses, could be traced back to a "dare."

Parental attitudes. There are parents who, instead of encouraging their offspring to respect the authority of the school and to attend regularly, undermine, through unreasonable criticism, the child's esteem and enthusiasm. It is either the "newfangled system of teaching" in general as compared to the methods used in the "good old time," some "mean" teacher against whom the mother or father happens to have a personal grudge, or the obligation, now commonly accepted, to share with the educators the right to mold the child's personality, that are resented more or less vigorously and verbosely. The pupil is more than apt to make these views his own and to take his attendance duties too lightly. Sometimes he is even supported in his practice of truancy by parents who will "help him out" by knowingly misrepresenting the facts in a note of excuse (usually on the ground of "sickness") written to the teacher.

There are parents who unintentionally foster truancy by their habit of keeping the child at home too often for reasons of personal convenience. The arrival of a visitor, house cleaning in which the child is expected to help, a pleasure trip which could very well be deferred until the weekend, the rumor of some contagious disease of a classmate or schoolmate, the need of aid in harvesting, husking corn, or sowing are sometimes considered sufficient reasons for having the child stay away from school. The greater the ease with which this is done, the better is the soil prepared for the youngster's "hooking" on his own iniative.

There are, finally, parents who, uneducated themselves, feel that the educational duty of the school is completed when the child can read, write, and add passably and that further instruction is superfluous. This attitude is found especially among immigrant laborers from Eastern and Southern Europe, negroes, and Southern hill folk. They withdraw their children from school and send them to work (and, in rare instances, to beg).

On the other hand, we have seen intelligent children whose behavior was beyond reproach and whose truancy was dictated by motives of laudable altruism.

We have, for instance, reference to a thirteen-year-old boy whose progress and conduct in school was very satisfactory and who worried considerably over the parents' poverty and undeserved unemployment. He went early in the morning to a grocery market and earned money first by delivering packages and later by selling shopping bags. He did not spend a penny for himself, walked long distances with sometimes heavy loads without ever being tempted to use the streetcar, and saved in the course of a few weeks a fair sum which he wanted to present to his mother as soon as he had thought up a plausible story. He was caught a few times, at other times the teacher informed his parents of his long absences. He refused to give explanations and silently accepted punishment. No one could understand why a quiet, clever, and dependable boy of a sudden had become a chronic truant. Even during the interview with the psychiatrist, it took a long time before the underlying facts could be obtained. The family was referred to a relief agency which paid their rent and supplied them with groceries. The child's attendance became very regular.

In a few instances, children stayed away from school because of *lack of proper clothing*, owing to the parents' poverty. Torn shoes, for the repair of which there was no money, figure not infrequently in the cases of truancy during the winter months.

Desire for exploration and adventure. Many school children, especially among those raised in the tenement and slum districts, lead a drab, monotonous life, devoid of any little joys and thrills. Some of them, lured by detective and adventure stories, try to obtain them by wandering the streets, where there is much to observe and to discover. They are mostly youngsters who are given no opportunity for recreational outlets. Roaming in parks and in the woods is a pleasure for which they are willing to suffer the punishment which is certain to follow. This is often the case with youngsters who, because of a discrepancy between capacity and class requirements or for some other reason, have developed a discontent with the school. A child with a good deal of imagination will surround his wanderings with the glamor of adventure and with a feeling of self-importance which the home and school do not permit to develop.

The danger of truancy lies not only in the act itself but also in the possible results. Discovery necessitates excuses and ingenious lying. Hunger during the excursions has caused many a child to resort to the stealing of food from stores and market stalls. Other children will yield to the temptation to "sneak" into a moving picture house. The truant youngster may make harmful acquaintances in the streets, especially in the slums. Theft, participation in gang activities, and prostitution not infrequently originate in this manner.

The therapeutic approach will depend on the etiological factors involved in the individual case. One will make sure that the child is physically healthy; pupils with visual difficulties are particularly apt to be unhappy in school. It is necessary to ascertain whether the child's intellectual endowment is suited for the grade work which he is required to do; if this is not so, proper adjustment must be made. A sympathetic teacher can do much to create a liking of the school. The desire for play and adventure can be used constructively by providing organized recreation with unobtrusive supervision; boys' and girls' clubs in the nature of the Y.M.C.A. and Y.W.C.A. or the Boy and Girl Scouts are splendid means of securing safe guidance, play, and the necessary thrills. Faulty parental attitudes must be corrected. Philanthropy must come to the rescue to provide proper clothing and food, wherever there is a need for it. Association with other truants must be prevented. Occasional group excursions with the school, club, or the parents will make it unnecessary for the child to look for adventure in devious ways. The patient will, in personal interviews, be given an opportunity to express his problems and views, and the corrective arrangement will be made with him as well as for him.

WANDERING AWAY FROM HOME

Children's escapades from home are as varied in their etiology as is truancy from school. They occur in psychopathological conditions and in youngsters who may grow up to be normal individuals. The attempt to collect them under the heading of "poriomania" is largely the result of the nineteenth century tendency to speak in terms of monomanias as loosely conceived nosographic translations into Greek of such acts as stealing (kleptomania), lying (mythomania), arson (pyromania), and women's promiscuous sex activities (nymphomania). They say just as much or as little as the English words, except that they imply two incorrect notions: they are often not "mono-" reactions since thorough investigation usually reveals the existence of additional personality difficulties; nor are they in most cases "manias" in the sense or irresistible drives. This, we trust, has become apparent in our discussions of lying and stealing.

In the large number of juveniles who came to our attention because of their running away from home, we felt justified in distinguishing between two groups: those who had left their homes intentionally and those who at the time of their escapades had no clear realization of what they were doing.

In the first group, it was relatively easy to establish the motive or motives, of which the commonest are listed below:

Running away as an emotional reaction to disagreeable home conditions.
1. Immediate response to an acute affect, especially fear, anger, and spite. A child receives a bad report from the teacher which he is to hand to his parents. He may have been promised severe punishment if he did not live up to the school requirements of good progress and conduct. He may, on previous occasions, have become acquainted with the painful results of

beatings with father's razor strap, deprivations of food and freedom, and continued parental hostilities. In his fright, he decides to run, with some excuse, to the protective grandparents or to a sympathetic aunt or, if these opportunities are not available, simply to stay away, with the feeling that any place and any hardship would be better than the home and the dreaded punishment. The same situation may arise if he has broken a treasured vase or committed, wittingly or unwittingly, any other kind of misdemeanor. He stays away because he is afraid to come home.

Another child may run away because he feels that he has been treated unjustly by his parents. He may have been beaten or scolded for something of which he is not guilty. He may have been denied a privilege granted to all the other children of the household. In his anger, he revenges himself on the family by staying away.

Children who are contrasted with their siblings or nagged constantly may run away in a reaction of spite, usually with the additional feeling that their disappearance will make their parents worry over them, recognize their good qualities and appreciate them better than they had previously. In the fantasies of unhappy youngsters who feel neglected or unwanted or unloved, the idea of going away often plays a considerable rôle as a daydream which may never be enacted. They may spin dramatic yarns around this preoccupation and, if the situation seems to become intolerable, they may actually run away.

2. Disappearance from home as a climactic reaction to domestic unhappiness. The child may, or may not, be personally involved in the unpleasant situation. He may resent the atmosphere of continual parental quarrels or the brutalities of an alcoholic father.

Leroy C., a somewhat retarded boy of ten years, had for more than three years been mistreated by a chronically intoxicated stepfather, who was also a wife beater and excluded from his cruelty only Elmer, one of the boy's two younger brothers, to whom he was particularly attached. Leroy decided to escape and to take James, the other ill-treated brother, with him. Out of consideration for his mother, he delayed his plan time and again until, after an especially disgusting scene, he carried it out. Both boys were apprehended and returned. Leroy, as the instigator, was whipped brutally and locked up in the house for several weeks (he had chosen the beginning of the summer vacation for his escapade because the idea of being all day with his stepfather looked particularly gloomy to him). On the first occasion, he again ran away. He stole a gun from a home where he knew there was one. This time, when picked up by a policeman and taken home, he aimed the gun at his stepfather (he did not even know whether or not it was loaded). He did that with the intention of being committed to a correctional institution which appeared to him to be a better place than his own home. All three boys were removed from the morbid environment and placed in boarding homes. This put an end to Leroy's desire for running away.

3. Occasionally, the escapade is the result of a protracted emotional attitude of ill-humor and irritability.

4. If children run away from summer camps, boarding homes, orphanages, or reformatories, this may be due to similar reasons. Even though conditions have improved considerably since the days of Oliver Twist, the

emotional needs and difficulties are often treated much more lightly than the physical needs. Unnecessary harshness and the installation of fear are still too frequently employed as disciplinary methods. To what extent home-sickness (nostalgia) is a part of the reaction, depends on the individual instance. Spoiled children are especially apt to be home-sick during the first days they spend in a new environment in which they do not manage to occupy the center of attention; it is then that the desire to go back home may become so strong that the youngster wanders off notwithstanding his lack of railroad fare.

Love of adventure is another common etiological factor, particularly if home life is too monotonous or when emotional difficulties are an added incentive. Many are the youngsters, usually intellectually retarded, who dislike the school responsibilities and the home routine and hide in freight trains or circus wagons until they are too far away to permit their instant return. Often the boys are driven by the altruistic wish to find a job somewhere in order to help to support their parents or prompted by the dream, fed by the many "success"-mad magazines, to "make a fortune." Sometimes two or three boys start out togteher, after having for a long time saved up some money and planned the affair minutely. The lure of the unknown and unexplored and the "something different" pushes aside the consideration of a loss of accustomed home comforts. Suggestions coming from books and moving pictures and persuasion by playmates contribute their share to the final elopement. The desire for adventure may lie altogether in the direction of a hunt for more amusement than is allowed by parents who are too strict.

The realization of economic distress drives some youngsters to go out and try to take care of themselves. In times of nation-wide industrial or agricultural depressions the migratory urge of children may assume the proportion of a great epidemic. According to recent statistics, not less than approximately two hundred thousand boys have taken to the roads in these United States in the course of the past two years of financial panic. It requires little sociological knowledge to be aware of the grave danger contained in a movement of such tremendous magnitude. In many of these cases the term "running away from home" is not quite correct since the youngsters leave with the knowledge and consent of their destitute parents.

While in many cases the love of excitement and activity, the desire for work, and the hope of attainment of economic independence are strong motives, in others the exact opposite is true. There are children who *like to drift*. They have, through training and parental example, failed to learn to appreciate the value of routine and regulated effort and of submitting to orders. They seem to follow what to them appears as a line of least resistance by simply wandering off, getting free rides from generous tourists, sleeping on freight trains, in empty houses, in the barns of hospitable farmers or, if the weather permits, in the open, begging their food and shabby clothes, and living the lives of tramps.

It is true that quite a few children who run away from their homes are psychopaths. Some turn out to be early schizophrenics. Others are epileptics. Most of them come from disorganized or unorganized homes. A considerable number is definitely feebleminded. But many can be reëducated to become stable citizens if proper mental hygiene is applied in the sense of adequate home management, timely economic relief, and supply of organized recreation.

The second group, composed of children who do not realize clearly the nature and consequences of their action, consists of those whose escapades are performed *in a condition of clouded consciousness* or who have never been able intellectually to appreciate the fact that they are wandering away. The latter is true of idiots. They have no intention to give up the home. They act more or less like the infants who get lost in department stores, attracted by some toys and then forgetting, at least temporarily, that they had strayed away from their mothers. The idiot strays away from the familiar block, following a dog or an organ grinder and, not finding his way back, keeps on walking aimlessly. When picked up in the streets or on the highway, he can give no reason for his straying. He just "wanted to go for a walk" or "does not know why he kept on walking."

Running away in a state of clouded consciousness is usually referred to as "fugue." The term has never been clearly defined. It does commonly not include the escapades of postencephalitic children and juvenile paretics. It may, or may not, be extended to the migrations of children suffering from the after-effects of cerebral traumatism. It is ascribed chiefly to the wandering in schizophrenia, hysteria, and epilepsy. The epileptic fugue (epileptic poriomania or dromomania) must be distinguished from a rare and peculiar form of epileptic attacks in which the patients run about ten to twenty steps forward before falling down (epilepsia procursiva, or dromolepsy). The epileptic fugue is followed by amnesia. Healy, with his wide experience, has seen only one case of an amnesic fugue in one thousand juvenile repeated offenders.

There are many dangers involved in all forms of children's migrations. The idiotic child is helpless when he has removed himself from home. Not knowing the fundamental principles of self-preservation and avoidance of danger, he may be run over by an automobile or by a street car or by a train. We have seen a child whose parents live not far from railroad tracks and whose mother complained that he was in the habit of running out and several times narrowly escaped being killed by approaching locomotives.

Stealing may precede or follow a child's escapade. The child may appropriate money and food and clothes in preparation of his planned trip. Or he may steal afterwards in order to provide the vital necessities. In the course of a short time, he may become accustomed to larceny and burglary or even robbery.

Great peril may arise especially in the sexual sphere. The idiotic girl may be taken advantage of by feebleminded adults or by hoboes. We have seen several such children, mostly little negresses, who had contracted gonorrhea in their aimless wanderings. The older and more intelligent girl may find in paid sex indulgences an easy means of supporting herself. An attractive girl of sixteen years who was turned out of the house a number of times by an alcoholic father (always together with her mother) finally decided to leave alone and of her own accord. She went to the home of a woman recommended to her by a chance acquaintance who had escaped from a girls' reformatory. There, a man was very attentive to her and finally persuaded her to have intercourse with him. He gave her five dollars. When the money was spent, she returned. She soon made a profession of selling her body. Boys may fall into the hands of homosexual adults. Those who take to tramping may sooner or later become the "sweethearts" of habitual vagrants who feed them for their services. Sometimes, several tramps share in the affections of a boy. Some boys have the same master for a long time, others abandon themselves to homosexual prostitution.

Many adult gangsters began their criminal careers when they ran away from home. On the other hand, there are numerous individuals in whom the escapade has remained a comparatively harmless episode in their lives to which they look back with a certain feeling of amusement.[1]

[1] We list only a few of the monographic presentations of vagabondage and wandering away from home:

Flynt, Josiah. Tramping with Tramps. New York. 1901. Wilmanns, Karl. Zur Psychopathologie des Landstreichers. Leipzig. 1906. Marie et Meunier. Les Vagabonds. Paris. 1908. Joffroy, A. et Dupouy, R. Fugues et Vagabondage. Paris. 1909. Pagnier, A. Le Vagabond. Paris. 1910. Stier, E. Wandertrieb und pathologisches Fortlaufen bei Kindern. Jena. 1913.

CHAPTER XXXIX

SEXUAL DIFFICULTIES

MASTURBATION

WE HAVE, in a previous chapter, dwelt upon the generic, personal, and conventionally determined sex differences and on the gradual evolution, during the years of childhood, of the anatomo-physiological, psychobiological, and educational-social sex characteristics, attitudes, goals, and habits. We have stated that the ideal approach to the entire topic is one of frankness and truthful satisfaction of the child's curiosity, graded according to his grasp and the type of his questions and handled as an intellectual rather than moral issue, with the constant aim of impressing upon the youngster's mind the natural trend towards family formation. Training in sexual matters is as far from ideal attainment as is child training in all other functions and activities, hygienic, nutritional, emotional, etc. This may be due to faulty environmental influences and to features inherent in the child's own personality not sufficiently modified by the elders or not sufficiently modifiable to begin with. It is hardly to be expected that the sexual sphere should alone be altogether exempt from minor or major deviations from a perfectly smooth adjustment.

The commonest complaint with which the physician and educator are approached by the parents with regard to children's sexual performances is that of masturbation[1] which, in popular diction, is termed "self-abuse" or "a nasty habit" or related more descriptively in the form that "he plays with himself" (frequent euphemistic expression) or that "he handles his privates." Nothing could give a better picture of the attitudes of the complaining parents than their own reports, of which we quote a few:

"He fools around with his person and has no sense of shame. I tell him he will go crazy if he continues to do it."

"I discovered while we were in China that she puts her hand where she shouldn't. She gets terribly red when she does it. I think there is some connection between her nightmares and this. Her daddy and I told her it would give trouble later, that she will suffer in later life."

"His teacher says he plays with himself in school. He opens his clothes and plays with himself all the time. The principal believes this will lead to insanity or criminality and has frightened the child. The teacher is much disgusted by his behavior and very unsympathetic. We have never seen him do it at home. I think he has learned it from boys in the neighborhood."

"He masturbated a year ago. We slapped him every time we caught him."

"I am constantly worried about the child because she has a bad habit. The doctors have called my attention to it and told me terrible things will happen to her when she grows up if she does that sort of thing now."

[1] From *manus*—hand, and *stuprare*—to defile.

397

"She seems to masturbate as soon as she is by herself. I imagine it is hereditary with her; I wonder if she is like her father."

Rohleder[1] distinguished four types of masturbation:

1. The usual manual form, practiced by the individual himself (*auto-masturbation*). It is most frequently performed in bed, either before going to sleep or after waking up in the morning. With some children, it becomes a regular ritual upon retiring. It is often also carried out during the day, with or without consideration of the environment. It is done through the clothes, or the trousers are unbuttoned for the purpose, or it is indulged through a hole in the pocket which has been discovered incidentally or prepared artificially. In girls, a pillow between the legs or the corner of a chair or a table may serve as a means of excitation. Thigh rubbing is another method sometimes employed by girls.

Mutual masturbation between a group of children who stimulate one another digitally. This occasionally takes place in boys' and girls' reformatories, in boarding schools, and among the members of boys' "gangs." Sometimes auto-masturbation is practiced in company with other children, often introducing an element of contest in which he is considered the winner who is first to have an orgasm. Many children have been in this manner initiated in the habit. Moll reports a veritable epidemic which was introduced to the pupils of a Berlin high school by an adult actor. The ten-year-old brother of one of our own patients had met daily a group of half a dozen coëval boys behind a garage (and in bad weather within the garage), where they masturbated mutually for over a year before the affair was detected by his mother; they even had set regulations as to which two boys should stimulate each other on certain days of the week.

3. *Instrumental masturbation* through the introduction of various objects into the vagina or, less frequently, into the male urethra.

4. *"Mental masturbation"* (a term coined by Hufeland), which consists in the production of orgasm without mechanical means through sexual fancies or through pornographic pictures or literature. It is most unusual in children since it is mostly preceded by many years of manual excitation. In the later period of childhood imagination of nude bodies or of the act of cohabitation plays a significant part in the process of mental masturbation.

The *time of onset* varies with different individuals. The handling of the external genitalia has been observed as early as during the first year of life. At that age, sexual significance can hardly be attributed to the practice, which need not differ from the other forms of habitual manipulations of the body, such as thumbsucking or earpulling. It would, as a matter of fact, seem rather strange if the infant, in his first manual explorations, did not incidentally come upon his genitals and play with them as he plays with the other protuberances and cavities of his body. It cannot be denied that stroking, rubbing, or pulling his fingers, ears, nose, lips, or penis or introducing the thumb into his mouth produces a sensation not obtained from the handling of his insensible toys and that the sensation is pleasurable. If one wishes, as does the psychoanalytic school, to call all these sensations sexual or libidinous, then it is understandable how, on this basis, the other

[1] Rohleder, Hermann. Die Masturbation. Zweite Auflage. Berlin. 1902.

forms of manipulation have come to be looked upon as *larvated masturbation*. A less prejudiced view will hesitate to draw analogies between the masturbation of later years, aiming definitely at orgasm or, at least, at erection, and the playful undifferentiated handling of parts of the body by the infant.

It is one thing to ascribe erotic values to the activities of the infant. It is another thing to state that eventually, in the course of the child's natural development, the originally undifferentiated habit may assume more and more the specific characteristics of the full-fledged self-gratification of the pubescent or adolescent youngster. This transition is one of several factors in the *etiology* of masturbation.

Local irritations of the genital and perianal regions give rise to scratching which, in turn, makes the child experience for the first time the sensations coincident with genital stimulation. After the itching skin affection (pruritus, prurigo, eczema, pediculosis pubis, intertrigo) has been remedied or the disturbing oxyuriasis or phimosis have been removed, masturbation may become a goal in itself. Sometimes the irritation may be produced by uncomfortable clothes.

The child may *learn the practice from others*. In ill-supervised boarding schools one "knowing" youngster may teach the habit to a number of other pupils. Even in private homes brothers or sisters sleeping together may learn from one another to indulge. Occasionally, servants, tutors, and governesses are responsible. One of our patients, a six-year-old boy, had received his instruction from a five-year-old girl in the neighborhood.

In more instances than is usually believed, children have *spontaneous erections* which may or may not be occasioned by local irritations or distension of the bladder. The erections and the sensations accompanying them draw the child's attention to his genital organs which he comes to stimulate artificially.

There exists a considerable number of children, especially those at the age of pre-puberty who, without any local irritations or erections and without being taught by others, *discover themselves the mechanisms and pleasures of masturbation*. This fact has been overlooked by many authors.

It is true that, as Boenheim[1] has emphasized, *domestic unhappiness and parental mismanagement furnish a large contingent of child masturbators*. Inquiries made by Exner and by Davis show that between sixty and ninety per cent of college trained men and women remember having practiced masturbation in their early years.[2] It is hardly conceivable that they all come from abnormal home situations. Yet Boenheim is nevertheless right, for he distinguishes clearly between relatively harmless occasional masturbation and the more serious form of habitual masturbation which indeed arises mostly in the midst of domestic unhappiness. The individual case history rather than statistical figures or a postulated frequency will help to make the distinction.

[1] Boenheim. Curt. Kinderpsychotherapie in der Praxis. Berlin. 1932.

[2] Exner, M. J. Problems and Principles of Sex Education. A Study of 948 College Men. New York. 1915.

Davis, K. B. Factors in the Sex Life of Twenty-Two Hundred Women. New York. 1929.

In the following, we give as examples the family situations of a few habitual masturbators:

Boy, eleven years, mentally retarded. His father was dead. An older brother masturbated for several years. The mother showed great consternation concerning the boy's habit because she was told that he was sure to lose his mind if he could not be stopped by means of an operation.

Girl, three years, seven months. Only child ("the only ray of sunshine in our home"). Parents quarrelled. Father hypochondriacal. Mother's "natural tendency to worrying and irritability" had been increased by much physical illness and many operations.

Girl, ten years, five months. Constantly nagged and threatened by her mother. Contrasted unfavorably with her brothers and sisters. She received poor hygienic care. After a week's training in a Convalescent Home she was considered there an "ideal child." Masturbation, nailbiting, and feeding problem were resumed immediately upon her returning home.

Boy, six years, one month; seriously retarded, thumbsucker. Both parents had many much discussed physical complaints. The child was maladjusted in school. His older sister used to masturbate "when she was quite young."

Girl, six years, ten months; superior intelligence. Psychopathic father, who spied on her incessantly, threatened her with the penitentiary, urged her to repent, and tyrannized over his wife. The child was not permitted to play with anybody. The father told her that her soul was lost because he learned she had played "husband and wife" most innocently with a twelve-year-old boy in the presence of the boy's parents.

Local results of excessive masturbation are observed mainly in girls. In boys, some redness of the foreskin may be seen at times; in the rare cases of introduction of cylindrical objects into the urethra, serious injuries may occasionally occur. One girl of our observation had at seven years an excoriation of the labia minora and a profuse vaginal discharge which had begun three years before after she had injured herself while straddling a chair with masturbatory intent. Another girl, at six years, had a purulent discharge from the vagina, a hypertrophied clitoris, and an inflamed vaginal vestibule. The habit resulted in a widely patent hymen in a seriously retarded girl of six and a half years. Sometimes the physician is called upon to remove from within the vagina hairpins, buttons, and other objects which had been forced into it by the children with the purpose of masturbating.

No other habit, however undesirable or injurious, has been surrounded with such a wealth of direst prophecies as has been the practice of masturbation. To this, Tissot gave the impetus with his famous work, *De l'onanisme ou Dissertation sur les maladies produites par la masturbation*, published at Lausanne in 1760. The worst possible future, the most dangerous and hopeless physical and mental diseases were predicted for the poor offenders. As a result, "sex education" was advocated which intended to warn the youngsters against ruining their lives and incurring the perils of early insanity and locomotor ataxia which were believed to be the common sequels of masturbation. These ululations continued and are still in our midst, relegated mostly to the uninformed laity but occasionally cropping out in the prognostications offered by medical men. Lallemand, in his work, *"Des pertes séminales involontaires"* (*Paris, 1836–1842*) added to the ominous forebodings put into circulation by Tissot. Rohleder, as late as in 1902, referred in his monograph on masturbation to the practice as a "vice" and called it in extra fat print one of the widest-spread popular diseases: "Yea, I go even further, the widest-spread by far . . . I claim, even syphilis and gonorrhea are not so wide-spread as masturbation". The habit may, according to Rohleder, have destructive effects on the various organs of the body and often on several organs simultaneously or successively; it may lead to something which he called "sexual cerebrasthenia (whereas excessive cohabitation was said to cause "sexual myelasthenia" and coitus interruptus to result in "impotentia psychica"). He distinguished three stages of progression: the stage of physical and psychical malaise and of a change in the total physiognomy; the stage of internal, especially nervous diseases; the stage of mild psychoses. Krafft-Ebing (*Allgemeine Zeitschrift für Psychiatrie. 1875, 31, 425*) went so far as to speak of cases of "insanity through masturbation." The habit has been declared by some authors to be the actual or exciting cause of hypochondriasis, depression, hysteria, epilepsy, and schizophrenia.

A better knowledge of the child and a better insight into his sexual development, together with a truer information about the frequency and possible effects of masturbation, did away with all these harmful misconceptions. It was almost to be expected that the pendulum should occasionally swing to the opposite extreme of disregarding masturbation completely or even considering it as a "physiological" occurrence. We are, after all, not indifferent with regard to such habits as breathholding or thumbsucking or tics, even though we do certainly not identify them with future psychoses or "cerebrasthenia." A child whose masturbation is frequent enough to interfere with his attention in school and at home, with his recreational activities, and with his preparation for normal heterosexual adjustment, is undoubtedly in need of treatment and training. He must be protected against injudicious beatings as well as against unrestrained indulgence. Lack of concentration, though certainly not a "result" of the habit in the sense of hyperirritability or weakening of some mythological brain center, is doubtless a part feature of the youngster's frequent masturbatory preoccupations. The need of hiding the performance of the practice from the elders leads naturally to secretiveness and isolation. Mutual and instrumental masturbation are certainly far from being "physiological." The person who instantly yields to the slightest sexual impulse is one who must be taught to abstain from the habit of following every one of his whims, to consider the tastes of others, and to develop better self-control.

The *treatment* of masturbating children must be directed in the first place towards the enlightenment of the patient and his family. Faulty notions must be corrected. There is a belief that strangers can tell by looking at a person whether or not he "abuses himself." Mothers have taken their offspring to the clinic because "dark rings around the eyes" suggested to them the possibility of masturbation. Sometimes it so happened that the child actually did have the habit, at other times the "diagnosis" was wrong. But the popular notion has made life miserable for so many a youngster, even though the practice was performed very rarely; it made him wonder in the street, in school, everywhere, whether this or that person "could tell by his looks," whether they despised him, whether their looking at him meant knowledge, whether, when talking to others, they discussed him and his habit. A child who goes about with that sort of an attitude must be reassured. His and the parents' consternation about impending ruin and insanity should be radically removed. Much alarm and worry, much morbid self-observation, many deep-rooted personality difficulties could be prevented or, at any rate, alleviated if such superstitions could be eradicated as soon as possible.

2' The introduction into the home of emotional balance, physical hygiene, and healthy sleeping arrangements constitutes the next therapeutic step. Mutually masturbating siblings or play groups must be separated or very closely supervised. Mechanical restraint is a hardship which usually has no satisfactory results because it is aimed at the habit and not at the child.

3' Sending a youngster to bed in punishment for some misdeed has, aside from other disadvantages, often the effect that he masturbates, having nothing else to do and replacing the worry over his humiliation with something which to him affords gratification; often, as a matter of fact, it is this type of punishment which gives to the child the first impetus to perform the act. The same is true of forcing a child to retire long before he is ready for it or letting him remain in bed in the morning unoccupied for a long time. The better regulated the child's activities are during the day, the less he is left to himself, the less the habit is made a topic of discussion, the sooner will

4' he overcome the urge to masturbate. Beatings and other punitive measures, shaming, teasing, nagging, pleading, bribing should be utterly discouraged.

5 The child should receive adequate sex information commensurate with his age, grasp, and degree of curiosity. A satisfactory division of work, rest, and recreation should be instituted over the twenty-four hours of the day.

6' Any local irritation in the region of the genitals should be promptly remedied. The clothes should be fitting. Excessive fondling and sexual stimulation on the part of the parents, siblings, or servants must cease. Erotic moving pictures, exciting literature left lying around in the house, "dirty" stories or jokes told backstairs are not wholesome for a child's eyes and ears, masturbator or no masturbator.

A youngster should never be "surprised" or "caught" masturbating. When he is found indulging in the habit, he should receive the same treatment as the thumbsucker or nailbiter. Without particularly referring to the act, he should be given some pleasant and interesting task or invited to play a game which will distract his attention from the genitals and interrupt his preoccupations in a manner which he has no occasion to resent. Close observation, however, is something entirely different from spying upon the child and expecting him *a priori* to masturbate. The child should not be given an opportunity to sense an atmosphere of fear, suspicion, or hostility.

If the parents tend to remain unreasonable in their attitudes, it sometimes helps, as Boenheim and Thom have pointed out, to ask them if they themselves have never had any problems with the same habit. The issue must, of course, be broached very tactfully. Occasionally it dawns upon the father or mother that they, indeed, had not lost their minds nor become criminals in spite of their own indulging in earlier years.

Where the home situation is disastrous and unmodifiable, one will have to arrange for the child's placement in a boarding home, not so much because of the masturbation itself, but because of factors much more serious and involving much more deeply the patient's entire personality formation.

HETEROSEXUAL INTERESTS AND ACTIVITIES

Children's sexual interests and performances range from natural and legitimate curiosity, common to all youngsters who are intellectually capable of any inquisitiveness, to the instances of coarse practices, known especially to the juvenile courts. Among the delinquency cases disposed by eighty-eight courts of the United States in 1930, a total of two per cent of the boys and not less than twenty-one per cent of the girls were arraigned because of sex offenses, mostly of an heterosexual nature. The age distribution was as follows:

Age	Boys %	Girls %
Under 10	2	11
10–11	1	9
12–13	1	15
14–15	2	22
16–17	3	30
18+	6	33

Proceeding from the normal and near-normal to the antisocial and pathological sex problems during the years of childhood and pubescence, one may perhaps build up a graded scale, of which the individual steps call for different handling and evaluation.

Sex curiosity, which, as has been pointed out elsewhere, requires wise and frank educational guidance in the sense of enlightenment adapted to the age and grasp of the child.

Sex preoccupations. They may dwell upon the contents of a normal curiosity which has not been satisfied or which has been even rudely rejected by the elders, the imposed secrecy and possible misinformation being added stimuli. The initiated youngster may indulge in coarse fancies with or without masturbatory activities. The daydreams may be soaked with romanticism featuring heroic deeds and rescues in honor of some existing or imagined Dulcinea. Boastfulness, "love poems", a certain degree of shyness and awkwardness in the presence of members of the opposite sex are more subtle outward manifestations of the erotic stirrings of the older child. The preoccupations sometimes lead to partial or more complete withdrawal and may interfere with attention in school.

Discussions with other children. Sex topics form a subject of conversation among schoolmates and playmates, especially when they are tabooed in the home. A well-trained group will, of course, use restraint and tactfulness. The child with an uncultured family background, one who has been raised in the slums, one who has been exposed to verbal obscenities, is apt to introduce an offensive terminology into the discussion. The relation of amorous adventures, real, exaggerated, or wholly invented, plays a significant part in the contents of the talks among boys and girls during the second decade of life.

Attachments and crushes. They begin at a much earlier age than is commonly believed. They may, in the beginning, have no conscious erotic meaning to the child. A teacher, an uncle or an aunt, even the father or the mother may hold a temporary fascination for the youngster. Sometimes these perfectly harmless admirations may be taken improper advantage of by some unwise or more or less perverse adult, with the result that a transient hero-worship is turned into a weighty affair of major proportions. At what age "love" enters into the life of a person, depends to a large extent on the degree of maturation, on sentiments existing in the home, on the books read and moving pictures seen, and on the child's general makeup. It is reported that Alfred De Musset "fell in love" at four years, Byron at eight, Dante at nine, Alfieri and Goethe at ten. While "love" in one child expresses itself in veneration and in another in the desire to be near the chosen one, it may sometimes, especially in the retarded or untrained, give rise to the first overt erotic urges and their satisfaction.

Peeping. The wide-spread custom of whole families sleeping together, a custom often made inevitable through dire economic necessity or due to indifference or parental overindulgence, gives the children an opportunity to watch, incidentally or intentionally, the nude genitalia of the members of the opposite sex. This may be not at all injurious and may contribute to the youngsters' information. But the opportunity is mostly accompanied by attitudes which make of the observation a forbidden act and are apt to introduce a strong element of spying. It is, in such a setting, hardly avoidable that sooner or later the child awakes to find the parents *in statu cohabitandi*. The situation, whether it be puzzling or understood, may cause the child to lie awake at night and wait for repetitions of the exciting spectacle. There are youngsters who go to the length of finding out when certain people in the neighborhood undress without pulling the shades down (a much too common occurrence) and peeping through the windows.

Irvin K., fourteen years old, of superior intelligence, was a spoiled child who was in the habit of obtaining his wants, with the aid of temper tantrums if it must be. He had played truant whenever he "did not feel like going to school." Following one of his whims, he had enlisted in the U.S. Army, giving his age as eighteen years. He was well developed physically and really looked much older than he was. Sex had been a topic in the home, since his father, an industrious and sober man, had been accused by his wife, probably without reason, of making advances to his nieces. Irvin had gone with a group of boys whose principal subject of conversation consisted of sexual obscenities. He slept in the same room with a maternal aunt and on one occasion tried to uncover her while she was sleeping. He noticed that a woman in the neighborhood undressed in a room the windows of which opened into a back yard. Every evening, he climbed up a tree and spied on her. After a time, he masturbated while watching her. Later on, he also masturbated at home, imagining that he observed the woman. After indulging for several months, he was detected and taken before the juvenile court. The domestic methods of overindulgence were remedied. He was transferred to another school to get him away from his undesirable schoolmates. Adequate recreational outlets were provided. He was given sensible information in sexual matters. The sleeping arrangements were changed. The best was made of his intellectual facilities. For the past three years, he has offered no problem of any kind.

Verbal annoyances. Ill-bred boys, especially when in groups, sometimes find pleasure in annoying little girls with more or less conspicuous sexual allusions. It is not too unusual for girls with a none too desirable domestic background to respond with similar word play.

Inspection and manual exploration. This may occur at a relatively early age. Play of this sort is, of course, encouraged very much if brothers and sisters are made to sleep together. It is hardly an exaggeration to state that more information about the configuration of the genitalia of the opposite sex is obtained in cellars, attics and haystacks than anywhere else. Wedekind's famous play, *Frühlings Erwachen*, furnishes a pertinent illustration. The issue becomes especially serious if the manipulations are forced upon another child against his will.

Donald D., ten years old, had a long series of personality disorders. He sucked his thumb until four years of age and wet his bed until six years. He was an extremely restless sleeper, with frequent somniloquy and occasional sleepwalking. He was afraid of the dark (a light was kept burning in the bedroom, in which his mother and sister also slept). His maternal grandparents separated. His father, alcoholic and brutal, ran about with other women and his wife left him when Donald was two years old. Donald was arrested for placing his hands on the genitals of a three-year-old girl. Her father found him on top of the child behind a clump of bushes. This followed the boy's conversation with playmates, in which "dirty things" had been discussed. At the age of nine years, Donald had been forced into an homosexual experience.

James T., thirteen years old, had an excellent family background with regard to economic status, decency, and home spirit. He was a spoiled lad, an only child, who was worshipped and overprotected by his parents. In school, he was impertinent, disobedient, and defiant. He cut classes and spent the time smoking in the lavatory. At one time, he stole $21.00 from the school teacher's desk. He was caught "placing his hands on the genitals" of an eight-year-old girl in an alley. He had asked her once before to "let him do it" but she refused. This time "she pulled down her bloomers and asked him if he wanted to do it." He did it.

Exhibitionism is the exposure of the genital organs to others without any attempt at intercourse or other contacts. A not uncommon type is "the mutual and perfectly voluntary exhibition of their genital organs by children, generally boys and girls together; in these cases the acts are determined rather by curiosity than by the sexual impulse" (Moll). The other type, that of deriving gratification from the display, is quite rare in children and occurs mostly in seriously retarded and in postencephalitic boys.

"Petting" is a term which covers a wide range of sexual practices preparatory to, but not usually ending in, actual intercourse. It includes various forms and extents of mutual manipulations, embraces to the point of orgasm, *immissio membri inter femora*, etc. It has become a widely indulged activity among adolescents, though in a lesser degree it certainly must be conceded to be an age-old custom, especially among couples engaged for a

long period of time. The previous attitude of wholesale condemnation has been replaced by many people by unreserved condoning. There is certainly no excuse for sanctioning or encouraging the custom, though moral indignation without understanding is equally out of place. Thom says: "There is no reason to believe that any large portion of those individuals who indulge themselves indiscriminately in what is now commonly called petting ...are actually getting what they are going after. All too frequently one or both of the parties involved find themselves unable to digest these experiences that may be aesthetically repulsive and therefore not emotionally satisfying. The question of why this type of activity is continued if it gives promise of so little satisfaction is not difficult to answer: In the first place, there is a group of individuals who find no conflicts either social, moral, aesthetic, or emotional, and they carry on their pastimes unhampered by any inhibitions. In the second place, sex activity of the type described is ofttimes a means rather than an end itself; it is regarded as the 'price of admission' for a certain popularity and for certain attentions which the girl and boy fear would otherwise be denied them. In the third place, sex indulgence, like alcoholic indulgence, becomes a habit; a physiological demand and appetite are created and these become strong enough to overcome the feeling of repugnance following each previous experience."[1]

Sexual intercourse. Juvenile Court experience as well as venereal disease statistics teach that at the ages of between nine and fifteen years, in colored children even a little earlier, cohabitation occurs and is often enough a serious problem. The situation is best illustrated by the following examples (for which white children only have been selected):

Kenneth L., eight years old, went with another boy and two little girls to see the other boy's uncle, hoping to get from him a nickel. They found the man in a state of alcoholic intoxication and in a compromising position with a drunken woman. Upon Kenneth's suggestion, the children went into another room and tried to imitate the uncle's sex act. Kenneth was the fourth of nine siblings. He had a pleasing personality, high average intelligence, did well in school and was well liked by his teacher and playmates. He was once caught stealing at seven years. He and his brother slept with their mother. His paternal grandparents were divorced; each remarried soon afterwards. His maternal grandparents were divorced because the man "ran around with women." His father, illiterate, lazy and shiftless, deserted the family on several occasions; he was once arrested for making sexual advances to his oldest daughter. His mother was in the habit of delivering herself of her babies in her children's presence.

Byron C., fourteen years old, with a mental age of twelve years, was apprehended while attempting intercourse with an eleven-year-old girl (as was later learned, upon her invitation), while two boys were watching. He had a history of truancy. His mother died when he was eleven years old. His father was a periodic drinker. His brother, aged twenty-six years, had a record of burglary and running away from a boys' reformatory. Another brother had had incestuous relations with his eleven-year-old sister.

[1] Thom, Douglas Z. Normal Youth and Its Everyday Problems. New York and London. 1932, pp. 70–71.

Lorraine F., thirteen years old, very seriously retarded in intelligence (I.Q. 62), was, at ten years, involved in a rape case; an old man tried to assault her and her sister in a public park, promising candy. At twelve, she and a companion spent a night at an hotel with two men. At thirteen, she submitted to intercourse with a man, "after he had threatened her," and was greatly upset by being paid only fifty cents instead of the two dollars promised. She was the illegitimate daughter of a luetic, ignorant, and irresponsible father and a luetic, feebleminded mother. Her sister, also born out of wedlock, had congenital syphilis and was an imbecile. A paternal aunt was in a psychopathic ward, diagnosed as "paranoid." Her maternal aunts all had questionable reputations. Lorraine had been tossed about between her parents and had been in several institutions and homes. The child was indifferent to everybody and everything.

Helen W., fourteen, normally intelligent, illegitimate child of an unknown father, whose mother died six years ago of tuberculosis, rejected by her stepfather, went to a boys' party and stayed there all night. She later married the boy who had had sexual relations with her.

Lillian K., fourteen, slightly retarded, left home to live with a married man who had seven children. The man posed as single and told her he would marry her as soon as he collected $6,000.00 from an inheritance. Under his influence, she stole a watch at her place of work (as a domestic) and pawned it for five dollars. When twelve years old, she had had intercourse with a man who had "forced it on her." Lillian was an only child of socially dependent, "incompatible" parents who separated several times. She had an unintelligent, worrying, nagging mother. Her maternal grandmother, a "noted spiritualist," used the child as a "medium" and "taught her to throw fits." She had lived a very seclusive life with her mother and grandmother and was not permitted to have friends.

Jeannette B., fourteen, physically healthy, somewhat retarded intellectually, was persuaded by a girl friend to run away from home and to go with her to another state together with two young men. When the four were apprehended in an hotel, the friend was pregnant and Jeannette, more fortunate, remained without child. A judge married her friend to the expected baby's father (who soon afterwards disappeared) and placed Jeannette in the custody of an older sister, not knowing that the custodian herself was promiscuous and had run away from her decent husband and two children to live with a good-for-nothing psychopath. The child's parents had separated six years previously. Her mother mistreated her children brutally and brought home and entertained men at all hours of the night. The family was known to practically all charitable and juridical agencies of the community. Alcoholic excesses, quarrels, mutual accusations of the vilest nature, arrests, temper outbursts, and evictions were matters of daily routine in the home. It was to the prostitute psychopathic and alcoholic mother that a wise court decreed the authority over her minor children! Jeannette resented being supervised, scolded, and beaten by a sister who made a practice of extramarital sex indulgences. She ran away from her. She was this time taken to the juvenile court and placed as a domestic at a denominational convalescent home where, for the past two years, she has done splendidly, fully appreciating the humane treatment which she receives there.

Mary R., thirteen, seriously retarded (I.Q. 66), has been for more than a year in the habit of frequenting vacant houses with boys with the purpose of having sexual intercourse. At the age of eleven years, a man had lured her into a vacant house and deflowered her. After this experience she became sexually aggressive. She stayed away from school, hunting for boys. She had no mercenary designs. When taken to the juvenile court, she had an acute gonorrheal infection. She found nothing wrong in what she had done; she felt that people "make a fuss over it because they ain't got nothing else to talk about." She was committed to a training school for feebleminded children.

These examples could be augmented *ad libitum*. They show plainly the settings in which the first full-fledged erotic experiences of children may take place. First in the order of frequency is the seduction of feebleminded children by irresponsible adults. Bad example in the home comes next. Other factors are parental cruelty, persuasion by friends, desire for adventure, and the hope of remuneration. Sexual precocity has often been named as a prominent etiological feature. But it stands to reason that even full attainment of nubility is not necessarily nor desirably a *carte blanche* for unrestrained cohabitation. Loose home standards and attitudes, unsupervised association with treacherous companions, faulty or lacking knowledge of the possible results are the main things which must be fought against with a prophylactic and therapeutic aim. In doing so, we naturally cannot afford to disregard the social texture of our environment. Some courts unfortunately do disregard it and prefer to work with abstract ideas and ideals. Crocodile's tears of an immoral and alcoholic mother, the false sentimentalism of a jury stimulated by the flowery oratory of a lawyer who has been paid for it, the attribution of adult reasoning to children, the rigid adherence of some of the judges to an impersonal "law" oblivious of potent human factors, have paved the road to disaster for many a first offender or even precipitated the first offense. We recall the case of a well developed, normally intelligent, and sensible twelve-year-old girl whom the father and a paternal aunt tried to remove from her mother's home. The mother armed herself with a good lawyer ("good" in the sense of being capable of persuasive oratory), with a flood of tears, with accusations against her husband and his sister, and with profuse promises, and "won the case." Soon afterwards (as a matter of fact, within the same week), she and an older daughter forced the child with brutal beatings to have intercourse with a drunken sailor who repaid them well. This is by no means a single occurrence. It is most fortunate that our juvenile courts know better how to handle children who are lucky to fall under their exclusive jurisdiction.

Prostitution in pubescent and even pre-pubescent girls is more common than one should like to believe and than the uninformed usually do believe. Again the feebleminded contribute a large contingent. The same factors are active that we mentioned in connection with the more episodic cases of sexual intercourse. A few illustrative examples may lead the reader into the midst of the problem.

Martha G., thirteen, was the seriously retarded (I.Q. 65) daughter of an alcoholic father and a feebleminded mother who, after separation from her husband, went to live with another man, also feebleminded, of whom she had one child. A brother was sent to a reformatory after running away from home. Martha had a history of temper tantrums. Her mother wanted her to "go" with a feebleminded boy who had seven court charges against him and who was repulsive to her. She left her home and sold herself to whomever wanted to buy her. She contracted a gonorrheal infection.

Lucy M., feebleminded daughter of an alcoholic, migrating laborer and a mentally retarded mother, one of the four survivals of eighteen pregnancies, expelled from school when in the fifth grade (at a mental age of seven years!), acquired at twelve years gonorrhea, necessitating bilateral salpingectomy and right oöphorectomy. She had a long record of sex delinquency, beginning at nine years. On several occasions she stayed away from home for many days during which she had promiscuous relations. She married at sixteen. Her sister married at thirteen, after becoming pregnant.

Alice O., daughter of an alcoholic loafer, gambler, and skirt-chaser and of a deaf, nagging mother, only slightly retarded, with a record of truancy and stealing (a watch and a ring), had been promiscuous since the age of eight years, preferably with sailors and married men. Her mother shielded her and blamed the men "for everything." Alice said: "I run away from home because I get devilishness in my head." Her sister was committed to a reformatory at thirteen because of sex delinquency.

Grace W., a healthy girl of average intelligence, had been dealt with very sternly at home by a temperamental father and an illiterate mother. At twelve, she was assaulted sexually by her seventeen-year-old brother. At thirteen she was found in a compromising position with a man in a parked automobile. She had been in the habit of flirting with bus drivers in public parks. She developed the habit of visiting (for pay) and having intercourse with two men to whom she referred as "Booze" and "Mitchie."

Anna A., a foundling, physically healthy, very unattractive, with left internal strabismus, was adopted and raised by an obscene bootlegger who was in the habit of calling her, "Dirty old cock-eye," and an equally immoral woman. Men and women, both white and colored, frequented the home at any time of day and night. The foster-mother forced Anna, when she was thirteen, to be "nice to men." She did not resent that (not knowing of any other standards), but when she was once mistreated she left the place and went to live with a young man with whom she had previously had relations in her own home. After a time, he told her that she was no longer wanted, and she began to pick up men in the streets. At fifteen, she gave birth to a child and a wise judge caused her to be married to the baby's (putative) father. The couple lived together for exactly twenty-five days.

Mildred H. and Ethel R., when seen at the juvenile court at the ages of fifteen and seventeen years, respectively, looked back to many years of prostitution in Baltimore, Philadelphia, Washington, and New York. Mildred had a brutal father, a heavy drinker, who beat his children and his deaf, paralyzed wife whom he enjoyed kicking out of bed and of her wheelchair. A paternal aunt was schizophrenic. A sister had an illegitimate child at fourteen and lived from the proceeds of selling her body. Mildred's mentor, Ethel, whose grandfathers both died from the effects of alcoholism, had a father who claimed to be a full-blooded Cherokee Indian; he was tattooed all over the body, had cerebrospinal syphilis, was socially dependent, and had spent several terms in jail, mostly for stealing. When confronted with his daughter's problems, he did not see anything at all offensive or harmful in her behavior and felt that "she acted just like any other girl."

Assault. It does happen, though fortunately quite rarely, that boys of poor training and poorest self-control attack girls brutally and force themselves upon them.

George L. fourteen, only son of a policeman, a badly spoiled boy of normal intelligence, set fire to a barn at ten years. He was committed to a reformatory where, through an assumed meekness and clever flattery, he won the hearts of the authorities so completely that they returned him to his parents after a few weeks. He broke into a store and again was sent to the correctional institution where, this time, he was treated less as a wronged angel. In revenge, he set fire to the mechanical shop and, in the general excitement, managed to run away. His father kept him at home for some time, during which he made restitution for the boy's occasional thefts. When George again attempted to burn a building, he was committed to a psychopathic hospital. From there he was discharged as "not insane." George, meanwhile fourteen years old, ran away from home soon after his return and went to "look for a job" in a middle-sized town. The next thing his parents heard was that he had been arrested for assaulting a girl sexually. He had learned that, in order to come home, she had to pass through a quiet, uninhabited alley. He lay in ambush and when she appeared he threatened her at the point of a pistol to keep quiet. He gagged her, cohabitated with her and went away. Luckily, the girl managed to rid herself of the gag and shouted, and George was arrested.

Incest. Sexual intercourse between parents and children and between brothers and sisters is comparatively infrequent but it does occur. In a few of the cases quoted above it has been a factor in the life of the patient or in his or her family. In the type of domestic situations in which foundations are laid for prostitution and other forms of abandon to a social and antisocial activities, incestuous relations are not always looked upon with the same disgust as in families with higher standards. I have had opportunity to deal with a considerable number of such instances. In every one of those cases which have come to my attention the home setting and parental influences were utterly disastrous. The act is fostered by the custom of letting brothers and sisters sleep together in the same bed. In one of my cases, a fifteen-year-old girl had a child from her own alcoholic and feebleminded father! It can hardly be judged how many such relations remain unknown, being kept secret by those involved.

HOMOSEXUAL ACTIVITIES

Homosexual "crushes," occurring in high schools, are usually as harmless as the transient heterosexual attachments, if handled calmly and with understanding. They are much more common in girls than in boys. A woman teacher or an older girl is admired with all the ardor with which other girls worship a male teacher or an older boy. The "crushes" usually fade away, if they are not mismanaged by provoking the child's resentment through ridicule or rudeness.

Overt homosexual practices are more serious and fortunately less fre-

Factors leading to

quent. Imitation of others, exposure to a homosexual assault by an adult, mutual masturbation with children of the same sex are the outstanding factors driving a youngster in this direction.

John S., thirteen years old, of low average intelligence, was the son of a man who for many years had spoken openly of his "sex failure," accused his wife of illicit affairs, and finally killed her and one child, injured the other children, and committed suicide, when John was eleven years old. John went to live with an older sister who resented his presence from the first and threatened to have him "put away" if he did not behave. He often pondered over the meaning of his father's "sex failure." At thirteen, he lured a six-year-old boy into the house, took off his trousers, attempted to have sex relations with him, and later put his penis into the boy's mouth. He had seen boys in the neighborhood do the same thing previously and thought that his not doing so was the first sign of "sex failure."

Harry S., fourteen years old, of slightly superior intelligence, an only child, untruthful, impudent to his mother who suffered from Addison's disease, and spoiled by his father who was subject to depressive episodes, was sent to the country at the age of twelve years to spend his summer vacation with his father's friends. A farm hand there initiated him into homosexual practices under terrible threats. When he returned home, he took to smoking and drinking (stealing the cigarettes and drinks from his father's drug store) and, with similar threats, intimidated a seven-year-old boy into letting him have sex relations with him. The affair was discovered incidentally after it had gone on for approximately eighteen months. The younger boy was so afraid of Harry's revenge that not until Harry's placement in a boarding home at some distance did he reveal the facts.

In these two and many other cases the theoretical question as to whether there exists such a thing as a congenital homosexual tendency is certainly of much less practical significance than the concrete facts which obviously led up to the boys' performances. Again, as in the problems of heterosexual maladjustment, the home standards and attitudes, the mode of child training, and the type of parental supervision are seen to be of paramount importance, in addition to more or less unpredictable, accidental experiences which may exercise a potent influence on a child's behavior. But wise management in the home will detect and remedy such influences earlier and better than carelessness or misplaced emotionalism.

Fellatio (immissio membri in os) is a surprisingly frequent form of boys' overt homosexual activities.

Charles A., a seven-year-old boy who also masturbated openly and frequently, had diurnal and nocturnal enuresis, and stole. Although his stepmother, eager to be rid of his care, grossly exaggerated his misbehavior, it remained true that he had approached boys from six to eleven years of age inviting them to perform fellatio with him. He had often been beaten up for it by the older boys but apparently found several boys who were willing to do it or frightened into doing it. Charles began this practice at the age of five years. He was described as being "like a girl" in his manners; he delighted in house cleaning, scrubbing steps, and washing dishes. The boy had normal intelligence. The home was pervaded with a tangle of lies, accusations, hostilities, peculiar financial arrangements and, above all, an inhuman stepmother's attempt to rid herself of Charles, trying to encourage his habits in order later to use them as "evidence" against him. Unfortunately, legal obstacles were in the way of removing the boy from his impossible home and giving him an opportunity for adequate training.

FETISHISM

A fetish, in the sexological sense, is "an object having no intrinsic significance of sex, but arousing erotic feelings" (The Winston Dictionary). Though in adults fetishism may assume the most peculiar and sometimes harmful forms, it rarely expresses itself in children in any other manner than the romantic keeping, kissing, or pressing to the heart of the beloved person's handkerchief or glove or a flower received from the admired girl. It is a harmless pleasure which I have never known to assume pathological significance below the age of adolescence. A perverted adult patient of Krafft-Ebing's recalled that since the fourth year of his life polished, shiny shoes produced in him a sexual excitement; such "early recollections," however, must be taken with the proverbial grain of salt.

BESTIALITY (SODOMY)

Sexual activities with animals as the objects occur sometimes in pubescent and adolescent children, especially those living in rural communities. Charles A., whose case we just reported, was accused by his stepmother of having relations with a dog, but this story turned out to be her invention. Ziehen cites the case of a girl who stated that she had cohabitated every evening with a male dog since the age of eight years; her foster-mother knew of the affair and assured her that it would do her no harm. The girl had temper tantrums, bit her fingernails, picked her nose, pulled her hair out, wet her bed until the age of ten years, stole, lied, ran away from home, masturbated frequently, and was in the habit of introducing into her vagina her six-year-old cousin's penis. A schizophrenic boy of our own observation practiced coitus with calves "ever since he could remember."

THE CHILD AS AN OBJECT OF SEXUAL PRACTICES

This is the title of a chapter in Moll's book (The Sexual Life of the Child. Translated by Eden Paul. New York. 1924. Pp. 219–245), in which the injurious activities, performed on children by adults, of an heterosexual ("pederastic," "pedophilic"), homosexual, sadistic, or masochistic nature are discussed. Some of the cases quoted above have already given the reader a taste of such occurrences. This is a side of our social life which should be known to every parent and educator. In every type of community, in every sort of residential section (less in the suburbs than in the slums, to be sure) there are men and women who are bent upon abusing children sexually, sometimes because they prefer children and sometimes faute de mieux. They lure the unsuspecting youngsters with pennies, sweets, or promises into their homes or into alleys and make them the objects of their desires. They often hang around schools and playgrounds, selecting and waiting for their victims. Threats and a feeling of guilt and shame prevent the children from reporting their experiences to their parents. Some people, after discovering the affair, fail to inform the police for fear of a "scandal," preferring to let the same offenders run loose and seduce more children. It is for this, if for no other, reason that early sex education is invaluable and makes the youngsters wary of the designs of such persons. It is for this reason that parents should know their children's associates and whereabouts and should be most careful in their choice of servants, tutors, and governesses.

CHAPTER XL

ATTACK DISORDERS

CHILDREN are subject much more frequently than adults to sudden and brief events of first magnitude, "attacks" or "seizures" or "spells" or "fits," which for a few seconds or minutes or hours involve the patients' total reactivity and exclude them wholly or partly from their usual adaptations and participations. It is perhaps unwise to combine under one heading, however broadly conceived, heterogeneous happenings, some of which occur on an infrapsychobiological level, while others are clearly exaggerated emotional responses, and still others occupy a place somewhere between those two categories. They do, however, have certain features in common which, chiefly for the purpose of organization, may justify an attempt to consider them together: their sweeping character, their suddenness, explosiveness, the relative shortness of their duration, and their tendency to repeat themselves. We have found it expedient to deal with a few of them in connection with other disturbances. Some of them are never or almost never encountered beyond the early years of life; this is true, for instance, of breathholding spells, the laryngospasms and convulsions of tetany, cyclic vomiting, and pavor nocturnus. It is interesting to note that, while night terrors usually disappear at or before puberty, the less explosive nightmares may be continued during adolescence and adulthood. Temper outbursts and sobbing spells, though largely reactions of childhood, are met with less often in people who have grown up physically but not emotionally. On the other hand, asthmatic episodes, migrainous seizures, and anxiety attacks are less common in children than they are in adults.

We have preferred to take up migraine, night terrors, anxiety attacks, and hysterical convulsions in some of the other chapters. Here we deal with the convulsive disorders, pyknolepsy, breathholding spells, and syncopal attacks.

CONVULSIONS

The first two years of life furnish the greatest contingent of convulsive phenomena. The frequency then decreases gradually. It has been noted that rachitic infants are more apt to have convulsions than non-rachitic ones. This is due to a large extent to the marked coincidence of rickets and spasmophilia.

Convulsions may occur in any condition in which there is cerebral tissue alteration. They may arise on the basis of cerebral birth injuries, intracranial hemorrhage, meningitis, encephalitis, hydrocephalus, thrombosis or embolism, abscess and tumor of the brain. They may follow concussions and skull fractures. They are met with in congenital lues, especially during the first months of life, in juvenile paresis, and occasionally in amaurotic family idiocy. They are seen in approximately one-third of all microcephalic children. They are an essential symptom of tuberous sclerosis.

414

Infectious, toxic, and autotoxic conditions are prone to set up convulsions in children. They are found in lead poisoning, in uremia, and in severe gastro-intestinal disturbances. They may occur at the beginning of pneumonia, scarlet fever, and measles. None of the contagious diseases of children is totally exempt from the possibility of convulsive complications, though they are peculiarly uncommon in diphtheria. They are comparatively rife in pertussis. In some children, any elevation of temperature may be accompanied by convulsions. As a matter of fact, many authors (e.g., Holt, Sachs) consider them as having the same value as the initial rigor or chill which ushers in a severe acute infection in the adult. There is no noticeable correlation between the height of the fever and the occurrence of convulsions.

Between the ages of about six months and two years, tetany is the commonest cause of infantile convulsions. On very rare occasions, hemorrhages into the suprarenal glands have been reported to result in convulsions in the newborn.

Asphyxia at birth has often been mentioned as an etiological factor. It is perhaps also responsible for the jerkings which are observed in a very small percentage of breathholding spells.

In addition to all these manifold causes and to the grand hysterical attacks which are discussed elsewhere in this book, there are convulsions and related phenomena (petit mal attacks, "absences," fugues, "equivalents") which cannot be objectively referred to clinically demonstrable cerebral lesions nor to bacterial nor toxic nor metabolic damage nor to more or less clearly recognizable psychogenic affections. It is customary to speak of them collectively as "genuine" or "idiopathic" epilepsy, or as "epilepsy" in short. Some authors prefer to use the plural, "the epilepsies," to indicate that they deal with a variety of clinically and etiologically similar, yet by no means identical conditions.

EPILEPSY

It has in recent years become more and more customary to get away from too rigid a distinction between the so-called symptomatic epilepsies with well-known structural or metabolic (e.g., febrile, hypoglycemic, etc.) disorders and the idiopathic epilepsies in which gross lesions cannot be demonstrated. The attack phenomena are a common denominator present and very similar or equal in both groups. The modern advances in brain surgery and in encephalographic diagnosis have tended to shift an appreciable number of cases from the idiopathic to the organic category. The whole series of convulsive conditions is perhaps one of the best advocates of the integration concept, in that it presents a thorough and inseparable amalgamation of events occurring simultaneously, successively, or vicariously on both the vegetative and the psychobiological levels of existence. There are many instances in which the pendulum swings clearly and obviously towards a definite and unmistakable predominance of the anatomo-pathological involvement; in others the psychopathological factors are decidedly in the foreground. A total disregard of either set of facts would frequently amount to unjustified and arbitrary abandon of material highly valuable from an etiological, symptomatological, and therapeutical point of view.

The attacks are usually divided into three classes, one or two or all of which may occur in the same patient:

1. Grand mal.
2. Petit mal.
3. Psychic equivalents.

Grand mal. The *major* or *grand mal attacks* are the convulsions *par excellence*, characterized mainly by abolition of consciousness, abnormal motor discharges, and termination in drowsiness or sleep.

The convulsions may be preceded or initiated by a prodromal foreboding or warning, the so-called *aura*. Gowers found it to be present in 57 per cent of epileptic adults; it is less common in children. It may be motor, sensory, visceral, or psychic. The *motor* aura, which is less frequent than the other forms, consists of various kinds of tremulous movements or jactations, often restricted to a circumscribed group of muscles, or of more complicated automatic performances, such as running or taking off the clothes. The *sensory* aura may manifest itself as localized pain or numbness or a feeling of warmth or cold or different sorts of visual, auditory, olfactory, or gustatory sensations or hallucinations. The *visceral* aura is most usually expressed in children as abdominal discomfort, located mostly in the epigastrium, or as a feeling of tightness in the throat; palpitations, vertigo, headache and head pressure are more apt to be found in adults than in children. The *psychic* aura, which is sometimes combined with one of the other forms, is either simply a vague presentiment that the attack is about to happen, or general restlessness, or an experience of fear, or a feeling of unreality in which things seem to be different, changed, not as they should be, or a mood disturbance with irritability, or an undetermined notion that something is about to happen, or the obtrusion of an obsessive idea. According to Vogt, psychic aura is especially prone to be met with in cases which offer an unfavorable prognosis. The duration of the aura varies from a few seconds to several hours or even days. It is sometimes so brief that the attack takes place at the very moment of its realization. Again, the child may have time to announce its presence or to run to the mother for protection or at least to lie down somewhere in order to prevent injuries which may result from the fall. Occasionally the parents report that they can predict a seizure many hours before it comes from the child's change of disposition, inattentiveness, and disturbed sleep. The longer the "warning" lasts, the more the little patient is bound to suffer, not so much because of the symptoms of the foreboding itself as because of the apprehensive knowledge that another seizure is inevitable.

The following is a selection of examples of aurae gathered from our case material:

"He sees the colors red, white, and blue in front of his eyes about ten minutes before the attacks."

"He says he sees things on the wall or on the ceiling."

"She said she had a black spot in front of her right eye and remembered no more. At another time she complained that her stomach hurt. Before another attack she said that her throat hurt and that she was sick. Mostly she comes to an adult and says that she feels sick (nauseated)."

"He complains that his eyes hurt before he has a convulsion."

"She has a swimming of her eyes and a feeling that she ought to shut her eyes."

"He complains of his stomach hurting him, then he shouts. Sometimes he knows the attacks are coming and is able to tell his parents. He says that right before the attacks he feels electric shocks through his eyes."

"She feels as if her eyes would pop out of her head before an attack."

"Sometimes he has an aura and sometimes not. The aura usually is in the form of frontal headache and a feeling of tightness in the throat. On one occasion he said, "I am having a convulsion,' just as his arms and face began to jerk."

"A typical attack is preceded by a peculiar feeling in the throat with dizziness. Once he felt like somebody pressed his throat and thought he would have a convulsion but it passed away without a spell that time."

"She can feel it coming on. Something comes up in her throat that chokes her."

"At the beginning she has a feeling like something coming up in her throat and she has to keep swallowing and swallowing."

"He complains of fright in his chest and pain in his stomach. Before the convulsion, he has a feeling that something hits him in the stomach, then goes up and chokes him, then he has the attack."

"She wakes up at night and says that she feels sick and wants to vomit. She throws up and soon afterwards her hands, feet, and eyes start to jerk."

"She always complains of pain in her stomach before an attack comes on."

"Before any type of attack and sometimes when no attack follows, she feels worried, as if something were going to happen."

"She used to feel like her stomach would be big and water bubbling in it and then she had a pain in her heart before the grand mal came on. When petit mals come on, she feels her throat jumping and her mother sees the movements of her larynx."

"On numerous occasions she has flushed intensely and been very much excited for a few minutes before the convulsions."

"He gets to giggling and laughing before he has a spell."

"She has no warning of the spell but laughs at the onset of her attacks."

A boy of six years associated his attacks in a peculiar manner with toothbrushes and toothpaste. He had the definite notion that the thought of a toothbrush brought on a convulsion. Yet he drew at the clinic upon request a toothbrush and when provided with one cleaned his teeth without anything happening. What really took place was that the aura assumed the form of an obsessive thought of cleaning the teeth. It is of interest that his mother reported that brushing her teeth made her gag.

The aura is suddenly terminated by *loss of consciousness*. Where there is no aura, the seizure comes altogether unannounced. There may be a shrill and piercing *initial cry*. At the moment of the loss of consciousness and as a result of it, the patient collapses. The fall is followed by the *stage of tonic spasms* in which the entire body is involved. The trunk, more often the head and face, may be turned to one side. After about thirty to sixty seconds, the tonic phase is replaced by a *stage of clonic convulsions* lasting from one to three minutes. They consist of jerking, kicking, irregular movements of the extremities and sometimes also of the head which may bounce on the floor. The trunk also may be thrown about. Participation of the diaphragm may cause the emission of rhythmical gasping or gargling noises. The tongue may move about in the mouth; it is often bitten owing to spasms of the muscles of mastication. The eyes frequently roll upward. The cutaneous and tendon reflexes may be diminished or, less often, exaggerated during the attack. The Babinski sign is positive and may remain so for some time after the seizure. The corneal reflex is abolished. The pupils are at first small, then become widely dilated and do not react to light. The pulse rate rises with the increase of muscular activity. The temperature is often elevated at the end of or after the convulsion. The pallor at the onset is soon replaced by redness and later by cyanosis as a result of spasms of the respiratory musculature. Occasionally involuntary defecation takes place; much more common is micturition during the period of unconsciousness. Salivation is often increased and the saliva either runs out of the oral cavity or forms a froth between the half-open lips.

The convulsion is mostly followed by a few minutes to several hours of profound sleep (the terms "stupor" and "coma" are less correct; real coma exists during and not after the seizure). Upon awakening, there may be a short time of drowsiness and weakness, and consciousness is gradually regained.

The attacks do not always take this "typical" course. Any number of variations is possible, though it can be said that, whatever form they may assume, they resemble one another in the same individual with almost photographical exactness. But even in the same patient, especially under therapeutic influences, they are reported to be different in their degree of severity. The simplest form is sudden pallor without aura, and collapse without motor or other disturbances. Binswanger described as *rudimentary attacks* all those in which there is only incomplete loss of consciousness or comparative brevity of the entire event or absence of either the tonic or the clonic component. *Epilepsia rotatoria* is characterized by seizures in which the patient, in a state of partially abolished consciousness, turns rapidly around his longitudinal axis. *Epilepsia procursiva* (*dromolepsy*) refers to a type of attacks in which the child suddenly runs a few steps forward before falling; it is to be distinguished from the running aura and from the wanderings in an epileptic fugue. In very serious and prognostically unfavorable cases several convulsions may follow each other so quickly that the next begins before consciousness has been recovered from the preceding one; this condition is designated as *status epilepticus*, in contradistinction to a *series of attacks*, as many as ten to fifteen in one day, in which the new seizure does not begin until the preceding one is completely over. The status is apt to be followed by paralyses, high fever, aphasia, and visual disorders. It is often enough fatal; upon autopsy one sometimes finds hemorrhages into the medulla oblongata.

The grand mal attacks rarely show a definite pattern of periodicity. The frequency varies with different individuals; in some patients they are as rare as once in a year or even rarer, in others they may occur daily. There are also considerable variations in the same person; there may be free periods of weeks' or months' duration succeeded by a cumulation of seizures.

The detailed observation of the convulsions sometimes furnishes a clue with regard to the presence and nature of organic involvement. The *Jacksonian type*, in which the motor phenomena are restricted to a circumscribed area or in which there is a localized aura, is suggestive of a focal cortical lesion. Usually a hand or a forearm is affected, less commonly a foot or a leg. Yet it must be remembered that the limited twitchings may quickly be followed by a generalized convulsion, that in some cases the attacks may begin in the same patient sometimes on one side and sometimes on the other, and that focal lesions may occasionally produce convulsions which are generalized from the beginning. In Jacksonian epilepsy consciousness is as a rule not as completely abolished as in "idiopathic" epilepsy. Visual aurae, especially those that are unilateral, are said to be indicative of an involvement of the occipital cortex. Auditory forebodings (noises, voices) are said to point in the direction of a participation of the temporal lobe. Olfactory aurae (peculiar odors) are considered as proceeding from the uncinate gyrus ("uncinate fits").

The grand mal attacks may occur at any time of the day, during waking or sleeping. The nocturnal convulsions sometimes go unnoticed and can be inferred only from a fresh injury to the tongue, from the bedclothes which are wet with urine, or from drowsiness, confusion, headache, or weakness in the morning. One of our patients sometimes rolled out of his bed during his nocturnal seizures.

There is complete *amnesia* for every attack. The children do, however, frequently remember the aura and are mostly in a position to describe correctly their own experiences and the activities of those about them during the warning. The attitudes and facial expressions of their parents may indicate to them afterwards that they had had an attack.

Petit mal. The *minor attacks* or *absences* (staring, dreaming, dopy, vacant spells) are characterized by very short lapses of consciousness without convulsions. Aura is rarely reported (as, for instance, in the child whose staring spell was preceded for about thirty seconds by abdominal pain). The patient interrupts for from two to ten or more seconds whatever he may have been doing and usually stares into the vacant space. He then resumes his activity as if nothing has happened and has no recollection of the event. A few typical complaints follow:

"If he does something, he would stop all of a sudden and then keep on walking or doing what he wants to do."

"He sits with a far-away look and pays no attention."

"At one time he had a spell while pouring milk; he kept on pouring and the milk ran over the table on the top of the glass. Sometimes in school he would raise his hand and when the teacher calls him, he would keep it raised for a few seconds and stare. He would stop in the middle of a sentence and then resume it with the same word as though nothing had happened."

"She becomes unconscious for about two seconds, falls over wherever she is, often hurting herself. She then gets up and acts as if nothing has happened."

"He would look or stare rather fixedly at some distant point and his eyes oscillate slightly. Sometimes he stands up, shakes his head and his eyes move back and forth. He keeps his little hands stiff but they shake, too. He used to wet himself nearly every day both at home and in school but during the past week since taking the medicine (luminal) he has not wet himself once. The bed was also wet in the morning very often but not during the last week. He has never fallen during the attack. Sometimes he has it when he is walking and I am afraid he will walk into a machine in the street. Last summer he had one in the street and the children in the neighborhood saw him and called him crazy. Since then I don't let him play with any children except his sister." During the examination, the child had two attacks. He stood quietly and stared upward and to the right and his eyes moved with slow lateral nystagmus. He did not answer when spoken to and had no recollection of the events when they were over. He stated that he can feel an attack coming on, "he feels a flush come over him."

"He has slight attacks of glaring and makes swallowing movements and his left hand shakes some. It never lasts more than a few seconds."

There is always a complete amnesia for the actions and occurrences during a petit mal attack. There are few components of the grand mal seizure that could not be occasionally observed in the minor spells. Involuntary micturition, tongue bite, rolling of the eyes, jerkings, the fall, and subsequent sleep or confusion have been reported in a relatively small number of cases. The characteristic cry, the succession of tonic and clonic convulsions, the cyanosis, and serious injuries are not seen in the absences. Those are right who consider the differences between the two types of events as being of a quantitative rather than qualitative nature; there are seizures offering features which make it difficult to make a definite statement as to the category in which one might want to group them.

The *secousses* and *salaam spasms* which we described in connection with the differential diagnosis of spasmus nutans are sometimes regarded as varieties of petit mal, while others set them apart as atypical epileptic attacks *sui generis*.

Epileptic psychic equivalents. There are occurrences in some epileptic persons, rather uncommon in children, which are manifested in the form of temporary clouding of consciousness with automatic motor performances which are not remembered by the patient. Some are of so short a duration that they cannot be clearly distinguished from unusual petit mal disorders.

One of our children who also had unmistakable absences sometimes exclaimed, "as though in a dream state": "Look at the swords!", or, "They are hurting me," or, "Come on, brother, hold these horses!" He did not recall afterwards what had happened.

A nine-year-old boy who had several generalized convulsions had episodes which were spoken of by his stepmother as "queer actions." Sometimes he suddenly got up and ran around the table purposelessly for several seconds. He had paroxysms of "wagging his head from side to side and fidgeting his shoulders." At times he "acted silly" for as long as half an hour without recollecting what he had done.

A nine-year-old girl who had both grand and petit mal attacks "sometimes performed actions while in a daze, such as suddenly breaking eggs in a store."

A seriously retarded six-year-old colored boy with frequent major and occasional minor attacks had episodes during which he wandered around the house aimlessly or tore his clothes or the curtains. Often "he gets up at night and wanders around, walks up and down the steps, then you'll find him upstairs on the third floor sitting in the dark. Early in the morning around three o'clock he gets up and starts walking into things. About a month ago, he backed up against the oil stove and burned himself."

A thirteen-year-old boy who had some sort of "spasms" for the first five years of life ("his eyes rolled up, his head was held back, his fists were clenched, he fell and was rigid"), had since the age of six or seven years paroxysms in which he performed impulsive actions followed by complete amnesia. During a typical attack, his face was red, he laughed, giggled, reached his hands out into space, and talked incessantly. The spells came very often, sometimes none for a week or even a month, at other times every day, even several times per diem. Twice he had them immediately upon waking in the morning. "I might be studying or doing anything, they may come on any time at all. They may come when I am playing or resting or eating. I never had them when sitting on the toilet. If I am in church, if I do it quick enough, I may manage to go out of the church, so I would not cause a disturbance. Before the attacks come, I have a dull pain in my throat. During the spell I do not know a thing that is going on. I might even get up at the offertory of the mass. I might hit a boy. Once in church, I threw a prayer book on the floor. After the spell is over, I feel all right, just like I never had one." The spells usually lasted three minutes. He did not remember anything that happened during them; he only knew what the others told him. But he always knew that he had had a spell because he remembered "the beginning" (the pain in his throat).

It is true that night terrors and temper outbursts are not uncommon in epileptic children. Cases have been reported in which pavor nocturnus was later replaced by characteristic convulsions. But one would go too far if one were to consider night terrors or tantrums as equivalents in every child who happens to have grand or petit mal seizures. It would be even more unjustified to postulate an epileptic character for every instance of pavor in youngsters who manifest no symptom of epilepsy. This consideration, however, does not relieve one of the obligation to think of the convulsive possibilities and to make sure whether or not they are really present in the patient.

The mere description of the main types of epileptic paroxysms has already made it clear that the psychopathological implications are of great importance. They are indeed far more numerous and complex than one might infer from the observation of the various forms of seizures alone. We shall try in the following paragraphs to point out the many possibilities of psychic involvement:

Psychic aura, described above.

Complete loss of consciousness during the grand and most of the petit mal attacks and clouding in the equivalents, confusional states, and fugues.

Postconvulsive sleep and drowsiness.

Amnesia for the events during the seizures with frequent recollection of the aura.

The psychic equivalents.

Confusional states which are either preparoxysmal, or postparoxysmal, or interparoxysmal. They usually do not appear until the epileptic condition has persisted for several years. The equivalents are looked upon by some authors as special types of interparoxysmal confusion.

Specific forms of epileptic confusion are the *fugues* or *twilight states* in which the patients perform complicated acts lasting usually much longer than the equivalents. There is a peculiar kind of clouding of consciousness in which the routine duties of everyday life are discharged without noticeable difficulty; the patients feed and dress themselves normally, take good care of their excretory needs and may answer questions correctly. Yet there is a certain automatism present in all activities. The children may wander away from home without having a definite goal (*epileptic ambulatory automatism*), do not know why and whither they are straying and do not seem to realize that they are doing anything out of the ordinary. At the same time they may know enough to stop an automobile on the road and ask for a ride, or to hop a freight train, or to beg for food and shelter. Food and other objects are often stolen during the fugue by youngsters who would not otherwise touch anything that does not belong to them. It is consistent with the nature of the automaticity that they do not try to conceal their actions and, when apprehended, offer no resistance. Disorientation as to place, time, and even as to person may seriously complicate the picture. Peculiar behavior during the migrations is most apt to call the attention of the public to the morbid state of the patients, who are rarely below the age of puberty; they may be seen throwing money away or they may enter a strange house and proceed to make themselves at home there as if it were their own. We have pointed out elsewhere that fugues occur also in hysterical, schizophrenic, and post-traumatic conditions and in feebleminded children.

A very rare form of epileptic confusional state is that known as the *Ganser syndrome* or *paralogia* which we shall discuss in more detail in connection with hysteria. It consists in giving answers which formally pertain to the questions asked but are not correct in their content. I have seen only one such case, an eight-year-old girl of low average intelligence, whose reactions in a condition of post-convulsive cloudiness strongly resembled the Ganser syndrome.

The intellectual faculties are often found to be impaired in epileptic children. There are said to be three types of relation between idiopathic epilepsy and feeblemindedness:

1. Intellectual retardation and epilepsy are coördinated. The individual is *a priori* intellectually inadequate and disposed to convulsive phenomena.

2. An originally feebleminded child becomes epileptic in the years of puberty.

3. Intellectual deterioration takes place in an originally bright child as a result of the epileptic condition. In this case many authors speak of *epileptic dementia* which is said to be progressive unless, through treatment or spontaneously, the attacks cease. The progression is said to depend on the frequency of the grand and petit mal seizures. According to Ziehen, it takes for an adult an average of nine years from the onset of the disorder until intellectual deterioration becomes apparent, while in children it is already evident after a period of from three to six years. He states that mild degrees of impairment are observed in at least sixty per cent and severe degrees in at least twenty per cent of all juvenile patients.

In comparing the intelligence quotients of one hundred cases of our own material (admittedly a small number), which belong to groups 1 and 3, we found the following conditions to prevail:

I.Q.	Number (%)
Under 30	2
31-40	6
41-50	9
51-60	10
61-70	11
71-80	13
81-90	24
91-100	13
101-110	6
Above 110	6
Total	100

It is true that a considerable proportion of the children was standardized less than three years after the onset of the convulsions. Even then it appears that the relative number of patients with quotients of below 70 is much higher, and that of patients with quotients above 90 is incomparably lower than the respective percentages of all the children referred to us for psychiatric consultation. Cases of "idiopathic" epilepsy only were considered. In the obviously organic cerebrogenic epilepsies the results are much more distressing and idiocy and imbecility much more frequent.

In the cases of progressive intellectual defect there is a *slowing of the mental activity*. Hahn has carried out association experiments on a number of juvenile epileptics and repeated them from time to time for a period of from two to four years. He found that there was a definite and gradually increasing prolongation of the reaction time and that sometimes a slight degree of perseveration could be observed. This slowing deserves consideration in giving intelligence tests to epileptic children, especially in those tasks which require certain time restrictions; it is of interest to know whether the child can do the requirements within the postulated time limit, but it is also very important to know whether they can be carried out at all. A mere minus score is in those instances therefore unsatisfactory. In addition to the slowing, there is often also a marked *impoverishment of contents.* In advanced cases, the range of interest and the stock of information are extremely limited. Thinking becomes monotonous and concerns itself only with the simplest everyday activities. Spontaneity and productivity are reduced to a minimum, excepting for impulsive acts of which we shall speak later. Speech becomes slow, heavy, sometimes even slightly inarticulate.

It is perhaps because most of our cases were examined and treated at an early period that the picture just painted has been seen by us less often than one would expect from the perusal of the literature. From the distribution of the intelligence quotients it appears that the greatest percentages are found in the borderline, dull normal, and low average groups and that even superior intelligence is not at all incompatible with epilepsy. (If further proof were needed, it is furnished by such outstanding examples as Feodor Dostoyevsky and Gustave Flaubert.) But it is equally obvious that intellectual retardation or deterioration does undoubtedly occur in epileptic children oftener than in non-epileptic ones.

Personality traits. Much has been said and written about the personality make-up of epileptic patients. Before entering into a discussion of the individual features, it is perhaps well to state that whatever character traits or behavior disorders one encounters must be considered from various angles rather than ascribed too readily and too exclusively to a morbid process or to innate tendencies. It should not be overlooked that both the child and the family are apt to react to the illness in some form or another which may make special inroads on the patient's personality development and that furthermore intellectual inadequacy, wherever present, may be responsible for certain modes of behavior. The feebleminded child does not worry about the paroxysms; if they have begun early enough, they are simply taken as passively and in the same matter-of-fact manner as any natural phenomenon is accepted, without particular concern or curiosity. The psychiatric problems then are largely the same as in any other feebleminded youngster, plus the need for specific treatment. If the attacks begin at a time when the child is able to reason and to wonder and if the patient is intelligent enough to take issue with the experiences of life, the realization of being subject to the paroxysms may have a decided effect on his attitudes and preoccupations. The occurrence of the convulsions often places him in an unusual position at home and in school. He may learn to fear their recurrence in public or while in the classroom or while with the playmates. Frequent attacks may necessitate unforeseen absences from school. He may brood over the nature of his condition; sometimes he will be affected by the tales of hospital commitments or deaths of epileptic relatives or other people. He may come to think of himself as being different from the other children and withdraw from contacts with them. He may learn to utilize his illness in order to obtain domestic privileges which would not be granted to him if it were not for his attacks. All the while, he is exposed to environmental attitudes which cannot but leave their marks on the formation of his character. Some children may pin undeserved adjectives on him (we have seen patients who because of their attacks were labeled "crazy" or "looney" or "goofy" or "fits") and make him excessively self-conscious and sensitive and either quietly unhappy or aggressively pugnacious, at first in what seems to him justified self-defense and later from sheer force of habit. The parents, naturally worried about the condition, may dispense with the usual methods of training, give in to all of his whims, and spoil him as a "sick child" in every way imaginable. He may be submitted to all sorts of superstitious procedures which are especially popular in the folk-treatment of epilepsy, fed patent medicines, and dragged to doctors, chiropractors, osteopaths, and faith healers. He may be made to feel that the neighbors shun him or pity him. All these things must of necessity exert their influence on the child.

Over and above all this, there are certain character traits which are observed in epileptic children more frequently than in others. Some authors feel that the convulsive phenomena of idiopathic epilepsy are specific psychogenic manifestations, regressive reactions to difficult life situations of persons who have *a priori* a definite personality make-up. Egocentricity, selfishness often hidden under a mask of shallow and verbose altruism, self-righteousness, a peculiar type of religiousness, a marked circumstantiality of speech and actions, impulsiveness, pugnacity, and emotional instability are said to be the outstanding characteristics. It was especially L. P. Clark who devoted much attention to the psychodynamics of epilepsy.[1] His psychoanalytic contentions have not been verified. One sees enough cases in which the above mentioned features are absent. Besides, parents often report that their epileptic children did not offer before the onset of their illness the personality difficulties which obviously developed later and which may be at least partly explained on the basis of the child's and the environment's reactions to the attacks. The most frequent of these complaints are restlessness, temper tantrums, a tendency to fight, and generally an "ugly disposition." Enuresis (other than the involuntary micturition during the paroxysms) was present in 24 per cent of our cases. The complaint of drastic outbursts of anger was offered in not less than 43 per cent. In a considerable proportion of cases the parents noticed that the children developed an almost insatiable appetite; in fully fifteen per cent, the patients' voraciousness was mentioned as a major feature.

Impulsiveness often not only shows itself in the form of frequent temper tantrums and of pugnacity upon the slightest provocation or with no adequate provocation whatsoever, but also may lead to serious antisocial acts dictated largely by cruelty. Raecke has made a special study of these cases. He stresses the occurrence of brutal mistreatment of other children, sometimes associated with overt sadistic tendencies.

We cannot leave the subject of personality difficulties of epileptic children without making sure that we correct the impression which the foregoing generalizations might have made on the reader. It is necessary to

---

[1] Regardless of whether or not one agrees with Clark's ideas, he deserves the credit for being the first to study the genetic-dynamic implications of the epileptic reaction forms. It is therefore most surprising to find that a recent book which deals with children's epilepsy and the "epileptoid character" (Gilbert-Robin. L'Épilepsie chez l'enfant et le caractère épileptoide. Paris. 1932) does not even mention Clark's work with one word. The author nowhere departs from a purely descriptive level of presentation.

state emphatically that there are and that we have seen quite a few children with "idiopathic" epilepsy who in spite of many years of grand mal or petit mal attacks or both have retained good intelligence and remained stable, alert, well behaved, and affable individuals, displaying at no time the slightest evidence of possessing the so-called epileptic personality make-up.

The *onset* of epileptic events in children has been studied systematically by Birk; he distinguishes three modes of development:

1. Attacks beginning in infancy and followed by a long interval after which the paroxysms recur. Usually there is only one convulsion during the first or second year of life, and the pause is of varying duration. Emotional difficulties are said to precipitate the recurrence in the majority of cases. In most instances the attacks come back during the seventh year of life, coinciding with the first school term. Birk found only one-third of these patients to be intellectually normal soon after the reappearance of the epileptic phenomena. In the interval, there are often marked personality difficulties, especially in the sense of emotional instability, temper tantrums, irritability, restlessness, and night terrors. Vogt feels that in children who have a history of one or two convulsions in early life the existence of these behavior disorders should make one suspect the possibility of later epileptic developments.

2. Attacks beginning in infancy and continued without remission throughout the years of childhood. The course, the nature, and the severity varies in individual cases. Grand mal seizures may become milder or more serious, they may be replaced or accompanied by petit mal attacks, and they may increase or decrease in number. A child may have major paroxysms throughout, or minor attacks only, or any sort of supersession or combination.

3. Attacks beginning in later childhood after a period of several years of perfect health.

From one-third to one-half of all epilepsies are said to begin in childhood. According to Gowers, 29 per cent of his cases began before the tenth year (32 per cent of Binswanger's material). The ages preferred for the onset are the first two years of life, the seventh year (beginning of school attendance), and the time of puberty. From recent tabulations by Calvert Stein it appears that of one thousand patients at the Monson, Massachusetts, State Hospital for Epileptics not less than 43.2 per cent were admitted between the ages of one to fifteen years inclusive (one to five years: 6.6 per cent; six to ten years: 16.9 per cent; eleven to fifteen years: 19.7 per cent).

Heredity has been said to play a prominent part in the etiology of epilepsy. Davenport declared it to be a Mendelian character due to a defect in the germ plasm. Recent studies have tended to reduce the assumed significance of the hereditary factor. Myerson has drawn attention to the fact that epilepsy is rarely observed to occur in brothers and sisters. Instead of taking sides in a controversy based on different kinds of material (institutionalized or ambulatory) and on different concepts of "heredity" and including different criteria (convulsions alone, or epilepsy and migraine, or adding alcoholism, psychoses, or adding or not adding paternal desertions or any number of other items), we may be permitted to let the facts speak for themselves by listing the personality disorders of any type in the families of fifty unselected, not institutionalized children suffering from "idiopathic" epilepsy:

1. Father epileptic since the age of 34 years. Paternal grandmother had paralysis agitans. Paternal aunt had petit mal attacks until 30 years old; she had an imbecile, microcephalic son. Mother had febrile convulsions at five years. Maternal grandfather had spells of aimless wandering; he had a schizophrenic brother. Two brothers and one sister had "teething spasms."

2. Father alcoholic, bootlegger, and wife beater. Paternal aunt was epileptic. Mother peculiar, used to take the patient into her bed and to make him "bounce up and down her naked body."

3. Mother walked in her sleep in childhood, bit her nails, and had facial tics; she was diagnosed as hysterical. Maternal grandfather alcoholic. Maternal grandmother had crying spells.

4. Stable family.

5. Father alcoholic, reached third grade only. Left family when the patient was a few months old. Mother hypochondriacal, very excitable, had occasional encopresis.

6. Stable family.

7. Father alcoholic; his half-sister, a deaf-mute, had severe convulsions. Maternal uncle died of epilepsy. Several maternal cousins had infantile convulsions. Of the mother's twelve children, six died in early infancy.

8. Father, a prominent lawyer and politician, was hypochrondriacal; he had a depressive episode at 24 years. Paternal grandmother very eccentric. Brother, now well adjusted at 17, had breathholding spells in infancy and enuresis until seven years old.

9. Father was under a physician's care for "nervousness." Brother in the fifth grade at 15 years.

10. Stable family. A third cousin was feebleminded.

11. Father tyrannical, used obscene language. A paternal cousin died in "spasms."

12. Stable family.

13. Stable family.

14. Stable family.

15. Father, paternal grandmother and five uncles diabetic. Father and paternal grandmother alcoholic. Sister had fainting spells until the age of seven years, now has diabetes. Brother had until six years of age spells of confusion lasting two to three minutes when awakened in the morning; they were followed by amnesia. Of the mother's 27 pregnancies (five pairs of twins, six miscarriages), only five children survived.

16. Stable family.

17. Father had violent temper outbursts. Mother had "spasms" in infancy; she "hollered when she was nervous."

18. Maternal aunt, now in her thirties, had convulsions between eleven and sixteen years.

19. Stable family.

20. Father alcoholic. Mother unintelligent, "shakes" when she has anything to do: "It runs in my family." Maternal grandmother "shakes all the time." Maternal aunt and two uncles very excitable.

21. Paternal grandfather "alcoholic." Mother easily excited.

22. Father disappeared several years ago after being arrested for bootlegging; he had a court record of stealing. Mother had two illegitimate chil-

dren. Maternal grandfather, alcoholic, never went beyond the third grade in school. Maternal grandmother, diabetic, reached the third grade. Maternal great-grandfather had several "spells of insanity." One maternal uncle epileptic, another schizophrenic, a third "queer" and a chronic invalid, an aunt had a pyschotic episode of an unknown nature. Brother feebleminded. Half-brother in State Training School for the Feebleminded. Information about the father's relatives could not be obtained.

23. Mother had "spasms" in infancy. Parents separated for five years.

24. Mother had temper outbursts.

25. Father had convulsions in infancy. Paternal grandmother had asthmatic attacks. Brother mentally retarded, had congenital nystagmus.

26. Stable family. Paternal cousin died from the results of alcoholism.

27. Father had convulsions until ten years old, reached the fourth grade only, had a violent temper. Three of father's siblings had convulsions until about six years of age. A maternal cousin had asthma.

28. Father "nervous and thin." Mother unintelligent, irritable. Both grandmothers diabetic.

29. Father deserted soon after the patient's birth; whereabouts unknown.

30. Stable family.

31. Mother "quick-tempered." Maternal grandfather, uncle, and aunt diabetic.

32. Father reached second grade only, had chorea at eight years. Paternal aunt had chorea. Mother syphilitic. Maternal second cousin epileptic and mentally defective. Sister, four years old, feebleminded, had night terrors.

33. Mother died in convulsions ten days after the patient's birth; said to have been unfaithful to her husband who doubted his paternity to any of her children.

34. Both parents illiterate. Brother enuretic at fourteen.

35. Father alcoholic, brutal. Mother married to him without obtaining a divorce from her first husband. Maternal aunt morphine addict. Sister died in childhood of convulsions complicating pneumonia. Another sister had an illegitimate child.

36. Mother easily excited. Maternal uncle had epileptic attacks until the age of 27 years. Paternal grandfather diabetic. Alcoholism rife in both branches.

37. Paternal grandmother had convulsions. Paternal cousin schizophrenic. Sister, ten years old, had temper tantrums. Half-brother enuretic at seventeen.

38. Father alcoholic. Mother and two maternal aunts had convulsions in infancy. Sister, eight years old, feebleminded, had convulsions between one and three years of age.

39. Maternal cousin had "spasms." Sister had convulsions with pneumonia at two years. Another sister had atresia ani.

40. Father alcoholic, "moody and grouchy." Maternal grandmother had "spells of aimless wandering." Sister had an illegitimate child.

41. Mother unintelligent, stubborn, superstitious. Paternal cousin schizophrenic.

42. Stable family.

43. Father had a "quick temper." Mother inclined to worry, oversolicitous.

44. Paternal aunt had "fainting spells."

45. Maternal grandmother spent two years in a State Hospital with a depression. A maternal great-aunt was paranoid, "always thought someone was after her." A maternal aunt was a deaf-mute.

46. Father deserted when mother was pregnant with the patient who was an illegitimate child. Mother feebleminded, totally illiterate. Sister imbecile.

47. Paternal uncle died of epilepsy. Paternal aunt, now 23 years old, had convulsions between four and twelve years.

48. Father alcoholic. Paternal grandmother alcoholic, ran a bootlegging establishment. Mother had "fainting spells" since childhood, alcoholic, had temper tantrums; married at thirteen. Two maternal uncles had police records for larceny. Two maternal aunts had illegitimate children from as many fathers as there were children. Brother, 8, enuretic, feebleminded, had temper tantrums and crying spells. Sister, 7, had defective articulation, was mentally defective. Brother, 4, had convulsions at one year associated with otitis media.

49. Mother, illiterate, feebleminded, had convulsions "when a girl."

50. Father alcoholic, had a "ferocious temper," but managed to hold a high municipal position. Paternal grandfather alcoholic.

Lennox and Cobb, in an excellent monograph published in 1928, summarized the facts and theories concerning the *etiology* of epilepsy and the physiological mechanisms involved in convulsions. It is mainly from their presentation that we cull the following data. There are investigators who hold to a purely cortical origin of the attacks, and others who claim that the clonic phase is localized in the cortex and the tonic phase in the basal ganglia. Others regard epilepsy entirely as an extrapyramidal syndrome. Some declared the medulla to be the origin of the seizures. "In fact," say Lennox and Cobb, "almost every division of the brain has at some time been held responsible," and they feel rightly that "too much anatomical schematization is unjustified." They distinguish four principle theories with regard to the neurological mechanisms:

The *irritation theory*, according to which convulsive phenomena always originate from irritation of the cerebral cortex.

The *release theory*, holding that convulsions come, not from stimulation, but from inhibition, "from a temporary suspension of function of the higher centers which allows the lower centers to discharge explosively."

The *short-circuit theory:* "A cortical lesion is considered capable of interrupting enough association fibers to check the normal spread of nerve impulses and cause them to take a shorter, abnormal route, leading to explosive discharge."

The *explosive theory*, holding that "a seizure arises as a general widespread change in brain tissue, not dependent upon spread of nerve impulses, but upon some sudden metabolic change—such as anaphylaxis, anoxemia or alkalosis."

Specific lesions of the central nervous system have not been demonstrated. Areas of degeneration have often been found in Ammon's horn on microscopical examination. Encephalographic roentgenograms have in some cases suggested brain atrophy, evidenced by increased accumulation of air in the subarachnoid spaces, and arachnoiditis, evidenced by the absence of air in the normal fluid pathways. "Concerning abnormalities in the body elsewhere than in the brain, the most constant is the inconstancy of physiological processes. For instance, there is a variation from day to day in such measurements as pH of the blood, oxygen consumption, blood sugar curves, activity of reflexes, vasomotor reactions, leucocytic formula, excretion of ammonia, evidence of instability of the sympathetic nervous system." Only a very small number of patients having seizures presents clinical evidence of endocrine dysfunction. In a small proportion of cases the presence of increased fibrinogen and speed of sedimentation of the red blood cells has been reported. Spinal fluid pressure is said to be abnormally high in approximately twenty per cent; the total protein content is increased in about an equal number. Artificially induced hypoglycemia may assist in the induction of seizures. During and immediately after convulsions, as a result of asphyxia and muscular contraction, there is a temporary condition of acidosis. Alkalosis induced in epileptics may be followed by attacks. Katzenelbogen found that there is in epilepsy a tendency (in eleven out of his eighty-six cases) to an increased permeability to calcium of the barrier between blood and spinal fluid and that there existed no relation between the calcium findings and the mental state of epileptic patients.

The *diagnosis* of "idiopathic" epilepsy should be made only after a very careful physical examination has excluded the presence of neurological or gross metabolic disorders. When no such disturbances are found, the condition must be differentiated especially from hysteria, fainting spells, narcolepsy, breathholding spells, and tetany.

Epileptic attacks are distinguished from *hysterical* seizures by the absence of the light reflex of the dilated pupils, the presence of the Babinski sign, the tongue bite, the lack of caution when falling, the occurrence of nocturnal paroxysms, the sleep and complete amnesia following the attack; enuresis may occasionally also occur in hysterical attacks. Some authors, feeling that hysterical and epileptic reaction tendencies may combine themselves in the same person or that some patients may present features common to both conditions, speak of such cases as *hystero-epilepsy*.

It is often a difficult task to separate *fainting spells* from epileptic convulsions. A history of petit mal phenomena sometimes clears the diagnosis. A typical syncope is usually preceded by a sensation of darkness before the eyes, and the profound pallor is in most cases not superseded by cyanosis. It is followed by a quick recovery without drowsiness or sopor. It never impairs the patient's intelligence.

Narcoleptic sleep is in no way different from normal sleep. The history of typical cataplectic phenomena and the characteristic electrical skin resistance readings help to assure their recognition.

Cyanosis does, and twitchings or jerkings occasionally may, occur in *breathholding spells*. But a correct description or personal observation of a "respiratory affect disorder" and the cessation during the second year of life easily reduces the possibility of diagnostic errors.

A means of establishing the differential diagnosis between epilepsy and some of the conditions just mentioned consists in some cases in the possibility to induce convulsions in persons subject to seizures through voluntary overventilation of the lungs. The method was first introduced in 1924 by Joshua Rosett. The patient is asked to expire forcibly for a period of ten minutes. In a small proportion of cases (from a few up to fifty per cent, according to various investigators), artificial hyperpnea is followed by a convulsion or its equivalent.

The convulsions of *tetany* (infantile eclampsia) are associated with some of the other symptoms of this condition: laryngospasm, carpopedal spasm, Trousseau's sign, Chvostek's sign, the peroneal sign, Erb's phenomenon, low serum calcium. In "latent tetany" (spasmophilia), Erb's sign is to be considered as especially pathognomonic. Even though the convulsions of tetany disappear during the second or third year, it should be mentioned that Thiemich described a form of "late eclampsia," "which develops on the soil of the spasmophilic diathesis and differs from the usual eclamptic attacks of early infancy only by its onset in later childhood," that is between the fifth and eighth years. It offers a favorable prognosis and can be recognized by the presence of other tetanoid symptoms. The convulsions themselves, both in early and late eclampsia, cannot be distinguished from epileptic seizures. There has been a good deal of discussion about the possible relations between tetany and epilepsy. Careful follow-up studies by Birk and Potpeschnigg have made it certain that children who have had undisputed tetanoid convulsions do not develop epileptic reactions more frequently than the average run of the population.

Bratz has described convulsions in "unstable" individuals, which are produced by emotional upheavals and resemble epileptic attacks, except that consciousness is not always completely abolished. They are said to occur in "neuropaths" and "psychopaths" with vasomotor instability, who are given to temper outbursts and to antisocial behavior. They do not affect the intellectual faculties. Bratz designated the condition as *affect epilepsy*. Some authors have accepted his isolation of this group from other cases of epilepsy, while others deny its specificity. The reaction has not been observed in children.

Unverricht has reported a rare hereditary condition known by the name of *myoclonus epilepsy*, which is more common in girls than in boys, usually begins in later childhood, and leads progressively to intellectual deterioration. It starts with epileptic nocturnal attacks. After about one or two years, myoclonic movements (clonic successive twitchings in an individual muscle or in a small group of adjacent muscles, not sufficient to produce noticeable excursions of the limbs) occur in daytime and become gradually more frequent, while the patient loses weight and is, in the final stage, emaciated, bedridden, and demented. There is sometimes a family history of epilepsy without myoclonus or of myoclonus without epilepsy. The organic pathology is unknown.

The *prognosis* of epilepsy is perhaps the most difficult task confronting one in the handling of a condition which offers so many other difficulties, etiological, educational, and therapeutic. When the first paroxysms appear in a child, any opinion about the possibilities of future development will, of course, hinge on the recognition of their nature. The outlook for tetany is usually favorable. So is that for febrile convulsions, though we find that patients presenting such a history have relatively often major or minor personality problems. A few examples may serve as illustrations:

A boy, eight years and four months old, had at six years a convulsion associated with mumps and one a few months later with acute tonsillitis. He had high average intelligence (I.Q. 110). He was brought to the clinic with the complaints of enuresis, temper tantrums, and inability to get along with other children.

A boy, eight and a half years old, had at five weeks convulsions with bronchopneumonia. He had an I.Q. of 109. The complaints were night terrors, hypochondriacal trends, vomiting when forced to eat, restlessness, nailbiting, poor progress in school.

A girl, aged six years and four months, had at one year a convulsion connected with an acute gastro-intestinal upset and one at three years "with moderate fever." She had low average intelligence (I.Q. 93). She was a spoiled child who would not eat, had temper tantrums, and masturbated.

A boy, nine years and two months old, had one febrile convulsion at one year, another at three years, and a third at eight years initiating measles. His I.Q. was 93. His main difficulty was a specific reading disability.

A badly spoiled boy of eleven years, of average intelligence, who at one year had a convulsion with pneumonia, had frequent temper outbursts, dominated the household, was disobedient, and would not eat.

A nine-year-old boy of normal intelligence had two convulsions immediately after tonsillectomy at four years. His behavior difficulties were poor progress in school, enuresis, and refusal to eat, all of which improved rapidly after adjustment at home and in school and after correction of his refractive error.

One may, of course, justly point to the fact that those children are not old enough to make one too certain that the danger of recurrence of the attacks has passed. Yet one gets the history of one or more febrile convulsions in many adults who have remained free from epilepsy. On the other hand, it is well to know that the occurrence of febrile convulsions does not make a person immune against the later development of epileptic reactions.

We have, for example, seen one boy of eight years who had two febrile convulsions at two years and six months and a third two months later and who at the age of seven and a half began having typical petit mal attacks. He was healthy physically, of normal intelligence, and offered no personality problems at the time of the examination nor before nor afterwards. A maternal aunt, now in her thirties, had had infrequent convulsions between ten and fifteen years of age.

The course of "genuine" or "idiopathic" epilepsy is so varied and so unpredictable that a generalized prognostication is practically impossible and one's expectations in the individual case depend largely on what has already happened, the patient's responsiveness to therapy, the finding of the type of treatment to which he might respond better than to others, the time at which treatment has been started, environmental factors, the ingrained personality assets and liabilities, the factors of general health, and so forth. The knowledge that therapeutic and even spontaneous recoveries do occur and that, on the other hand, in spite of all effort progressive deterioration often cannot be checked should cause one to abstain equally from absolute pessimism and unlimited optimism. It has been said that epilepsy which develops after a long interval in a person who has had but one convulsion in infancy offers a particularly unfavorable outlook. It has also been said (e.g., by Thiemich) that quick recovery casts a doubt on the correctness of the diagnosis or on the permanency of the freedom from future attack phenomena. The frequency of intellectual retardation cannot be disregarded. It should, however, be remembered that the gloomiest views on prognosis come from authors whose contact with epileptics has been limited to institutional material. The epileptic status must always be regarded as ominous. It has been estimated that approximately ten per cent of all children who have had convulsions in infancy, including those of organic origin, febrile, etc., become epileptic in later life.

In approaching the *treatment* of epileptic children, the first task is that of creating in the patient an optimal condition of responsiveness to any therapeutic plan. All physical defects, regardless of whether or not they have a direct bearing on the paroxysms, should be remedied. The family's full coöperation should be secured, in order to be sure that all recommendations will really be carried out.

The treatment itself consists of a combination of several measures, one or the other of which may gain prominent significance or will have to be omitted in the individual case. The measures are:

Medicinal.
Nutritional.
Surgical.
Domestic.
Scholastic.
Vocational.
Custodial.

There is hardly a drug that has not at one time or another been tried in the treatment of epilepsy. For a long time *bromide medication* has been in the lead and still justly occupies a very prominent place. In recent years, especially under the influence of Ulrich's observations in an epileptic colony in Switzerland, the administration of bromides has often been combined with a restriction of chloride intake, since it was found that some of the bromide replaced body chloride and was more effective in checking attacks. The bromides have received a strong rival in *luminal* (*phenobarbital*). It is given in doses of one-fourth of a grain three times a day in children under three years; at a later age, the same amount is given at the beginning and increased, if necessary, up to one and a half grains per day as the average dose for adolescents. Sodium luminal is more soluble than luminal but has a greater degree of toxicity. In some cases which do not respond to either bromides or luminal separately, a combination of the two often has more satisfactory results. The quantity of either drug necessary to control the paroxysms must be tried out in the individual case and may have to be changed from time to time. The tolerance especially for bromides is variable, and overdosage (that is, intake surpassing the tolerance of the individual) may have untoward results (drowsiness, staggering gait, confusion, acneous eruption, delirium); Wuth's method, later modified by others, of determination of the bromide contents of the blood has been said to offer help in establishing a measure of the patient's tolerance. *Potassium borotartrate* has been found successful in some cases in which bromides or luminal did not help; the dosage is ten grains three times per diem in children below five and fifteen grains in older children; it may be combined with either of the two other drugs.

Constipation, which is often found to be associated with epilepsy, calls for special attention.

The forms of *dietary management* may be divided into the following categories:

Restriction of chlorides in connection with bromide medication.

Fasting has been found to result frequently in an interruption of seizures which, however, return upon the resumption of the normal diet.

Ketogenic diet, with the object of producing acidosis. "In practice," according to Peterman, "this amounts to feeding not more than fifteen grams of carbohydrate, and in some cases less than ten grams of carbohydrate daily, with not over one gram of protein for each kilogram of body weight, and enough fat to make up the required calories. These diets should not be started abruptly, or they may not be tolerated. After a few days on less rigid carbohydrate restriction, however, they can be instituted without harm, if due attention is paid to vitamins and salts in planning menus." The treatment may be combined with medication. It is said to have especially satisfactory results in petit mal attacks which do not yield to luminal and to bromides. It is more successful in children than in adults.

Dehydration. It has been pointed out that fasting, ketogenic diet, and acidosis have in common the effect of removing large quantities of water from the body and in children there is a relation between the frequency of convulsions and the state of hydration (McQuarrie). It has been possible to produce convulsions in dogs and also in epileptic children through the excessive administration of water. These experiences have led to the introduction of dehydration through rigid restriction of fluid intake as a form of treating epilepsy. The results are not so satisfactory as those obtained from ketogenic diet.

Surgical interference has proved helpful in some cases of "symptomatic" epilepsy of traumatic cerebrogenic origin. The method of cervical sympathectomy is too recent to permit of definite conclusions.

All these methods of treatment are directed toward an abolition or reduction of the epileptic paroxysms. Although this is undoubtedly the outstanding goal in any approach to the problem of epilepsy, it is highly important to *deal at the same time with the child as a personality*. It will be most desirable to create and maintain a domestic atmosphere which will not only secure parental coöperation with regard to medication or dietary arrangements but will also help the child to develop satisfactory behavior. If it is really true that, as many hold, there is such a thing as an innate epileptic personality make-up with unhealthy characterological potentialities, then one is under even greater obligation to train the patient in a manner which would prevent these potentialities from being converted into dangerous actualities. However this may be, the epileptic child certainly deserves the benefit of a training as sensible and constructive as that which should be given to any other youngster. It is natural that parents should be concerned over their offspring's illness. But they must be educated to realize that they should not pile on the convulsive difficulties other handicaps resulting from lack of proper discipline and habit training. The current popular fallacy that convulsions invariably lead to insanity should be corrected. Superstitious notions should be intelligently dispelled. The child should, wherever possible, be reared in a calm, stable, patient environment in which he would have an opportunity to develop proper conventional manners and an adequate degree of self-dependence and ability to get along with people. He has a right to the best that mental hygiene can offer. He can often obtain that at home; where this is not possible, placement in a boarding home will have to be considered.

The *school adjustment* will depend on the child's intellectual capacity, the frequency of the paroxysms, the time of day and the place of their occurrence, and the patient's general disposition. An epileptic youngster, just as any other, should not be pushed in school beyond his ability, yet should not be denied educational facilities accessible to others. Many children never have an attack in school. Mild "staring spells" usually go unnoticed by the classmates. But if major convulsions occur during lessons or recess periods in school, then consideration for the other children and the effect upon them of witnessing the seizures demands the patient's exclusion from school. Some of the more progressive communities provide for such children home teachers who visit them at regular hours and instruct them privately. In others, the parents must assume the financial burden of paying for tutoring at home. Sometimes children who are intelligent enough to go to school and do not have convulsions during class hours are nevertheless undesirable pupils because of their interparoxysmal impulsiveness and mischievousness and general restlessness or because parental oversolicitude, spoiling, lack of habit training, and the ever-ready assertion that the patients should not be "crossed" have helped to drive them in the direction of what has been called the "epileptic character." These children require specific disciplinary measures, if necessary, custodial.

It is obvious that the children should be prepared only for such occupations as are in keeping with their intellectual abilities and which are not too hazardous. Children of wealthy parents may be fitted for some suitable and supervised mechanical or horticultural activities; if they do not measure up to the expectations, the occupation may be changed or interrupted, since the question of earning a living is not paramount. But children from the middle and laboring classes, who do not require institutional care, offer indeed very serious problems with regard to vocational adjustment. Supervised farm work offers perhaps the best chances, both because of the smaller danger of accidents and because of the greater simplicity and quietude of rural life.

It often becomes necessary to commit to *institutional care* seriously deteriorated epileptics or those whose domestic environment is not conducive to successful treatment or those whose behavior is dangerous to the environment. The choice of institution depends on the finances of the parents, the type of problem, and the facilities offered by the commonwealth. Some states have utterly neglected the important question of the custodial care of epileptic children, while others offer excellent opportunities. The demented patients will find their way into institutions for the feebleminded. Antisocial acts will land others in correctional places. The best arrangements can be made in those states which have special colonies for epileptics; there, medicinal and dietary treatment can be adequately combined with proper habit training and, wherever feasible, with vocational preparation for useful occupation outside or at least within the colony.

The treatment of convulsive conditions has been summarized very lucidly and with sound criticism by Lawson Wilkins. We cannot refrain from quoting verbatim the last paragraph of his paper: "In most cases of epilepsy treatment is still far from satisfactory. Where localized cerebral lesions exist, surgery offers possibilities. Where sympathetic imbalance is suspected, sympathectomy has been suggested, although its efficacy is perhaps questionable, owing to the anatomic difficulty of interrupting all pathways. In the majority of cases, treatment must be directed toward decreasing the nervous irritability. Above all, as emphasized by Talbot, it is important that the patient himself be treated, and not merely the epileptic seizures. Constipation and all physical defects must be corrected and necessary psychological and environmental adjustments must be made. The sedative drugs, such as bromides and phenobarbitals, still must be relied upon in the majority of cases. The reports in the literature indicate that the ketogenic diet has given better results than any other treatment. Bridge believes that it should be preceded by a fast of five days. It should be tried for at least six months before it is judged ineffective, as favorable results are sometimes late in occurring. Some patients who have been rendered free from attacks have gradually returned to unrestricted diets without recurrences. The dehydration régime, on the whole, has yielded less satisfactory clinical results than the ketogenic diet. Instead of ketogenic diet, a high fat 'borderline' diet (with a fat-carbohydrate ratio just insufficient to produce ketosis) may be combined with fluid restriction in some cases. The addition of sedative drugs to the ketogenic diet controls seizures in some patients who are not helped by either treatment alone. The treatment by either ketosis or fluid restriction requires a very rigid régime and the patient must have the intelligence, the willingness and the financial ability to coöperate to the fullest extent. It is to be hoped that a better understanding of the physiological and chemical mechanisms underlying the 'convulsive tendency' may eventually lead to simpler and more effective means for its control."

The *management of the individual convulsion* can be summarized in one sentence: "Leave the patient alone!" Mustard baths, blowing one's breath into the child's mouth, slapping and shouting are not uncommon among the laity; the family often feels that something drastic should be done to "bring the child out of the attack." These activities should be discouraged. If an aura indicates the imminence of the seizure, it will be well to place the youngster in a position on a couch or on the floor in which he is least likely to sustain an injury. Tongue bite can be prevented by placing a folded handkerchief between the teeth. The child should not be left alone during the attack. The sleep following a seizure should not be interrupted. The status epilepticus, on the other hand, calls for heroic measures; large doses of bromides or luminal, enemas, and chloroform narcosis have been especially recommended.[1]

PYKNOLEPSY

M. Friedmann, in 1906, described for the first time a condition which in many ways resembles epileptic petit mal reactions, yet differs from them in several significant respects. He believed them to be related to narcolepsy and spoke of them as "frequent, non-epileptic absences or small attacks" (*gehäufte, nicht-epileptische Absenzen oder kleine Anfälle*). Later, upon Schröder's suggestion, the name of pyknolepsy has been generally adopted.

At the ages of between four and nine years, the child more or less

[1] Selected Bibliography:

Binswanger, O. Die Epilepsie. Wien und Leipzig. 1913.

Birk, Walther. Über die Anfänge der kindlichen Epilepsie. Ergebnisse der inneren Medizin und Kinderheilkunde. 1909, 3, 551–600.

Bratz. Das Krankheitsbild der Affektepilepsie. Allgemeine Zeitschrift für Psychiatrie. 1906, 63, 509.

Bridge, E. M., and L. V. Iob. The Mechanism of the Ketogenic Diet in Epilepsy. Bulletin of the Johns Hopkins Hospital. 1931, 43, 373.

Clark, L. Pierce. Psychology of Essential Epilepsy. Journal of Nervous and Mental Disease. 1926, 63, 575–585.

Davenport, C. B. and D. F. Weeks. The First Study of Inheritance of Epilepsy. Journal of Nervous and Mental Disease. 1911, 38, 641–670.

Hahn, R. Assoziationsversuche bei jugendlichen Epileptikern. Archiv für Psychiatrie und Nervenkrankheiten. 1913, 52, 1078–1094.

Katzenelbogen, S. The Distribution of Calcium Between Blood and Fluid and the Carbon Dioxide Content of the Blood in Epilepsy. Journal of Nervous and Mental Disease. 1931, 74. 636–644.

Lennox, William G., and Stanley Cobb. Epilepsy from the Standpoint of Physiology and Treatment. Medicine. 1928, 7, 105–290.

McQuarrie, I., and C. M. Husted. Epilepsy in Children: The Relationship of Water Balance to the Occurrence of Seizures. American Journal of the Diseases of Children. 1929, 38, 451.

Myerson, A. The Inheritance of Mental Diseases. Baltimore. 1925, pp. 57–72.

Peterman, M. G. Ketogenic Diet in the Treatment of Epilepsy. American Journal of the Diseases of Children. 1924, 28, 28–33.

Potpeschnigg, Karl. Zur Kenntnis der kindlichen Krämpfe und ihre Folgen für das spätere Alter. Archiv für Kinderheilkunde. 1908, 47, 360–416.

Raecke, Julius. Über antisoziale Handlungen epileptischer Kinder. Archiv für Psychiatrie und Nervenkrankheiten. 1913, 52, 961–980.

Rows, R. G., and W. E. Bond. Epilepsy. A Functional Mental Illness. London, 1926.

Stein, Calvert. Hereditary Factors in Epilepsy. American Journal of Psychiatry. 1933, 12, 989–1037.

Strohmayer, W. Die Epilepsie im Kindesalter. Altenburg. 1902.

Talbot, F. B. The Treatment of Epilepsy. New York. 1930.

Thiemich, Martin. Funktionelle Erkrankungen des Nervensystems. In: Die Krankheiten des Nervensystems im Kindesalter. Edited by Thiemich and Zappert. Leipzig. 1910, p. 208.

Vogt, Heinrich. Die Epilepsie im Kindesalter. Berlin. 1910.

Wilkins, Lawson. The Present Status of Epilepsy. International Clinics. 1933, 2, 265–279.

suddenly begins to have short attacks, lasting a few seconds only, in which he interrupts his regular activities and, for all practical purposes, appears unconscious and irresponsive. Neither the patient nor the persons of his environment have any means of noticing the approach of the individual spell, which comes wholly unexpected and unannounced. During the absence, the child remains standing or sitting in a rather limp fashion, the eyes are turned upward, voluntary movements and the ability to speak are suspended. The child never falls during the attack; one case has been reported, in which one of the absences occurred while the patient was climbing up a tree without dropping down. The hands do not lose their grip of objects which they happen to hold; but the child is not conscious that the objects are taken away from him. There is an amnesia for what has gone on during the episode, but after its termination the child knows that it has taken place. The onset of the condition (but not of the later attacks) is usually preceded by strong excitement.

The outstanding features, in distinction from petit mal attacks, are the mildness, great frequency, and uniformity of the seizures, their occurrence in individuals who are otherwise healthy physically and mentally and remarkably free from serious personality problems, and the fact that they more or less abruptly disappear at the time of puberty or early adolescence. The daily number varies from five to more than one hundred. They are said to be more apt to come during school hours and especially while the child is reading than at any other time. They resemble each other very closely, not only in one person but also in any number of children. They have no damaging effect upon the patient's health or development. They are never associated with convulsions; the only movements ever noticed are the upward motion of the eyeballs and a casual slight flickering of the eyelids. The child's native intellectual endowment is in no way impaired. The average duration of the condition is approximately three or four years; no case is known in which it extended beyond the nineteenth year.

Pyknolepsy is an extremely rare condition. Many instances cited in the literature have either been diagnosed incorrectly or are at least very doubtful. They have most often been confused with epileptic and post-encephalitic disorders. Their differentiation is by no means always easy. The surest diagnosis is that made after the cessation of the attacks.

The etiology is not known. Several theories have been propounded. There has been a tendency to follow Friedmann's example and think of pyknolepsy, narcolepsy, and cataplexy as closely allied reactions. Ratner has claimed for all these conditions as well as for affect epilepsy and certain hysterical and manic-depressive features the common basis of an hypothetical constitutional inferiority of the diencephalon; since objective evidence of such an assumption has not been brought forth, his "diencephaloses" are just another addition to the many neurologizing speculations which have tended to deter so many practically-minded physicians from occupation with psychiatry. Others regard pyknolepsy as an atypical form of petit mal attacks, and still others like to think of it as an hysterical manifestation. Some investigators deny the existence of a pyknoleptic entity and feel that a differentiation from other forms of petit mal is not justified.

In a number of cases, Mann found the presence of galvanic responses typical of latent tetany.[1]

The *prognosis* is always benign. Yet it is always advisable not to exclude too readily the possibility of an epileptic nature of the attacks. There is no safer diagnosis than that made *post factum*.

The *treatment* consists mainly of alleviating the parents' fear of epilepsy and of physical and mental deterioration. Where the attacks are so frequent that they interfere with the regular class activities, competent home teaching seems preferable to school attendance. Activities, such as crossing streets and swimming, may involve dangers which should be obviated by close supervision.

BREATHHOLDING SPELLS

There are episodes in the course of the first four or five years in the lives of some children, in which, mostly in the midst of violent crying, they suddenly cease breathing and do not resume respiration for the length of about a minute, or a little less or more. During this period, the patient almost always becomes cyanotic, especially around the lips and the face; in severe cases, he may show signs of apnoeic distress, throw his arms and legs around helplessly, and look about him with an expression of utter despair. Sometimes the eyeballs turn upward. There may, on rare occasions, be twitchings and jerkings of a localized or generalized character. If breathing is not reëstablished quickly enough, the child may become unconscious and fall over, usually backward, but at times forward. The body is in most instances rigid, in other cases it may be limp and lifeless. In unusually severe attacks, full-fledged convulsions have been observed. The head is often thrown backward and held in opisthotonos fashion during the beginning or the total duration of the episode. When the attack is over, the child who has not been unconscious continues to cry, otherwise he may be weak and exhausted for a short time.

These very dramatic events are known as "breathholding spells" or "holding breath spells." The parents, in their complaints, refer to them either with these terms, or as "fits," "spasms," "fainting spells," "attacks," or even "convulsions." One usually gets good descriptions from the informants, except that the duration is apt to be greatly exaggerated. The popular German designations are *Wutkrämpfe* (anger spasms) or *Wegbleiben* (going off or staying away; compare the name "absences" for petit

---

[1] Friedmann, M. Über die nichtepileptischen Absenzen oder kurzen narkoleptischen Anfälle. Deutsche Zeitschrift für Nevenheilkunde. 1906, 30, 462. Zur Kenntnis der gehäuften nichtepileptischen Absenzen im Kindesalter. Zeitschrift für die gesamte Neurologie und Psychiatrie. 1912, 9, 245.

Heilbronner. Über gehäufte kleine Anfälle. Deutsche Zeitschrift für Nervenheilkunde. 1907, 31, 472.

Schröder. Die Bedeutung kleiner Anfälle (Absenzen, petit mal) bei Kindern und Jugendlichen. Medizinische Klinik. 1917.

Ratner, J. Beitrag Zur Klinik und Pathogenese (Zur Begriffsbestimmung der Diencephalosen). Monatsschrift für Psychiatrie und Neurologie. 1927, 64, 283.

Mann, L. Über die Beziehungen der Narkolepsie zur Spasmophilie. Zeitschrift für medizinische Elektrologie. 1911, 13, 82.

mal seizures). Ibrahim has introduced the very fitting name of *respiratorische Affektkrämpfe* (respiratory affect spasms).[1]

They are indeed almost invariably the result of an emotional upheaval in the sense of fright or anger. It seems of interest to quote some of the parents' observations with regard to the circumstances under which the breathholding spells take place:

"When he falls or when he is angry." "When things don't go to suit him." "When his playmates take something that he wants." "When she cries after being hurt or crossed." "When he is startled or when he has a temper." "Whenever he is provoked." "When she is denied something or when she has been hurt." "Whenever he is crossed or told not to do something." "When he is not given his way." "When she has a fit of temper." "When we refuse to give her anything she wants." "After a fright or when she is angry." "Precipitated by anything which displeases him and causes him to cry." "Every time she sees me (the mother) go away; if I tell her I will be back soon, she does not have them." "Whenever he is scolded or hurt or does not get his way." "When his wishes are not complied with." "Mostly when he is angry, but at times also when he is sitting quietly alone." "When he is startled or angry; they are brought on by irritation, agitation, and defecation" (the child is constipated). "Every time someone hits her" (child had a typical attack when an attempt to get a Chvostek was made). "If she wants something and would not get it." "With the least little scare or bump." "The usual spell starts if you want him to sit in the high chair or anything like that and he does not want to do it." "Elicited by bathing."

The *onset* often coincides with a fall or some other frightening experience:

"It began with a fall which frightened her considerably." "It started immediately after the second injection against diphtheria." "Two months ago he had a fall from a sofa; his mother heard him cry and found him apparently unconscious on the floor. He remained so for about two minutes. He seemed weak for the next five or six minutes. Two weeks later he burned his finger on a radiator, and the same thing happened. Since then he has had about fifteen attacks, brought on by fear or anger." "The first time he had one of those spells was when he was aggravated when he hit himself very lightly with a rattle."

The age at onset is usually the first half of the second year of life. In our group of forty-four unquestionable cases of breathholding spells, the earliest date at which the attacks began was at five and a half months. In nineteen cases they started some time in the second half of the first year. In none of them did they make their appearance later than at the end of the second year. They hardly ever extend beyond the termination of the fifth year.

One very retarded girl with a mental age of five years still had them at nine years and nine months; she was infantile in her behavior in many other respects (fear reactions, temper tantrums, feeding difficulties, restlessness); both parents, her sister, and a paternal uncle had "violent tempers."

The spells also persisted from early infancy in a twelve-year-old boy (mental age of nine years), who was seen because of enuresis, temper outbursts, masturbation, and disobedience; he came of an emotionally unstable family.

[1] Ibrahim, J. Über respiratorische Affektkrämpfe im frühen Kindesalter (das sogenannte "Wegbleiben" der Kinder). Zeitschrift für die gesamte Neurologie und Psychiatrie. 1911, 5, 388–413.

His father, alcoholic, abusive, was divorced on the grounds of cruelty and non-support. His mother was hypochondriacal, excitable, and unintelligent; an older brother was enuretic at sixteen. His sister wet the bed and "shook" at fourteen years.

The frequency of the individual attacks varies from very rare incidence to several episodes in one day. There are usually long intervals at the beginning, becoming much shorter within a few months, and again getting longer before the ultimate cessation of the spells.

Twenty-five of our breathholders were boys, and nineteen were girls. There was only one negro child among them. Nineteen were only children, and sixteen were youngest in their families. All of them were badly spoiled.

It is very interesting that in five of our cases a definite *relation to pertussis* existed. In four of the children the whooping cough stridor was apparently the child's first apnoeic experience, which was then, even after recovery from the primary illness, repeated in the form of reactive breathholding spells, occurring only when the children cried. One little patient, who vomited a good deal during his seizures of pertussis, kept throwing up every time he had a breathholding spell afterwards. Another child had for three weeks what seemed to be typical episodes of holding her breath when she developed a regular whooping cough, at the end of which the spells disappeared entirely.

Parental mismanagement in the sense of overindulgence, oversolicitude, and overprotection, and emotional instability in the family are frequent findings in the cases under observations.

A study of the *personalities* of the patients themselves shows that in a considerable number there are other behavior disorders besides the breathholding spells.

These are a few examples:

Boy, two years and six months. Developmental level of less than eighteen months. The child was deaf. He had temper tantrums, and was destructive. He said a few words only. Bowel control not established.

Boy, two years and nine months. Premature baby, birth weight a little less than three pounds. Icterus neonatorum from the second day until the age of six months. He did not form words until the age of two years. Rickets, recurrent jaundice, dental caries, tonsillar hypertrophy, mild left internal strabismus. Slow in walking and talking. He stuttered, wet the bed, was afraid of strangers, and a restless sleeper.

Girl, eighteen months. Poor appetite. Mild rickets. Had the habit of biting the chairs, otherwise normal development and behavior.

Girl, when first seen at ten months, a week after the onset of the breathholding spells, was restless and reported to sleep poorly. Serious feeding problem at two years.

Boy, five years. Breastfed for fifteen months. Always "mischievous." Hypochondriacal. Feeding problem. Enuresis. Was given strong tea and coffee to drink.

Boy, four years and ten months. Phimosis, internal strabismus, undescended testes, generally underdeveloped. Mental age of less than three years. Talked baby talk, stuttered, bit finger nails, regurgitated food, disobedient, fearful, restless sleeper.

We had an opportunity to study breathholders a number of years after the termination of the attacks. It is of particular interest to note the frequency of temper tantrums, which are in most instances a direct continuation of the breathholding spells.

Girl, only child, with congenital stricture of ureter. Onset of breathholding spells at seven months, kept up until two years. At four, the child had temper tantrums, enuresis, feeding difficulties, and stuttered. She was badly spoiled by her mother, whose occasional training efforts were immediately frustrated by in-law interference.

Girl, nine years, had breathholding spells in infancy. Normally intelligent. Undernourished. Temper outbursts took the place of the spells. She was afraid of the dark, kidnapping, and riding in automobiles. She bit her fingernails. She "shook awfully" when asked to recite in school. Mother had attacks of despondency with crying spells, always complained of "run down condition" and "stomach trouble." Paternal grandmother, who lived with the family, was "very nervous and worrisome."

Boy, eight years, an only child, had temper tantrums ever since he ceased holding his breath. He also had crying spells "when he didn't get his way." During the past year he developed the habit of holding his fingers before his mouth and breathing out suddenly. He had nightmares and slept poorly. Superior intelligence. Referred for psychiatric consultation "because he seems to be a perfectly healthy child in process of being ruined by poor management." He bit his fingernails. He held back his urine "to the last minute." He presented a feeding problem. Father very restless, "just moving all the time," had tremors and tics. Mother hypochondriacal, did not sleep well, "cannot sit still." Both grandmothers excitable and hypochondriacal.

An unusual case was that of Paul C., seven years old, intellectually retarded (I.Q. 66), who had breathholding spells until the age of three years. When last seen a few months ago, he was undernourished, had an epigastric hernia, a refractive error, and chronic tonsillitis. He was badly spoiled, afraid of dogs, darkness, and negroes, "shaking and whiny." The remarkable feature in this case consisted in the fact that both parents and all five children had histories of breathholding spells in early childhood; an older brother, now fourteen, had them until the age of seven years. The father deserted the family five years ago and contributed insufficiently to their support; he was a gambler, a skirt chaser, "high strung and irritable." The mother suffered from "nervous chills," had an episode of depression with crying spells and insomnia, and at night she had spells of "choking in her throat." The patient slept with his mother.

The family usually becomes alarmed over the occurrence of the spells, which are often responsible for a considerable increase in the over-indulgence already present in most instances before the onset of the breathholding. Fear that the child may die in the attack and the success of any sudden interference introduce as routine measures the practices of shaking or slapping the patient, throwing cold water on his face, applying mustard plaster to the skin or spirits of ammonia to the nose, or picking him up, and almost always giving in. One mother was in the habit of constantly running after the baby with a glass of cold water ready to throw it on his face at the slightest indication of an approaching attack; on visits, she immediately dashed into the kitchen for a glass of water. Her primary thought was to prevent the child from being crossed. She hovered around him every moment, trying to anticipate his slightest wish.

All rash methods of *treatment* are successful; as a matter of fact, the individual attack ceases without any treatment whatever. But the family's distress, the drastic manipulations and, above all, the ensuing satisfaction of the child's wishes, though seemingly helpful for the moment, soon may teach the patient that he has in his breathholding spells a valuable tool for dominating the household and obtaining his wants. Thus the shaking and the showers with all that precedes and follows them prove to be of dubious value; the attack itself will terminate without them as well as with them, and their employment is apt to, and mostly does, become an incentive for further and more frequent episodes. It is true that the first attacks are practically always involuntary and surprise the child as much as the parents; this is why we discuss the breathholding spells together with the other personality difficulties of an involuntary and more or less unconscious character. But later on they may come to have a more specific and purposeful meaning in the life and daily habits of the child as gainful emotional outlets.

Therefore, the treatment which intends to obtain permanent rather than momentary results will select methods that work for a better stability in the child, who must learn that holding his breath is by no means a mode of securing compliance and indulgence. It is best to ignore the attack calmly. This, of course, can be expected of the parents only after they have been assured that the spells involve no danger of any kind. No child has ever died or been injured in a breathholding spell. The prognosis as to life and the outcome of the individual episode is always good, that of the patient's development of desirable emotional habits depends largely on management of the attacks themselves and of the child generally.

The *diagnosis* offers no difficulties in most cases. The attacks must be differentiated from a number of other respiratory or convulsive phenomena:

Congenital laryngeal stridor is noticed during the first days of life. It is apt to occur during sleep as well as in the waking hours. It is more permanent in character. It has little, if any, connection with emotional disturbances. It is produced by the obstruction of the narrow glottis through sucking into it of loosened folds of the mucous membranes. It usually ceases before the end of the first year. It is rarely dangerous.

Laryngismus stridulus, or *tetanoid laryngospasm*, is much more apt to be mistaken for breathholding spells, and vice versa. As a matter of fact, most French authors still regard breathholding spells as mild forms of laryngospasms, which they call "internal convulsions" (*convulsions internes*). It was Neumann who, in 1905, first separated the two conditions clearly and emphatically.[1]

[1] Neumann H. Über das Wegleiben kleiner Kinder. Archiv für Kinderheilkunde. 1905, 42.

The main differential-diagnostic points are given below:

Breathholding spells	Laryngospasms
1. No signs of latent tetany.	1. There are practically always symptoms of latent tetany (spasmophilia): Erb's sign (increased excitability to the galvanic current of the peripheral nerves), Chvostek (twitching of the orbicularis oris or orbicularis oculi muscle upon tapping the facial nerve in front of the ear), Trousseau (production of tetany by constricting the upper arm), and low serum calcium.
2. No typical inspiratory crowing.	2. Characteristic inspiratory crowing sound.
3. Always affect-determined.	3. Not affect-determined, but sometimes aggravated and occasionally precipitated by strong emotions.
4. Prognosis always good.	4. Fatalities are very rare, but their possibility must be kept in mind.
5. Easily influenced by proper educational handling.	5. Controlled by large doses of calcium bromide plus adequate physical and mental hygiene.

The *whooping cough stridor* is easily distinguished from breathholding spells; the possibility of the coincidence of such spells with pertussis must, however, be kept in mind.

Especially in the severer cases with twitchings or convulsions one must be careful to exclude *epilepsy*. The epileptic attack is less apt to occur in the midst of crying. The typical breathholding is absent. Drowsiness or sleep are prone to follow the epileptic seizure. Besides, the evolution of the entire picture may serve as a valuable guide for differential diagnosis.

It must be added that breathholding spells may sometimes develop in the subject of congenital stridor, tetanoid laryngospasms, or stridor of pertussis.

Stier, in an elaborate monograph, has tried to explain the mechanism of breathholding spells on the basis of vasomotor disturbances.[1]

It is of historical interest that one of the earliest references to breathholding spells is contained in an American textbook of pediatrics.[2]

FAINTING SPELLS

There exists one not at all unusual type of attack disorders, occurring in the second half of the years of childhood, which has been commonly neglected by the authors of most pediatric textbooks. They are occasionally mentioned briefly and perfunctorily as symptoms of "neurasthenia" or "neuropathic constitution." They are sometimes considered in connection with the differential diagnosis of epilepsy. We refer to the "fainting

[1] Stier, E. Die respiratorischen Affektkrämpfe des frühkindlichen Alters. Jena. 1918.

[2] Meigs, J. Forsyth. A Practical Treatise on the Diseases of Children. Philadelphia. 1848.

spells" and related attacks of "dizziness" or "giddiness," which have been drawn by Gowers into the "borderland of epilepsy" together with vagal attacks, vertigo, migraine, and certain sleep disturbances. They have been studied and excellently presented by Stier, Rohde, and Husler.[1]

Contrary to the common belief and to the conditions in adults, syncopal attacks occur in boys not less often than in girls. The first faint rarely happens before the onset of school age. In Stier's eighteen "diagnostically clear" cases the ages at the first attacks were:

Age of onset	Number of cases
3 years	1
5 years	1
6 years	3
7 years	2
9 years	6
10 years	2
12 years	1
13 years	1
14 years	1

Among the conditions in which fainting spells are most likely to take place, fatigue and exhaustion predominate, especially when heat, hunger, and poor ventilation are additional factors. Children are often seen to collapse after standing still or marching in formation for a long time in parades and school festivities or in crowded churches attended before breakfast. Reports of the particular frequency during girls' confirmation ceremonies point in the direction of an emotional etiology. More or less direct affective causes can be found in approximately one half of all syncopal episodes. Prominent among them are fear, disgust, and anger. Well known are the faints upon the sight of blood, during vaccination, when a drop of blood is obtained for hemoglobin determination or for a cell count, or when a blood specimen is taken for a Wassermann test. Fear of punishment to be executed immediately, the discussion of accidents in the child's presence, the excitement of active participation in public performances have occasionally resulted in syncope. One of our own patients had her first faint when, at the end of an especially exerting school session with two decisive tests, she was to give an art demonstration to the whole class. She had been preoccupied for several days with the anticipated affair, had been "keyed up" too much to have breakfast that morning, and was exhausted from excitement, the tests, and hunger when her turn came to give her talk. When about to begin, she felt as though all the children looked at her intently, their eyes growing larger and larger, some

[1] Gowers, W. R. The Borderland of Epilepsy: Faints, Vagal Attacks, Vertigo, Migraine, Sleep Symptoms and Their Treatment. Philadelphia. 1907.—Stier, Ewald. Über Ohnmachten und ohnmachtsähnliche Anfälle bei Kindern und ihre Beziehungen zur Hysterie und Epilepsie. Jena. 1920.—Rohde. Zur Genese von "Anfällen" und diesen nahestehenden Zuständen bei den sogenannten Nervösen. Zeitschrift für die gesamte Neurologie und Psychiatrie. 1912, 10, 473 (case material consists of adults only).—Husler, J. Zur Systematik und Klinik epileptiformer Krampfkrankheiten im Kindesalter. Ergebnisse der inneren Medizin und Kinderheilkunde. 1920, 21, 624.

of her classmates seemed to laugh, then everything became vague, "swam before her," then it was dark around her, and she fainted. One of Stier's patients collapsed every time that a certain place on his chest was pressed which had been slightly hurt a few months before when he had fallen upon it while playing. Sometimes no plausible direct cause can be detected; the child swoons soon after waking in the morning (while dressing, at the breakfast table, or while still in bed) or at meal times later in the day. We found the majority of those youngsters who faint in the morning to be intellectually retarded and to both dislike and fear school.

The children disposed to fainting spells usually show evidence of a labile and inadequately balanced autonomic nervous system. They are mostly gracile, thin-boned, sensitive, touchy little persons with shining eyes, large pupils, the proverbial "rings under the eyes," a fine, transparent skin which shows the cutaneous veins; the hands and feet are cold and sometimes also moist. Dermatographia is often present. They blush and pale easier and have a greater tendency to perspire than normal, non-fainting youngsters. They react readily with intense dislike, nausea, or even vomiting to unpleasant odors and tastes and to changes in the equilibrium of the body (swinging, merry-go-round, streetcar, railroad). Sleep is often restless; night terrors are not uncommon. Most of the youngsters subject to fainting spells are shy, timid, easily frightened, irritable, and cry easily. The prevailing affective tone is one of unhappiness and dissatisfaction.

The single attack is ushered in gradually. The child is aware of the slow waning of consciousness. There may be aura-like experiences of darkness before the eyes, of things seeming far away, of various sorts of paraesthesias. The most conspicuous objective symptom at the beginning is extreme pallor and a progressive loss of muscular tone. Then the patient collapses. Consciousness is completely abolished at the height of the faint. Enuresis is rare. Tongue-bites never occur. The attack lasts from a few seconds to a few minutes, but sometimes durations of a half hour and more have been reported. The children "come to" gradually; the common custom of pouring water over the patient's face, a vigorous slap, or calling his name loudly may hasten the recovery, which is followed by general weakness, at times by headache, and often by profuse perspiration, never by sleep as in epileptic seizures. Tonic or clonic convulsions are always absent.

Alcoholism, psychoses, epilepsy, and idiocy or imbecility do not figure in the family histories more prominently than in those on non-fainting children. In not less than approximately one-third of the cases, there is a record of fainting spells in close relatives (parents or siblings). If one also considers the more distant branches of the family tree, then one finds an especial frequency of headaches, migraine, and breathholding spells.

The same situation does not always give rise in the same child to a full-fledged syncope with total loss of consciousness. Often the patient responds only with nausea, giddiness, marked pallor, or partial loss of muscular tone. Stier refers to these conditions as *abortive fainting spells*. The same author also calls attention to cases of *local syncope*, related to Raynaud's disease, in which there is alone, alternating with, or preparatory to, general faints a feeling of numbness in a finger, toe, arm, or leg.

The frequency of syncopal attacks varies in different individuals. Some children only have one faint throughout their lives, in others they repeat themselves in short intervals, yet almost never more than once in the course of the same day. In contrast to epilepsy, where usually there is a long pause between the first and second seizures, the second faint often follows the first within a few days.

The individual syncope (in all cases discussed here, the faints of anemic children and of those suffering from cardiac illness have not been included) needs no special treatment other than calmness on the part of the environment and rest after the faint. More important is the general regulation of the patient's life and daily routine, the establishment of a proper balance of work, play, and relaxation, avoidance of emotional upheavals in the family, adequate feeding régime with particular emphasis on a satisfactory breakfast, good ventilation at home and in school, good school adjustment wherever necessary, and the creation of a kind, calm, and happy atmosphere through association with coëvals and through the supply of the little thrills which every child desires and needs.

Husler has described as *orthostatic epileptoid* a group of four children of normal intelligence, ranging in their ages between six and fourteen years, who had fainting spells and occasionally even convulsions whenever they were forced to stand for a long time or after getting up in the morning. Upon these occasions (and only then) albumin was found in the urine. The children felt the urge to sit or lie down, and if they could not satisfy this urge, extreme fatigue was felt and soon followed by an attack. All four patients were found to have the same instability of the autonomous nervous system and the same personality features as those disposed to the syncopal attacks described above.

CHAPTER XLI
THE MINOR PSYCHOSES
(Psychoneuroses. Merergastic Reaction Forms.)

"THE PSYCHONEUROSES, or minor or merergastic or part psychoses are," according to Adolf Meyer, "not mental disorders of a sweeping character but rather conditions of a relatively normally behaved personality with certain reactions or episodes still supposed to be the prerogative of the normal in contrast to the definitely and sweepingly psychotic. They are more or less definitely substitutive reactions, i.e., alternatives of the normal, without adequate structural or even neurophysiologically well defined foundations for the disorders. They are nevertheless euphemistically styled 'nervous' because of the traditional medical psychophobia and what goes with it, and because they do indeed quite frequently suggest affections of the nervous system, central or sympathetic, conditions like paralysis or contracture or anaesthesia or tremor or weakness (hence the term psychoneuroses or neuroses); but after all on close analysis (in contrast, for instance, to the more truly neurological disorder, chorea) are part-affections preëminently of the psychobiological field, and also of special organs and their functions, but only psychobiologically intelligible."

If we sort out all those personality difficulties which go with structural or metabolic disturbances of the body, if we further set aside certain attack disorders, the intellectual inadequacies, and the major psychoses (schizophrenia, thymergastic reactions) which are exceedingly rare in children, then all the other anomalies of behavior in childhood could be united under the heading of "minor psychoses:" the anger, jealousy, and fear reactions, the faulty feeding habits, the sleep disorders, abnormal sexual adjustments, certain antisocial trends, the habitual manipulations of the body, stuttering, tics, the psychogenic dysfunctions of the gastro-intestinal, circulatory, respiratory, and genito-urinary systems, obsessive tendencies, hypochondriasis, and hysteria. Dr. Meyer once remarked that, if one wanted to create a new term, one could allude to the rank and file of children's psychopathological performances as *"poikilergasia"* (from Greek *poikilos*—manifold, multifarious, and *ergasia*=performance). Out of the vast and variously combined number of individual varieties, certain groups were singled out on the basis of some common denominators. Scholz used personality traits as indicators of resemblance and as starting points for his elaborate classification which is remarkably free from terminological bias; he thus came to speak of the sensitive child, the timid, or restless, or seclusive child, and so on. The outstanding trait served as the caption under which youngsters presenting it were discussed together.

Popular usage has for a long time comprised most of those personality difficulties which did not appeal to the laity as being outright "crazy" or "bad" in an ethical sense, under a term which is still employed a good deal in the intercourse between physicians and patients and which is often utilized by various authors as a broad indicator of general uneasiness, restlessness, fidgetiness, and emotional instability. We have in mind the word *nervousness*. Some writers, having the justified desire to treat of the common behavior disorders of childhood under a short and fitting subject-heading, speak sensibly of "the nervous child," without wanting to allocate the one or the other symptom to "nervousness" as a diagnostic entity. Others could not abstain from circumscript definitions, creating more or less artificial distinctions between nervousness, neuroses, neuropathies, neurasthenia, psychasthenia, and similar terms. Cramer contrasted a "pure simple, endogenous nervousness" with "complicated nervousness," without making clear the nature of the contrast or the need for establishing it. There is no doubt a constitutional tendency in some children to respond with hyperactivity, irritability, excitability, fatigability, general ill feeling, and somatic reactions throughout life or especially during convalescence or whenever things do not go too well at home or in school. They differ in this respect from the average, "non-nervous" child who is well-balanced and does not stray too markedly or too frequently from a healthy equilibrium of composure, satisfaction, and kinetic economy. It is therefore quite practical, though not absolutely necessary, to use the term "nervous child" collectively for all those children who fit the above description and whose behavior disorder is not specific enough to warrant a more distinctive designation. The same consideration applies to the adjectives "neurotic," "psychoneurotic," and "neuropathic," except that they are often used loosely for artificial differentiations. (See the chapter on "Diagnostic Synthesis.")

Out of the mass of the not essentially organic and not specifically oligergastic, parergastic, or thymergastic reaction patterns, a number of more or less circumscribed groups has been singled out, of which the outstanding are:

Neurasthenia.

Anxiety attacks (which we described together with the other fear reactions).

Psychasthenia; obsessive-ruminative tension states.

Hypochondriasis; invalid reactions.

Hysteria.

So-called motor neuroses, such as tics, stuttering, nodding spasms, general hyperkinetic restlessness, etc.

Neurasthenia was first introduced into the literature as a clinical syndrome by Beard in 1880. As the name indicates, it was supposed to be based on an irritable "weakness of the nervous system." Its symptoms were said to consist of easy fatigability, both physical and mental, general irritability, forgetfulness, poor concentration, a tendency to bodily complaints, headache and head pressure, increased tendon reflexes, lack of appetite, sleep disturbances, oversensitiveness to noises, strong lights, and difficult life situations (frustrations, disappointments). Various causes were claimed to be responsible by different authors: inherited constitution, excessive masturbation, autointoxication, autosuggestion, emotional perturbation, and overwork or, on the other hand, idleness and boredom. A little

German verse was coined which was supposed to contain the etiology and
prophylaxis in a nutshell: *"Haste nie,—doch raste nie,—dann hast du nie—
Neurasthenie."* (Never hasten and never be inactive, then you will never
have neurasthenia). It has been said that neurasthenia is characterized by
a minus, i.e., inability to do things (to eat, to sleep, to concentrate, to go
through with one's work), while "nervousness" implies that all these functions may well be performed with satisfactory results, yet with the subjective experience of tension, inner unrest, and general discomfort. Adolf
Meyer states: "The last word is not said concerning the internal working
of these conditions, the range of justification of the exhaustion theory and
the disappointment theory for the general frame and the rôle of the part-
phenomena and share of the special organs, and the origin of the neurasthenic or generally asthenic constitution, the autointoxications and
other vicious circles."

Psychasthenia is a term which had been used by several authors for
different purposes but was elevated by Pierre Janet to the rank of a special
clinical entity in his classification of the psychoneuroses. He included in
his psychasthenic category largely episodic states of fear, doubt, imperative ideas and acts, fatigue, and inability to cope with difficult situations.
He worked with the concept of "nervous tension" or "psychological force"
which he claimed to be generally lowered in psychasthenia. He felt that
this reaction had some relation to epilepsy, of which it perhaps presented
a milder form. Incapable of following Janet's psychological hypotheses
which are based on abstract reasoning rather than on concrete facts, we
prefer to deal with the personality difficulties which he united under the
caption of psychasthenia under the more objective headings of "fear reactions" and of "obsessive-ruminative tension states."[1]

OBSESSIVE-RUMINATIVE TENSION STATES

Obsessions are ideas which keep obtruding themselves irresistibly and
distressingly upon a person's consciousness, interrupting the orderly sequence of thought or action, are felt by the patient as something foreign
to him and unrelated to his usual behavior, and yet cannot be cast off by
him in spite of his realization of their unnaturalness. The first definition
was formulated in 1878 by Westphal, who understood under obsessions
(compulsive ideas, imperative ideas, *Zwangsvorstellungen*) "ideas which in
persons of otherwise unimpaired intelligence, independently of an effective
or emotional condition, step into the foreground of consciousness against
and contrary to the patients' volition, cannot be banished, hinder and cross
the normal train of thought, are recognized by those affected as abnormal
and alien and contrasted by them with their healthy consciousness."

Several attempts have been made to subdivide and classify the various
forms of obsessive preoccupations and ruminations. Pitres and Régis distinguished between obsessions which do not transcend the realm of ideation (*obsessions idéatives*) and those which are connected with a forcible
urge to overt motor manifestations (*obsessions impulsives*). It has become

---

[1] Janet, Pierre. Les Obsessions et la Psychasthenie. Vol. i. Paris. 1908.—Janet,
Pierre, et F. Raymond. Les Obsessions et la Psychasthenie. Vol. ii. Paris. 1911.

customary to reserve to the former the designation of obsessions *sensu strictiori* and to refer to the latter as *compulsions* or *imperative acts*. Ziehen has three groups: 1. *Disparate* obsessions, simple, trivial disconnected ideas obtruding themselves again and again more or less painfully; they are mostly memories of actual experiences of a pleasant or unpleasant nature (*Zwangserinnerungen*), such as an engaging melody or the sight of an accident. 2. *Connected* obsessions, more complex and having a richer content, such as the notion that the door has not been locked properly, or that the homework has not been done correctly. 3. *Incitomotor* obsessions, displaying a tendency to perform acts which to the patient himself seem utterly absurd, such as the compulsion to do things by threes, to walk on cracks, to omit cracks, to touch people, to skip stones, or to wash the hands incessantly.[1]

Another, less consistent, grouping is concerned mainly with the contents of obsessive phenomena or with the situations in which they arise. The ideational contents are often divided into thoughts, doubts, and phobias. It is, in the face of terminological confusion, important to state that not all fears of children are obsessive phobias. If a youngster is afraid of the dark because he has been told that ghosts or robbers lurk there or because an older sibling has the same attitude, the fear to him seems justified and a natural reaction. A phobia shares with the other obsessions the feeling of strangeness and unreasonableness and the strong desire to be rid of the unwanted, not understood, and utterly disturbing sensation. Under the influence of French and, to a smaller extent, of German authors, the psychiatric vocabulary has been heavily endowed with many names for the various shapes which an obsession may assume. Some of these terms are listed below, partly because they are frequently used in the literature and partly because their enumeration offers a repertoire of the commoner obsessions and compulsions.

A. Contents of obsessive thoughts, doubts, fears, and actions, as characterized by specific names:

Arithmomania: Obtrusion of certain numbers of combinations of numbers, or urge to do things a certain number of times.

Onomatomania: Obtrusion of certain words or sentences.

Folie du doute (Legrand du Saulle): Obsessive doubting whether certain acts have been carried out at all or carried out satisfactorily (door locked, lights turned off, match extinguished, the truth told exactly, windows closed, etc.).

Grübelsucht (Griesinger), *Fragesucht:* Brooding over trifling matters, compulsion to ask irrelevant questions without being especially interested in the answers ("Why does a table have four legs?" "Why is the sky blue?" "Why is snow white?" "Why is God in Heaven?").

Délire de toucher (Legrand du Saulle): Obsessive fear of touching objects or persons.

Mysophobia (fear of contamination): Fear of soiling oneself through con-

---

[1] Westphal, C. Zwangsvorstellungen. Archiv für Psychiatrie. 1878, 8, 735.— Pitres et Régis. Les obsessions et les impulsions. Paris. 1902.—Ziehen, Theodor. Die Geisteskrankheiten im Kindesalter. Berlin. 1926, pp. 372–390.

tact with anything which possibly might be dirty or dusty or contagious.

Pyrophobia: Fear of causing a fire through negligence.

Aichmophobia: Fear of pointed objects (needles, pencils, sharp edges).

Erythrophobia: Fear of blushing.

Paralipophobia: Fear of precipitating disaster by having omitted or forgotten something.

Taphephobia: Fear of being buried alive.

Phobophobia: Fear of being afraid of something.

Pamphobia (Pantophobia): Multiple obsessive fears of practically everything (being run over by automobiles, infection, catching cold, falling, drowning, being asked embarrassing or difficult questions, etc.).

B. Situations in which obsessions may arise, as indicated by specific terms:

Agoraphobia: Obsessive fear of open spaces, crossing the street, being in a crowd. It is rather rare in children.

Claustrophobia: Fear of being shut in or isolated in the classroom or in a theater or in the bathroom or in the compartment of a railroad train. The fear may be associated with the idea that in the case of a fire there will be no opportunity for escaping or that it might be difficult to satisfy a sudden urge to urinate or to defecate. One of our patients became extremely agitated at the mere question what she would do if the office door were to be locked.

Homilophobia: Constant tormenting idea that, while together with other people, they might find something wrong with the patient's looks or clothes or behavior.

This vocabulary could be, and has been, augmented *ad libitum*, without exhausting the terminological possibilities. One might add *hypochondriacal obsessions* and the obtrusive notions that the patient might have sinned against religious prescriptions or that his actions might arouse all sorts of suspicions in other people. They differ from similar paranoid delusions by their obtrusiveness and by the patient's recognition of their morbidity and lack of justification in reality. In rare instances, obsessions may manifest themselves in the form of hallucinatory experiences, usually in the shape of hearing one's name called or receiving short commands; they are, in contradistinction to delirious or schizophrenic hallucinations, not believed by the patient to come from without and he fully realizes their pathological nature. They were first described by Séglas as *obsessions hallucinatoires*. Obsessions may be restricted to one particular form or may be multiple.

Obsessive and compulsive phenomena are most frequently encountered in individuals who are extremely overconscientious, shy, pedantic, punctual, painstakingly addicted to the minutest orderliness and love of symmetry, people who are not satisfied until everything is "just so," who may be quite lenient in their expectations with regard to others but perfectionistic when it comes to the evaluation of their own performances. The history or geography lesson must be studied over and over again, the child must be overheard by the parents or older siblings a number of times, and even then there is tense uneasiness and doubt as to whether the result will be satisfactory in school. A child may be conciliatory and handle the play-mates with the utmost generosity and politeness, yet may afterwards worry for hours that he may have offended some of them.

The consequence of the obsessive state is often a tendency to withdraw from the association with other children. In addition to the often inherent timidity and the unhappiness due to the inability to throw off the disturb-ing thoughts or impulses, the criticism on the part of the parents to quit talking or acting nonsense and especially the desire to be unobserved when yielding to the uncontrolled urges are apt to drive the patient into solitude and seclusion. A thirteen-year-old girl was kept away from school by her parents because of her "nervousness" which consisted of a variety of obsessive trends. She soon refused to leave the house because she felt, against her better judgment, that the people outside suspected her of playing truant. She knew that it was not so and tried to "reason it out of herself" but could not manage to get rid of the feeling which kept forcing itself upon her. This made her so disconsolate that she even spoke of suicide. A fifteen-year-old farmer's boy felt compelled to do things by threes (three morsels or spoonfuls, then pause, then again three morsels or spoon-fuls; opening or closing the door three times in succession; three words, then pause, then again three words; every statement or question had to contain three or six or nine sentences). He was constantly preoccupied, reviewing his activities and becoming agitated at the mere thought that somehow he may not have lived up to that ritual, an omission which to him spelled disaster. He lay awake for many hours each night going over the last day's events with the same ruminations and fears.

Most authors differ with regard to the frequency of obsessions in chil-dren as compared to adults. According to some, they are very unusual be-fore puberty. According to others, fifty per cent or more of all adult cases can be traced back to the years of childhood. It is a fact that children before the fourteenth or fifteenth year are rarely brought to one's atten-tion with the complaint of obsessive tendencies. It is also a fact that ritualistic games with rules similar to compulsions coming from within are often played by children. In some localities, groups of playmates enter upon an agreement obliging them to carry with them green leaves, stones, or other objects and to produce them upon a given sign. In some places, straw hats of the passers-by are counted; if one hat is missed (every count must be "sealed" by a specific gesture), any witnessing child who partici-pates in the game "takes away" from the defaulter the total number which he has accumulated. It is not unusual in the streetcars to observe groups of two or three children who have enjoined upon each other the task of count-ing the passing automobiles or taxicabs and to compare notes from time to time. Many children are apt to make their decisions dependent upon some incidental and unrelated events (which one of the raindrops will first reach the bottom of the window-pane; which bird of a flock will fly away first). From such beginnings obsessive thinking may occasionally de-velop but usually they do not transgress the character of a game. It is therefore not quite in order to refer to them as *rudimentary obsessions*, as has sometimes been done. Nor is one always fully justified in considering them as an early onset of later obsessive developments.

The following cases may serve as illustrations of infantile obsessions. They were taken from the material of the dispensary of the Henry Phipps Psychiatric Clinic and studied by Dr. Esther Loring Richards:

Helen C. was first examined at the age of twelve years and eleven months. Her mother had been subject to anxiety attacks throughout her life, most outspoken during her pregnancy with Helen, who was the eldest of three children. In those attacks she thought that she was dying and that her blood stopped circulating, called for help, and the physicians who were called to her bedside, mostly by Helen, gave her hypodermic injections, electric treatments, and various medicines. The other members of the family were well adjusted. Helen weighed only $3\frac{1}{2}$ pounds at birth. She was an excitable baby and cried easily. She had temper tantrums until the age of five years. At six, upon entering the first grade she stuttered for a short time. She had night terrors. At seven, she was hit by a police patrol wagon and was unconscious for a few seconds. She was spoiled by her parents and slept with them until she was eleven years old. She was healthy physically. When first seen, she had a mental age of not quite ten years (I.Q. 77); she was in the low fifth grade, having spent two years each in the first, second, and fourth grades. Her younger sister had caught up with her and was held up to her as a model. There was a history of some masturbation and slight worry over it.

When she was ten years old, a playmate told her to keep away from a certain woman in the neighborhood because she would "put spells" on her. One day, this woman rang the doorbell. Helen went to open the door and was very much frightened because she had "touched the doorknob which the visitor had touched," and felt that she must wash her hands. Since then she kept washing her hands almost incessantly, so much that the skin became red and bleeding. Some time after that, a dirty coal dealer sat in one of the chairs and she felt the compulsion to wash her hands whenever she happened to touch that chair.

A few months later, her grandmother took her for a visit to New York and went with her to call on an old woman who gave them a meal that did not satisfy the usual standards of cleanliness. During the next four or five weeks, Helen held at arm's length all groceries and cooking utensils and anything else which had to do with food.

Then, for about three months, she walked backwards wherever she went in the house. After that, she developed a tendency to count by drumming with her fingers on the table and repeating, "One, two, three, four, five. . . . One, two, three, four, five. . . . "

When she was twelve years old, she experienced a "conversion" in a Holy Roller revival meeting, joined the church, talked a good deal about forgiveness of God, wanted to talk in religious gatherings, and felt the compulsion to say, "Amen," on inappropriate occasions (shouting it or whispering it in school, at home, and during play). She had the greatest difficulty in connection with her meals. Before she sat down at the table, she had to go upstairs to talk out loud to herself, repeating many times, "Amen. I won't promise to do anything." Sometimes one such excursion sufficed, but often she had to go through the same procedure two or three times in the course of a meal. She would excuse herself by saying that she wanted to go to the bathroom or that she needed a clean handkerchief. In order to avoid the distressing ritual, she refused to eat more than one meal a day.

Helen fully realized the unreasonableness of her compulsive performances and tried in vain to rid herself of them. Her unhappiness was aggravated by her father's attempts to "beat her out of her ways." She often remarked, "Oh, I cannot stand it," or, "I feel terrible." She withdrew from her friends, gave up her previous recreational interests, and became very seclusive.

She was placed in a girls' convalescent home with the idea of changing her environment and protecting her against the eternal arguments and whippings and parental yielding to everyone of her whims. But, not getting her way for the first time in her life, she ran away from there, was picked up on the road, and taken home by her family. Proper school adjustment in an ungraded class was arranged, the parents were instructed to desist from reproaching her or otherwise causing embarrassment. Her condition improved markedly. Upon termination of school, a position was secured for her, which was suited to her interests as well as abilities (cutting shirts). At eighteen, she was married to a stable motorman. Helen is now well adjusted and has not been bothered by her obsessions for several years.

Paul M. was a physically healthy, intellectually superior, but emotionally unstable boy of Italian-German descent. His mother was excitable and had "choking spells" when Paul was nine years old. When he was a little boy, he ran fearfully away at the sight of blowing or falling leaves; he was also afraid of feathers at that time: "In the store on the corner where they sold chickens he used to stand around the chicken coop and the minute a feather flew he ran away." He was enuretic until the age of ten years. At nine, he became preoccupied when not playing outdoors; he would sit looking into space and when asked what he was thinking of, he said, "Oh, nothing." At eleven, he was told by a classmate that if you got acid on your hands, it would eat holes in them. He kept thinking about that and feared that he might get acid on himself. Three weeks later he returned from the movies in a state of collapse and could not get his breath. He then had daily anxiety attacks with choking sensation and fear of death. Soon after that, he was asked to take a "poison tablet" to his father's fruit store for a helper who had hurt his hand. From then on, he washed his hands incessantly. He fought desperately when his mother tried to put salve into his nose, declaring that the fumes would get into his lungs and that the specks on the tube would poison him. Every day he had crying spells for which he would give no reason. If his mother went out in the evening, he would beg her to stay at home, cling to her and cry. He had previously helped his father by selling fruit in the street. Now he refused to sell "seconds" in bananas and tomatoes for fear the spots would kill the people who ate them. When he received money, he wept bitterly and thought that the coins might be covered with poison. He would not clean his teeth for fear that he might swallow some of the tooth paste. His parents sent him to visit an aunt in Philadelphia; while there, he was sent to look for a box of candy in a closet and came upon a bottle marked, "Poison." He became extremely agitated, begged to go home, and finally had to be taken back by his father. He had always been fully aware of the absurdity of his notions and had not dared talk about them. He was given an opportunity to discuss his difficulties freely without being criticized or ridiculed. His recreational outlets were broadened. He went to a Boy Scout Camp for two weeks. His obsessions slowly disappeared and did not return. His father stated enthusiastically, "He has been a different boy since he came back from that camp he went to."

Charity S. was the daughter of Russian immigrants. Her father, a steel mill worker, changed to working as a presser following pneumonia. Both parents were originally Greek Catholic but about a year before Charity was born they were converted and became ardent Baptists. The conversion apparently had a good effect on the father, who gave up entirely his former habits of drinking and gambling. Charity developed well physically and intellectually. Her mental age was slightly above her chronological age. At nine months, she alarmed the family by swallowing a number of "liver pills" which her father had given her to play with; for about three years that followed she was considered sickly on the assumption that the pills had harmed her. At two years, she was frightened by the noise made by a stone crusher working on the road nearby; since then she was upset by the sight of funerals, the mention of accidents, and anything else that was out of the ordinary. At six years, she once became so agitated in school that her teacher carried her to the open window, sent a pupil for a drink of water, and asked the school nurse to take her home.

At the age of nine years, Charity was brought to the Henry Phipps Psychiatric Dispensary with the complaint that, whenever she saw anyone hurt or bleeding or whenever she was present when another child was beaten, she became sick and pale, trembled in her knees, felt her heart beat rapidly, and could not sleep in the following night unless her mother took her into her bed and caressed her. She had a fear of everything dirty or sticky and washed her hands constantly. If she went on an errand to the grocer's, she worried all the way there and back thinking that she might lose some money and counted the change over and over again on her return trip. She worried all the time that her mother would die and ran home from school as soon as she could to reassure herself that her mother was still alive. (Hermann Berger, *Über einen Fall von Zwangsvorstellungen und Zwangshandlungen bei einem zehnjährigen Kinde, Archiv für Psychiatrie, 1887, 18, 872–876,* reported a ten-year-old girl, the only child of a paretic father and migrainous mother, who had a history of two convulsions in infancy, temper tantrums and grimacing and who was distressed by the compulsion to kill her mother.) In addition, Charity had many hand-twisting movements and a trick of blowing repeatedly. She described her obsessions with these words: "I get things on my mind and cannot get them off."

Charity was described and impressed one as serious-minded, over-conscientious, very clean, fastidious with her clothes, punctilious in personal matters, exceedingly impressionable, and having a keen sense of responsibility. Her teachers spoke of her as a "lovely child and an exceptionally good pupil." It was learned that her parents were very active in religious missionary street meetings, in which her father played violin and her mother the cornet and Charity and her two sisters, Faith and Hope, sang hymns and recited Bible verses. The high-pitched emotionalism of these gatherings and public exhortations and the parental eagerness to show her off and push her into sainthood evidently were too much for this child who was perfectionistic to start with and created in her an unhealthy tenseness, which gave rise to the obsessive manifestations.

With the consent of the coöperative parents, the child was removed from the setting of missionary zeal and emotional display and placed in a boarding school where she soon adjusted herself remarkably well and lost her difficulties. When she was fourteen years old, her teachers had this to say about her: "She loves beautiful things, is very neat and prompt, can assume more responsibility than formerly, is happy, and a joy to those around her."

One often finds in the families of children with obsessive-compulsive reactions histories of similar or dissimilar personality disorders, particularly fears and depressions. For this reason, *heredity* has been proclaimed as one of the prominent etiological factors. Several investigators assumed a specific *constitutional predisposition.* Thus Soukhanoff (*Sur la pathogénie des obsessions morbides. Revue neurologique. 1903, 11, 860-861*) spoke of a *constitution idéo-obsessive.* Ziehen distinguished between *obsessive psychoses* on one hand and an *obsessive psychopathic constitution* on the other; as criteria for the innate, non-psychotic tendency he considered a trend towards "theoretically corrigible but not really supressible obtrusiveness," abnormal persistence of fear responses, and the frequency of vago-sympathetic attack phenomena. Obsessions are sometimes continuous as long as they exist, but occasionally they appear in the form of episodes of varying duration (*obsessive crises*). The cases of Helen C. and Paul M. show how these conditions may be precipitated by special life experiences (Ziehen's *Anknüpfungserlebnisse*). Obsessions are slightly more frequent in girls than in boys.

The psychoanalytic school tries to explain obsessions on the basis of *displacement.* The unpleasant memory of a sexual trauma has been repressed and is kept from reappearing in consciousness by the permanent rumination on some indifferent and seemingly unrelated topic or by the constant repetition of an apparently meaningless act. The disturbing memory is "displaced" by some other disturbing thought or fear or action, the choice of which is usually determined by some previous life experience.

Many of the obsessions of children are benign and transient, especially those which are built up on playful activities. On rare occasions, they may be precursors or early part manifestations of depressive or schizophrenic reactions. The very mild forms hardly ever come to the physician's or even to the teacher's or parents' attention.

The *treatment* will hardly be successful if it is directed toward the obsessions themselves. Explanations to the child that the notions or compulsions are unreasonable are useless because the patient himself realizes that better than anyone else and has usually already tried in every way possible to argue with himself and to shake them off. It is far better, as the outcome in the quoted cases demonstrates, to proceed on the basis that the youngster has those difficulties and must learn to live with them without giving up healthy associations and recreations. At the same time, all tensions must be relieved and the emotional and environmental problems adjusted. The child should be given an opportunity to talk freely about the obsessive urges without having to fear argumentations or ridicule. Removal from the home is often helpful because it provides for a new environment with the need of new adaptations, lifts the patient out of the rut which had been formed, and gives him new contacts and interests. It is remarkable how the obsessive-compulsive trends often fade away within a few weeks or months under such régime.

We may say in conclusion that compulsions that may sound very dangerous, such as the urge to kill someone, to jump out of the window, to cut other children with a knife, and the like, have never been known to result in the actual performance of such things. Harmless urges, such as touching people or washing the hands, are yielded to much more readily. The compulsive nature of certain habits of stealing has, in our opinion, been grossly exaggerated.

HYPOCHONDRIACAL TRENDS

The organs located in the region of the hypochondrium were once regarded as the seat of depression and of bad mood in general. The Reminders of this old view are still to be found in the original meaning of several terms describing unpleasant feelings or temperaments and connected etymologically with the viscera in the upper abdomen. The adjectives, "bilious," "choleric," "spleeny" have been relegated to lay language, whereas "melancholy" and "hypochondriasis" still figure in medical terminology. Hypochondriasis, in some of the standard dictionaries, is identified with depression and interpreted as "a condition of extreme melancholy" or "a morbid state of mind, characterized by general depression, melancholy, or low spirits." The word has, however, come to assume a more specific meaning in modern psychiatric literature; it refers to a mode of reaction consisting in the patient's centering his attention on the functioning of one or the other organ or several organs of his objectively healthy body, or exaggerating unreasonably minor or minimal ailments or sensations, and constantly and habitually complaining about his somatically unfounded aches and pains. Like many other psychiatric reaction pictures, hypochondriasis used to be considered as a separate "disease," and it is worthy of note that both Bleuler[1] and Ziehen[2] (the latter on two occasions) in their textbooks find it necessary to emphasize the fact that a disease named hypochondriasis does not exist. Ziehen states that there is no psychosis which may not occasionally present hypochondriacal delusions and that in children they occur chiefly as hypochondriacal melancholia, hypochondriacal neurasthenia, as part feature of obsessive thinking, and, where the complaints are the result of parental education, as *folie imposée* (imposed or induced insanity).

In dealing with hypochondriacal trends in children, we are forced to assume a much broader attitude, similar to the one adopted by Richards[3] and most satisfactorily outlined by Kehrer.[4] It is a matter of common observation that many people, not necessarily psychotic, not often even "neurotic," are prone to respond to life's difficulties, worries, frustrations, disappointments, discontent, boredom, etc., with bodily sensations and complaints of varying location, degree, intensity, quality, and duration. They are more or less conscious substitutions for unpleasant experiences or anticipations. They express themselves most frequently in the form of headaches, backaches (especially in women), dizziness, and digestive discomfort. They are emotionally and situationally determined. They are in no manner merely "imagined" or "simulated" or invented in order to harass the family or the impatient physician, who fails to discover any pathological substratum; they are actually felt and may be most annoying to the patient. High intelligence and even good medical knowledge are no bar. Once they

---

[1] Bleuler, E. Lehrbuch der Psychiatrie. Zweite Auflage. Berlin. 1918. p. 121.

[2] Ziehen, Theodor. Die Geisterkrankheiten im Kindersalter, einschliesslich Schwachsim und psychopathische Konstitutionen. Berlin. 1926. pp. 370, 499.

[3] Richards, Esther Loring. The Significance and Management of Hypochondriacal Trends in Children. Mental Hygiene. 1923, 7, 43–69.

[4] Kehrer, Ferdinand. Hypochondrie. In Karl Birnbaum's Handwörterbuch der medizinischen Psychologie. Leipzig. 1930, pp. 224–227.

have established themselves, it is only natural that the sufferer should look for a "cause." He observes his somatic functions more closely and devotes much of his time and thoughts to the "study" of his "symptoms." He consults popular health books and gives heed to the folkloristic notions of friends and neighbors. He becomes "cautious" about what he does and what he eats, consumes large quantities of patent medicines which a sympathetic druggist is only too glad to recommend, and becomes convinced that he is the victim of some more or less severe malady. He has no confidence in his physician who, unable or unwilling to detect and discuss the actual state of affairs, exhausts his diagnostic and therapeutic resources with the conclusion that there is absolutely nothing wrong with the patient, the prescription of a tonic or sedative (even though there is "nothing wrong"), and possibly the suggestion of a "change of climate."

In children, hypochondriacal attitudes may arise from a variety of sources. Prominent among them is the *imitation of observed adult patterns*, resulting from real illness or of the type just described. The gains and privileges derived during actual sickness may prompt the child to continue complaining, so that he may not lose the attention and consideration which he received while ill. Unhappiness at home or in school, ill-treatment, overwork with no recreational outlets, solitary life, parental oversolicitude, a feeling of insecurity, medical mismanagement, fear of punishment, anticipated failure to be promoted to a higher grade, home sickness may all contribute to the development of somatic complaints. If they are permitted to entrench themselves more or less permanently and treated on a physical basis, they may assume the proportions of a hypochondriacal reaction. The occasional complaint of a headache in the morning of a day when a difficult examination or test is expected in school is not at all uncommon. Nor is a casual stomachache when the hated spinach appears on the dinner table. This can hardly be alluded to as hypochondriasis. *Hypochondriasis is a chronic complaint habit.*

Often it is the parent who has the habit of complaining about her offspring's health. It is primarily not the child's hypochondriasis, but hypochondriasis of the mother centered on the child's somatic functioning instead of (and sometimes in addition to) her own. It is, therefore, essential to obtain a report of the complaint and its development both from the parent and from the child.

Helen K., twelve years old, came of a family in which every member's attention was centered permanently on his own bodily functioning and on that of the others. The conditions of heads, backs, and stomachs were the incessant topics of conversation and concern. Mr. K. had been operated on for bilateral hernia and for stricture in the rectum; four years ago he broke his leg in two places; he always felt badly and was always complaining; he suffered a great deal of pain from neuritis. Mrs. K. was taken out of school at eleven years (while in the third grade) because of chorea and never returned; she complained of severe temporal headaches; she had had stomachache and backache ever since an operation for appendicitis 14 years ago. A sister, 24, was taken out from school because of chorea (while in the first grade) and never went back; she stuttered until her marriage. A brother, 3, had acute nutritional disturbance with convulsions. The maternal grandmother and a maternal aunt did not go to school because of their "nerves" and chorea. A maternal uncle "lost his mind" and died in a State Hospital. Both the paternal and maternal grandmothers died of Bright's disease. The paternal grandfather died of spinal meningitis. If anything happened in the family, a headache, or a complaint of poor appetite, the "symptom" was discussed by all and a "diagnosis" made. The mother gave the following report of Helen's condition: "Helen complains of spine bone hurting her. The pain never lets up. Once in a while, she has a sudden pain in her back, like a knife cutting into her back, and she cannot move. She had headaches quite often, sometimes sudden pain in her head, always on the left side of her forehead. She has sick headaches about once in two weeks; just gets sick in the stomach, never throws up. She has backache also at night. She never sleeps painless. She complains with her stomach every once in a while, just pains her. She is very restless at night, generally goes to sleep towards morning. Her speech is bad; she stutters terribly; she makes me nervous listening. She keeps chewing her fingernails. She is easily frightened, afraid of the dark, of everything. She worries a great deal over everything and is very sensitive." Physically, she had marked lordosis, visceroptosis, and a large spina bifida on top of the sacrum; when first seen, she was 13 pounds underweight. She did a great deal of daydreaming. Helen was told of the nature of her aches and pains. The parents were persuaded that her complaints were not the symptoms of a hopeless malady; they were made to give up their anxiety about her. She was to sleep alone instead of with the parents, who were ready, at any given moment, to "turn her over" at night because her backache prevented her from doing it herself. Because of her undernutrition, she was sent to a convalescent home. On her return, she was caused to join a girls' club, and other recreation was also provided. The school situation was adjusted; she was no longer kept at home whenever she expressed the slightest complaint. Her fears were allayed. After nine months, her hypochondriasis had entirely disappeared; her daydreaming was reduced to normal proportions; her stuttering was hardly noticeable. But a new difficulty had arisen within the family. The mother, thinking of Helen's approaching menstruation, began to worry about the many alleged dangers connected with it. The problem was discussed both with her and with Helen, who at present is a tall, healthy, noncomplaining girl of fourteen, well adjusted at home and in the vocational school which she attends; she speaks rather quickly and stutters only very seldom.

The contents of the hypochondriacal complaint or complaints depend largely upon the following factors:

The child's own experiences may supply him with the complaint pattern. An acute indigestion or a cough has caused him to be kept out of school, which he happens to dislike, to be treated with gentleness and special consideration, to enjoy the suspension of the regular daily routine with its sometimes not too well liked demands. In the case of later distress or strain, the gastric discomfort or the cough may become an actually felt, though not organically justified expression, more or less conscious, of the desire for relief of a similar nature.

In the greatest majority of instances, the pattern is furnished by the environment. Where the father or mother or any other adult in the home reacts to emotional or other difficulties with headaches or backaches, the hypochondriacal child is apt to complain of headaches or backaches. But his imitation of symptoms is not necessarily limited to that of psychogenic pains and aches of his elders; real illness in his surroundings may provide him in equal measure with source material for his complaints.

Fear of heredity is another item contributing not infrequently to the type and contents of the complaint. In our case material, it was particularly the fear that the child might inherit, or might have inherited, cancer, Bright's disease, or epilepsy, with which some member of the family has been afflicted. Every slightest indisposition is looked upon with alarm and instantly connected with the disease which is anticipated on the basis of "heredity."

In one instance, a neighbor's statement that the child "looked so much like the epileptic aunt, especially under her eyes" was enough to create an atmosphere of worry and dread in the home, leading to "staring spells" of more than one hour's duration; needless to say that they had nothing in common with petit mal attacks; they could be interrupted easily by an invitation to go out for a walk or by the offer, made routinely, of a piece of candy.

A spoiled five-year-old boy, whose mother had a morbid fear of inheriting her father's carcinoma and who responded to this attitude with gastric complaints, saw her vomit once; he said, "Mother, don't do that. I'll never do anything like that," and promptly had a vomiting attack, the first of a long series, which made his parents feel that he also was doomed.

A similar effect is reached by the custom of attaching diagnostic labels to any sort of complaint, no matter whether it is organically or situationally determined. This is done by some parents, neighbors, and even physicians. In our own community, the populace is treated to the peculiar and certainly not medical term, "a touch of. . ." A child with a cough may have no bronchitis; he is then adorned generously with the "diagnosis" of having "a touch of bronchitis." Thus we come to see almost daily patients with all sorts of "touches." To the child and to his parents, of course, the "touch" is as much of a label as is the bronchitis itself. There is another term which is handed out in proper recognition of the problem, yet which has done untold harm in many cases. We have reference to the diagnosis of nervousness which is used much too liberally in the presence of children. To many little patients "nervousness" means a disease which does not differ from any other disease. The minute he has been told that he is "nervous" he ties his complaints up with this "diagnosis," in which he sees an objective justification for his aches and pains. He has been advised by medical or parental authority that, translated into his own mode of thinking, he suffers from a sickness called nervousness; hence it is something in his body, his nerves, which is fully responsible for his complaints.

The vast variety of hypochondriacal complaints may be illustrated by a few citations from our case material.

"Headache and hot flushes like a person who has high blood pressure." The father was a chronic invalid on a hypochondriacal basis, complaining of headaches and hot flushes which he ascribed to high blood pressure.

"She suffers with her back and her stomach. She has headaches when she rides in street cars (so does the mother). She gets pains in her stomach about once a week, and then she gets giddy." She was somewhat retarded intellectually, did not progress well in school, and was continually contrasted with her younger and brighter sister.

"He sometimes gets a pain in his heart when his teacher talks to him."

"I have pain in my stomach. It keeps me from going to school occasionally." A very ambitious fourteen-year-old girl, considerably retarded, whose wish to go to high school was thwarted by lack of capacity and economic distress.

"I can hardly talk to you about it. It is things that you can see and hear but not talk about. She has headaches, terrible headaches, and backaches. I thought it is her kidneys but Dr. S. told me that her kidneys are all right but he found a very high nervous tension." Her mother had "terrible headaches" and backaches. The paternal grandfather and a paternal aunt died of Bright's disease, and the family had decided that that was what the child had.

"I do not know where to start. Which pains do you mean? It feels like pins and needles all over me. My legs hurt a little, I can't hardly move them, I guess it is the calves, that is where it pains. Sometimes all my muscles hurt, my arms, my legs, and everything. Sometimes, in school, my head seems to throb. I have a backache when I write a long time or when I am leaning forward." This boy also complained of sleeplessness. He had pain in his shoulders with "cramp in the arm" during arithmetic lessons only. According to his mother, "he evidently must be suffering somewhere, or else he would not act this way. There is something somewhere that the doctors did not find out. I can't imagine that a child could put on so much."

Speaking of girl twins, eight and a half years old, a mother said: "Every once in a while they complain of their stomachs hurting them. They complain about their legs hurting. Sometimes they say their shoulders hurt. Usually they complain of the same things at the same time. They both have headaches once in a while."

Complaints of headaches, dizzy spells, needles sticking in her heart, weak spells, choking sensations, shortness of breath, pain in her jaw (since the time when her mother had a dislocation of the mandible) in a girl of 13 years, 7 months, who, with a mental age of three years below her chronological age, was expected to live up to the family tradition of being first in her class (she was "only" second). Her nosebleeds were treated by a chiropractor. A physician had told her that she had a "leaky heart," which was not true.

An eight-year-old boy, raised with the notion that he was nervous, with serious intellectual retardation, resenting the fact that his younger brother had overtaken him in school, had "attacks" when the second and third fingers of his right hand become stiff. They occurred either in school or at home, always while he was writing. During the episodes, he would "fool around" with these fingers and say, "Look, my fingers are stiff!" As soon as he was excused from further writing, they became "all right again." During the interview, he stretched his fingers forward several times, shook them vigorously, and when nothing was said to him, he volunteered: "See, I am nervous, I ain't shaking it. I wouldn't shake it. They didn't tell you

I am nervous, did they?" He had been kept out of school for several months, during which he took "medicine for his nerves." School adjustment in an ungraded class plus removal of the "nervousness" label caused the "attacks" to disappear.

The children's attitudes with regard to their hypochondriacal complaints vary considerably. Some are quite despondent and worry over their supposed illness. It is often striking to observe how some really existing ailment is totally disregarded or minimized by the patient and his family, while everybody is kept agitated over the hypochondriacal pains and aches. It is at times most difficult to obtain the consent for a badly needed tonsillectomy or treatment of dental caries, while the whole family clamors for a gastric analysis or even an appendectomy because of a situationally determined stomachache. It is not at all unusual to see husky children carried or wheeled into the office and displaying most pathetic physiognomies. There are, on the other hand, little patients who take great delight in relating their ailments and proclaim their "sickness" with the most radiant facial expression and a great deal of eloquence.

Lena T., 12 years, 4 months old, began her story with the stomach. "I came here for my stomach. Sometimes, when I eat something, it sticks right by my chest. It sticks right here in my throat, and I can't swallow. When I weigh myself, I never gain. One week I weigh 63 (incorrect!), and the next week I still weigh 63. When I bend down to pick up something, I vomit a little bit. And every time I go to the lavatory, I throw up a little bit. I have a headache. I have pain in my leg; I think it is the left; when I go to the lavatory, it gets real tired." All this was told with a good deal of unconcealed pleasure. Specific inquiry revealed considerable suggestibility, or rather unwillingness to abandon the pleasure of reporting pain in any organ. But finally she became suspicious. When questioned whether she had pain in her arms, she said, after some hesitation, "No." On second thought, she added, "Not so much." After another pause, she said, "Sometimes it hurts me." A little later, "You know, sometimes I have a real bad pain." Another pause. Then, "Something like rheumatism." And finally, as a climax, very pathetically, "You know, doctor, I think I have rheumatism in my arm."

Even in the case of Lena, where the diagnosis is obvious, a thorough physical examination is indispensable. The presence of some organic condition does not always exclude hypochondriasis and the absence of demonstrable findings does not always justify the diagnosis of hypochondriasis. There are, in prodromal states or in convalescence, complaints which may well arise from a physical source which cannot be immediately detected. On the other hand, a low percentage of hemoglobin or a refractive error does not explain the combination of backaches and stiffness in the fingers during writing only. To make sure that the nature of the complaints is understood, the investigator must add to the physical exploration a study of the child's personality and the environmental setting. The diagnosis of hypochondriacal trends is complete only if the entire psychobiological background is clearly recognized and can be used for the establishment of a therapeutic plan.

If the patient is properly treated, the *prognosis* is good. Mismanagement

may so fixate and make a permanent habit of the complaint and the reactions thereto, that the feeling of sickness may seriously interfere with the
child's adjustments to the demands of everyday life. He will then slide
into a chronic invalid reaction which will make him an unfit person for
the necessary occupational and social adaptations. He will become a slave
to his somatic preoccupations and self-indulgences. He will become, as
Richards has put it, a chronic "benchholder" in physicians', osteopaths',
chiropractors', and faith healers' waiting rooms, in hospitals and dispensaries. The physician has it in his hand to prevent or to foster such a development. He may further it by means of faulty diagnostication, by failure
to recognize, or if he has recognized it, to explain to the child and his
family the mechanisms involved, by prescribing drugs and thus strengthen-
ing the child in the belief that he is sick and by advising "rest cures" and
taking the child out of school. The very fact that a "rest cure" was considered necessary, the prescribed medicine (which is usually a placebo),
and the enforced idleness, together with the parental anxiety, are just the
soil in which chronic invalidism grows best.

In the *treatment* of children's hypochondriacal trends, the first step,
after careful history taking and investigation, is a frank discussion, devoid
of any professional lingo, with the child and with the parents, with an explanation of the nature of the complaints. To do this, it is unnecessary
and unwise to display roentgenograms and microscopic pictures; positive
and negative findings could not be distinguished by the layman, who depends on the physician's knowledge. If the latter does not have the required authority, the parading of X-ray pictures will not help. The principal postulate for successful treatment is the patient's and his family's
conviction that the complaints are not based on organic pathology but on
the psychobiological factors found to be active.

The second therapeutic step is the situational adjustment. As far as
possible, the specific disappointments or reasons for unhappiness or boredom should be remedied. Necessary school adjustments should be arranged. Parental overindulgence and solicitude must be discouraged and
substituted by adequate methods of training. Above all, it will often be
advisable to have the hypochondriacal parent or sibling or whoever had
furnished the complaint pattern examined with the aim of doing away with
any example that can be, and has been, copied.

The third step consists in a regular follow-up work with the child, who
is to learn through judicious home management and medical advice that the
hypochondriacal pains are an unhealthy, undersirable, and unprofitable
expression of improper adaptation. They should be replaced constructively
through social and recreational outlets and through utilization of the child's
assets.

HYSTERIA

The frequency with which hysteria is diagnosed in children depends
largely on what forms of reaction the individual investigators want to
include in the concept. Some authors, not unlike the lay public, use the
term so loosely as to apply it to any kind of emotional instability with
major outbursts, to any sort of hypochondriacal habits, to any mode of

simulation. Others, desirous of a clearer formulation, limit the designation to a behavior pattern well distinguished from other abnormal sets of performances by means of its clinical manifestations and its essential psycho-pathological background. It is for this reason that one finds in the literature all gradations from the assertion that hysteria is an everyday occurrence in children to the statement that it is most unusual. It is for this reason that the observation made by Sachs that "it is rare enough in adults, it is rarer still in children," has been ridiculed (unjustly) by Bruns as "peculiar." These discrepancies, however, have their roots not only in the underlying diagnostic criteria but also to a considerable extent in geographical and chronological factors. It is generally conceded, and a perusal of the literature compels one to conclude, that cultural advances with the incident taming of unchecked emotional responses have tended to diminish markedly the occurrence at least of the grand hysterical attacks in the more enlightened countries. The cooler and more self-controlled Germanic races and those people of other lineage who have lived in their midst for many generations are said to be much less liable to display hysterical symptoms.

On February 22, 1888, Charcot, in one of his famous Tuesday lectures, presented to his audience a fourteen-year-old boy with grand hysterical attacks. Even though hysteria in children, seen singly and in epidemics, had been reported before that date, Charcot's demonstration resulted in a veritable flood of further communications. The subject became a favorite topic of theses and dissertations, and case descriptions poured into the medical periodicals in an almost unending stream. But the establishment of the fact, long doubted by many physicians, that children may display hysterical reactions similar to those which are more common in the adult, was confused by the eagerness of numerous investigators to label as hysteria almost any behavior difficulty which may be encountered in the years before puberty. It became fashionable to treat under this heading of temper tantrums, easy crying, chronic invalidism, fantastic lying, enuresis, and other personality problems more or less rife among youngsters. This tendency still exists in certain quarters and is responsible for the strange fact that the indices of some pediatric and psychiatric clinics abound with records of "hysterical" children while others, more circumspect and adhering more closely to certain leading criteria, have only very few cases on their files. Bézy suggested that the future development of a child should decide whether early convulsions and "simple nervousness" before the age of two years should be diagnosed (retrospectively) as hysterical

The first monographic publications on infantile and juvenile hysteria began to appear in 1880. During the following thirty-five years, approximately thirty-five theses, pamphlets, and books were issued on the subject, and then the tide receded almost abruptly. The articles in medical journals show an almost identical curve of frequency. The oldest monograph dealing with children's hysteria is probably that written by Landor.

In the following we try to give a complete list of books and monographs devoted to hysteria in children:

1873.

Landor, H. Hysteria in Children as Contrasted with Mania. London.

1880.

Guiraud, G. Essai sur l'hystérie précoce se développant chez les jeunes filles avant la puberté. Paris.

Paris, H. De l'hystérie chez les petites filles considérée dans ses causes, ses caractères, son traitement. Paris.

1884.

De Casaubon. De l'hystérie chez les jeunes garçons. Paris.

Schaeffer, S. Über Hysterie bei Kindern. Stuttgart.

1885.

Peugniez, P. De l'hystérie chez les enfants. Paris.

1887.

Riesenfeld, P. Über Hysterie bei Kindern. Kiel.

1888.

Clopatt, A. Études sur l'hystérie infantile. Helsingfors.

Goldspiegel, H. Contribution à l'étude de l'hystérie chez les enfants. Paris.

1890.

Von Tietzen-Hennig, H. Über Hysterie bei Kindern. Freiburg i. B.

1891.

Burnet, J. F. Contribution a l'étude de l'hystérie infantile, au dessous de l'âge de cinq ans. Paris.

Holz, A. Über juvenile Hysterie beim männlichen Geschlechte. Jena.

1893.

Bardol, A. De l'hystérie simulatrice des maladies organiques de l'encéphale chez les enfants. Paris.

1895.

Wolze, W. Über einige Fälle von Hysterie im Kindesalter. Göttingen.

1896.

Conturie, J. Sur l'hystérie chez les jeunes enfants. Paris.

Hopp, R. G. G. Kasuistischer Beitrag zur Kenntnis der hysterischen Lähmungen bei Knaben. Greifswald.

1897.

Bruns, L. Die Hysterie im Kindesalter. Halle.

Loeser, L. Beitrag zur Lehre von der Hysterie der Kinder. Heidelberg.

1898.

Bibent, V. L'hystérie simulante les affections organiques chez l'enfant et l'adolescent. Toulouse.

Geisler, O. Beiträge zur Kasuistik der hysterischen Psychosen im Kindesalter. Tübingen.

1899.

Jacob, A. Über einen Fall von Hysterie im Kindesalter mit Mutismus, Blepharospasmus und Astasie-Abasie. Erlangen.

Kaler, A. L. Contribution a l'étude de l'hystérie chez les enfants. Nancy.

1900.

Bézy, P., et V. Bibent. L'hystérie infantile et juvenile. Paris.
Nolen, W. Hysterie bij kinderen. Leiden.

1901.

Sonneville, F. D. La chorée arhythmique hystérique chez l'enfant. Lille.

1902.

Saenger, A. Neurasthenie und Hysterie bei Kindern. Berlin.

1903.

Le Ridant, J. L'hystérie avant l'âge de deuz ans. Toulouse.

1904.

Bassenco. Ein Fall von hysterischer Aphasie im Kindesalter. Berlin.
Weill. Le développement de l'hystérie dans l'enfance. Paris.

1905.

Eulenburg, A. Die Hysterie des Kindes. Berlin.

1907.

Schmidt, H. Zur Prognose und Symptomatologie der Kinderhysterie.
Tübingen.

1909.

Alary, A. Considérations sur l'hystérie infantile. Toulouse.

1910.

Pietrkowski. Beiträge zur Hysterie der Kinder. Kiel.

1913.

Tobias, A. Zur Prognose und Ätiologie der Kinderhysterie. Berlin.

1914.

Dessecker, K. Zur Genese hysterischer Anfälle bei einem neunjährigen
Knaben. Berlin.

1915.

Madin, G. L'enfance de l'hystériques. Paris.

All these publications had two outstanding beneficial results. They informed the medical world of the fact that hysterical phenomena do manifest themselves before puberty.[1] At the same time the arbitrariness with which every imaginable form of children's behavior disorders was attributed to hysteria prepared the way for a growing demand for a clarification of the concept, to which Bernheim, Charcot, Freud, Janet, and others made valuable contributions.

Perhaps the clearest condensed characterization of the reaction is given by Adolf Meyer: "As hysterical dysmnesic-dissociative we designate the non-organic areflexia of cornea and pharynx, the globus, nausea and disgust complexes, anaesthesias and hyperaesthesias, limps, paralyses, astasias-abasias, contractures, convulsions, fits and tantrums and deliria and somnambulic amnesic states and certain multiple personalities. They can be shown to be dysmnesic substitutions which follow the type of more or

---

[1] Probably the first author to mention infantile hysteria was Carolus Lepois who, in 1617, said: "Enim vero experientiae fide, multae puellulae vivunt hystericis tentatae symptomatibus ante duodecim aetatis annum."

less unconscious self-suggestion. i.e., a suppression or repression of incompatible experiences, with substitutive reactions, the connection of which tends to be 'forgotten' and which, themselves, are often unheeded or accepted with indifference and complacency, or with actual satisfaction (Freud's *Krankheitsgewinn*), but great emotional lability. . . . The typical hysterical is rather indifferent and carefree between paroxysms."

Since the symptomatology is so manifold that it may include in its realm practically every human reaction, it is necessary that it should be organized sufficiently to avoid confusion and bewilderment. It has long been customary to divide the hysterical manifestations into sensory, motor, and psychic features. Attempts have also been made to distinguish between leading essential, authentic, more or less pathognomonic symptoms, the so-called hysterical stigmata, and incidental, superimposed, additional disorders which may be observed also in non-hysterical patients and which "may resemble anything." We shall take up the principal features under the following three headings:

1. Somatic manifestations, or part-dysfunctions.

2. Episodic performances or states, involving conspicuously the entire organism.

3. The hysterical personality.

The *somatic part-manifestations* may be sensory, motor, visceral, and vasomotor, and may combine themselves to form countless individual patterns.

The *sensory disturbances* which, if present, are quite characteristic of hysteria and are of especial differential diagnostic value may involve any kind of sensation: touch, pain, temperature, muscle sense, vision, audition, taste, and smell. They may be the only or essential feature of the complaint (numbness, blindness, deafness, pain) or discovered incidentally in the course of the examination (anaesthesias, scotomata). They may be isolated and independent phenomena or accompany motor disorders or episodic states. They may last a long time or have a relatively brief duration, with sudden dramatic onset and an equally abrupt cessation.

The *disorders of cutaneous sensation* are either in the nature of diminution or complete abolition, hyperacuity, or qualitative alterations. The tactile, algetic, and thermic perceptions may be involved in equal measure or in different degrees. The characteristic feature of all hysterical anaesthesias or hypoaesthesias is the type of their regional distribution. They do not follow the course of a cutaneous nerve and the area supplied by it but affect a certain division of the body in the sense of common popular usage unburdened with the knowledge of anatomy. The naïve lay representation of the body and not the segmentation of the central nervous system supplies the pattern for the configuration and extent of the involved area, which may be the hand, the foot, the forearm, the thigh, the breasts, or the face, regardless of the nerve supply. If a limb or a part of it is affected, the anesthesia is invariably circular; e.g., the arm is anaesthetic on its radial, ulnar, anterior, and posterior surfaces. The border between the sensible and insensible parts is a sharp circular or straight line. The designations, *glove anaesthesia* and *stocking anaesthesia*, have been characteristically applied to the type of insensibility which in the upper and lower extremities extends over surfaces covered usually by a glove or a stocking. If the entire half of the body is involved (hemi-anaesthesia), the border follows exactly the midline or a line very near and parallel to it. In some instances, the sensory disorder appears in spotted areas throughout the body, again irrespective of the segmental innervation. The anaesthesias are never associated with atrophy of the muscles and rarely with abnormal reflex responses.

The hyperaesthesias and hyperalgesias are rather narrowly circumscribed. The joints, the epigastric region, the areas over the ovaries or, in boys, over the center of the inguinal ligaments, the breasts, and the middle of the back are places of predilection. The slightest touch or pinprick may produce excruciating pain or occasionally even major hysterical attacks. Ziehen suggested the term *topalgias* for these "topical" pains called forth in those regions to which the French allude as *hysterogenetic zones*. Both the anaesthesias and hyperaesthesias may be influenced by suggestion in the sense that the insensibility may be transferred from one place to another (*transfer phenomenon*) or that, for instance, the hypersensitive spinous processes of the lumbar or dorsal vertebrae may be made to vary in number and in their upper or lower limits in the course of the same examination. The topalgias are usually elicited by external stimulations but may at times occur spontaneously. During sleep, the cutaneous sensibility disturbances do not exist; the patients respond normally to pinpricks applied to the anaesthetic areas and are not unusually sensitive to excitation of the so-called hysterogenetic zones. Whereas insensibility is quite frequently linked to motor disturbances, hyperalgesia is, at least in children, hardly ever encountered in a paralyzed part.

Anaesthesia of the mucous membranes often leads to the pathognomonic absence of the pharyngeal gag reflex and of the conjunctival reflex. Sometimes the corneal reflex is abolished.

Visual disorders play a considerable part in hysterical individuals. Most of them are usually discovered only during the examination. Hemianopsia and scotomata have been reported, the former mostly together with hemianaesthesia and hemi-paresis. Diplopia, polyopia, micropsia, and macropsia have been known to occur. Color vision may be affected in the direction of achromatopsia (all objects appearing colorless, gray) or dyschromatopsia (other, usually complementary, colors being seen instead of the real ones). Photophobia and blepharospasms are sometimes seen. Hysterical amblyopia, or blindness, has been said by most authors to be so rare in children as to be negligible. We have, however, had the opportunity to observe a comparatively large number of cases. It is transitory in most instances, but apt to recur. It is best characterized by the *triad of Dieulafoy:*

1. Suddenness of onset.
2. Absolutely normal ophthalmoscopic findings.
3. Normal pupillary reactions to light and accommodation.

Abt described an interesting case of hysterical blindness in a three-year-old girl so vividly that we can do no better than render his report verbatim:

"Early one morning, after having been reprimanded by her mother, she complained of sudden blindness and pain in both eyes. Upon arriving at the house I found that the terror-stricken family were grouped in a darkened room, all weeping and gesticulating, and the child was crying that she was blind. The pandemonium was indescribable. After clearing the room of every member of the family except the child and holding her before the bright daylight I observed that her pupils responded. I assured her that she could see, and very soon she and I were discussing the sights on the streets below. Her vision was restored."[1]

We add a few cases from our own material:

In the section on stealing, we had the occasion to cite the case of Sybilla, an hysterical shoplifter, whose attack of sudden blindness lasted three months and, upon the suggestion of the family physician, disappeared just as suddenly at the onset of menstruation.

Alice F., fifteen years old, had an attack of blindness in which she was unable to read or see pictures, following a diving episode in which she hurt her head. Examination revealed normal neurological and ophthalmological findings. The nature of the reaction was typically hysterical. A little later, following a wake, she had a delirious experience during which she was hallucinated (spoke of seeing a child and a white woman), had laughing spells, and kept talking to herself in a confused manner; she wandered away from home and was picked up on the road; she often screamed and both her arms were "cold and stiff."

Margaret H., thirteen years old, was the oldest of four girls, all of whom were bedwetters. She was ten pounds underweight but otherwise in good physical health. She had a mental age of almost twelve years (I.Q. 85). In October, 1930, she was pushed by a boy and fell "real hard" on the back of her head and "acted dazed" for a few hours without losing consciousness. In October, 1931, she had another fall following which her right knee was in a cast for some time. Since then she had spells in which her right knee "gave away" and she fell. For the past year, she had had attacks of pain in her eyes and dimness of vision recurring in fairly frequent intervals. At night she sometimes thought that she could not close her eyes but was relieved at once by rose-water placed in her eyes by her stepfather. One night she woke up suddenly and complained that her eyes hurt her when she tried to close them. Her first episode of visual disorder occurred while she was in school. The teacher was reading a story and from time to time would ask questions. Margaret was afraid she would be asked. She felt sick, her eyes were hurting, she could not see, and put her head on the table. The teacher then sent her home. The spells came back about every other month, whenever she was confronted with school difficulties. They always resulted in her being permitted to go to rest in the nurse's room. The last "blind spell" occurred in September, 1932. It started near the end of the morning session after she had finished the spelling test. She came home feeling nauseated but had her lunch. She went right back to school. That afternoon she did not do any work but put her head on the desk and "slept" through the geography, arithmetic, and history periods. The attack began with her eyes starting to get blurry. It felt "as if someone were trying to knock my eyes out way back there and then they got blurry." Shortly after that, the fingers of her left arm commenced to become numb, then the

[1] Abt, Isaac. Hysteria in Children. Medical Clinics of Chicago. 1915, 1, 477–487.

sensation spread through the entire arm. Because of her illness, she did not have to stay after school as she usually did to work out extra problems. When she reached home, the arm felt all right but her fingers were still numb; the vision was restored but the eyes still hurt. She was pale and her mother sent her up to bed. She came down for supper and went to bed again. After supper, she was perfectly well.

Total *hysterical deafness* is much less frequent than minor degrees of impairment of hearing and a sort of selective deafness limited to the class hours or even to certain subjects or to certain teachers. *Olfactory and gustatory disturbances* are extremely rare in children.

The hysterical *motor disturbances* may assume the form of peculiar postures with alterations of the entire body configuration (*Änderung der Körpergestalt;* Homburger), such as torticollis, scoliosis, kyphosis, strange contortions, etc. They may manifest themselves as anomalies in the performance of movements in the shape of tremors, myoclonic contractions, choreiform excursions, ataxic features, tics, and various kinds of jactations. Or they may, most frequently, appear as diminutions of motility. The *hysterical paralyses*, like the anaesthesias, depend in their extent on the lay conception of such functional units as "an arm," "a leg," "a hand," or "a foot," that is, on gross external segmentation rather than on segmental innervation. The paralyses may be spastic or flaccid. The reflexes fail to show the changes corresponding to similar organic conditions. There may exist a hemiplegia, paraplegia, or monoplegia, but an isolated muscle paralysis is never observed in hysteria. The affected part is never atrophied, except secondarily from long disuse. Gordon, Chaddock, and Oppenheim phenomena are always absent, knee and ankle clonus have been reported in exceptional cases only. The areas supplied by cranial nerves (other than the spinal accessory) never participate in hysterical hemiplegias, which are conspicuously free from facial nerve palsies or third, sixth, and twelfth nerve involvement. On the other hand, the paralyses are very frequently associated with anaesthesias having an identical distribution, and with hemianopsias; this, however, is seen more often in adults than in children. The complications seem to be proportionately related to the patient's experience and to the number and nature of preceding examinations. As long as a child does not "know" that a paralyzed limb is in any way supposed to be insensible, the anaesthesia fails to appear; at a later period, when he is sufficiently "informed," pinpricks may cease to be registered. Hysterical contractures are relatively rare before puberty.

A not so uncommon hysterical symptom is the so-called *astasia-abasia*, the inability to stand and to walk in spite of the fact that the lower extremities are capable of performing other voluntary movements. When the children are sitting or reclining, not the slightest sign of a motility disturbance is evident; the patient may swing his legs, resist passive movements, kick objects, and perform any kind of complex and coördinated activities with the legs in a normal manner. The functions of standing and walking, however, are entirely eliminated. The children act as though they had completely forgotten or never learned how to make steps. If they do make attempts at locomotion, they behave like infants in their first walking efforts. Occasionally one sees hysterical youngsters with an outspoken

abasia who swim quite well (case reported by Charcot) or are capable of
jumping or climbing. Bruns has divided the forms of hysterical astasia
and abasia into three goups:

Paralytic form; the children collapse when put on their feet.

Spastic form.

Shaking or *choreatic* form, in which the patients tremble so long and so
vigorously that they ultimately drop to the floor ("stuttering of the legs").

Astasia-abasia is said to be ten times as frequent in children as it is in
adults.

Among the *disturbances of speech*, aphonia and mutism predominate. The
children do not speak above a whisper, though they may cough, weep, and
even sing loudly. Or all verbal expression may be absent. Hysterical mutism,
also not quite correctly alluded to as aphasia, differs distinctly from analogous reactions produced by organic conditions. Henderson and Gillespie
suggest that the two types of speech disorder have to be distinguished

  1. by their completeness—every phonated word and sound is lost in hysteria;

  2. the absence of any intellectual disorder;

  3. the preservation of the ability to communicate by writing or by signs;

  4. the absence of paralysis of the lips and tongue;

  5. the vocal cords can be seen to be fully adducted in inspiration.

One may add as a sixth criterion that the hysterical child makes absolutely no effort to speak.

Hysterical stuttering usually is more bizarre than stuttering in non-
hysterical patients. The onset is usually sudden. The children often repeat
the first word of a sentence a number of times but then have no difficulty
in continuing and completing a long statement. There is in most cases no
disturbance in the economy of respiration.

The *visceral disorders* may involve any organ system. Aside from the
globus which we have described elsewhere and which is counted among the
"stigmata," they are mostly regarded as secondary, incidental, not necessarily pathognomonic symptoms. It is, as a matter of fact, often difficult
to decide whether a functional constipation, a psychogenic cough, or a non-
organic polyuria is "hysterical" or whether these not uncommon forms of
children's personality problems just happen to be present in an hysterical
child, as they are so often seen in non-hysterical youngsters, though it
may be readily conceded that the former is more apt to avail himself of
any of these modes of reaction. If we keep this in mind, we are not compelled to take sides in the peculiar controversy about enuresis, the majority
of authors asserting that bedwetting is rare in hysteria, while others maintain that it is an exquisitely hysterical manifestation. Feeding difficulties
(anorexia) occurring in hysterical children are much more serious than in
others, since with their common tendency to "massiveness," of which we
shall speak later, they are prone to carry their refusal of nourishment to a
point of alarming inanition necessitating radical therapeutic measures.

It would lead too far and occupy too much space if we were to exemplify
all possible visceral disorders of an hysterical nature. They are too multi-
form and vary too much in different individuals. We are therefore limiting

ourselves to two illustrations in which disturbances of deglutition are the prominent manifestations.

Harry B., a normally intelligent boy of almost twelve years, was brought to the dispensary with the complaint that he had "difficulty in eating; things catch in his throat and won't go down." His dysphagia was accompanied by fright. It had begun suddenly three weeks after Christmas; he had always presented a feeding problem and his father used to beat him severely whenever he would not eat properly. Following one such scene, Harry could not swallow his food. His dysphagia was still present in the following October when medical aid was finally solicited. He could take liquid and semi-solid nourishment only. He was, since the onset of his swallowing difficulty, well treated by his parents who were worried that he might have some serious throat disease. There had been a slight temporary improvement during the summer vacation from school. He had lost eleven pounds. The child was found, upon physical examination, to have a rather large head, slight internal strabismus, occult spina bifida, stigmata of rickets, and dental caries. The pharyngeal gag reflex was absent and the deep reflexes were somewhat diminished. His mother had "fainting spells" and his grandmother had "spells of weakness" which the boy had occasionally copied. Harry, after a better home management had been secured, readily accepted the interpretation of his deglutition disorder as non-organic. Since the father had become less stern and the various "spells" of the female elders had disappeared, the home atmosphere became more pleasant. The purpose which the dysphagia had served more or less unconsciously no longer existed. The symptom vanished almost over night. It is probable that a preceding tonsillectomy had furnished the pattern.

Cecelia R., seven years old, of low average intelligence, came with the following story: "Her tongue went down her throat on Wednesday evening, and yesterday (on Thursday) several times. She could not put her tongue in her mouth for fear it would go down her throat again." The child reported that on Wednesday she did not want any supper, was not hungry. She had eaten macaroni out in the back yard. She then had come into the house, swept the floor, put the dishes into the sink, and gone out to play. When she felt hungry, she came in and asked her mother for bread. When she went to the ice-box for butter, she suddenly began to cry because her tongue went down her throat. Her mother could not see her tongue and screamed. Her father came and gave her water. The water made her feel better. Next day, the family went on an excursion by boat, which she enjoyed very much. When they got off the boat, she felt her tongue was drawing in and she stuck it out to keep it from going down her throat. This was repeated in the following night when she lay from twelve to five o'clock with her tongue kept pressed tightly between her lips, groaning, clenching her hands, and unable to speak. It is significant to know that two years befor she had her tonsils and adenoids removed and her uvula clipped and that her oversolicitous mother worried "that she has never been well since." At five years, she had developed enuresis after moving into another home which she disliked. She had always been afraid of the dark and a light was kept burning in her room all night. She fussed about her food, was described as "sulky, nagging, whining, nasty." When asked how she was treated at home, she said, "My mother is very good to me when I am sick."

The *vasomotor and trophic disturbances* are as a rule not so outspoken and "massive" as the other disorders. Dermatographia is not uncommon.

Edemas have been reported in a limited number of cases. Whether or not erythemata, ulçers, and blisters are artefacts or produced by auto-sugges- tion, is a question which has called forth a good deal of controversy. Disuse atrophy of paralyzed limbs depends on the duration of the paralysis.

It is characteristic of practically all somatic manifestations of hysteria that they are not present during sleep; the rigid limb relaxes, the anaesthet- ic arm responds to painful stimulation, the hyperaesthetic zone does not react to mild irritation, there are no spontaneous topalgias. It is further typical that the physical handicap does not usually endanger the patient; unlike the frequent records of burning the hand or arm in syringomyelia, the hysterical insensibility does not lead to similar injuries; blindness or hemianopsia does not keep the patient from avoiding perilous obstacles. Though hysterical symptoms may "resemble anything," their semeiology hardly ever is fully identical with that of the conditions which they re- semble. There is usually something in the distribution, in the reflexes, in the symptom combination, etc., that differs from the neurological or other organic syndrome which is suggested and that makes the physician mindful of the possibility of the existence of an hysterical reaction.

The somatic symptoms of hysteria may be episodic in nature, beginning and leaving suddenly and lasting from less than one hour to several years. The cases of amblyopia or amaurosis, the instances of dysphagia and of tongue swallowing described above have occurred as transient events. Yet they appeared to the observer, before further examination and analysis, to happen on an infra-psychobiological level, involving only a narrowly circumscribed part of the personality. Even then it often becomes evident at first glance that psychic factors may be at play; there are hysterical paralyses which exist only so long as the patient does not look at the af- fected limb; if he watches it, he can move it freely. Yet there are reactions which immediately impress the observer as performances much more sweep- ing in character, carried out by the individual in his entirety, easily recog- nized as dysfunctions of the total personality. In this sense, they are com- monly referred to as the *mental or psychic symptoms* of hysteria, though one must, of course, always keep in mind that the bodily manifestations are not less mental or psychogenic or, as Ziehen expresses it, *ideoplastic*.

These "psychic" episodes are major attacks or fits, fugues, paralogia states, deliria, and the rare instances of double or multiple personalities.

The *hysterical attacks*, which seem to have been quite frequent in former centuries, are very unusual in our time and environment. There are busy psychiatrists and pediatricians who confess having witnessed but very few in the many years of their experience. It has been customary, since Charcot, to divide the seizures into a number of stages. But either all or only a few or even only one of them may be present; their succession may vary; the picture of the individual stages may differ essentially not only in different individuals but even in several attacks had by the same patient. The stages are:

Prodromal stage, characterized by visual (flashes, colors) or auditory (various kinds of noises, buzzing, ringing, whistling, thunder) experiences, the globus sensation, spells of unchecked laughing or crying, or less dramatic moods of depression or hilariousness, headaches, or an aura with pelvic, abdominal, or thoracic pain, or backache.

Epileptoid stage with rigidity, various forms of twitchings, clonic or tonic convulsions; in contradistinction to epilepsy, the tongue is not bitten, sphincter control is usually preserved, the pupils react normally, there is no froth at the mouth, and consciousness is not so completely abolished. Injuries are rarely sustained as a result of the fall.

Stage of peculiar postures and grimaces. Arc de cercle, in which the back is bent to the extent that the occiput may touch the heels, with opisthotonos; various forms of awkward rotating, kicking, incoördinate movements ("clownism").

Stage of affective attitudes (*attitudes passionnelles*) with features and postures expressing terror or rapture or love or hatred, with clouding of consciousness and more or less coherent verbalizations.

Delirious stage, which sometimes may occur alone as a rudimentary attack; orientation is impaired to a larger or lesser degree, and the delirium is usually not followed by amnesia, whereas most of the experiences in the other stages are not recalled.

The attack may last from ten to fifteen minutes to several hours. In spite of the sometimes violent motor discharges, the patient emerges from the episode without any signs of exhaustion.

Allen R., twelve years and ten months old, with a mental age of nine years, had at eight years an attack in which he ran wildly for several hundred yards into the fields and then fell over, apparently unconscious. At that time he was given treatment for worms. Four years later, he again had "running spells," occurring once in two days to twice daily. After about one month, he began to have "drawing spells," described as attacks beginning with a drawing sensation at the top of the head, into the shoulders and back, accompanied by severe pains and by quivering and twitching of the limbs; they were ushered in by "a curious feeling in the head." One spell was followed by blindness of his right eye and paralysis of his left leg, which cleared up spontaneously after one week. On the next day, he was examined in the dispensary. In the afternoon, while at home, he said that he had queer feelings in his head ("It draws me double; it carries me over several times") and that he was going to have another attack. When a physician was called, he found the boy lying across the bed and, quite suddenly, grabbing his feet, arching his back, and thrashing about on the bed. He then began to turn quite quickly in a spinning fashion, his head on a pillow. His eyes were turned upward and to the left. From time to time, the patient made chewing movements without biting his tongue and tried several times to bite the physician when any attempt at restraint was made. On having his fingers put between his teeth, he very gently chewed on them. He was allowed to roll about on the bed as he desired but did not fall out of it. About forty-five minutes later, the patient, quite suddenly, opened his eyes, was clear, talked nicely, said he had been asleep, realized someone had taken his stockings off, but stated that he did not know when the physician came into the room.

In the *fugues* or *twilight states* (*Dämmerzustände*) consciousness is sufficiently impaired to make the patient's performances appear as having no connection with the immediate reality of the surroundings. They can therefore not be understood by the observers. They are, however loose and seemingly disconnected, held together as events or series of events replete with affective drives and experiences not dependent on the moment nor on the actual environment. They resemble the pictures obtained in sleepwalking or night terrors, in that all three are governed by something going on within the performer and followed by a more or less complete amnesia. It seems to us, however, that the term somnambulism is not well chosen for the hysterical act and better reserved entirely for the condition of sleepwalking of the type which we discussed together with the other sleep disorders. It seems preferable to use the designation of "vigilambulism" suggested by Sollier.

An interesting case was seen at the Henry Phipps Psychiatric Clinic (record number 4003); it was used as an illustration of hysterical fugues in the Text-Book of Psychiatry by Henderson and Gillespie (London. 1927, p. 433). Eugene W. was admitted to the Clinic at the age of fourteen years. While attending a military school, he was repeatedly picked up miles away, sometimes clad very scantily. On one occasion he was found at a place sixty miles from the school, walking with his eyes half closed but capable of avoiding dangers and obstacles, and unable to give any information other than telling his name. During his residence in the Clinic he had similar episodes, occurring suddenly both in daytime and at night; sometimes the event was preceded by his falling on the floor in the state of complete flaccidity, lasting for a few minutes, after which he would rise and attempt to leave the hospital. Questions remained unanswered but when given a pencil and a piece of paper, he automatically, with his eyes closed, wrote fairly legibly the following words (the spelling has not been changed): "Doctor plase find out my trouble so I can go back to school. I wish I hadn't let that man hypnotize me last year. I keep thinking of him all the time. he seems to be near me all the time. I've thought of him every since he hypnotized me last year at school. he seems to keep telling me to fall and do what ever he tells me to. His name is Valpriso, and if he as any control over me please try and get me natural again because I want to go to school so bad. I wish I hadnt been hyponotized I cant seem to stop thinking of him." It was then learned that he had been hypnotized by a traveling showman before the onset of his fugues and that he had been told that if he would return six months later to the same place he would be released from the hypnotizer's power. If he did not return, he would remain permanently under the man's influence. The boy also had a slight speech difficulty, consisting in lisping and a mild degree of stuttering.

Paralogia (syndrome of approximate answers; the Ganser syndrome) is a specific form of hysterical twilight reaction. Its occurrence has been reported also in epilepsy, schizophrenia, and in organic cerebral conditions (arteriosclerosis; lues cerebrospinalis; parietal lobe tumor). It was first observed by Moeli in 1888 and more elaborately studied by Ganser in prisoners. Although Jolly once stated that it is "especially frequent in hysteria of children," the only case that we have been able to find in the literature is that of a twelve-year-old blind boy cited by Hey in his monograph.[1]

---

[1] Moeli. Über irre Verbrecher. Berlin. 1888.—Ganser. Über einen eigenartigen Dämmerzustand. Archiv für Psychiatrie. 1898, 30, 633.—Jolly F. Allgemeine Neurosen. Ebstein und Schwalbe: Handbuch der praktischen Medizin. Vol. IV. 1900, p. 769.—Hey, Julius. Das Gansersche Symptom und seine klinische und forense Bedeutung. Berlin. 1904, pp. 12-15.

For this reason it is not uninteresting to quote a case of our observation, to our knowledge the youngest child ever known to present the picture of paralogia. The syndrome consists of a tendency, lasting for from several days to two weeks, to answer questions in a way which shows an understanding of their meaning but narrowly misses the correct reply.

Dorothy M., six years old, was the daughter of a shoemaker who had a history of psychogenic "cramps in his stomach" and a mother who had several mild depressions. She was youngest of four girls all of whom bit their fingernails. Dorothy was also in the habit of biting her toenails. Frances, thirteen, only in the fifth grade, bit her toenails until school age. Helen, eleven, "nervous," had been "broken" from her lefthandedness. Anna, ten, was "delicate and nervous" and only in the third grade. Dorothy, at the age of one year, in the course of pneumonia, became rigid and rolled her eyes for about two minutes. Since the age of approximately four years, she presented feeding difficulties. She had always been extremely restless. She had frequent temper outbursts and screaming spells; the latter began when her sister, Frances, cut her finger with a broken ring and screamed in pain; Dorothy joined her and afterwards screamed "whenever she wanted something and could not get it." In one of her tantrums she fainted but was immediately revived by shaking. She cut short another "spell" by remarking, "Mother, look at them Indians fighting." For the past two years, she had had quite regularly, almost every morning, when sitting in the bathroom to empty her bowels, peculiar attacks, lasting from three to eight minutes, in which she suddenly burst out laughing or ran wildly from room to room. When asked what the trouble was, she would complain about the stomach. At other times, always in the morning, she would become rigid, without falling or frothing or biting her tongue, and not respond to her parents' questions. She had been taken from one doctor to another and given all sorts of diagnoses and medicines. Masturbation had been a problem of long standing with her. In the school (kindergarten) she fought a good deal with the children, was very contrary, and did just the opposite of what she was told. On May 9, 1931, her mother asked Dorothy to go out to play. When she looked out through the window, she saw the child sitting in the gutter in an awkward position. When she went to her, Dorothy was rigid and her head moved rhythmically from side to side. Dorothy remained in that position for eight hours, in the course of which an ambulance took her to the Harriet Lane Home. When she awoke, a transient right hemiparesis existed for about twenty-four hours. For the following sixteen days, she presented the characteristic picture of paralogia. Some of the questions and answers are recorded below:

Q.	A.
What kind of place is this?	Plain house.
What does that mean?	It is painted.
Have you ever been in a hospital?	Yes.
When?	Next Monday.
How old are you?	Three months.
When are you going to go home?	Five years.
What is the name of this place?	Two hundred.
How many fingers have you?	Three.
Count them!	(Counts.) Five.
Well, how many fingers have you?	Six.
(Asked to count 17 squares.)	Fifteen.
(Asked to count them again.)	Eighteen.

How many chairs do you see in this
room? (There were three.)   (Counts repeatedly): Four.
Color of grass?   Green.
Color of snow?   White.
Color of the sky?   Yellow.
Is ice hot or cold?   Hot.

On the ninth day, at the dinner table, she put a torn toy balloon into her
mouth and pointed to her stomach. She said that she had stuffed her mouth
with the "blower" because she had a stomachache.

She cleared up rather suddenly on May 25, except that for a time she
playfully kept giving her age as five years instead of as six years and then
correcting herself either spontaneously or when told that that was wrong.

In the course of the ensuing year, under a régime of indifference, the
child had no more "spells" of any kind. She was a "different child," according to her mother. Masturbation and temper tantrums had ceased. Instead
of taking off her stockings several times during the day in order to bite her
toenails as she used to do, she "only" bit them off once a week after she
had her bath. She, however, developed the habit of putting her earlobes
into the external meatus. Sleep and appetite were satisfactory. She still wet
her bed about once or twice a week as she had always done. She went to
school regularly and got along quite well with the other children.

There exist all sorts of transitions from the twilight states to the hysterical *delirious and stuporous reactions*. The delirium is not followed by amnesia. The disorientation is more profound, and hallucinations are more
frequent. The contents are usually more coherent and less fleeting and
changeable than in the anergastic and dysergastic deliria.

The phenomenon of the *dual or multiple personality* is characterized by
the fact that the dissociation is more complete than in the other hysterical
episodes. It has been most painstakingly studied by Morton Prince.[1] The
two dissociated "personalities" exist, as it were, independently in the Dr.
Jekyll and Mr. Hyde fashion. The patient is at times her own natural self,
at other times she is in all of her actions and attitudes someone else, mostly
an infant. We have never observed the phenomenon in a child.

Much has been written on the difference between the hysterical reaction
form in children and that seen in adults. The outstanding features are
listed below:

Hysteria in children has been said to be *monosymptomatic*. This is true
of some cases, but certainly not of all. Dorothy M., in addition to her peculiar spells, indulged in various forms of manipulations of the body (biting
her fingernails and toenails, pulling her ears, masturbation), had dramatic
temper tantrums, was enuretic, and refused to eat. It is, however, a fact
that usually only one of the "stigmata" is encountered at a given time.

The French have pointed out that the hysterical symptoms of children
are characterized by their *massiveness*. The paralyzed arm is incapable of
any sort of movement. The anaesthetic limb has no sensation whatever.
Any type of hysterical manifestation of a child impresses the layman and
even the physician as complete, serious, eminently acute.

Janet, in discussing somnambulism, has distinguished a *monoidetic* and

[1] Prince, Morton. The Unconscious. New York. 1914, pp. 299–302.

a *polyidetic* form according to the scantiness or richness of the content. It may be said that in children, who are more naïve and less experienced than adults, all hysterical symptoms are comparatively poor in content and impress one as either monoidetic or, at best, oligoidetic.

Children seem *more suggestible* than adults and for this reason offer a better prognosis.

The factor of *imitation* seems to play a more significant rôle in children.

The knowledge of the hysterical symptoms and their diagnostic evaluation is undoubtedly of paramount importance. But aside from the recognition of a visual disturbance or a fugue as being hysterical, it is necessary to learn something about the general make-up of the individual who is capable of such manifestations. Are there, in other words, any personality features and reaction tendencies and emotional patterns common to all or to a majority of hysterical children? Do we have to depend in our diagnosis solely on the absence of the gag reflex or on similar "stigmata" or is it possible to obtain more intrinsic criteria expressing themselves in the patient's character and the quality of his everyday performances? Full-fledged temper tantrums, convulsions of all sorts of etiology, the transformation into somatic complaints or symptoms of affective events or states ("dysphorias") are so frequent in children, that these factors themselves are in no manner typical of hysteria, certainly much less so than in adults.

Many investigators have attempted to depict the essential traits of the *hysterical character*. As far as children are concerned, no one has succeeded as excellently as Homburger. It is from his enlightening presentation that we abstract the following particulars. "True love and attachment, gratitude, loyalty, naïve fulfilment of duties, truthfulness, reliability are substituted by artificial, feigned, consciously or not quite consciously falsified sentiments and performances which are invented, thought up, decided upon, and carried out largely to produce the impression of, and to derive satisfaction, from one's own excellence which is fully or partly believed and more or less efficiently acted. Devotion, unpretentiousness, modesty, moderation, sympathy, tenderness, impressionability, amiability are pretended by shrewd hysterical children with great perfection. Superficial, dependent on moods, incalculable, and often hardly understood likes and dislikes for children and elders dominate the psychic life of these patients often enough from early years and cause innumerable conflicts." There exists a marked desire for ostentation, a studied coquettishness which shows itself when confronting the teacher, visitor, or physician, when asking a passer-by for the correct time, or when reciting a poem. At home, in school, among strangers, in the street car, the child finds or creates opportunities to attract attention by fair means or foul. Instead of the natural shyness, reserve, and feeling of immaturity in the presence of adults, there is a display of assumed poise, "putting on airs," ready judgments which are either enthusiastic endorsements or disdainful disapprovals. All this is linked with an emotional lability, with a lack of affective equilibrium. The expressions of love, hatred, anger, pain, despair, repentance, etc., are carried to extremes, being out of proportion to the importance of the exciting cause in their boundless massiveness and violence. Ill-explained sadness alternates suddenly with equally unmotivated periods of elation. In the midst of vivid play with other children, in which the patient is more active than the rest, he may abruptly withdraw and appear listless; or he may all at once advocate a change of games, though up to that moment he has seemed highly interested and absorbed. A long and vigorous temper outburst or crying spell may be cut short unexpectedly without further concern over the original cause. Imitation, which plays a significant part in the life of every child, is a leading factor in hysteria. Dorothy M.'s screaming spells began when she witnessed her sister's reaction to cutting her finger with a broken ring; the screaming was copied, exaggerated, and utilized for other purposes. Many of the essential symptoms originate in the imitation of observed, discussed, or formerly experienced real illness, and a chain of reactions is established, the principal links of which are imitation, exaggeration, and more or less unconscious purposive utilization. Suggestion or auto-suggestion often takes the place of imitation.

A girl of fifteen averted with her right hand her boy friend's repeated attempts to touch her genitals; she experienced a good deal of conflict between her desire to comply and the much stronger moral considerations; she developed a rhythmical, diurnal, violent shaking of her right arm which was diagnosed as electric chorea and made to disappear by means of salvarsan injections. Her mother's illness and death threw the entire household responsibilities upon her. Her father's constant criticism and comparison with how much better her mother had done made her very unhappy. She had an older sister who had considerable musical talent and was away from home, being trained in a famous conservatory; she had already given several public concerts and was hailed as a genius by her family and in her home town. Goldie (the patient) had been denied an adequate education and considered herself a martyr to her sister's career. Following her sister's visit to attend her mother's funeral, the shaking returned and was this time not influenced by salvarsan, massages, and other forms of treatment. The only time her arm did not shake was when she played the piano or prepared a certain kind of soup which her father had said was her specialty. The child was made to recognize the connections. A housekeeper was engaged. Goldie went back to high school. She was given piano lessons. Her shaking disappeared permanently. She later, of her own accord, married her boy friend and became a happy and healthy mother. This case shows the great complexity of factors which may be active in the formation of an hysterical symptom.

It would require a special volume to go into the details of all the theories that have been advanced with regard to the *etiology* and nature of hysteria. Etymologically, the term is derived from Greek *hysteron* (the uterus) because of the notion which the ancients had that the condition is due to the womb's migrating about the body. For this reason, it was believed that the reaction occurs in women only. We know to-day that this is not so, though it must be conceded that it is far more frequent in the female than in the male. In smaller children, there seems to be an equal distribution between the sexes. At the age of puberty, however, girls are said to be affected twice as often as boys. The question, of course, arises what becomes of these little boys in later life, and a follow-up would be very instructive. It is, on the other hand, true that in later years the hysterical features make their appearance more frequently in girls in whom they had not been in evidence in early childhood.

Hereditary factors have been made responsible by various authors, who consider all other etiological moments only as *agents provocateurs* (Charcot, Guinon). Homologous transmission is said to be predominant; "hysterical parents have hysterical children." Bruns, however, feels that "especially under the influence of Charcot's school too great importance has been attached to pure inheritance of nervous diseases in general and of hysteria in particular." If one adds the statement that heterologous heredity is also to be blamed and that psychoses, alcoholism, epilepsy, peculiarities and eccentricities, and even tuberculosis (Ziehen) in parents, grandparents, siblings and their offspring must be considered, then there are few individuals, indeed, who are not disposed to hysteria. Our own attitude has been expressed in the chapter dealing with the "Constitutional Factor."

In predisposed individuals, *strong and sudden emotions* are said to precipitate hysterical reactions. Many examples are quoted in the literature illustrating the rôle which fear and fright may play in the production of hysterical symptoms.

Charcot taught that hysteria, which he believed to be an inherited degenerative condition, is based on a loss, on a *dropping out of certain conceptions*, that the patient has forgotten how to use his paralytic arm, how to feel with the insensible limb, how to stand and how to walk. At the same time, he emphasized the part played by imitation; it was Charcot who called hysteria *la grande névrose imitatrice*.

Bernheim came to consider hysterical symptoms as the *results of suggestion*. Babinski claimed that everything that is hysterical may be caused by suggestion and can be removed by persuasion; he coined for the reaction the term *pithiatisme* (from Greek *peithain*, to persuade, and *iatos*, curable). At the same time, he declared the vasomotor symptoms to be of reflex origin, referable to disturbances of the vegetative nervous system.

Janet saw the main factor in a *disturbance of the synthesis of the personality*, characterized by a restriction of consciousness and a tendency to dissociation. Certain functions and ideas are "split off" from the conscious personality. The more they have been involved at the moment of a major affective experience, the more are they apt to become dissociated. (Compare the rhythmical shaking of Goldie's right arm which had been active in the repulsion of her boy friend's sexual overtures).

Freud referred hysterical manifestations invariably to forgotten or *repressed psychic traumata* of a sexual nature. The emotional material is lodged in the "unconscious," according to him, and later appears in the disguised form of the symptom, the selection of which depends on the mental factors involved and which represents a symbolic substitution or *conversion* of repressed ideas in the form of somatic manifestations. The functional disorder, at the same time, is the expression, again symbolical and disguised, of an unconscious wish, the fulfilment of which gives to the patient an emotional satisfaction, even though he may not be aware of this. He, unknowingly, solves a conflict and derives a gain (*Krankheitsgewinn*) from his illness.

There is some truth in all of these theories. Constitutional features certainly cannot be left out of the account. The significance of acute emotional upheavals, stressed especially by Déjerine, can hardly be denied in a considerable proportion of cases. That the pattern for the symptom can be copied from others, is an observation which has been made countless times. Suggestion and auto-suggestion are strong forces in hysteria, especially that of children. The dissociation concept is most helpful and appears very obvious in its extreme forms, such as fugues and double personalities. Freud's genetic-dynamic approach and his substitution idea have contributed substantially towards the understanding of the reaction.

To summarize: Hysteria is a *dissociative* (i.e., characterized by a splitting off from the personality of certain functions or episodic function compounds), *dysmnesic* (i.e., incompletely forgotten, affect-loaded material forming the basis for the symptoms), *substitutive* (i.e., ideas, wishes, emotions being transformed into somatic manifestations), *hypobulic* and *hyponoic* (i.e., according to Kretschmer, carried out on a lower level of volition and consciousness) reaction form, often *monosymptomatic* and *monoidetic* in children, developing on a more or less evident constitutional basis, influenced in the choice of symptoms by environmental factors, imitation, suggestion, past life experiences, and by a more or less realized purposive utilization.

In the *therapeutic approach*, a number of results must be aimed at:

The removal of the symptom or symptoms.

Adjustment of the patient by training him to respond more adequately to the demands and opportunities of his environment.

Creating, through proper modification or complete change, an environment in which the desired adjustment of the patient can be made possible.

Various methods have been recommended for the removal of the symptom. We have discussed their applicability and their therapeutic wisdom in the chapter devoted to specific aids in the psychiatric treatment of children's personality disorders. To avoid unnecessary repetition, we enumerate them here without further comment:

The method of surprise, advocated by Bruns.

The method of deception; the physician acts as though he believes that the symptom has an organic pathology and prescribes a pharmacal or mechanical or electrical placebo which is to "cure" the "sick" organ.

The methods of waking and hypnotic suggestion.

The method of ignoring the symptom.

The first two modes of approach should be definitely discarded, the one because of its rudeness and because initial failure instantly discredits it in the eyes of the patient, the other because of its obvious dishonesty. The question as to whether suggestion or ignoring should be adopted, depends on the age and intelligence of the child, the nature of the symptom, and the coöperation to be expected on the part of the elders. No approach, however, can be considered satisfactory if it does not go beyond the limited attention to the isolated manifestation of a motor, sensory, or episodic character. It may, in the eyes of the perplexed parents, teachers, neighbors, and the patient himself, be indeed a remarkable medical feat if of a sudden the lame youngster who has distressed everyone with his astasia-abasia gets up and walks across the room or if the child's lost vision is suddenly restored. The surprise method may sometimes accomplish that. So may a a placebo or a hypnotic session. So may a pilgrimage to a famous shrine or a chiropractor's "adjustment of a displaced vertebra." So may the cessation of the school term or an anticipated birthday party. So may the superstitious procedure of going silently at midnight to a cemetery and touching the paralyzed limb with the hand of a skeleton. Yet one would certainly hesitate to recommend those tricks as medical and logical devices for the treatment of hysteria, no matter how "miraculous" and effective they may prove to be in individual instances.

We have, after all, learned to work with people rather than with detached organ dysfunctions, especially where we are confronted with expressions of a personality disturbance. It is well to regard the disappearance of the symptom as a test of our therapeutic skill. But we have come to realize that our approach should be broader and directed towards the patient as a whole and towards those who take an active part in the molding of his character and reaction patterns. After a thorough study of the individual case, it is our duty to impart the insight which we have gained to the child and to the family in a manner fully adapted to the grasp of those to whom we speak and in a form which is acceptable to them. Thus we proceed to correct faulty notions and attitudes and harmful educational principles and practices. After explaining to the parents the factors and situations which we have found to be at play, their consternation based on the assumption of a serious organic involvement and the ensuing oversolicitude and overindulgence are removed from the setting. This alone contributes towards the child's improvement, because one of the main gains, the family's attention, has been removed and the symptom therefore has lost one of its essential *raisons d'être*. At the same time constructive work with the youngster is begun. He is built up physically. All existing bodily handicaps are remedied. Infected teeth and tonsils, visual defects, chronic constipation, malnutrition are treated. New avenues of interest are created which would give to the child at least as much satisfaction as that derived, knowingly or unknowingly, from his hysterical reaction. It has been said that a person "once hysterical, is always hysterical." This is not necessarily true in the sense that a child who has once reacted to a difficult situation with an hysterical manifestation will always do that. We know, on the other hand, that such a child usually has certain character traits which will dispose him to more or less drastic responses. These traits can be used educationally by giving gifted youngsters an opportunity to find legitimate emotional outlets in little plays and recitals and dramatic clubs, where they learn simultaneously to moderate their desire for too much of a display and where they are taught that exaggerated acting is bad acting.

If, in the setting of parental emotionalism of hysterical, alcoholic, feeble-minded, or other origin, the home environment offers no hopes for an adjustment, removal from the home is the logical alternative. But then it is not enough to arrange for a few weeks' sojourn at a camp or with relatives or in the country, letting the patient come back to the same situation at the end of that period. We have to decide whether or not the child's home is modifiable. If it is, then we have to employ our best persuasive methods to make the parents provide a more stable and balanced home for the returning child. If this cannot be accomplished, then a more permanent placement in a suitable boarding home must be planned.

CHAPTER XLII

THE MAJOR PSYCHOSES

PARERGASTIC REACTION FORMS

(Schizophrenia. Dementia Praecox).

OF THE psychopathological reaction forms of the adolescent and adult, none has within the past thirty or forty years received greater attention on the part of psychiatrists, sociologists, and the public in general than has the behavior, the fate, and the communal care of the schizophrenic person.

Kraepelin, in 1896, isolated from the various "insanities" which he attempted to classify a large group of morbid mental states which he called *dementia praecox*. He saw clearly that the disorders which he thus united under one heading bore essential resemblances which warranted a distinction from other groups, especially from that which he described as the manic-depressive psychoses. Not satisfied, however, with the appreciation of similarities, he went a significant step farther and declared dementia praecox to be a pathological unit, a circumscribed disease entity with a uniform etiology, organic pathology, and a common and inevitable course. The term "dementia" was to indicate an irresistible and incorrigible trend towards progressive mental deterioration; the adjective "praecox" alluded to the early onset during the years of adolescence.

Bleuler, in 1911, introduced for the same group of psychotic manifestations the designation of *schizophrenia*, or splitting of the mental processes. In doing so, he turned away from the prognostic implications contained in the term "dementia praecox," feeling that a hopelessly pessimistic attitude was not, or at least not always, justified; the disturbance, so he stated, "may come to a standstill at any stage and some of its symptoms may clear up to a large extent or altogether, but if it does progress, it leads to a dementia of a specific type." His designation also does not hinge on a "precocious" onset; numerous cases, indeed, do not display the characteristic features of the disorder until after maturity has been reached.

Adolf Meyer, fully acknowledging the fact that "schizophrenia" is "a less finalistic formulation of Kraepelin's nosological entity", realized at the same time that it implies "still definitely an entity with nosological pretense, somewhat more broadly conceived than Kraepelin's 'dementia praecox'." In conformity with his genetic-dynamic formulation of the problems of psychopathology, he was the first to turn his back to any rigid etiological, pathologic, or prognostic strait-jacket methods of classification and to any speculative assumptions of unproven cerebral or glandular lesions or dysfunctions as being "the" cause of every kind of behavior which might be considered as belonging in this group. Meyer's integration concept (discussed in the second chapter of this book) made it possible for him to recognize "the structural disorganizing impingement of the condition and process where it can be demonstrated"; but, instead of stopping there and indulging merely in descriptions of the fully developed mental pictures, he stressed the significance of the constitutional factors and life experiences leading to the development of the personality disintegration. He thus came to formulate the condition as a "habit disorganization on constitutional ground." It is not a "disease" which, like scarlet fever or acute encephalitis, comes upon the patient regardless of his constitutional and biographical background, but an abnormal reaction form which certain types of individuals may develop as an inadequate adaptation to the total life situation. He states: "In the main, we can say that 'dementia praecox' in Kraepelin's nosological-prognostic sense 'has' the patient; it makes the patient a specific case of a special group. It is an identification with the whole person and it favors the formula, 'One person, one disease.' There are, however, cases in which we do better to say the person 'has' a certain disorder or disease, if you wish, or several disorders, but also retains an identity apart from the disease. This certainly holds for long periods in many cases and particularly for the beginnings and is the formulation which allows one to work with the patient." Meyer bases his grouping of psychopathological reaction patterns on the principle of observable performance ("ergasia"), including overt and implicit activity. We have had an opportunity to familiarize the reader with the anergastic, dysergastic, oligergastic, and merergastic sets of reactions. To these, Meyer added the *parergastic reaction patterns*, constituting "the more odd and archaic types" of behavior and involving the "general activity, scattered or set, daydream or fancy born."

The outstanding characteristic of the parergastic reaction form consists of an odd, bizarre, incongruous, unintelligible mode of thinking and acting, utterly foreign to the waking life of the normal individual and somewhat reminiscent of the notions and manners of the primitive, archaic stages of human evolution.

There is a marked *withdrawal from the environmental realities* or, perhaps better, a more or less complete disregard of life's actualities and their subordination to, and interweaving with, dream-like, fanciful, disconnected or loosely connected ideas and experiences. Not only do the wishfulfilling and compensatory fantasies, such as we encounter in daydreams, in artistic, and poetical creations, and in folklore and mythology, manage to push aside any consideration for logical everyday contacts and adaptive needs, but they are also often conceived and expressed in the form of unrecognizable symbolizations which the patient accepts as his dominant realities. This is one of the reasons why it is so extremely difficult for the family or even for the physician to be *en rapport* and on common ground with the patient. Another reason is that the incongruity of thinking is linked up very closely with an incongruity of affect.

There is *general emotional blunting*, sometimes to the point of absolute indifference and failure to participate in the minor and major concerns of the environment. Where emotional responses do exist, they are either out of proportion to the external situation or a half-hearted, not quite genuine, superficial sort of reaction or apparently unmotivated explosive outbursts of laughter or crying or anger.

The *discrepancy between mood and thought* is often very striking and highly characteristic of the schizophrenic disturbances. Ecstasies or tortures may be imagined or reported without the slightest outward sign of happiness or suffering.

The fancies may take the form of more or less systematized, changeable, dramatic, complex "plots" in the shape of *delusions*. The patient may believe himself persecuted by real or imagined persons or groups or he may, in addition or separately, come to think of himself as being someone else, Napoleon Bonaparte or Jesus Christ or the devil or some animal.

Ideas of reference are not infrequent; the patient, suspicious of his surroundings, may feel that people are talking about him, that newspaper items make special allusions to him, or that certain events in the community have been caused to take place for his benefit or in order to annoy him.

There are sometimes peculiar *feelings of being influenced* in the sense of believing that one's mind is being read or that unaccountable thoughts are being put into one's brain or that one's own thoughts are being drained or that one is being made to do things like an automaton.

Such influences may not only be "sensed" but vividly projected on the environment in the form of mostly auditory, often visual, and in rarer instances olfactory, gustatory, and tactile *hallucinations* which may, or may not, seem to be related to the delusional contents.

The disorders of ideation and affect may show themselves in a variety of *queer performances* of a nature which often immediately impresses the the observer as "insane" or "crazy." The entire body posture may be affected; awkward positions may be assumed and maintained for a long time; there may be general muscular rigidity with or without periods of relative motionlessness. The movements may be manneristic and grotesque, entirely incompatible with the conventional standards of one's use of the body. Crawling, walking backwards, grimacing, weird movements of the head or arms or legs, monotonous repetitions of stereotyped performances may be a part of the picture. There may be an automatic submission to various suggestions without the slightest criticism or, on the other hand, a negativistic resistance to all kinds of demands and a refusal to perform the most natural and sometimes even vitally important acts, such as answering questions or even talking spontaneously (mutism), eating, going to the toilet, dressing, or washing.

The verbal expressions may be incoherent and irrelevant; sometimes new words are formed by the patient, either through the chopping up of existing words or throught the condensation of several other words or through the creation of entirely new words (*neologisms*). The disconnection of speech may go so far as to consist of a string of apparently unrelated words, often repeated a number of times (*verbigeration, "word-salad"*).

It is essential to know that it is not the presence or absence of one "symptom" or another that is to be considered as pathognomonic or as a *conditio sine qua non* for the diagnosis or exclusion of a parergastic reaction picture. Emphasis must be placed on the total behavior, the general oddity and incongruity of thinking, feeling, and acting, the discrepancies between thought and mood and between ambition and performance, rather than on the existence and nature of certain delusions or hallucinations or motor or linguistic disturbances. It is furthermore true that there are often strong affective admixtures which would cause serious differential diagnostic difficulties if we were to adhere strictly to the notion that we deal with "a disease" which must by all means be kept apart from other "diseases." Meyer warns against "making diagnoses merely out of an agglomeration of . . . fragments. We should speak of a diagnosis of schizophrenia . . . only when we have a fair picture of a broader consistency of the events, a fair etiological accounting, and an understanding of the factors determining the developments."

Among the various schizophrenic reaction forms, there are some in which certain features stand out sufficiently to lift them out somewhat from the total group. Henderson and Gillespie are right when they state that, "if we wished, we could form almost as many groups as there were individuals." Nevertheless, it has been customary to distinguish four principal varieties, but again one must keep in mind that an almost unlimited range of combinations is possible and that in the course of the illness there may be a succession of different pictures in the same patient. The four varieties or subdivisions are:

The hebephrenic type is characterized by considerable scattering and incoherence, superficial emotional responses, frequent spells of laughing and crying when the external situation does not justify such behavior, and sudden, explosive outbursts of violent anger. Mannerisms, gesticulations, tic-like movements are frequent. The delusions, if present, are unusually grotesque, changeable, without any degree of systematization. "Voices" may call the patient's name, curse and insult him, accuse him of crimes and sexual offenses. He may "see" God, the devil, faces, masks. There is a good deal of symbolic interpretation. Vague "messages" may be received through the air, over the radio, through the chirping of birds. The outstanding feature of this group is the "silliness," fluctuation, senselessness, incoherence, and scattering fragmentation of thinking and performance.

The catatonic type. In contrast to the hebephrenic looseness and fragmentation, a general state of tenseness and rigidity predominates. The chief characteristics lie in the field of psychomotor disturbances. Awkward positions may be maintained for hours or days or weeks or even much longer periods; they often represent symbolical expressions of internal conflicts or strivings; the patient may believe that the balance of the planets or the happiness of mankind depends upon his uninterrupted fixation in a certain attitude of the body. There may be strong resistance to passive movements; in other cases, or in the same case at other times, the patient not only yields readily to passive movements "like a figure of wax" (*flexibilitas cerea*) but also keeps the impressed posture for a long time without displaying signs of fatigue (*catalepsy*). Certain motions or words or sentences may become detached from their original meaning and be repeated monotonously (*stereotypy*); a patient may keep saying, "I want to go home" almost incessantly, yet when invited to leave will not make the slightest attempt to do so and still go on saying, "I want to go home." *Negativism* is a striking symptom of the catatonic reaction; it shows itself in refusal to speak and to eat and to respond to excretory urges and in doing the opposite of what is requested. The patient, when told to open his eyes, keeps them tightly closed; when asked to show his teeth, he clenches his jaws with all his force. Paying no attention to his surroundings, not even responding to painful stimuli, motionless, he gives the appearance of being in a profound *stupor*. Instead of contrariness, there may sometimes be an automatic obedience in which the patient's personality does not seem to participate. He does everything that he is told to do with the apathy of a robot, repeats actions seen (*echopraxia*) and words heard (*echolalia*) without seeming to attach any meaning to them. At times, the patient may present a much better formal behavior, when he is communicative, eats and dresses well, gives a fair account of what had gone on during the stuporous period, gives expression to his inner experiences of a feeling of omnipotence or of other delusions and mystical notions. At other times, however, he may suddenly burst out in a violent excitement in which he is extremely dangerous to himself and expecially to others; his actions then are quick and explosive, and utmost vigilance becomes necessary.

Kahlbaum, in 1894, described catatonia or "tension insanity" (*Spannungsirresein*) as a specific "clinical form of psychic disease." Kraepelin, however, noticed that most of the individuals so afflicted presented many features of his "dementia praecox" group and that many ended in complete mental deterioration. He therefore included catatonia as a special subdivision under the heading of dementia praecox.

The paranoid type. Here delusional experiences predominate. They are of a highly fantastic nature, inconsistent, illogical, bizarre, with a good deal of mysticism (excursions into the stars, communications with supernatural forces), persecutory and grandiose notions, and various hallucinations. The contents are not clearly systematized and hang together most loosely or not at all. This form of schizophrenic reactions rarely starts before the third decade of life.

The simple deteriorating type. Kraepelin, after uniting the hebephrenic, catatonic, and paranoid groups under the dementia praecox heading, later added as a fourth type one which is characterized by "impoverishment and devastation of the whole psychic life, which is accomplished quite imperceptibly." There is no marked scattering, no predominance of psychomotor disorders, no prevalence of delusional contents. The main feature consists of a gradual loss of interests and ambitions, a slow withdrawal from playmates and from family contacts, and a persistent sliding into general listlessness and apathy. The patient loses all initiative and pride in personal appearance and achievements and follows the line of least resistance. He stays away from school, wandering aimlessly about the streets. He sits quietly in a corner when others discuss topics of general interest or enjoy athletic games. He may take to tramping, procuring his food through begging and stealing. Henderson and Gillespie state: "We are all familiar with this type of individual. These are people who at one time have looked as if they might develop into something much better. They are quiet, pleasant individuals who gradually sink more and more into themselves, and who never fulfil the promise of their earlier days."

As regards the *course* and outcome of schizophrenic developments, the best summing up comes from Adolf Meyer. We can do no better than quote it verbatim: "The course occasionally may present an actual clearing up or at least remissions, especially often in the stupors, less in the scattering and paranoid forms . . . Quite a number of those states are amenable to a far-reaching readjustment but oftener there is a gradual or step-like drifting into dilapidation and indifference. In any of the forms one is apt to meet as a terminal state an apathetic self-absorption and deterioration, often with remarkably well-preserved but erratic memory, and with really correct, but at times strangely distorted interpretations and complicated 'double' or 'multiple orientation' as to person, situation, and time, i.e., a striking refusal of the inconsistencies to exclude each other, a facile assumption of various simultaneous interpretations of persons, places, times, with simultaneous inclusions of the correct grasp. Catatonic reactions may pass into paranoid compensatory states which in turn may fade into indifference. Sometimes one finds a remarkably smooth superficial behavior, with an astounding confusion as soon as the patient writes or tries to explain or argue a point. The more or less outspoken types of 'terminal dementia' produce the greatest proportion of the lasting asylum population. It does, however, seem to me that the old concept of 'terminal dementia' was prematurely assigned to but a single nosological group. There are very similar 'terminal states' in widely different processes. But the majority of the cases of terminal dementia is undoubtedly furnished by individuals showing from the start parergastic or schizophrenic reaction sets or indications thereof. Unless an acute attack leads to exhaustion, longevity is usually not interfered with; only tuberculosis seems to have a strong hold especially in the catatonic cases."

A constructive and objective genetic-dynamic formulation does not exclude legitimate curiosity with regard to the *somatic features* of the schizophrenic patients. But it makes three significant reservations. First, it postulates actual demonstrations instead of mere hypothetical assumptions. Second, it shrinks from applying to all cases the observations made in a limited number. Third, it does not immediately jump to the conclusion that casual findings of endocrine or cerebral or other disturbances must be correlated with the etiology or even with the exclusive etiology of the total reaction. It follows with the greatest interest, examines critically, and encourages studies, both clinical and post mortem, of the physical conditions of the patient. So far, the results and claims have been contradictory and far from conclusive. Kraepelin assumed the existence of an auto-intoxication based on some metabolic disturbance and especially on disordered secretion of the sex glands. Mott found deterioration of the gonads with arrest of spermatogenesis and atrophy of the cells of the testicular tubules as well as lipoid alteration of the nerve cells. Nolan D. C. Lewis saw atrophy of the procreative glands and aplasia of the circulatory system. Other workers centered their attention on focal infection from the teeth, tonsils, and gastrointestinal tract (Cotton, Bayard Holmes, Reiter). It is only natural that the central nervous system should have been made the object of painstaking study. It would lead too far to outline here the many investigations carried on for the past twenty-five years, particularly in Germany and in the United States, under the leadership of Alzheimer (abundance of ameboid neuraglia cells), Nissl, Sioli, Southard (patches of induration in the cortex), von Monakow (disorders of the choroid plexus), Spielmeyer, Josephy, Bouman, and many others. Charles Dunlap, in a paper published in 1924, summed up his thorough and critical work with the statement that he failed to find any constant fundamental or characteristic changes of nerve cells and that those found by other authors were reactions to different somatic conditions plus post mortem and technical factors.

All these investigations are undoubtedly very valuable and call for further elucidation. A uniformity of findings has obviously not been reached and is, indeed, hardly to be expected if one properly considers the huge variety of modes of onset, of behavior pictures (often changing in the same patient), and of outcomes encountered in people united under the diagnosis of dementia praecox or schizophrenia. Again we quote Adolf Meyer: "In the main, there is undoubtedly a tendency towards a more or less clearly organic fixation of the deterioration (through the ringing in of endocrine factors and toxic or metabolic disorders?), but quite different as to lesions and manifestations from the real autonomously destructive defect-processes. The character of the tissue-damage is more like deficits of the balance of anabolism and catabolism than any autonomous tissue disease. In harmony with this largely incidental character of the lesions, one occasionally meets with remarkable rehabilitations during acute illnesses which arouse vital interests of self-concern and natural appeals to the family and to reality, and this is occasionally used for therapeutic purposes."

We move on much safer ground if, without losing sight of the somatic implications, we center our attention on the more easily obtainable and practically helpful psychobiological integrative features of the development and progress of the condition in the individual case. We are then confronted mainly with the following questions:

What are the known facts of the patient's family background? Heredity plays an important part. In a large majority of cases, but not in all, serious maladaptations are found in close relatives, often reaching the degree of full-blown psychoses. The personality disintegration has a tendency to appear at an earlier age in the descendants than in the antecedents. On the other hand, one does see schizophrenic developments in persons coming from relatively stable and well adjusted stock.

What are the known facts concerning the patient's ingrained personality difficulties? Meyer sums up his experience with the following words: "The entire picture makes it very probable that congenital or infantile incongruities tend to the formation of reactive tendencies which may develop gradually or more or less suddenly on exposure to new demands after a protected phase of life. . . . Many of the individuals present defect-types from childhood; others are unusually precocious or prematurely conscientious types, with extremes of undesirable tendencies and exalted ideals; many are worth the strongest efforts to save them, by heading off the specially great tendency to shyness and unprofitable comparisons, to daydreaming and withdrawal from contacts, to complex fixations, to one-sided preoccupations, to flight into fancy, etc."

Kretschmer found that many schizophrenics are of an asthenic or athletic body configuration.[1] The reaction may develop in people with any degree of intellectual endowment. If it is engrafted on a feebleminded individual, the German literature is, since Kraepelin, accustomed to speak of *Pfropfschizophrenie*[2] (which Bleuler, in a footnote in his textbook, considers as possibly being a disease *sui generis*). Since Meyer's emphasis on the significance of the constitutional make-up in the etiology of mental disorders in 1903,[3] growing attention has been paid to the pre-psychotic personality characteristics of schizophrenics. The type of person who is more apt than others to be driven into a parergastic disorganization has been variously termed as ingrowing (Meyer), shut-in (Hoch, who found from fifty to sixty per cent of all schizophrenics to have belonged in this group prior to their illness), introvert (Jung), schizothymic (Kretschmer), and schizoid (Bleuler). These designations, though referring more or less to the same withdrawing, self-centered, over-imaginative, yet uncommunicative, not reality-bound type of personality, are nevertheless not regarded as synonymous, since some of them imply too readily a connection with certain somatic configurations (Kretschmer's schizothymic being linked too closely to an asthenic build) or with a rigid division of mankind into two groups (Bleuler's schizoid and syntonic) and too narrow a relation to certain mental diseases.

Kraepelin has studied the childhood characteristics of a large number of his adolescent and adult patients and observed mainly four groups of pre-psychotic personalities:

Quiet, shy, retiring children, inclined to live solitary lives of their own.

Irritable, sensitive, excitable, nervous, stubborn children, especially girls, given to religious preoccupations.

Lazy, inactive, unstable, mischievous children, mostly boys, who sometimes become tramps and delinquents.

Manageable, good-natured, anxiously overconscientious, industrious model children, mainly boys.

Homburger has put together the following childhood traits of persons who in their adolescence or adulthood have become schizophrenic:

As to basic affective tone: serious-minded, surly, peevish, sober, uninteresting, without appreciation of humor, rarely laughing; moody.

As to mental alertness: quiet, disinterested.

As to emotional activity: irritable, excitable, easily angered.

As to expressive urges: shut-in, taciturn, uncommunicative, secretive, unsociable, quiet.

As to reactive direction: timid, sensitive, bearing grudges, suspicious, easily offended.

As to productive tendencies: careless, flighty, indolent, lazy, inert.

As to persistence of emotions: bearing grudges, easy-going, unreliable, indifferent, superficial.

As to persistence of interests: jumping from one thing to another, lacking endurance, obstinate.

[1] See the chapter on "The Constitutional Factor."

[2] Pfropf means plug.

[3] Meyer, Adolf. An Attempt at Analysis of the Neurotic Constitution. American Journal of Psychology. 1903, 14, 354–367.

As to ability to get along with people: unsociable, quarrelsome, unable to compromise, unyielding, stubborn, incorrigible, dogmatic.

As to self-assertiveness: imperious, domineering, ambitious, vain, proud, arrogant; selfish, jealous, niggardly; pleasure-seeking; fussy, pedantic.

As to relation to environment: unfeeling, cold, malicious, unkind, incapable of tenderness, rude; bigoted, superstitious, self-righteous.

What are the life experiences which have led up to the development of a parergastic reaction in persons with or without specific hereditary backgrounds and with whatever personality make-up they were found to possess? We are, in this book, primarily interested in children. It would be most valuable to follow the destinies of a large number of children from their earliest days, especially of those who stand out because of poor hereditary background, early personality and habit difficulties, or unhealthy environmental influences. But this has not been done on a large scale because it has been only in recent years that a consideration of habit deteriorations has been included in the study of schizophrenia and because such work would require at least two decades of close contact with a multitude of cases. Besides, fortunately for those children who have come to the attention of psychiatrists at an early age, they have received the benefit of prompt treatment and readjustment with mental hygiene methods intended to prevent rather than to wait for more serious personality disorganizations. Another source of information consists of the data obtained from the biographies of individuals who have developed parergastic reactions. However, the literature contains very little in this respect. Mrs. Gladys Terry has kindly placed at my disposal an unpublished study of the genetic-dynamic aspects of schizophrenic reaction patterns, based on one hundred cases examined at the Henry Phipps Psychiatric Clinic. She has found that in fifty-eight cases mothers or mother-substitutes were said to be "neurotic," domineering, possessive, overattentive or oversolicitous, overindulgent, eccentric or psychotic. In an additional number of cases the mothers or parents did not inflict their oversolicitude and domination aggressively but fell too readily into such rôles as imposed upon them by the instabilities of the patients themselves. Following these cases along into adolescence and early adult periods, one observes striking histories of maladjustment on the basis of an inability to emancipate from parental emotional fixations and from clinging states of dependency on the family. Still other cases presented pictures of faulty preparation and training in sex matters, when families with set and unintelligent attitudes have made it difficult for corrective factors to work in a timely manner and paved the way for brooding fears and guilt reactions to early and pubescent arousals and the later attempts at active socializable fulfilment. It is interesting to note that sixty-one patients had held a solitary position in the family, i.e., were only children, oldest or youngest children, or only sons or daughters, and that sixty-four "scored a positive for such childhood irregularities as neuropathic habit traits and disorders; convulsions, spasms; striking asocial tendencies; backward mental development; delicate, sickly physical conditions."

Parergastic reactions are very infrequently seen to develop before the age of puberty. But such cases undoubtedly exist. Ziehen states that in

extremely rare instances he could trace the development of typical schizophrenia back to the seventh year of life. In most of the pre-pubescent cases
the onset lies beyond the tenth year.

Heller, in 1908, published six cases of what he termed *dementia infantilis*,
a condition which Zappert, in 1922, described as having the following
characteristics: The illness begins between the third and fourth years of
life in children who theretofore had been absolutely normal in their physical
and mental growth. Very soon speech disturbances make the parents aware
of the existence of an abnormal condition. At first the little patients
mutilate words which they had been well capable of pronouncing before.
Then echolalia sets in. This is followed by an increasing loss of capacity
for articulation until the child regresses to the babbling form of vocal
expression. Finally spontaneous speech is lost entirely, and also the comprehension of words heard suffers a progressive impairment. The children
are very restless and given to strong fears and to episodes of excitement
which sometimes may assume an hallucinatory character. Within a few
months, they become completely demented without, however, showing
their intellectual defect in their facial expressions; they often lose control
over their excretory functions and are not amenable to educational influences. Their motility is mostly unaltered and the clinical neurological
findings remain normal throughout. The dementia becomes stationary
without in the least interfering with the physical health. By 1930, Heller
had collected twenty-eight cases, Zappert had reported thirteen, and
Montesano had described two cases. Heller was in a position to follow the
destinies of some of his patients whom after many years he found to be
totally demented, mute, unable to grasp anything said to them, incapable
of learning even the simplest type of occupation, sometimes displaying
tics and stereotypies, yet always looking outwardly more intelligent than
the idiots with whom they happened to be housed together in institutions.
Some authors originally thought that one deals with a very early form of
schizophrenic development. But now practically all investigators agree
that dementia infantilis or Heller's disease is an illness *sui generis* and
should not be identified with schizophrenia.[1]

At about the same time when Heller published his first communication,
Sante de Sanctis reported a case of what he designated as *dementia prae-
cocissima*. This report was followed by similar observations by himself and
by other Italian investigators, and a few reports came from France, Germany, and Switzerland. (Oskar Diethelm, in a paper to be published soon,
gives an excellent bibliographical review, a critical discussion of the case
material found in the literature, and contributes many well-selected cases
of his own in illustration of schizophrenic reactions and allied mental ab-

[1] Heller, Theodor. Über Dementia infantilis (Verblödungsprozess im Kindesalter).
Zeitschrift für die Erforschung und Behandlung des jugendlichen Schwachsinns.
1909, 2, 17–28. Über Dementia infantilis. Zeitschrift für Kinderforschung. 1930,
37, 661–667.—Zappert, Julius. Dementia infantilis (Heller). Monatsschrift für
Kinderheilkunde. 1922, 22, 389–397.—Montesano, Giuseppe. Beitrag zum Studium
der Dementia infantilis. Zeitschrift für die Erforschung und Behandlung des
jugendlichen Schwachsinns. 1922, 8, 254–269.

normalities in childhood.) Children who had previously developed normally or may have been somewhat retarded to start with were noticed to show abrupt or more insidious personality changes, sometimes as early as at the age of three years. Catatonic symptoms become very pronounced; fixed postures, mannerisms, stereotypy, negativism, refusal to speak and to eat, unprovoked anger outbursts, echolalia, and emotional blunting dominated the picture; marked intellectual deterioration was the outcome in most instances, though in single cases a fair adjustment under relatively simple life situations could be arranged. De Sanctis, in his textbook (1925), mentioned as etiological factors: (1) Hereditary predisposition, chiefly paternal alcoholism; (2) Acute or chronic toxic diseases, such as pertussis, intestinal infections, pleurisy, and rickets. (Strangely enough, he did not hesitate to number "psychic traumata" among those "toxic diseases.") (3) Factors inherent in children's development.[1]

In referring etiologically to factors inherent in children's development, De Sanctis refers to Weygandt, who emphasized the fact that many low grade idiots present motor disturbances which are closely related to those observed in catatonia: abnormal postures and attitudes, abnormal motions of a rhythmical character, abnormal mimical expressions (grimacing), abnormal verbal expressions (verbigeration), echolalia and echopraxia, and negativism. Weygandt felt that all of these motility disorders may be seen (in a much milder form, to be sure) in infants as a normal phase of their development: "In one child or another some of the above mentioned symptoms may appear in an especially pronounced manner without ever leading to deterioration after this early developmental stage has been passed. A certain fixation of that phase of infantile language is found in various nursery rhymes where one often meets with a putting together of nonsensical words and sounds. One must therefore assume that the uncoördinated movements and oral expressions which normally form a transient step in the development of children become fixated in some idiots and exhaust their expressive possibilities. In catatonics, because of their apperceptive deterioration, they retrogressively take the place of conventional language and coördinated movements."[2]

Most of the early childhood schizophrenias are said to be predominatingly catatonic in their character. Hebephrenic pictures are second in frequency. Paranoid developments are exceedingly rare.

Diethelm makes a distinction between the parergastic reaction forms encountered during the first decade of life and those beginning during puberty. Experience teaches us that such a distinction is quite justified, considering the fact that the schizophrenic disorganizations occurring in the first half of the second decade resemble much more closely those taking

[1] De Sanctis, Sante. Sopra alcune varieta della demenza precoce. Rivista Sperimentale di Freniatria. 1906, 32, 141–165. Neuropsichiatria infantile. Rome. 1925, pp. 623–661.

[2] Weygandt, W. Idiotie und Dementia praecox. Zeitschrift für die Erforschung und Behandlung des jugendlichen Schwachsinns. 1907, 1, 311. Idiotie und Imbezillität. Aschaffenburg's Handbuch der Psychiatrie. Spezieller Teil. Zweite Abteilung. Leipzig und Wien. 1915, pp. 211–215.

place during adolescence and adulthood and show much more clearly the dynamic connections with the patient's life experiences. Paranoid admixtures, sexual ruminations, obsessive phenomena, and hypochondriacal trends stand out much more frequently and prominently.

The following case illustrations were taken from the records of the Henry Phipps Psychiatric Clinic.

William H. was the son of an aggressive, inconsistent, emotionally unstable man who had frequent temper outbursts and periods of mild depressions; when William's father was about twelve years old, he was "dazed completely for many days, depressed and worried, about what I do not know; I am also prone to become dazed when I meet difficult problems or have business arousals; I suffer mentally more than I would if I were actually physically ill." During his "depressive" episode at twelve he had not talked for several days but recovered quickly after being sent to a farm. William's mother, twenty-three years younger than her husband (who was 48 years old when the patient was born), reached the fifth grade only and is said to have always been "very nervous." She was Catholic, while her husband was Protestant; their two children were brought up in the Catholic faith. William's sister, three years younger than he was, wet her bed until she was ten years old. A paternal uncle, who died in infancy, had a cleft palate. A paternal aunt was queer and "read deep books" most of the time. The maternal grandmother spent several months in a State Hospital with a "recoverable psychosis." William's father had been divorced twice before his marriage to William's mother.

William was born July 23, 1918. Birth was normal. He was breast fed for not less than sixteen months. At three years, he developed the habit of jerking his head and a peculiar facial tic. He had always "thrown his hands about" in a peculiar fashion. As a baby, he was fretful and cried almost constantly. He wet his bed until he was nearly five years old. He had many temper tantrums; at the age of ten years, he threw knives and scissors at his sister. A few weeks after starting school at six, he was taken out by his parents and spent the rest of the term at home because "he would twitch his shoulders when with a crowd" and his mother thought that he had St. Vitus's dance. In spite of good intelligence, he was always inattentive, restless, and preoccupied in school. He failed in the third and fifth grades. It took him a long time to put on his clothes in the morning; he was therefore dressed by his mother until he was eight years old, and even later "required a good deal of coaxing"; he was late nearly every day for his classes. He presented a feeding problem, dawdling over his meals. He always was afraid of the dark; at night, scared by the reflection of the street lights on the ceiling or of the shapes of hats, etc., on the walls, he called his mother and went back to sleep as soon as he heard her reassuring voice. Upon retiring at night, he was in the habit of covering his eyes with his hands or putting his head under the bed clothes.

He was a seclusive youngster who preferred to play alone; he did not care nor was he encouraged to associate with other children. He, like his aunt, liked to "read deep books." Without ever having had instruction in music, without being able to comprehend any rhythm, he liked for hours to discuss movies and operas, especially since the age of about ten years. Since that age he seemed languid, complained often of being tired, was more preoccupied and irritable than he had been previously, and frequently amused himself by dressing himself in various costumes and singing and acting before the mirror. He had always been considered as a "queer" and "different" child.

William was raised in the midst of constant parental quarrels. His father was untrue to his wife; whenever his infidelity was detected, he broke down and sobbed. All this went on in the children's presence. After many highly dramatic scenes, the mother left her husband because he did not support her adequately and kept going with other women. William was in his eleventh year then. He felt his parents' separation as a deep disgrace. Court procedures, mutual threats, and repeated verbal and manual fights added to his disgust. In February, 1930, he witnessed an especially tantalizing fight between his parents; early in the morning, his father appeared in his wife's house and demanded the photographs of one of his mistresses; when she did not produce them, he threw her down and held her by the throat. She, scared for her life, shouted for the police. When a policeman arrived, the man had disappeared. William and his sister lived with their mother, who spoiled her boy in every respect. The more sullen and peculiar he became, the more she indulged in his whims. She even slept in the same bed with him. Whenever his father saw him, he kept persuading William to help him bring about a reconciliation with his mother and painted verbal pictures of how happy they would be if they had a home together again.

In July, 1931, William spent two weeks of his vacation with his father who kept harping on the matrimonial situation. On July 25, he was strongly impressed by the moving picture, "Son of India," which he had asked to see. He returned home to his mother on the same day. He was not in any way unusual until July 28, when around midnight he woke his mother by a burst of crying and asked her: "Mother, is there a Heaven? Do take me to a priest. I want to do the right thing. I want to be a singer. I want opera, divine music." He kept talking excitedly about music, religion, the Orient, and "the higher things in life." During the next day he was very quiet, brooding, and looked sad and absorbed. He was preoccupied with the problems of his parents. In the following two nights, he acted as he had the night before. He was admitted to the Clinic on July 31. He was excited, overtalkative, his speech was poorly connected, vague, and full of abstractions. "I will be a great singer," he said; "I will help mankind; I am the Redeemer; I will die on the cross." "I am Dracula" (reminiscences of a moving picture he had seen). At times he cried, knelt, and prayed. He assumed postures of a mysterious, religious, or patriotic character, imitating the facial expression of angry Hindu demons, displaying gestures of prayer and benediction, posing as the Statue of Liberty, followed by glorification of France which gave the Statue to America and by recitation of the Star Spangled Banner. He slept poorly in spite of sedatives and hydrotherapy. Early in August, he was heard praying in a whining sentimental tone, telling God that he wanted to make others happy, that he felt God gave him the gift to compose sacred music, that he was the Savior of the World, that he was going to be like John McCormack. There were often rapid changes from laughter to tears. He once addressed another patient as "Dear Lord," offered him a pack of cards on a checker board as a sort of sacrifice, then prostrated himself before him, lying full length on his abdomen and sobbing bitterly for two minutes. He thought that he heard bells ring and pictures of opera stars talk to him. He saw men's faces on the wall and once said that he saw red eyes outside the window watching him. He insisted that his body was being pommeled, while he lay passively in bed, exhibiting no sign of pain or struggling. At night he often cried out that his father was killing his sister and himself. During the months of

August and September he was at times markedly cataleptic. After a period of excitement and destructiveness, he calmed down and became more and more indifferent. In September, he masturbated frequently, exposed his genitalia to the nurses, and occasionally defecated in his clothes. He sometimes moved his lips as if in conversation without speaking out loudly, staggered about, hopped on one foot, or walked on tiptoes. He expressed the fear that he might be turned into a toad. He felt that he was hypnotized and compelled by mysterious forces to tear up several books. He called himself St. Thomas and William H. (his own name) alternately. He said he was "born by the astrology sign." He refused his breakfast saying that it was poison. He picked waste, dirt, and paper from the bathroom floor and kissed it, giving as an explanation that "I am God." He related that he heard "echoes of breakers and hammers, of men pounding with hammers." He said: "There are too many serpents in the room. One gave me a pill that it held in the mouth. It looked up at me." When asked for a mood description, he said, with an empty expression in which there was not a trace of a smile, that he was happy.

He was transferred to a State Hospital, where he still resides. He has failed to make an adjustment even in the protected and supervised hospital environment. He is usually indifferent, listless, lazy, apathetic, takes no interest in his surroundings, masturbates frequently, has to be guarded against homosexual assaults on other patients, and has occasional outbursts of violent anger.

Sidney W. was fourteen years old when admitted to the Clinic on March 21, 1926. His father was a conscientious, ambitious, and industrious merchant. His mother, who until the age of thirty-two years was a happy, cheerful person, reacted to a robbery by negroes of her husband's store with brooding, continuous crying, and worrying that they might be robbed again. She became depressed and spent three months in a hospital. A week after her discharge she took poison and died soon afterwards. The five children, all boys, were scattered among relatives. Sidney, who was six years old then, went to live with a cousin and her husband. He had developed normally and always been healthy, except for chronic constipation; his parents had never succeeded in making him take laxatives. He sometimes remained for two to three hours in the toilet without having a movement. His cousin, who at the time of Sidney's coming to stay with her had no children of her own, spoiled the boy in every way imaginable. His father used to go there and find that his cousin prepared an excellent chicken dinner especially for Sidney, who would refuse to eat it, wishing some food from the delicatessen store; the cousin immediately went out and got it for him. He received no habit training and was permitted to rule the house and obtain all his wants by means of temper tantrums. He was stubborn and contrary and quite sensitive.

When Sidney was ten years old, his father remarried and the family reunited. The stepmother, a short, unattractive, slovenly dressed woman, was genuinely and sincerely desirous of making the children contented but so wrapped up in her husband's business that she had little time to provide for any but their physical needs. Sidney tried to transfer his habits from his cousin's to his new environment. He would not eat eggs and veal unless they were fried. He was angry when certain foods which he disliked were given him and his parents would coax and scold, trying to force him to eat. They indulged every one of his whims and treated him differently than his brothers to such an extent that he occasionally asked his father why they paid more attention to him than to the others.

At school, he was quiet and seclusive, easily abstracted, and spent considerable time daydreaming. He showed good scholastic and mechanical abilities; in the manual training classes he did not concentrate and would stand about in a detached manner. He did not mix well with other children. He was always shy and self-conscious when reciting and always "afraid of girls." When eleven years old, "my mother told me to mind my little baby sister (half-sister) while she was getting a diaper. Once in a while, she wore torn clothes, and it showed out. Thoughts came to my mind that women are superior. Their system is superior." Following this experience he began to play less and spent all his leisure time reading. He became increasingly seclusive and irritable. He began to masturbate at twelve but stopped after about one year. Since then he became more and more preoccupied with sexual topics. He felt that other people knew about his masturbation. He began to wonder if people could read other persons' minds. He would sit in school with his arms folded, so as to concentrate better and read the girls' minds.

In the summer of 1925, he wanted to be sent to a boys' camp. Instead, his stepmother took him and the other children to her cottage in the Catskill Mountains. There, he would not join the activities of the others but went off by himself and stood gazing up at the sky for several hours at a time. He refused to eat anything but dry bread. He had had no desire for food several months before but his appetite had improved after tonsillectomy. His stepmother, alarmed, returned with him home after ten days in the mountains. At home, he seemed as usual externally, except for his extreme irritability. When he returned to school (eighth grade) in September, he was absorbed by his sexual preoccupations. He felt that he could see the genitalia of the girls by means of "eye-sight, by my sense of power, brain power." He began to puzzle whether he was a boy or a girl. He wondered whether it would not be better to have female genitals which seemed "superior" to him. He now definitely felt that he could read people's minds and that they showed by the expression of their faces that he had been able to do so. He also felt that others had the ability to read his thoughts. "I cannot go downtown on the street car because I think of the people on the car. They know what I think. They give me a sign of it. They might be making signs and funny faces at others." He thought that he had the power to prevent people from doing certain things by looking at them. A person comes into the store. Slamming the door annoys him, so he thinks this person should not slam the door and this prevents the person from doing so. He was preoccupied with what he spoke of as "bad," "dirty," "sweet," "tender" things, adjectives which he used synonymously and interchangeably; they had something to do with "Gus," one of Sidney's schoolmates. He had many "dreams of tenderness"; "Lots of them. I don't mean skinny—seems sweet. I don't want to kiss them. I never dream about girls, more about boys."

Early in November, he suddenly refused to go to school, without giving any reasons for it. When persuaded to attend, he did fairly well, but quit on December 9. His father threatened to send him to the House of Detention. Sidney, becoming rather excited, begged his father to send him there. He said he was "crazy" and wanted them to "shut up his mind." During the excitement, he spoke of his mother whom he had never mentioned for years. He said that she had not wanted to live and neither did he, as everybody hated him. He kept repeating that his mother had no right to bear him and talked of killing his half-brother and half-sister to save them from suffering. He said that his teachers and classmates disliked him and that he feared they would lick him. He had violent outbursts of anger whenever the possibility of his going back to school was mentioned. He pointed to his right temple and said: "My mind seems to be clogged right here. I want my mind clogged, so the bad part will not come out. That keeps me from knowing what is happening." In February, 1926, he became enuretic. He talked of committing suicide.

Upon admission on March 21, he was alert and communicative. When taken into the ward, he screamed at the top of his voice and did not want to stay, but became calm after about two minutes and displayed good formal behavior for the next few days. He complained that he was too girlish, that his mind was not clear and he could not think, that he was different from other children, that he sat and worried over trifles, that he was troubled by "thoughts" and by "absurd and illogical notions." He occasionally emitted peculiar hissing sounds when he was not talking. He said that he was directed by an inner voice: "There is a voice that talks within me. It directs me. It might do me some good, but I think it hurts me. It says, 'I am dumb.' I am saying it all the time to myself. It's myself trying to explain everything." He kept repeating his old ruminations about the "superiority" of women and about being a girl: "I'd rather be a girl any time. I'd be better off. If I am a boy, my system (he always said "system" for sex organs) is taken away. If I am a girl, it is not." "I just had a funny idea. I thought I was a fifteen-year-old girl and had a boy's system at my side." "If that idea of taking away my system stopped, I'd be all right. It's a silly idea but I like to think about it." "It seems to me I was a girl in Heaven." "If I think I am a girl, maybe in the future I'll be a girl. But I am satisfied to be a boy. But if I say I am satisfied, I still keep on yearning and yearning and yearning and I get nervous. It's not possible to have a girlish mind and still be a boy." He once dreamed that his "system was exactly like a woman's system" and men were "trying to stick knives into it." He could not stand the sight or thought of pointed objects: "What really hurts me is to think of those piercing instruments, hatchets, tomahawks, all those instruments." "When I see a pick strike, it hurts me as if it struck me. Anything pointy, anything sharp, anything that can rub against, hurts me. I can't stand tearing."

After one week of good behavior in the ward, there was a decided slump. He no longer was alert but seemed mildly depressed. Thinking was at times slow and uncertain. He kept asking at the dinner table what he should eat next. He often sat motionlessly for hours, sometimes mumbling to himself. His answers were rambling and scattered. His clothes were untidy, his hair was unkempt. When told by the dentist to brush his teeth three times a day, he puzzled just how to time these operations. One way was the "northern way" while to brush his teeth after breakfast, after lunch, and before going to bed was the "southern way." The northern way also symbolized men, and the southern way meant women. These symbolizations were very important to Sidney: "I am worrying myself to death and I'll never settle these trifles." In April, he expressed an "eager desire" to devour everything, including feces. He felt compelled to fold his cap and put it into his coat sleeve which in a vague way represented a vagina to him. Later in the month, he seemed somewhat happier. He began to express compensatory ideas of grandeur: "I am the luckiest boy in America. I consider myself one of the healthiest. I have got the most blood. The girls are afraid of me. They used to admire me. I used to appear gigantic in their eyes. I mean, I was a hero in their eyes." He became growingly disinterested, assuming an attitude of distant hauteur. He was discharged to his parents upon their request on May 16, 1926, and was soon committed to a State Hospital, where he still resides.

Elsie C. had a childhood bereft of much longed for maternal attentions. Her mother was an invalid and left her entirely to the care of nurses; her death was met by ten-year-old Elsie with considerable emotional upheaval. The child's exclusive companion was a feebleminded sister in whose behalf she reacted sensitively and protectingly to the fun-poking taunts of the schoolmates. A puritanical governess instilled exaggerated ideas of right living and thinking and of God's punishment for wrongdoing. Elsie responded with early habits of thumbsucking, nailbiting, fear of the dark and night terrors to her various difficulties. The sight of a urinating uncle and the chance discovery of her sister's self-exposure to little boys upset her greatly. At thirteen, coincident with the onset of menstruation, the facts of sex as presented to her by her pregnant stepmother roused in her feelings of disgust and horror. The world at that time changed for her from an idealistic to an "unclean, animal" one. At the same time, however, an obsessive interest in the sex topic affected her with embarrassment and a fear of all males, including her father and brothers. She showed increased awkwardness and withdrawal and became forgetful and careless of her personal habits. She developed a feeling that she was different from others, that her presence made others nervous. Expansion of these ideas concerning herself gradually came to replace the disturbing sex ruminations. She became fascinated with thought of herself as being peculiarly endowed with a "psychic energy" that affected others unpleasantly. When in the company of people, she was compelled to experiment with this "power," at the same time feeling the urge to check it. Her notions accounted for certain motor accompaniments, such as rubbing her head and forehead "to brush these thoughts away" or putting her fingers in her ears "to hold the energy in." Her condition improved gradually in an institutional environment. She was reported to be more comfortable in her social activities at eighteen and less agitated and disturbed by her imaginations which, however, were still present. Elsie had one brother who was very unstable and irresponsible, and a maternal cousin who had gone through a schizophrenic psychosis.

Even these few examples show clearly that the schizophrenic difficulties did not come upon the patients out of a clear sky as the result of some cellular destruction or abscessed teeth or endocrine disorder or what not. There is a "story" to every case, a life story in which persons with certain make-up and backgrounds and experiences are actively and passively involved. Many children, it is true, have the capacity for living through parental quarrels and separations, early sexual stirrings and repentances, domestic mismanagements, and inadequate social situations without turning away completely from adaptive efforts and from attempts at a healthy orientation or reorientation. Even though minor or major disturbances may arise in the process, they do not in the majority of instances lead to a wholesale crumbling up of the functions of the personality. Yet there are individuals who are so constituted and whose habit training has been so deficient that, lacking proper guidance, they get lost in the turmoil of external mishaps and inner conflicts. The ultimate schizophrenic dilapidation often appears clearly as the cumulative result, in certain types of personality, of a long period of misdirected gropings, unchecked and sometimes inculcated misconceptions and misinterpretations, and continued ruminations, with final withdrawal from the disturbing realities and total surrender to a fancy-governed, inactive, inaccessible existence.

Where dilapidation has set in, the *treatment* can do little beyond protection against violence and self-destruction through suicide or persistent refusal to eat. Wherever possible, an adjustment to the environment on a simpler level and under careful supervision will be attempted, relieving the patient of initiative and planning of which he is not capable. All the while, one will prepare and wait for signs of a remission in which the patient would be approachable to a more direct attack of his problems. In many cases, this will have to be done in an institution. Sometimes, when there is no danger to the security of the patient and of others and when the standards of formal behavior and conventional living are not perceptibly impaired, it is possible to provide for an extramural occupation of a kind to which he can adapt himself under constant guidance and observation with a minimum of friction and conflict, preparing for commitment to a hospital whenever this may become necessary. All physical illness or irregularities found to be present should be promptly remedied. "The most important help," Meyer says, "lies in attempts at gaining rapport and a gradual hold on some reconstructive interests." There exist in puberty and early adolescence parergastic upheavals which do not keep the patient from returning to a level which had been his normal mode of reacting prior to the onset of his illness; Ziehen aptly refers to such episodes as *hebephrenic modifications of the puberty crisis*. Recoveries have been observed to occur in the schizophrenias of childhood (Vogt, Brill,[1] and others) and of later years.

As long as schizophrenia was looked upon as a doom, as an uncontrollable catastrophe, the inevitable result of some metabolic or structural alteration, the idea of prophylaxis could not take root in the minds of physicians. You can do very little to a "gliosis" even if you are sure of its existence. You can do even less to prevent any damage to cerebral tissues, the existence of which is more than doubtful and, where present, certainly not specific and not etiological. The enthusiasm in some quarters with regard to the supposed beneficial effects of the removal of focal infections has dwindled away in the face of many failures. We are, however, in a position to study the early evidences of faulty interpersonal relationships, adjustment difficulties, and withdrawal tendencies of children. We do really have an opportunity to learn almost daily in our pediatric and psychiatric and educational work of the daydreaming preoccupations, seclusive trends, oversensitiveness, and peculiar behavior of certain children and we fortunately can do something about them. Without being under the obligation to join the ranks of the prophets and to predict for any of these youngsters an ominous schizophrenic future, we have it in our hands to modify at an

[1] Vogt, H. Über Fälle von Jugendirresein im Kindesalter. Allgemeine Zeitschrift für Psychiatrie und psychiatrisch-gerichtliche Medizin. 1909, 66, 542.—Brill, A. A. Psychotic Children: Treatment and Prophylaxis. American Journal of Psychiatry. 1926, 5, 357–364.

early date their undesirable reactions and to recognize and steer into useful channels unhealthy potentialities which, if mishandled, may, or may not, become fixed in a pathological manner. We shall, wherever indicated, wean those (or any other) children away from nurturing ambitions which are unfulfillable because of physical, intellectual, social, or other handicaps, replacing them actively by adequate vocational guidance. We shall be sure to make the child somatically fit by remedying all infectious, metabolic, or other disturbances which an objective examination has found to be present. We shall try to eliminate, through work with the child and with the family, domestic disturbances as much as this is possible. We shall attempt to help the child, as soon as we can and as soon as this becomes necessary, to gain a proper perspective of the problems of sex and to keep away from the pitfalls of masturbatory, erotic, religious, or other ruminations. We shall be aware of parergastic possibilities without, however, being too eager to interpret all kinds of performances too one-sidedly as the danger signals of schizophrenia. Good physical hygiene has contributed a great deal towards the prophylaxis of tuberculosis by emphasis on fresh air, good food, sufficient muscular exercise, and adequate rest rather than by exclusive attention to the tubercle bacillus. Good mental hygiene will help individuals by emphasis on sound habit training in well-adjusted homes, proper vocational adaptation, and early education in controlling their emotions and getting along with people rather than by wanting, through some specific techniques, to prevent this or that mental disease. Of course, in those cases where the potentialities have developed so far as to become probabilities, one will have to be the more wary and resourceful and, without becoming oversolicitous or polypragmatic, employ his best constructive abilities in order to save the patient from sliding into schizophrenic disintegration.

THE THYMERGASTIC REACTION FORMS
(Affect Disorders. Manic-Depressive Psychosis. Circular Insanity)

The second group of the so-called "functional" major psychoses is characterized by abnormal moods in the direction of either protracted and situationally not justified elations or endogenous depressions not adequately explained on the basis of environmental influences. The elations have been known for a long time as *mania*, the depressions have been designated as *melancholia*. The term "mania" has been used, particularly by the French, for a variety of heterogeneous reactions; in some instances it was made to serve as an indicator of certain urges or drives (kleptomania, pyromania, poriomania, etc.), but mostly it was employed as a general descriptive name for all modes of strong excitement. For this reason, many cases of "mania" in children reported in French literature have in reality nothing to do with the conditions which we are about to discuss; they represent either delirious reactions or the more violent types of temper tantrums or excitements with religious implications, often of an hysterical nature ("religious mania"). Ever since 1851 (the older Falret; Baillarger), the close relation between elations and depressions has been recognized more and more clearly, owing chiefly to the observation of their frequent occurrence in the same person. Different names were coined for the alternating types, such as *folie circulaire* (the younger Falret; 1879), *cyclothymia* and *circular insanity* (Kahlbaum; 1882). In 1896, Kraepelin broadened the concept by comprising in his *manic-depressive psychosis* all endogenous elations and depressions, regardless of whether they appeared in one form only or alternated or presented "mixtures" of both in the same attack. This was doubtless a remarkable step forward. At the same time, Kraepelin's insistence that he dealt with a definite nosological entity created difficulties similar to those which we have mentioned in connection with his dementia praecox concept. Meyer, therefore, in accordance with his tendency to speak of reaction patterns rather than "diseases," preferred to fit the affective disorders into his provisional classification scheme based on behavior or performance as *thymergastic reaction forms* (from *thymos*— mood, and *ergasia*); *hyperthymergasia* refers to the deviations in the sense of an acceleration and increase of overt and implicit activity, the elations; *hypothymergasia* alludes to the disturbances which show a slowing and a decrease of mood and performance, the depressions.

Each of the two forms of mood disorder is characterized by a triad of abnormal reactivity, the single points being exact opposites if the two forms are contrasted with one another:

Hyperthymergasia (Mania. Elation)	Hypothymergasia (Melancholia. Depression)
1. Exaggerated happiness, hilariousness.	Profound sadness, downheartedness.
2. Acceleration of thinking, flight of ideas.	Slowing of the thought processes.
3. Increased psychomotor activity.	Decreased psychomotor activity.

The *manic* patient is in good spirits throughout. He is unusually happy, optimistic, elated, amused by the least remark or event. He has an inflated opinion of himself, his character, and his abilities. If delusions are expressed, they are of a grandiose nature and represent playful self-aggrandizements rather than fixed convictions. The thought processes are greatly accelerated; the patient jumps quickly from one topic to another, so that the stream of talk seems often to be disconnected (*flight of ideas*). The attention cannot be held for any length of time because the push from within and outside influences furnish the patient with ever new stimuli to which he instantaneously responds (*divertibility, distractibility*). He talks almost incessantly, interrupts others constantly, giggles, laughs, makes witty or sarcastic remarks, and puns and rhymes come to him easily. He has a quick and keen observation and immediately espies in the actions, speech, and dress of those about him some weakness or peculiarity which he does not hesitate to ridicule. Every impulse is promptly translated into overt performance. The patient is restless, always on the go, never still, talking, moving about, maintaining any goal for a few seconds only. The total behavior therefore lacks deliberation, planning, uniformity, and direction. The mood itself does not always remain on the same level; interference with the patient's actions, sometimes even the slightest criticism may result in angry outbursts or childish pouting. The degree of elation may vary from mild hypomanic states with not too markedly increased push and merriment to extreme excitement with often destructive violence, obscenity, and complete abandon of all conventional considerations.

The *depressed* patient is downcast and sad throughout. He feels unusually and painfully unhappy, pessimistic, saddened by many things which normally would make little or no impression on him. He has a poor opinion of himself, his character, and his abilities. If delusions are expressed, they are of a self-depreciatory nature; the patient is tormented by the belief in his sinfulness, unworthiness, poverty, poor health, and constantly accuses and reproaches himself. The thought processes are markedly retarded; thinking becomes difficult and labored and adheres monotonously to the depressive contents; poor concentration is complained of. Indecision adds to the subjective suffering and results often in the passage of long intervals between some trifling desire to do something and the action itself. Fears of an almost obsessive character may complicate or even dominate the picture; fear of impoverishment, of disaster to the family, fear that the patient's soul is lost, that he is too much of a burden to his environment, that preparations are made for his punishment by means of unspeakably cruel torture, or that he himself might be driven to dangerous deeds. In order to terminate his sufferings, to rid the world of so monstrous a sinner as he believes himself to be, or to administer self-punishment, or for no particularly specified reason, the patient may be preoccupied with the idea of committing suicide. The impulse to self-destruction is a real danger, especially at the periods before the height of the depression has been reached and after the first signs of improvement have made themselves perceptible. The sadness and the retardation are not always maintained on the same level; there is usually a *daily mood variation* in the sense that the patient feels somewhat better in the late afternoon and evening than he does towards the end of the night and in the early morning hours. Sleep and appetite are always seriously impaired. The degree of the depression may vary from mild despondency ("the blues") with but slight influence on the routine activities to extreme agitation with desperate suicidal inclinations or stuporous brooding with no heed to even the most vital functions.

Both the manic and depressive conditions have a tendency to *periodical recurrence*. The duration of the intervals varies from a very short time to many years or even decades. The attacks may be manic only or depressive only or the two forms may take alternate turns in the same individual. The chronological succession may differ in any possible manner:

Manic phase—depressive phase—interval.
Depressive phase—manic phase—interval.
Manic phase—interval—manic phase.
Depressive phase—interval—depressive phase.
Manic phase—interval—depressive phase.
Depressive phase—interval—manic phase.

Kraepelin's *mixed states* represent conditions in which the two triads of essential symptoms are shuffled irregularly, resulting in a manic state with depressive features, and vice versa. Thus we obtain pictures, such as manic stupor, depressive mania, akinetic mania, unproductive mania, agitated depression, and depression with acceleration of the thought processes.

These "mixtures" may be apparent throughout a single attack, but more commonly they form transitional stages during the change from one "pure" phase to another.

The *duration* of the individual phase differs from a few weeks to several months or even one to two years. It is a rule, which has many exceptions, that the recurrent excitements or depressions tend to last longer than the earlier ones. If well supervised, the single phases are practically always recoverable. Unsupervised or insufficiently supervised patients may succumb to exhaustion, exposure, starvation, or suicide. The possibility of a recurrence must always be kept in mind, but the time of the event cannot be foreseen even approximately. In the intervals, the patients appear as normal as they had been before the onset of the affective disorder. The person with the profoundest suicidal slump will pursue his usual activities, both occupational and social, in a manner typical of his previous personality adjustments. The wildest maniac will return to his pre-psychotic mode of general adaptation. The intellectual faculties usually remain unimpaired. It must, however, be stated that thymergastic reactions may sometimes be complicated by schizophrenic features, just as parergastic reactions may be complicated by manic-depressive episodes.

The hereditary factor plays a highly important rôle in the *etiology* of the thymergastic reactions. Elations, depressions, suicidal attempts, and successful suicides are found quite frequently in the ascendancy and among the siblings of the patients. Bleuler estimated the frequency of hereditary involvement at about eight per cent. In Vogt's cases of manic-depressive psychosis, not less than 22.2 per cent had psychotic parents and not less than 35.2 per cent had psychotic siblings. Rehm's study of the children of thymergastic patients shows that a large number of those children displayed personality disorders at a very early age. Of the offspring of a manic-depressive mother, one child was epileptic, one hysterical, and one blind. Of the six children of a sick father, one became manic and two depressive. Of the three children of a sick mother, one was epileptic and one feebleminded. A manic-depressive mother in whose family this condition was rife had four healthy children, two manic-depressive daughters (one of whom was feebleminded), and six children died of convulsions in infancy. Only in two of the nineteen families examined by Rehm (44 children) was the offspring entirely normal at the time of the investigation.[1]

Women are more apt to develop affect disorders than men. According to Kretschmer, persons having a pyknic body configuration are especially predisposed. Bleuler feels that the manic-depressive conditions represent extremes of the so-called "syntonic" personality make-up. The type of individual who is apt to become morbidly elated or depressed was studied by Meyer, Hoch, and Kirby. "The manic-depressive disposition is one in which the affect swings from states of elation to states of depression in people who are generally recognized to have frank, open personalities. They are either bright, talkative, optimistic, aggressive people, who make

[1] Rehm, Otto. Die Untersuchung von Kindern manisch-depressiver Kranker. Zeitschrift für die Erforschung und Behandlung des jugendlichen Schwachsinns. 1910, 3, 1.

light of the ordinary affairs of life, or else they take a gloomy outlook, bewail the past, make mountains out of mole-hills; or there is a combination of the above moods, rendering the person emotionally unstable and variable" (Henderson and Gillespie).

Full-fledged thymergastic disturbances are exceedingly rare before the fifteenth or sixteenth year of life. The manic-like excitements occurring sometimes in chorea and in delirious states, the peculiar euphoria seen in the advanced stages of tuberculosis, and the sadness and suffering which occasionally accompany the obsessive-ruminative tension states are of a different nature. Kasanin and Kaufman found among about six thousand patients admitted to the Boston Psychopathic Hospital in the years 1923, 1924, and 1925 only four cases of manic-depressive psychosis which developed before the age of sixteen years; in all four, the disorder had begun after the fourteenth year of life.[1] Ziehen observed manic excitement in girls of between twelve and fifteen years, in whom menstruation which had normally started and been repeated a few times suddenly failed to make its appearance.

Homburger has justly emphasized the fact that slight variations in mood are often observed in normal and healthy children. In certain youngsters, fluctuations are known to occur in the course of every day. There are different types of moodiness during the waking period. Some children are vigorous and frolicsome in the morning, become calmer towards noon, and are quiet later in the day. Others get up with difficulty in the morning, are slow and languid during the hours of the forenoon, are at the height of happiness and playfulness about noon, and again calmer in the evening. Other children are morose at the beginning of the day and slowly work themselves up to a higher and higher pitch of vitality which reaches its peak in the evening. Still other youngsters have their "good days" when they are amiable, obedient, communicative, and playful, and their "bad days" when they are irritable, whining, irresponsive, and listless. All these fluctuations are well within the normal limits and more or less typical of the child in question. Again there are youngsters, known as *live wires* or as *enfants terribles*, who are always slightly above the line of average push and activity, who are "full of mischief," "always up to something," of whom "you never can tell what they will do next," who are inclined to practical jokes, witty, restless, hyperactive, with a tendency to "butt in," to interrupt the elders, to shift quickly from one game to another. Their counterparts are slow, timid, "lazy," inert, slightly below the line of average push and communicativeness, worrisome, serious-minded, taking the minor or major family troubles very much to heart, brooding over trifles, with a trend to obsessive punctiliousness. One may say in general that the latter mood deviates more from the normal attitude of children than does hilariousness and unbridled bustling about during play, which would be decidedly abnormal and hypomanic in the adult. None of these reactions can in any way be used for prognostic purposes, since they often tend to even themselves out during puberty and adolescence.

[1] Kasanin, Jacob, and Moses Ralph Kaufman. A Study of the Functional Psychoses in Childhood. American Journal of Psychiatry. 1929, 9, 307-384.

The *treatment* of the severe and full-fledged elations and depressions requires hospitalization in every instance. In the institution, protection against destructiveness and suicide can be afforded much better than at home. Sedatives and hypnotics should be administered liberally though judiciously in order to secure sound sleep and to counteract the danger of exhaustion from manic hypermotility. Attention should be paid to the patient's general physical condition. Feeding often presents a specific problem which can be handled more satisfactorily in a hospital than at home. Wet packs and continuous baths often have a soothing effect. The milder cases, strange as it may sound, are sometimes more difficult to handle. The physician usually hesitates to advise admission to a hospital, especially since he realizes that the parents would hardly give their consent. Yet he must at least arrange for strictest supervision. The hypomanic boy or girl of fifteen or sixteen (below that age the condition is so rare as to be negligible) may easily be led to give unchecked vent to his or her sexual urges, incur excessive expenses and debts, and get into all sorts of difficulties because of his or her aggressiveness, uncontrolled adventurousness, and lack of inhibition and self-criticism. Even in the mildest forms of depression, the suicidal risk should not be ignored. It is the physician's duty to point out to the family the dangers involved and to recommend the most effective modes of preventing them.

CHAPTER XLIII

CHILDREN'S SUICIDES

ONE USUALLY thinks of childhood as a period of what the Germans call *Lebensbejahung*, a positive will to live and to enjoy life, an eager desire to get the most out of existence and to venture with bold unconcern into the unknown future. Growing curiosity is nourished by the continuous supply of newness and expanding orientation, building up and maintaining ever new interests and expectations. There is always something to look forward to, above all the great mystery and promise of becoming "grown-up." Even the unhappiest and most badly mistreated youngster commonly dreams of the days when he will be an adult and independent and do remarkable things. He may in the meanwhile react to the environmental difficulties in various ways, some wholesome and some unhealthy, but it is against the nature of children to think seriously of self-destruction. It is true that boys and girls may include in their daydreams the play with the notion that they are dead and their parents miss them now that they are gone. Such fancies are apt to arise especially after unkind criticism or punishment or when the child feels that he is not properly appreciated or that he is unwanted. Sometimes there is an element of revengefulness in these yarns, in the sense that the family is pictured as regretting its attitude toward the poor youngster who (in the daydream) has been driven to suicide. It is however much more frequent that the fantasies assume the form of running away from home than that of ending one's life.

Nevertheless, real suicide does occur during the years of childhood. A survey of the data furnished by the United States Mortality Statistics, gathered by the Department of Commerce, Bureau of the Census, shows that in this country from thirty to fifty-five children under fourteen years of age lose their lives annually through self-inflicted deaths. The toll was forty for 1926, fifty-three for 1927, thirty-six for 1928, and thirty-three for 1929. All occurred between the ages of ten and fourteen years, none under ten years during that period, except for one case in Iowa in 1929 not included in the above registration. In 1923, there were four suicides in the five-to-nine year group. Of the 162 cases reported in the period from 1926 to 1929, only nine were of the negro race; 106 were boys and 56 were girls. The methods used for self-destruction were, in order of frequency: firearms (79); hanging or strangulation (44); corrosive substances (14); drowning (8); poisons, not including corrosives and gas (8); poisonous gas (5); cutting or piercing instruments (2); crushing (1); "other means" (1). In 1929, the State of Illinois offered the highest figures (six), then followed Ohio and Pennsylvania (four each).

Ziehen tabulated all cases reported in Prussia for the twenty-four years from 1890 to 1913. There was a total of 1822 suicides during the entire period (an average of 76 per year); only sixty (46 male and 14 female) were committed by children below ten years of age, all others by youngsters between ten and fourteen years. Of the whole number, 1453 were boys and 359 were girls. According to Rehfisch (1893), Prussia, France, and Denmark led in the number of juvenile suicides; England, Switzerland, and Italy presented the lowest figures. More recent statistics, however, give the lead to Saxony, with 5.3 suicides per 100,000 boys of from ten to fourteen and 2.6 per 100,000 girls of the same age group. It is remarkable that jumping from the window which plays a prominent part among the methods of choice in most other countries is not at all represented in the United States of America; this may be due to some extent to the housing conditions in this country with a vast majority of not more than two story dwellings as contrasted with the four to five story apartment buildings in most of the European cities, surrounded by paved yards instead of by unpaved grounds. For this reason, the suicidal attempts by jumping from the home window in this country are apt to be unsuccessful and would therefore not be registered in the mortality statistics.

The figures, obtained from brief police reports, coroners' inquests, and newspaper items, contain little, if anything, that might be helpful in the evaluation of the motives. The Prussian statistics covering the period from 1869 to 1872 attributed ten per cent of boys' suicides to the non-contributory term *taedium vitae* (state of being tired of life), ten per cent to mental diseases, twenty per cent to remorse and shame, and not less than sixty per cent to "unknown motives"; the figures for girls were remorse and shame in fifty per cent and "unknown motives" in the other half.

The statistics further fail to account in any manner for the attempted suicides which did not result in death. Besides, some of the cases of self-destruction listed in the literature as "suicides" were really the unfortunate outcome of accidental acts of children who did not realize the danger involved in what they did. We had an opportunity elsewhere to mention the boy who playfully turned on the gas jet and crawled into the baking oven without the slightest intention to harm himself.

Full-fledged mental illness in the form of schizophrenic or depressive psychoses is responsible for children's suicides only in a very small minority of cases, largely because, as we have seen, it is exceedingly rare before the fifteenth year of life. Its importance should, however, not be underestimated. Many children may show more or less characteristic peculiarities long before the nature of the reaction is clearly recognized. Any profound unhappiness in a child, whether or not it is a symptom of genuine depression, calls for a thorough investigation and for remedial measures. It is unnatural for a child to be disgusted with life. An unhappy child, psychotic or not psychotic, is not a well child and requires judicious psychiatric handling. It is in an atmosphere of gloom and fear that the soil is prepared for thoughts of self-destruction; especially the dread of failure in school with ensuing ridicule and punishment on the part of strict and unrelenting parents, the fear of the brutalities of an alcoholic and tyrannical father, and misconceptions about the prophesied ill results of masturbation have been known to make children sufficiently desperate to wish to end their lives. A number of suicidal attempts could be traced to spite reactions in emotionally unstable feebleminded children. Some of the highly intelligent, solitary and educationally misguided children living in an eccentric environment with artificial "aesthetic" standards, undigested belletristic sentimentalism, and false romanticism are apt to breed unwholesome notions of *Weltschmerz* which, however, are found more frequently in the adolescent than in the child. Sometimes obsessive-ruminative tension states render the patient so unhappy that he entertains suicidal ideas. In all these instances, the understanding of the child's problems and a proper therapeutic program will not only prevent the danger of suicide but also help the patient to regain the normal joy of living of which he had been deprived.

Many "suicidal attempts" of children are fortunately only staged without the real goal of death. Hysterical children occasionally alarm the family by cutting themselves slightly or by means of other tricks, with the aim of attracting attention and being talked about.

One of our patients, Agnes C., a fourteen-year-old girl of low intelligence, whose mother had died six years ago and whose father had deserted his offspring, had been told by her aunt to return early in the evening. One time she did not come home until half past ten o'clock and was scolded. She stayed awake praying all night. In the morning, her aunt took the patient's little sister to school. When she came back, she found Agnes with an empty iodine bottle in her hand and her lips painted brown. She immediately administered milk and egg white and took the child to the clinic, where the gastric contents were found to be entirely free from the drug and the mucous membranes of the mouth and the saliva showed no trace of iodine. The girl did not complain of burning sensations but when the questions made her aware of this possibility, she told on her second visit a mournful tale of how her throat had hurt her. Agnes had, among other hysterical features, complete absence of the pharyngeal reflex.[1]

[1] There exists a vast bibliography with regard to the problem of suicide. Monographs on children's self-destruction are comparatively numerous. We mention only a few: Baer, A. Der Selbstmord im kindlichen Lebensalter. Leipzig. 1901.—Eulenburg, A. Schülerselbstmorde. Berlin. 1907.—Redlich und Lazar. Kindliche Selbstmörder. Berlin. 1914.—Proal, L. L'éducation et le suicide des enfants. Paris. 1907.—Barbaux, G. Étude médicopsychologique sur le suicide chez les enfants. Paris. 1910.—Moreau, J. Du suicide chez les enfants. Paris. 1906.—Rehfisch, E. Der Selbstmord. Berlin. 1893. Some of the statistical data used in our chapter were taken from Miner, John R. Suicide and Its Relation to Climatic and Other Factors. American Journal of Hygiene. Monographic Series No. 2. Baltimore. 1922.

NAME INDEX

A

ABRAHAM, 252
ABT, 469, 470
ACHARD, 162
ADIE, 365
ADLER, 8, 199, 238, 317
ALARY, 467
ALZHEIMER, 164, 489
AMMAN, 304
ANTON, 186, 199
APPEL, 162, 163
AQUAPENDENTE, 214
ARETAEUS, 152
ARISTOTLE, 63, 315
ARNDT, 165, 188, 190
ASAL, 259, 260
ASCHENHEIM, 215

B

BABINSKI, 481
BABONNEIX, 172
BAER, 510
BAILEY, 176, 177
BAILLARGER, 502
BALDWIN, 38
BARBAUX, 510
BARDOL, 466
BARKER, 153, 161
BASSENCO, 467
BEACH, 174
BEARD, 449
BECHTEREV, 4
BEERS, 9, 10
BEHM, 238
BERGER, 456
BÉRILLON, 336
BERNADON, 251
BERNFELD, 7
BERNHEIM, 467, 481
BERNSTEIN, 189, 190
BERZE, 367
BEVERLY, 266
BÉZY, 465, 467
BIBENT, 466
BIELSCHOWSKY, 144
BINET, 50, 52, 62
BINSWANGER, 237, 367, 418, 426, 437

BIRK, 426, 437
BISSELL, 238
BLANTON, M. G., 311
BLANTON, S., 311
BLEULER, 85, 164, 179, 458, 484, 491, 505
BLEYER, 146, 147
BLUEMEL, 311
BLUMBERG, 164
BOAS, 219, 220
BOENHEIM, 150, 151, 399, 402
BOGEN, 211
BONCOUR, 249
BOND, E. D., 162, 163
BOND, W. E., 437
BONHOEFFER, 186
BOUCHUT, 267
BOUMAN, 490
BOURNEVILLE, 145, 194, 206
BOUVERET, 213
BRAID, 315
BRAINERD, 148
BRATZ, 431, 437
BRIDGE, 436, 437
BRILL, 202, 501
BRISSAUD, 70, 250
BROCKBANK, 215
BROUSSEAU, 148
BROWN, 163
BROWN-SÉQUARD, 215
BRUNACCI, 212
BRÜNING, 215
BRUNS, 124, 465, 466, 472, 481, 482
BUCURA, 74
BÜHLER, C., 105
BÜHLER, K., 49, 50
BULWERS, 304
BUNKER, 166
BURGER, 365
BURNET, 466
BURR, 190

C

CAMERER, 152
CAMERIUS, 304
CAMERON, 174, 209
CAMPBELL, 137

SUBJECT INDEX

THIS BOOK

CHILD PSYCHIATRY

FIFTH PRINTING—1947

By

LEO KANNER, M.D.

was set and printed by the Collegiate Press of Menasha, Wisconsin; lithographed by the W. A. Krueger Company of Milwaukee, Wisconsin; and bound by The Boehm Bindery Company of Milwaukee, Wisconsin. The type face is 10 on 11 Monotype 31E. The type page is 27 x 46 picas. The text paper is 50-lb. White Offset Wove.

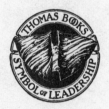

With THOMAS BOOKS *careful attention is given to all details of manufacturing and design. It is the Publisher's desire to present books that are satisfactory as to their physical qualities and artistic possibilities and appropriate for their particular use.* THOMAS BOOKS *will be true to those laws of quality that assure a good name and good will.*